On Bypass

Current Cardiac Surgery

Mehmet C. Oz, MD, and Michael Argenziano, MD
Series Editors

On Bypass: *Advanced Perfusion Techniques*, edited by *Linda B. Mongero,* BS, CCP, *and James R. Beck,* BS, CCP, *2008*

On Bypass

Advanced Perfusion Techniques

Edited by

Linda B. Mongero, BS, CCP
Division of Cardiothoracic Surgery
Clinical Perfusion
New York Presbyterian/Columbia College of Physicians and Surgeons
New York, NY

James R. Beck, BS, CCP
Division of Cardiothoracic Surgery
Clinical Perfusion
New York Presbyterian/Columbia College of Physicians and Surgeons
New York, NY

Humana Press
Totowa, New Jersey

999 Riverview Drive, Suite 208
Totowa, New Jersery, 07512

www.humanapress.com

This publication is printed on acid-free paper. ♾

ANSI Z39.48-1984 (American National Standards Institute) Permanence of Paper for Printed Library Materials.

For additional copies, pricing for bulk purchases, and/or information about other Humana titles, contact Humana at the above address or at any of the following numbers: Tel.: 973-256-1699; Fax: 973-256-83411; Email: humanapr.com; or visit our Website: http://www.humanapress.com.

ISBN 978-1-61737-687-0 e-ISBN 978-1-59745-305-9

10 9 8 7 6 5 4 3 2 1

Foreword

In *On Bypass: Advanced Perfusion Techniques*, editors Linda Mongero and James Beck have distilled the complex field of extracorporeal circulation and intraoperative mechanical support down to its most basic and important components. By identifying the critical pieces of the complex puzzle that is cardiopulmonary bypass and having these presented by a truly all-star cast of contributing authors, *On Bypass* represents a comprehensive, in-depth compilation of the current state-of-the-art in cardiopulmonary bypass technology and techniques.

In chapters dedicated to engineering, cannulation, blood flow, prime solutions, and ultrafiltration, the reader is exposed to detailed descriptions of the foundations of cardiopulmonary bypass technology. Other chapters illuminate the nuances of perfusion in special situations, such as pediatric, minimally invasive, and aortic surgery. Extension of extracorporeal support beyond the operating room is covered expertly in a chapter on ECMO and long-term pulmonary support. But this book goes beyond the traditional boundaries of a perfusion manual, and it is significantly strengthened by clinically oriented chapters dedicated to separation from cardiopulmonary bypass, the inflammatory response, and echocardiography. Finally, the editors draw upon their more than 50 years of experience as cutting-edge perfusionists in a chapter on policies and procedures, which constitutes required reading for anyone managing a perfusion program.

In sum, *On Bypass* represents an authoritative compendium of the most recent and best knowledge in every area relevant to cardiopulmonary bypass and perfusion. It is certain to become a trusted and well-worn resource on the shelves of clinical perfusionists, cardiac surgeons, anesthesiologists, and all others involved in the care of patients requiring extracorporeal perfusion.

Michael Argenziano, MD
Mehmet C. Oz, MD

Preface
Cardiopulmonary Bypass: Attractive, But Harmful?

With the introduction of cardiac surgery more than five decades ago, and the use of the heart–lung machine for open heart surgical procedures granting the surgeon unlimited time in which to operate inside the heart, a complex task has been given to the perfusionist.

Initially, cardiopulmonary bypass was so deleterious to the patient, and knowledge of bypass was so limited, that the unknown was balanced mostly by trial and error. Once extracorporeal support became feasible in man, a great need for skilled perfusionists sparked authors Charles C. Reed and Diane Clark to write *Cardiopulmonary Perfusion.* This basic textbook is surely on every perfusionist's shelf, and is useful as an adjunct to training personnel.

The next phase of cardiopulmonary bypass enhanced the skills of the perfusionist and enabled cardiac surgery to grow by leaps and bounds. Because of the complexity of artificial circulation and the importance of the science of perfusion technology, we have gained respect in the surgical arena, but at the same time our task is regarded as insidious, owing to its effect on inflammatory response.

The aberrations of normal physiology associated with cardiopulmonary bypass often bring criticism to its use; however, the fact that some patients have no ill effects from the procedure complicates this perception. After years of clinical investigation and publication, cardiopulmonary bypass has been deemed necessary in a controlled environment involving perfusionists, surgeons, and anesthesiologists.

Our library was limited to a varied selection of medical surgical textbooks until Joseph Utley et al. published a comprehensive textbook for perfusionists and clinicians addressing both practical and reference needs. We continue to develop new strategies to enhance our patient care. Along the way, innovations lead us to challenge present technology.

Today, it seems that the surgeon and patient would dream to have all procedures done OFF of cardiopulmonary bypass, thereby ameliorating its perceived deleterious effects. However, the nearly 650,000 procedures that require cardiopulmonary bypass and a perfusionist created a need for the development of a textbook that investigates advanced perfusion techniques that are currently being practiced; hence, *On Bypass: Advanced Perfusion Techniques.*

We hope that this collection of techniques and protocols will add to your repertoire and that your patients' care will be enhanced. We paired a perfusionist and a surgeon for each chapter in an effort to share a team approach to difficult and immediate decision making in the operating room. In fact, our practice depends on it.

Linda B. Mongero, BS, CCP
James R. Beck, BS, CCP

Contents

CONTRIBUTORS

SANJEEV AGGARWAL, MD • *Division of Cardiothoracic Surgery, New York Presbyterian/Columbia College of Physicians and Surgeons, New York, NY*

SANDHYA K. BALARAM, MD, PhD • *Division of Cardiothoracic Surgery, St. Luke's-Roosevelt Hospital Center, New York, NY*

JAMES R. BECK, BS, CCP • *Division of Cardiothoracic Surgery, Clinical Perfusion, New York Presbyterian/Columbia College of Physicians and Surgeons, New York, NY*

ELLIOTT BENNETT-GUERRERO, MD • *Department of Anesthesiology, Duke University Medical Center, Durham, NC*

BEN F. BRIAN, PhD • *Vice President, R&D Radiant Medical Inc.*

KEVIN A. CHARETTE, BS, CCP • *Division of Cardiothoracic Surgery, Morgan Stanley Children's Hospital of New York Presbyterian/ Columbia College of Physicians and Surgeons, New York, NY*

JONATHAN M. CHEN, MD • *Division of Cardiothoracic Surgery, Morgan Stanley Children's Hospital of New York Presbyterian/ Columbia College of Physicians and Surgeons, New York, NY*

LINDSEY A. CLEMSON, MD • *Department of Surgery, University of Texas Medical Branch, Galveston, TX*

EDWARD DARLING, MS, CCP • *SUNY Upstate Medical University College of Health Professions, Syracuse, NY*

RYAN R. DAVIES, MD • *Division of Cardiothoracic Surgery, Morgan Stanley Children's Hospital of New York Presbyterian/Columbia College of Physicians and Surgeons, New York, NY*

JOSEPH J. DEROSE, JR., MD • *Division of Cardiothoracic Surgery, St. Luke's-Roosevelt Hospital Center, New York, NY*

MARC L. DICKSTEIN, MD • *Department of Anesthesiology, New York Presbyterian/Columbia College of Physicians and Surgeons, New York, NY*

ROBERT J. FRUMENTO, MS, MPH • *Department of Anesthesiology, Duke University Medical Center, Durham, NC*

TERENCE GOURLAY, PhD • *Professor of Medical Diagnostics, Bioengineering Unit, University of Strathclyde, Glasgow, Scotland*

JERROLD H. LEVY, MD • *Department of Anesthesiology, Emory University Hospital, Atlanta, GA*

JAMES E. LYNCH, BS, RRT • *Department of Surgery, University of Texas Medical Branch, Galveston, TX*

JOHN MARKHAM, MS, MBA, CCP • *Chief of Perfusion, Director, Biomedical Engineering, St. Luke's-Roosevelt Hospital Center, New York, NY*

LINDA B. MONGERO, BS, CCP • *Division of Cardiothoracic Surgery, Clinical Perfusion, New York Presbyterian/Columbia College of Physicians and Surgeons, New York, NY*

RALPH S. MOSCA, MD • *Division of Cardiothoracic Surgery, Morgan Stanley Children's Hospital of New York Presbyterian/Columbia College of Physicians and Surgeons, New York, NY*

DAVID Y. PARK, BS, CCP • *Division of Cardiothoracic Surgery, Clinical Perfusion, New York Presbyterian/Columbia College of Physicians and Surgeons, New York, NY*

JAN M. QUAEGEBEUR, MD, PhD • *Division of Cardiothoracic Surgery, Morgan Stanley Children's Hospital of New York Presbyterian/ Columbia College of Physicians and Surgeons, New York, NY*

TIPO QURESHI, MD • *Imperial College, London, England*

BRUCE SEARLES, BS, CCP • *SUNY Upstate Medical University College of Health Professions, Syracuse, NY*

JACK S. SHANEWISE, MD • *Department of Anesthesiology, Division of Cardiothoracic Anesthesiology, New York Presbyterian/Columbia College of Physicians and Surgeons, New York, NY*

ROMAN M. SNIECINSKI, MD • *Department of Anesthesiology, Emory University Hospital, Atlanta, GA*

ALLAN STEWART, MD • *Division of Cardiothoracic Surgery, New York Presbyterian/Columbia College of Physicians and Surgeons, New York, NY*

BRITTANY A. ZWISCHENBERGER, MD • *Department of Surgery, University of Texas Medical Branch, Galveston, TX*

JOSEPH B. ZWISCHENBERGER, MD • *Department of Surgery, University of Texas Medical Branch, Galveston, TX*

1 The Engineering of Cardiopulmonary Bypass

Ben F. Brian, PhD

CONTENTS

SUMMARY

Cardiopulmonary bypass (CPB) has reached "gold standard" status in cardiovascular surgery for obvious reasons. In the same breath speaking of respect for its capability, there are often cries for its elimination. The absence of controlled clinical studies significantly powered to demonstrate or refute improvements in the CPB systems in use today has left perfusion practice fragmented. Recently, there has been a heightened interest in minicircuits that eliminate the conventional venous reservoir. There are glimpses of what mini-CPB systems could provide in terms of benefit, but the current systems, assembled largely from components designed a decade ago, are far from optimized. Six degrees of engineering separation are presented, which separate what CPB "is" today with what CPB "should be." With these improvements, CPB can once again be an enabling technology, this time for the next generation of minimally invasive surgical, as well as nonsurgical, procedures.

Key Words: CPB; extracorporeal circulation; minicircuits; microair; membrane oxygenator.

From: *Current Cardiac Surgery: On Bypass: Advanced Perfusion Techniques*
Edited by: L. B. Mongero and J. R. Beck © Humana Press Inc., Totowa, NJ

INTRODUCTION

With apologies to Daniel Handler *(1)*, if you were expecting a technical review of all the engineering accomplishments and historical improvements in the tools that have enabled cardiopulmonary bypass (CPB) from the days of Dr. Gibbon *(2)*, leading to a placating thesis of how the engineering of CPB has a rosy future in the capable hands of the current product suppliers, then you have come to the wrong place. If that is your interest, you would be well advised to pick up something else *(3)* to occupy your intellect, or at the very minimum skip this chapter altogether.

At the time of the preparation of this manuscript, there were 1767 published US patent applications containing the words cardiopulmonary bypass *(4)*. For every application aimed at engineering an improvement, there were at least 10 applications aimed at engineering its elimination. This is not entirely new, as the conduct of CPB, at least for coronary artery bypass graft (CABG) surgery, has been under an engineering and marketing attack for more than a decade with the development of "off pump" revascularization platforms *(5–7)*. Even from within the walls of the surgical suite, the vast extracorporeal circuit assembly and equipment used to assume the function of the patient's heart and lungs has been an easy mark *(8–10)*. The perfusionist has often been assumed guilty by association *(11)*. Today, this attack continues to fuel alternatives to CPB for coronary revascularization, and has aggressively expanded with companies racing to develop platforms for percutaneous repair and replacement of heart valves *(12–14)*. It is not worth debating what the ultimate fate of traditional CPB will be, but it is safe to assume that funding will continue to stimulate innovation aimed at engineering its elimination. As bleak as the future sounds, thankfully (for the patient), there is enough evidence in the scientific literature that CPB "best practices" should be sufficient to stave off these alternatives *(15)*. With some fundamental reengineering and extension of these practices, the conduct of CPB could become an enabling technology once again in the development of surgical (and nonsurgical) approaches that are truly minimally invasive. Exploration of this path is the primary intent of this chapter.

CARDIOPULMONARY BYPASS TODAY

Historical Perspective

The strengths of traditional CPB require little explanation. Nearly 50 years of continuous use has demonstrated the ability of CPB to enable the practice of cardiac surgery. There have been significant efficiency improvements in the components that comprise the CPB circuit during this time, but few advances have been attempted in developing new and more efficacious systems. The first major breakthrough in cardiac surgery came in the early 1950s, when the roller pump and the bubble oxygenator were developed. In the 1960s, the disposable bubble oxygenator expanded procedural capabilities. Early versions of the membrane oxygenator, and the first commercially available centrifugal pump, were introduced in the early 1970s, but it wasn't until a decade later that these products were refined enough to begin to gain market acceptance. Even then, it took an additional 10 years for the market to convert to the use of membrane oxygenators *(16)*, and centrifugal pump usage today remains less than that of the roller pump by almost 2 to 1. The major development of the 1990s was in the area of biocoatings, along with a much clearer understanding of the causes of postoperative morbidity. In the first half of the current decade, the innovation has shifted to the concept of minicircuits, which will be explored in more detail. Nonetheless, these developments have resulted in improvements in blood handling and reductions in blood trauma and the morbidity associated with CPB. Excellent reviews of the engineering accomplishments that have led to the circuits in use today can be found in other sources *(17–19)*.

Market Dynamics

The absence of significant system change is curious, given the body of scientific evidence of the numerous areas in which standard CPB contributes to postoperative patient morbidity. That research defines several causative relationships between hemodilution, shed-blood reinfusion, microair, large foreign surfaces, and quantifiable patient morbidity. The persistence of standard CPB can be attributed to the absence of proven safe, effective, and convenient alternatives. The lack of development of these alternatives has had more to do with economics than engineering challenge. Prices for CPB disposables are at an all time low, as multiple companies compete not by technical advantage, but by price and convenience *(20)*. The need to customize a tubing set to go with the components, and assemble that set all in one package, different for every customer, takes the gross profit margin on product to 30% for most companies, which is roughly half of the minimum threshold expected for medical devices. In this environment, research and development dollars have been shifted to rounding out product lines and getting manufacturing costs out of the current products. The advent of beating heart surgical stabilization products creates an interesting paradox for some companies, as revenues are better spent cannibalizing the traditional CPB market share for the higher profit margin stabilization platforms. The market dynamics have led to the perfusion companies defending their position in the field by consolidation, and ultimately posturing strategies against, rather than for, innovation in CPB.

Cardiopulmonary Bypass: The "Gold Standard"

Cardiopulmonary bypass is the recognized gold standard for coronary revascularization against which all other approaches are compared *(15,21)*. However, there is a problem with the generalization of CPB, in that all circuits are not created equal. The myriad of systems and protocols in use tend to be lumped generically together in a lowest common denominator (LCD) form. Any new technology, like those enabling beating-heart approaches, can look like a dramatic improvement by structuring a comparative study with the LCD of CPB. It is often very hard to find adequate detail in the publications on the specifics of the CPB used in the control arms of these studies. Some of the evidence-based differences in the circuits in use today need exploration before further steps in the engineering of CPB can be discussed.

Tissue Factor and Shed Blood

Ten years ago, you could look at the extracorporeal circuit and make bold claims that the intrinsic, or "contact activation," side of the coagulation cascade was the genesis of thrombin formation, and all that was bad with CPB rested solely on the large foreign surface area exposure. The scientific advances in the field of analytical biochemistry simply do not support this view today. The extrinsic or endothelial-based pathway begins with the release of tissue factor (TF), which is expressed when blood contacts subendothelium. When expressed in this manner, TF quickly combines with the serine protease Factor VIIa to form a potent complex that directly activates Factor X in the common pathway and Factor IX in the intrinsic pathway *(22)*, leading to thrombin production. Once thrombin is produced, there is enough feedback to get the coagulation cascade firing on both cylinders. Studies have demonstrated that the largest impetus for clot formation in the application of CPB actually comes from the surgical wounds, and not the extracorporeal circuit *(23)*.

TF levels are the highest in pericardial drainage, and studies on the level of activation and the pro-inflammatory content of shed blood are alarming *(24–27)*. The beauty of TF is that it is designed to be a local response to injury. However, in the LCD of CPB, this highly activated blood pool is spilling out of the pericardium and getting sucked up (in the name of blood conservation) and dumped right back into the relatively quiescent venous side of the extracorporeal circuit through a cardiotomy filter, which is most often integral to the open venous reservoir. With each revolution of the arterial pump, the local reaction becomes a systemic disorder, and direct reinfusion in this manner at any time point can have dramatic consequences on the associated morbidity of the surgical procedure.

Shed blood scavenged from the surgical field is best processed through a cell saver so that the activated components may be washed from the red blood cells before those cells are returned to the patient's circulation. Even with the obvious caveat being those circumstances where the volume of blood scavenged from the surgical field is unusually high, such that the beneficial effects of removing the undesirable contents of shed blood are superseded by the impact of the plasma loss, patients may be better served by transfusion over the alternative.

Venous Reservoir

Conventional open venous reservoirs with integral cardiotomy filters fueled the ease of use adoption of membrane oxygenators in the 1980s, but today they account for the largest volume and surface area of bio-incompatible materials in the circuit: air and silica powder/silicone oil–based antifoam *(28)*. Without the return of shed blood, the integral filter material in these reservoirs functions to generally process left vent blood and to remove air that is often entrained in the venous line. There is a unique open reservoir with separate compartments for venous and cardiotomy blood *(29,30)*, allowing the user to isolate the cardiotomy and assess the need for further processing and/or return to the circuit. With a relationship between the number of microemboli detected during CPB and the incidence of postoperative brain injury *(31,32)*, air handling of circuits has been the subject of renewed interest. Much of the air that enters the extracorporeal circuit was thought to be readily handled by the venous reservoir; however, significant performance differences exist between devices, and performance is either unknown or degrades considerably at low fluid levels or extended use *(33,34)*.

The application of vacuum to open venous reservoirs is a relatively recent development, which has allowed closer positioning to the patient and the use of smaller venous lines and cannula *(35,36)*. Vacuum-assisted venous drainage (VAVD) must be approached with some level of caution *(37–39)*. Despite the potential issues, many centers have incorporated VAVD into their standard practice with positive results.

As an alternative to the open reservoir, a closed venous reservoir bag has typically been considered more biocompatible *(40,41)* because of the elimination of the large air interface and the minimization of antifoam exposure, but market use is low for adult CPB. Until recently, vacuum assistance for closed circuits was difficult, but new circuits may enable broader use *(42,43)*. Today, the reservoir choice is a balance between the convenience and better air handling of open circuits and the biocompatibility improvement potential with closed circuits. Several centers incorporate the latter into effective approaches for blood conservation *(44)*. However, the choice of a venous reservoir today is overshadowed by any decision to add shed blood to it, and, as we will see shortly, elimination of this component in CPB is a primary goal of future systems.

Priming Volume

Approximately 20% of blood transfusions in the United States are associated with cardiovascular surgery *(45)*. With all the volume squeezed out of the membrane oxygenator, attention has been shifted to the tubing setup and minimizing priming volume by decreasing the interconnect lengths. The overall goal has been to reduce the dilution of the patient with the volume it takes to fill the circuit so that hemoglobin levels can stay above a minimum threshold and blood product usage can be decreased. There are several circuits that have taken existing components (venous reservoir, centrifugal pump, membrane oxygenator and arterial filter) and combined them in a pre-connected "frame" *(46,42)*, modeled in a fashion similar to the "Fallen Cassette," illustrated in Fig. 1. The Fallen Cassette has been marketed for several years in Japan, where a premium is paid for CPB technology and priming volume reduction is a dominant focus. By preconnection of the components in a frame, the interconnect tubing can both be minimized and standardized, a benefit to both the patient and the manufacturers (vs. custom sets). What is left is the connection to the patient, and with the application of VAVD, this volume can be reduced as well. With the prospective benefits of closed reservoir circuits, at least one circuit has modified the cassette concept with a closed venous reservoir, which can be used in vacuum-assist mode *(42)*. These circuits can get the priming volume to less than a liter with demonstrated reductions in postoperative blood product utilization *(47)*, and with appropriate design features can facilitate antegrade and retrograde autologous priming techniques.

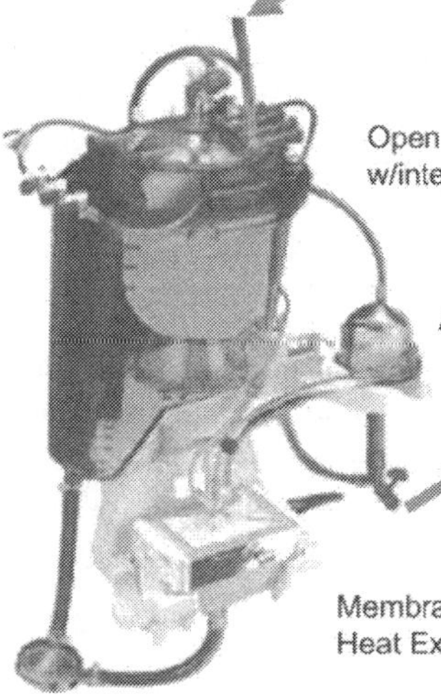

Fig. 1. Preconnected mounting of the components in the fallen cassette.

Biomaterials

Modifications of the engineering materials used in extracorporeal circuits (ECCs) for improved biocompatibility or biopassivity have held practitioner's interest since the early 1980s. There have been more clinical studies directed at proving efficacy than any other categorical aspect of extracorporeal technology. From the top four suppliers of perfusion products, six different coatings are offered. Three are based on heparin, two are based on hydrophilic/hydrophobic microdomain polymers, and one is based on a platelet membrane phospholipid. Each has their merits, and a biochemical marker study can likely be constructed to prove any one of them superior to the others. Heparin coatings have been the most studied, with little to differentiate the various offerings. There is a mechanistic rationale for complement benefit with heparin coating, as heparin binds directly to the C3b site for Factor B *(48)* and potentiates the down-regulation effect of Factor H *(49)*, thereby reducing the activation of the alternative pathway. Heparin effectively "consumes" complement, and the decreases in the associated markers of activation are the most commonly demonstrated benefit. Heparin is an effective drug, but it is not without consequences

(50). The direct platelet-activating and immunological aspects aside, the worst thing that can happen to the complement cascade of a patient is the administration of protamine sulfate for heparin reversal *(51)*. With the most bioincompatible surface in the circuit being air, it is not surprising that the most compelling use of these coatings comes from studies using closed venous reservoirs, no return of shed blood, and reduced systemic heparin levels with the associated reduction in the amount of protamine *(52)*.

If a "gold standard" practice of no shed blood return, minimal air interface, biocoatings and minimized circuit surface area/volume are incorporated in the conduct of CPB, then the necessary anticoagulation regime can safely be reduced and the true benefit of biocoatings realized, as well as outcome-related clinical benefits. It would be an interesting study to assess benefits of alternative non-CPB approaches to coronary revascularization and, in time, heart valve repair against this standard. However, before launching into a discussion on the further engineering of CPB, it is important to recognize that this gold standard is not practiced by a majority of centers today.

ENGINEERING OF CARDIOPULMONARY BYPASS

What improvements can be made to CPB? There have been several developments in recent years with minicircuits that give a glimpse of the potential however; the collective system engineering is far from optimized, and the circuits on the market are not yet ready for prime time. If we operate on the assumption that what CPB "should be" is somehow connected through a chain of interrelated developments to what the gold standard of CPB "is," then we can operate on the thesis that there are no more than six degrees of separation between the two systems. These separations are discussed in more detail below.

Extracorporeal Volume

For decades there has been a focus on minimizing hemodilution, primarily through the reduction in priming volume of the circuits in use for CPB, as discussed previously. The impetus was provided by the untoward effects of priming volume on the need for postoperative blood transfusions. However, recent studies provide a glimpse of just how far-reaching the impact of hemoglobin levels common with CPB currently is *(53,54)*. A decrease in the circulating amount of hemoglobin is now understood to place major organs at risk. The problem is compounded with the standard of care in monitoring the adequacy of perfusion, creating a blind spot for the perfusion team. Depending on the distribution of flow mainly to the brain and kidneys, a mixed blood gas in the circuit may provide a false sense of security. Worse yet, if there is not real-time blood gas monitoring, then the signal may be missed entirely.

To combat this blind spot, several centers have utilized cerebral oximetry to evaluate the incidence of renal failure and postoperative neurological events after open-heart surgery *(55,56)*. To use this monitoring technique in a feedback control method of perfusion parameters *(55)*, the saturation of oxygen in the cerebral cortex was proactively maintained at 40% or higher in a set of patients. "Interventions" used to increase readings included increased pump flow, elevated perfusion pressures, augmenting CO_2 levels, and transfusions. Of the available factors, adding blood to the circuit to increase the hematocrit had the most dramatic effect on cerebral perfusion by this measure. Cerebral monitoring can provide a stopgap in clinical practice today in respect to the brain, but other organs are not guaranteed adequate perfusion and protection. Patients may be better served getting blood on bypass at a much higher transfusion threshold than relying on adequate perfusion taking place.

The focus of discussion of circuit volumes needs to be shifted from priming volume, which is relevant at one time point in the procedure, to total extracorporeal volume at "steady state". With conventional venous reservoirs (open and closed), the ability to separate and remove air is compromised significantly at the low levels used at the initiation of bypass. Not only should these devices be run with as much blood in them as possible, they inherently will be throughout the course of the procedure. With volume shifts to decompress the heart and lungs, pressure or other indices will be reacted to and volume will be given to the patient. Cardioplegia will add volume and, before long, the optimized liter of initial priming volume has expanded to an extracorporeal volume of 3–5 L, with the snowballing cascade of hemodilution in full swing.

There are numerous case reports where a particular patient has been perfused on a conventional circuit with little to no change in hemoglobin over the case *(57)*. This has to be the foundation of any redesign of the CPB circuit, as the concept of increasing intraoperative blood product utilization is not an option in today's environment. Maximizing the amount of circulating hemoglobin on pump is critical to minimization of the circuit and a giant first step can be made by reducing the extracorporeal volume through the next degree of separation: elimination of the conventional venous reservoir.

Elimination of the Conventional Venous Reservoir

During the same period in which manufacturers have squeezed the last bit of prime out of the membrane oxygenator, venous reservoirs have gotten larger and larger. Priming volume has gone down and extracorporeal volume and surface area have gone up. The performance of CPB without an extracorporeal reservoir is not a new concept *(58)*. Ventricular assist devices, extracorporeal membrane oxygenation circuits, CPS circuits, and liver and major vascular circulatory assist circuits all work without the use of a large, capacitive reservoir. The paradigm mandating the use of a large reservoir during CPB is that the blood volume of the heart and lungs needs to be removed from the patient's body to provide adequate cardiac decompression and a dry surgical field. Circuits without a venous reservoir in line have been used for the most complicated pediatric procedures for nearly a decade and are emerging as viable CPB circuits for adult cardiac surgery today.

The circuit with the most clinical use is named after the concept itself of mini extracorporeal circulation (MECC) *(59)*. Initially developed for coronary artery bypass procedures, it consists of a heparin-coated, closed centrifugal pump circuit and standard components as in Fig. 1, with the simple omission of the reservoir. Combined with cell saving (no shed blood return) and Calafiore *(60)* blood cardioplegia (minimal surface area and added volume), clinical results have been impressive with the MECC system, and capability in more complicated surgeries has been demonstrated *(61)*.

With direct connection of a centrifugal pump to the venous cannula, minicircuits are at a much higher risk for venous line cavitation and subsequent air entrainment. The centrifugal pump affords some level of protection (by depriming) if a large bolus of air enters, and an arterial filter is added to mitigate any air that gets by the pump and membrane oxygenator. However, centrifugal pumps are known to "shred" smaller amounts of air into microbubbles that the downstream components cannot efficiently remove *(62)*. The clinical use of the MECC system to date demonstrates the potential benefit, but minicircuits will be for research only, without replacement of the air removal function of the venous reservoir *(63)*.

Venous air removal (pre pump) for minicircuits was suggested as early as 1993 *(58)* and was implemented in pediatric practice circuit several years later. The "venous pull" system developed at Miami Children's Hospital *(64)* incorporates a separate bubble trap in the venous line before the centrifugal pump with a bubble detector upstream. With the vent line of the bubble trap connected through a roller pump to a cardiotomy reservoir, the pump can be operated intermittently based on the bubble alarm to "actively" remove entrained air from the circuit. The venous pull system has been used successfully since 1997 in over 1,000 pediatric cases. A closed venous reservoir bag that allows for kinetic assisted flow has been developed *(42)* with an automated version of this type of air purge, in which the sensor is used to feedback control a pump or solenoid valve on the purge line to vent air, only when air is present. These early innovations in active air removal were taken one step further with the development of the integrated air removal chamber within the Cardiovention (CORx™) circuit, which combined the air removal, centrifugal pump, and a membrane oxygenator into one device aimed at minimal extracorporeal volume *(65)*.

With the introduction of the Cardiovention circuit, data was first presented *(66)* that air removal in a minicircuit could be equal to or better than the air removal of a traditional open reservoir circuit. This data was generated from the traditional method of a controlled infusion of air into the venous line and arterial side ultrasonic bubble counting (Hatteland). The output of the Hatteland is a bubble count versus bubble size from 10–90 μm in 10-μm increments. The total counts (adding up the 9 size ranges) are plotted for each condition (level of air infusion) and device in Fig. 2 from test results with bovine blood at the "standard conditions" *(67)*. Fig. 2 illustrates the micro bubbles counted in the arterial line with the Cardiovention circuit (no arterial filter) at a high venous air infusion rate, compared with a conventional reservoir-based circuit, as well as comparative data at lower infusion rates from a minicircuit as described earlier (with an arterial filter). In addition to the efficiency of air removal by the Cardiovention circuit, Fig. 2 illustrates the issue with direct centrifugal pumping of the venous line with small amounts of entrained air, and the moderate protection afforded by depriming of the centrifugal pump with larger air infusions in a minicircuit without active air removal. The concept of minicircuits without compromise in air removal safety was born *(68)* in a small compact circuit with an adaptable "standard" tubing set *(69)*, which solved many of the issues with translocation of volume. With positive and negative sides of the pump connected via a bypass loop, an empty IV bag (or other flexible reservoir) could easily be used for volume storage. Blood could be moved back and forth to the patient

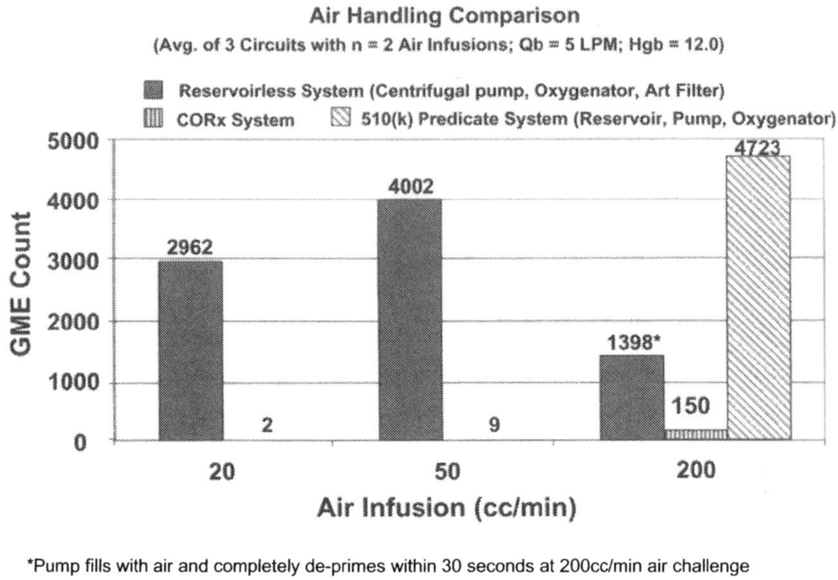

Fig. 2. Venous line air clearance comparison of three CPB circuits.

by adjustment of clamps, allowing access to the positive or negative pressure sides of the circuit.

With the Cardiovention circuit no longer available *(70)*, two minicircuits built on this concept have been introduced recently. The Medtronic Resting Heart™ system *(71)* automates the air removal in a bubble trap similar to the venous pull system. The circuit combines the bubble trap, standard pump, oxygenator, and arterial filter mounted in a frame similar to the Fallen Cassette. The Sorin group (Sorin/Dideco/Cobe) has introduced their Synergy™ System *(72)*, which has a bubble detector with air sensor on the venous line to automate the removal of air from the vent. This circuit has the added feature of the arterial filter being integrated into the outlet manifold of the membrane oxygenator and integration of the pump housing. The testing of these systems is in the early stages; however, it is likely that multigenerational improvements will be required for significant market acceptance. These additional degrees of separation start with further integration and automation of the motor control for improved safety.

Hardware Integration

If minicircuits are to be the future of CPB, then they need to become minisystems. More automation will be required for safety, and to ultimately justify the higher cost to the end user. However, to be proven safe, the circuits must first be tested with more applicable air challenges. A proposed air challenge set-up is illustrated in Fig. 3, in which a venous cannula is sealed within a large bore section of venous line. The negative pressure in the venous line can be adjusted by the pinch clamp shown in the figure, and a set of 30-gauge syringe needles, which are opened to atmosphere after the circuit has stabilized, are placed between the clamp and the cannula. With increasing negative pressure, the amount of air entrained through the needle holes will increase. This test set-up challenges the device in a more clinically relevant way, as high-negative line pressures can occur in the venous line with these circuits. In a similar manner to the data in Fig. 2, air counts in the arterial line of the Cardiovention minicircuit were quantified with bovine blood using this air entrainment model. The total counts (adding up the 9 bubble size ranges) are plotted in the left side of Fig. 4 versus venous pressure for two different dual-stage venous cannula (292902 and 293702) at 4.5 LPM of blood flow.

Fig. 4 illustrates the alarming effect of venous pressure on the amount of air that might exit these closed circuits with a smooth cannula transition in the venous line. The more negative the pressure

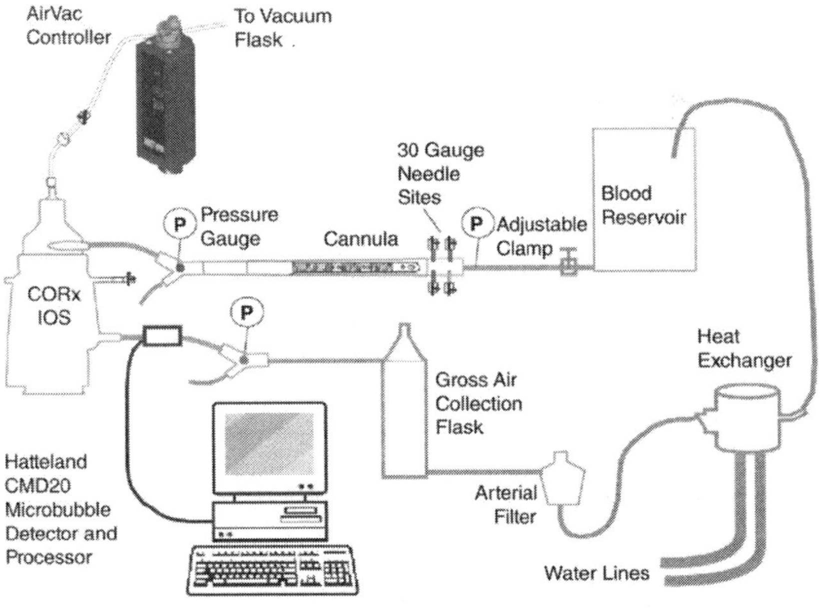

Fig. 3. Venous line air entrainment test model.

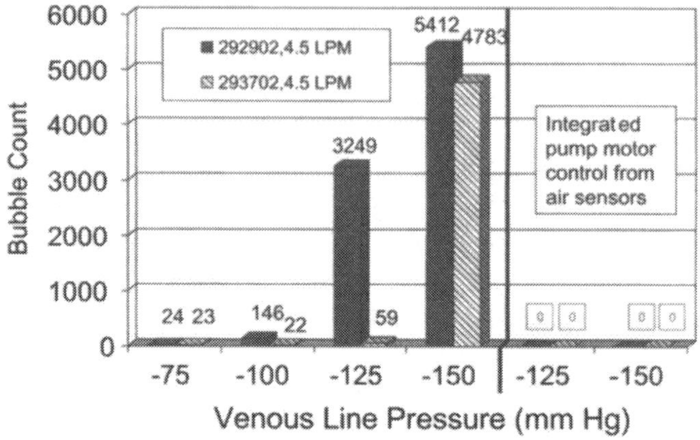

Fig. 4. Effect of venous line pressure and cannula size on the entrained air clearance of a minicircuit with and without automated flow control.

and the more tortuous the path to the air evacuation device is, the worse these results will likely be. Unfortunately, this type of data is part of the learning curve in developing these systems, and was the genesis of a major second generation upgrade to the Cardiovention circuit *(73)*. Feedback control was added to the centrifugal pump from three inputs: a) an air sensor with added intelligence to quantify the amount of air being entrained; b) a redundant bubble sensor in the venous line; and c) venous line pressure monitoring. A unique software algorithm was developed, which would react to the inputs and reduce the motor RPMs in a safe operating mode without stoppage of forward flow to the patient. Very small changes in the pump RPMs in these systems can have dramatic impact on the venous pressure and the resulting entrainable air. With this integration, the Cardiovention minicircuit became a minisystem, and the right-hand side of Fig. 4 demonstrates the safety and efficacy of the automatic flow control at the same inlet conditions that generated the microair previously. Note that the venous pressure algorithm was disabled for this testing to allow the same high negative pressures as tested on the left-hand side. Unfortunately, the performance characteristics of each minicircuit are going to be unique and what it takes from the hardware standpoint to improve the system safety will take time to understand, and design improvements to carry out.

The next steps in integration can then use the air-handling systems and motor control to automate the priming sequence and, with additional solenoid clamps, the volume relocation within the system. Negative pressure in the venous line can be used for left heart venting, and the positive pressure side used to provide blood for concentrated cardioplegia delivery, with the simple addition of a micro or syringe pump *(60)*. For coronary revascularization, stopping the heart can be avoided altogether with these systems, as discussed later. Combine integrated blood gas sensing, electronic gas blender, voice activation, etc., and the automatic pilot version of this type of system can be a reality. However with the immediate need for automatic flow control added to the air removal technology taken care of, there are a few degrees of separation in the circuit that should be addressed first.

Membrane Oxygenator Design

For practical purposes all membrane oxygenators in use today are of the blood outside the hollow fiber design. This is the most efficient use of the membrane material itself in a static design to introduce mixing *(16)*. Adult devices range from 1.8 to 2.5 m^2 of surface area in a variety of configurations, and some are rated as high as 7–8 LPM of blood flow. Surface areas decreased through the 1970s and 1980s from 3–4 m^2, reaching a low of 1.7 m^2 until the reintroduction of larger area designs, which started a puzzling trend back toward higher surface areas in the name of increased oxygen transfer. The oxygen content in blood will increase in proportion to the hemoglobin concentration in CPB with any of the oxygenators, and what tends to be lost in the shuffle is the impact of hemoglobin on the necessary flow rate to maintain a patient's metabolic demand. No system on the market today has been optimized for running higher hemoglobin blood, and there are two important factors to consider: required surface area and appropriate blood film thickness.

Blood activation from extracorporeal circuit materials increases with the surface area of contact *(74)*. Current adult membrane oxygenator designs have much more surface area than is necessary if they are to be successfully integrated in an optimized minisystem. As an example, the Cardiovention membrane compartment at 1.2 m^2 of area was designed to have the same oxygen transfer as the leading devices with the one caveat that running this oxygenator in a minisystem would result in hemoglobin values 10% higher than a traditional reservoir system. Clinically, the difference with these systems is much larger, meaning there is plenty of transfer reserve. This case in point is illustrated by comparison of clinical perfusion data from the Heart Center in Leipzig, where automated feedback control of arterial PO_2 has been practiced for several years through the use of a neural network program and arterial PO_2 electrode with outputs to an electronic blender and the pump motor controller *(75)*. A pilot study was conducted comparing the automated pump run for an arterial PO_2 set point of 200 mm Hg using a minicircuit (1.2 m^2 membrane area) with that of the standard open reservoir system having a 1.9 m^2 surface area. The pertinent data is summarized in Table 1 for the five patients run on each system. These results demonstrate the capability of arterial PO2 control with the Leipzig system and illustrate the significant reduction in pump flow necessary for the same effective patient oxygen transfer, even with a surface area that is 50% lower. This powerful impact of hemoglobin on the amount of oxygen delivered to tissue is not surprising, given the transfer equations and the required flow rate decrease with the mini-system is roughly equal to the hemoglobin increase on a percentage basis. This is an important benefit for the operation of minisystems, as venous line air entrainment will be reduced with lower required flows. It is safe to say that the current systems for CPB expose the patient's blood to 0.7 to 1.5 m^2 of unnecessary membrane surface area and compound this exposure with increased flow rates that go up in proportion to the level of hemodilution.

As the membrane priming volumes have been decreased with each new design, devices have become more efficient by squeezing blood through tighter and tighter spaces. The membrane devices of the 1980s had film dimensions on the order of 150 μm. Several leading designs in use today are half that size *(16)*. At this level, it doesn't take too many platelet layers to create a significant increase in inlet pressure *(76,77)* and a dramatic increase in shear stress. The bovine model was used in the early days of membrane compartment development and with approx 4 times the platelet count in a larger volume of blood, transient pressure increases varied dramatically with packing densities and manifold areas to "weed out" designs. If the devices on the market today require pharmacological intervention *(78)* or biocoating *(79)* to mitigate transient pressure increases due to dimensional changes in the flow path subsequent to platelet adhesion, then it is questionable that these devices are optimal for running the significantly less diluted blood capable in minisystems.

Membrane redesign may come from outside the current suppliers. There have been several attempts in the past to develop a pumping membrane oxygenator *(80,81)*. The original impetus was that active mixing of the blood and fibers would allow dramatic reductions in

Table 1
Comparison of the Clinical Perfusion Parameters Between a MiniCPB System and a Standard Open Reservoir CPB System with 50% More Membrane Surface Area

	Perfusion Parameters						Patient Size		
Patient	*Qb (LPM)*	*Vsat (%)*	*paO2 (mm Hg)*	*Gasflow (LPM)*	*FiO2 (%)*	*Hct (%)*	*Ht (cm)*	*Wt (kg)*	*BSA (m2)*
MiniCPB System, 1.2 m^2 membrane area, No Venous Reservoir (264 data points total)									
1	3.9	81.1	199.7	2.2	59.6	38.8	170.0	80.0	1.9
2	4.0	78.5	199.6	3.0	58.3	38.6	176.0	80.0	2.0
3	4.3	80.0	199.7	3.0	53.0	30.5	179.0	83.0	2.0
4	2.6	74.9	201.0	1.9	44.9	36.1	187.0	94.0	2.2
5	3.8	73.6	200.8	3.9	60.6	30.2	189.0	96.0	2.2
Avg	**3.7**	**77.6**	**200.2**	**2.8**	**55.3**	**34.9**	**180.2**	**86.6**	**2.1**
Standard CPB System, 1.9 m^2 membrane area, Open Venous Reservoir (661 data points total)									
1	5.1	82.1	199.6	4.0	37.9	21.2	168.0	73.0	1.8
2	4.9	83.3	198.4	3.1	39.3	21.9	164.0	77.0	1.8
3	5.1	77.1	198.7	3.5	47.9	28.5	186.0	86.0	2.1
4	5.6	67.9	199.2	3.1	61.1	27.3	182.0	113.0	2.3
5	5.3	79.9	199.4	3.1	48.1	28.3	181.0	80.0	2.0
Avg	**5.2***	**78.1**	**199.1**	**3.3**	**46.8**	**25.4***	**176.2**	**85.8**	**2.0**

*$p < 0.01$

surface area. With minicircuits feasible at 1.2 m^2 or less, this is not the issue it once was. However, micro air will continue to be a challenge to minisystems, and one major benefit of spinning a membrane bundle is that you can generate sufficient force to collect and potentially remove this air. Development of a pumping membrane is active once more with Ension, having been "spun" out of the McGowan Institute at the University of Pittsburgh *(82,83)*.

For the CPB circuit to be completely benign with respect to the patient morbidity in any surgical approach, there can be no compromise on surface area or volume minimization. With the large membrane area devoted to gas exchange reduced there is separation that remains with the remaining circuit components.

Further Circuit Optimization

Venous Cannula

Overall, venous cannula use today has changed little since the inception of CPB. As evidenced by Fig. 4, a venous cannula can impact the nature of entrained air significantly, and a design that can limit the increase of negative pressure in and around the access site is almost a necessity when running a minisystem. A catheter has recently been introduced that has significant potential advantages over the existing devices. The "Smart Canula™" *(84)* is an expanding metallic mesh design which maximizes hole surface area and minimizes the wall thickness to optimize flow rate and vascular access to the patient *(85,86)*. The design is based on the fundamentals of fluid flow that a short segment of a tube with a narrow internal diameter will not significantly impede flow through the tube. This has been the basis for Venturi meter *(87)* flow measurements in tubes for over 200 years. A cannula having a narrow diameter only in the insertion area and where dictated by anatomy within the vasculature would be expected to have much better flow rate characteristics than one having a semi tapered diameter small enough to fit within the narrowest points. With the emerging application of reservoir-less closed loop minisystems, the resistance to flow of the venous access device, as well as susceptibility to occlusion, are more important to an optimized perfusion system than ever.

Heat Exchange

The debate on optimal perfusion temperature for adult CPB continues with no definitive conclusion *(88)*. Generally, clinical papers favor the utilization of normothermic CPB when the outcome measures are related to cardiac function and bleeding. When the outcome is a measure of neurological function, the results tend to favor moderate hypothermia *(89)*. A novel catheter system designed to cool the brain and warm the body was recently developed and a feasibility trial completed *(90,91)*. Heightened awareness and discussion fueled by this system and neurological protection *(32)* have shifted the balance in perfusion temperatures more toward moderate hypothermia (32–35°C). All membrane oxygenators have integral heat exchangers that were designed when cooling and warming rates were at a premium. With several plastic fiber designs in use with areas greater than $0.5\,m^2$, there again is too much surface area devoted to heat exchange in today's systems.

Extracorporeal based heat exchange is not ideal to begin with. Upon weaning from bypass there can be significant temperature gradients within the patient. An improvement would be the incorporation of heat exchange technology that would be able to move with the patient through the recovery room and ICU to eliminate postoperative thermal regulatory problems which are associated with increased bleeding *(92)*. A nonextracorporeal methodology would allow much more gradual return to normothermia without extended CPB times and the occupation of OR to insure normothermia is maintained at least until the patient is more stable. Both surface *(93)* and endovascular technologies are available *(94,95)*, but in today's cost environment, the market is unwilling to bear the incremental cost with the extracorporeal device already there. As the nonextracorporeal devices are proven in other therapeutic areas, companies looking to provide the complete solution for optimal patient care in CPB will need to consider nonextracorporeal heat exchange technologies.

Arterial Filter

Although arterial filters date back to the earliest days of CPB, they remain a proven safety feature in today's systems *(96,97)*. Once used to filter matter and remove air, their purpose today is almost exclusively for the latter. This is especially true for systems with no direct return of shed blood. However, with minisystems any air entrained needs to be removed prior to the pump, as the arterial filter offers only moderate defense against micro bubbles *(32,60)*. This redundancy of air removal in the minisystems in use today is a requirement until the air handling capability is proven and/or upgraded. With a completely closed system that has air removal and automated flow control as discussed above, the arterial filter is not necessary, or at the minimum is on the wrong side of the pump. With the active air removal device on the venous side of the pump, it is straightforward to integrate 40-micron filtration for equivalent blood filtration to current systems.

Vent, Suction, and Cardioplegia

Much of the attention herein has been focused on the arterial pump circuit for obvious reasons. Miniaturization of this aspect alone addresses only one of the pumps in the huge mass of hardware used to conduct CPB today. Elimination of a pump for vent return by intermittent use of the negative pressure in the venous line is more than feasible if the air handling limitations of current systems are resolved. Removal of any access point in the venous line without clamping, as might be common with vent lines, would create a venous inlet full of air that would likely overwhelm the air handling system without the benefit of automated flow control. The additional two pumps dedicated to suction can be eliminated using vacuum based cell salvage devices. The CardioPAT™ *(98)* system originally designed for orthopedic surgery *(99,100)* is small enough to be pole mounted and moveable with the patient into the ICU. Finally, cardioplegia technique should be based on a system with minimal surface area and dilutional volume. Variations of the Calafiore method, whereby warm blood is taken from the oxygenator and intermittently injected into the aortic root, with concentrated potassium added by means of a syringe pump, have tremendous popularity in Europe. With elegant simplicity, minimal surface area, minimal added volume, and proven myocardial protection *(60,101)* these methods are ideal for the minisystems.

With these changes a system can be built around the minicircuit that looks like it came from this century and the large equipment footprint can go by the way of the museum. The disposable circuit has been integrated with the hardware for absolute minimization of surface area and extracorporeal volume. The only degree of separation left is optimal usage of such a system.

Cardiopulmonary Support

With coronary artery bypass graft (CABG) procedures making up the vast majority (70–75%) of cardiac surgical cases performed worldwide, it is curious that CPB technology more amenable to the "closed-heart" CABG cases has not evolved separately from traditional CPB. Rather, the concept of "beating-heart" surgery was developed to avoid the deleterious impact of the CPB on the patient. Although beating heart approaches are viable and the early results promising, the technique itself is difficult and usage has reached a plateau. If clinical studies are someday powered enough to convince the scientific community of the merit of beating heart approaches *(102)*, this merit will not have been derived from elimination of an optimized CPB circuit, but rather from the benefits of avoiding the cardioplegic arrest of the heart: elimination of the aortic cross clamp *(103)*, continued perfusion of the lungs *(104)*, and prevention of the associated reperfusion injury *(105)*.

The sixth degree of separation from the current CPB systems is that the minisystem can ideally be utilized for cardiopulmonary "support" in addition to "bypass", and as such can be an enabling technology, this time for the adoption of less invasive surgical approaches. The most applicable procedural category in this case today is "assisted" beating heart surgery. This procedure would combine stabilization with the minisystem as an assist device to "off-load" or decompress the heart. The heart is beating but the wall tension is substantially reduced, improving myocardial perfusion. The minisystem can seamlessly provide maintenance of hemodynamic stability when the surgeon needs to manipulate the heart for difficult to reach target vessels (lateral or posterior sides of the heart). In this manner the minicircuit enables additional grafts to be performed, allowing more complete revascularization. This hybrid approach is ideal for the majority of surgeons who wish to provide the benefits of beating-heart surgery without compromising the level of safety associated with stopped heart procedures *(106)*. The minisystem as described would be no more obtrusive than conceptualized in Fig. 5, and would enable expansion of the beating heart market and obviate the need for high end disposable stabilizers.

Similarly there is a significant push in the development of endoscopic approaches to CABG surgery fueled by robotic assistance *(107)*. There are significant challenges with this approach that have slowed progress from the initial inception. Improved manipulation systems and adjunctive stabilization products have enabled some progress, but many shortcomings remain. Closed chest valve repair is also feasible *(108)*; however, the advances in percutaneous valve approaches will likely supplant the endoscopic methods over time. Regardless of whether the procedure is a valve or CABG, percutaneous or endoscopic, volume needs to be removed from the heart and space created for device deployment. Minimally invasive surgical approaches could be significantly enabled with a minicircuit placed at the foot of the table with femoral access to provide safe support, and creation of the necessary space within or around the heart.

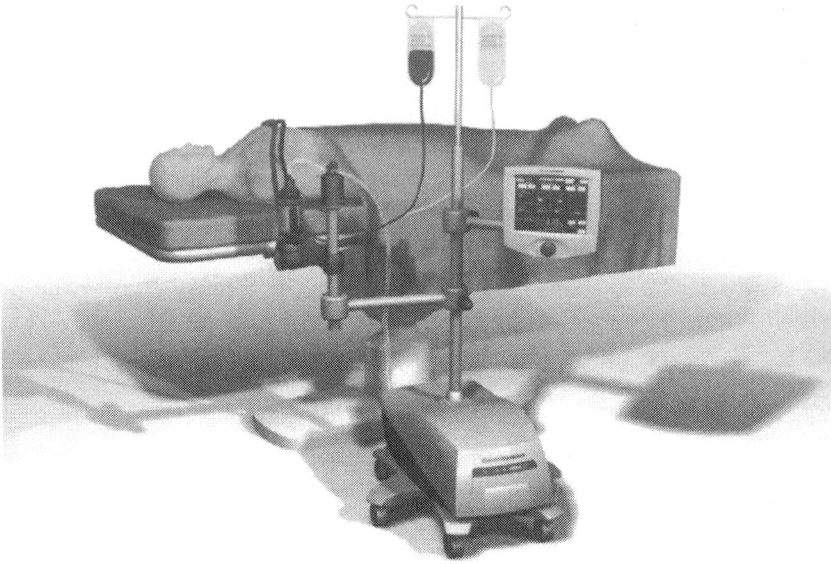

Fig. 5. Conceptualized cardiopulmonary support system.

CONCLUSION

Cardiopulmonary bypass has reached "gold standard" status in cardiovascular surgery for obvious reasons. In the same breath of respect for its capability, there are often cries for its elimination. The absence of controlled clinical studies significantly powered to demonstrate or refute improvements in the CPB systems in use today has left perfusion practice fragmented. In recent years, there has been a heightened interest in minicircuits that eliminate the conventional venous reservoir. There are glimpses of what mini CPB systems could provide in terms of benefit, but the current systems, assembled largely from components designed a decade ago, are far from optimized. Six degrees of engineering separation were discussed that separate what CPB "is" today with what CPB "should be". With these improvements, CPB can once again be an enabling technology, this time for a next generation of minimally invasive surgical, as well as nonsurgical, procedures.

REFERENCES

1. Snicket L. The Bad Beginning. HarperCollins Publishers, 1999.
2. Gibbon JH Jr. Application of a mechanical heart and lung apparatus to cardiac surgery. Minn Med 1954;37:171–180.

3. Oz M, Roizen MF. You the Owner's Manual. New York: HarperCollins Publishers, 2005.
4. Patent Application Full Text and Image Database [cited 2005 May 17]. Available from: http://appft1.uspto.gov/netahtml/PTO/search-bool.html.
5. Benetti FJ, Matheny RG, Taylor CS. Surgical devices for imposing a negative pressure to fix the position of cardiac tissue during surgery. US Patent Appl No 603328, 1996 Feb 20. (Issued as US Patent 5,727,569; assigned to Cardiothoracic Systems, Inc).
6. Ferrari RM, Taylor CS, Lasersohn JW, et al. Methods and devices for minimally invasive coronary artery revascularization on a beating heart without CPB. US Patent Appl No. 752741, 1996 Nov 14. (Issued as US Patent 5,875,782, assigned to Cardiothoracic Systems, Inc).
7. Delevett P. New surgical technology a cut above. Silicon Valley/San Jose Business Journal. February 13, 1998.
8. Pfister AJ, Zaki MS, Garcia JM, et al. Coronary artery bypass without CPB. Ann Thorac Surg 1992;54:1085–1091.
9. Edmunds LH Jr. Why CPB makes patient sick: strategies to control the blood-synthetic surface interface. Adv Card Surg 1995;6:131–157.
10. Roach GW, Kanchuger M, Mora-Mangano C, et al. Adverse cerebral outcomes after coronary bypass surgery. N Engl J Med 1996;335:1857–1863.
11. Borger MA, Peniston CM, Weisel RD, Vasilou M, Green REA, Feindel SM. Neuropsychologic impairment after coronary bypass surgery: effect of gaseous microemboli during perfusionist interventions. J Thorac Cardiovasc Surg 2001; 121:743–749.
12. Lambrecht GH, Liddicoat J, Moore RK. Cardiac valve procedure methods and devices. US Patent Appl No: 700167, 2000 Jan 27. (Issued as US Patent 6,896,690 assigned to Viacor, Inc.).
13. Spenser B, Benichu N, Bash A, Zakai A. Implantable prosthetic valve. US Patent Appl No: 270252, 2003 Oct 11. (Issued as US Patent 6,730,118, assigned to Percutaneous Valve Technologies, Inc.).
14. Seguin J. Device for replacing a cardiac valve by percutaneous route. US Patent Appl No: 130355, 2002 Nov 26. (Issued as US Patent 6,830,584).
15. Sternberg S. For heart patients, bypass might be best; Study: they live longer than with angioplasty. USA Today 2005 May 26;A1.
16. Voorhees ME, Brian BF, 3rd. Blood-gas exchange devices. Int Anesth Clin 1996;34:29–45.
17. Galletti PM, Mora CT. CPB: the historical foundation, the future promise. In: CPB: Principles and techniques of extracorporeal circulation. Mora CT, editor. Springer, New York, 1995.
18. Edmunds LH Jr. The evolution of CPB: lessons to be learned. Perfusion 2002; 17:243–251.
19. De Somer F. Strategies for Optimisation of Paediatric CPB [dissertation]. Groningen (Netherlands): Rijksuniversiteit Groningen; 2003.
20. Stammers AH, Mejak BL, Rauch ED, Vang SN, Viessman TW. Factors affecting perfusionists' decisions on equipment utilization: results of a United States survey. J Extra Corpor Technol. 2000;32:4–10.
21. Bainbridge D, Martin J, Cheng D. Off pump coronary artery bypass graft surgery versus conventional coronary artery bypass graft surgery: a systematic review of the literature. Semin Cardiothorac Vasc Anesth. 2005;9: 105–111.

22. Boisclair MD, Philippou H, Lane DA. Thrombogenic mechanisms in the human: fresh insights obtained by immunodiagnostic studies of coagulation markers. Blood Coagul Fibrinolysis 1993;4:1007–1021.
23. Philippou H, Davidson SJ, Mole MT, Pepper JR, Burman JF, Lane DA. Two-chain factor VIIa generated in the pericardium during surgery with CPB: relationship to increased thrombin generation and heparin concentration. Arterioscler Thromb Vasc Biol 1999;19:248–254.
24. Chung JH, Gikakis N, Rao AK, Drake TA, Colman RW, Edmunds LH, Jr. Pericardial blood activates the extrinsic coagulation pathway during clinical CPB. Circulation. 1996;93:2014–2018.
25. Philippou H, Adami A, Davidson SJ, Pepper JR, Burman JF, Lane DA. Tissue factor is rapidly elevated in plasma collected from the pericardial cavity during CPB. Thromb Haemost 2000;84:124–128.
26. Brooker RF, Brown WR, Moody DM, et al. Cardiotomy suction: a major source of brain lipid emboli during CPB. Ann Thorac Surg 1998;65:1651–1655.
27. Spanier T, Tector K, Schwartz G, Chen J, Oz M, Beck J, Mongero L. Endotoxin in pooled pericardial blood contributes to the systemic inflammatory response during cardiac surgery Perfusion 2000;15:427–431.
28. Daniel S. Review of the multifactorial aspects of bioincompatibility in CPB. Perfusion 1996;11:246–55.
29. Fini M. Combined device comprising a venous blood reservoir and a cardiotomy reservoir in an extracorporeal circuit. US Patent Appl No: 888777, 1997 Jul 7. (Issued as US Patent 6,287,270 assigned to Dideco, S.p.A.).
30. Albes JM, Stöhr IM, Kaluza M, et al. Physiological coagulation can be maintained in extracorporeal circulation by means of shed blood separation and coating. J Thorac Cardiovasc Surg 2003;126:1504–1512.
31. Stump DA, Rogers AT, Hammon JW, Newman SP. Cerebral emboli and cognitive outcome after cardiac surgery. J Cardiothorac Vasc Anesth 1996;10:113–118.
32. Stump DA. Embolic factors associated with cardiac surgery. Semin Cardiothorac Vasc Anesth 2005;9:151–152.
33. Jones TJ, Deal DD, Vernon JC, Blackburn N, Stump DA. How effective are CPB circuits at removing gaseous microemboli? J Extra Corpor Technol 2002; 34:34–39.
34. Mitchell S, Wilcox T. Bubble generation and venous air filtration by hard-shell venous reservoirs: a comparative study. Perfusion 1997;12:325–333.
35. Cosgrove DM, Foster RC. CPB system using VAVD. US Patent Appl No: 911870, 1997 Aug 15. (Issued as US Patent 6,315,751 assigned to Cleveland Clinic Foundation).
36. Cambron R, Vijay F, Knight R, Litzie K. Vacuum-assisted venous drainage reservoir for CPB systems. US Patent Appl No: 938058, 1997 Sept 26. (Issued as US Patent 6,017,493 assigned to Baxter International Inc.).
37. Jones TJ, Deal DD, Vernon JC, Blackburn N, Stump DA. Does vacuum-assisted venous drainage increase gaseous microemboli during CPB? Ann Thorac Surg 2002;74:2132–2137.
38. Cirri S, Negri L, Babbini M, Latis G, Khlat B, Tarelli G, et al. Haemolysis due to active venous drainage during CPB: comparison of two different techniques. Perfusion 2001;16:313–318.
39. Jegger D, Tevaearai HT, Mueller XM, Horisberger J, von Segesser LK. Limitations using the vacuum-assist venous drainage technique during CPB procedures. J Extra Corpor Technol 2003;35:207–211.

40. Schönberger J, Everts P, Hoffmann J. Systemic blood activation with open and closed venous reservoirs. Ann Thorac Surg 1995;59:1549–1555.
41. Hessel EA II, Edmunds LH Jr. Extracorporeal circulation: perfusion systems. In: Cardiac Surgery in the Adult. Cohn LH, Edmunds LH Jr, editors. McGraw-Hill, New York; 2003:317–338.
42. Tamari Y. Soft shell venous reservoir. US Patent Appl No: 141960, 1998 Aug 28. (issued as US Patent 6,337,049).
43. Barringer C, Fallen D, Rainone M, Umbach SR. Heart bypass system incorporating minimized extracorporeal blood circulation system and related method of use. US Patent Appl No: 653522, 2003 Sept 2.
44. Lilly KJ, O'Gara PJ, Treanor PR, Reardon D, Crowley R, Hunter C, et al. CPB: it's not the size, it's how you use it! Review of a comprehensive blood-conservation strategy. J Extra Corpor Technol 2004;36:263–268.
45. Shander A, Moskowitz D, Rijhwani TS. The safety and efficacy of "bloodless" cardiac surgery. Semin Cardiothorac Vasc Anesth 2005;9:53–63.
46. Fransen EJ, Ganushchak YM, Vijay V, de Jong DS, Buurman WA, Maessen JG. Evaluation of a new condensed extra-corporeal circuit for cardiac surgery: a prospective randomized clinical pilot study. Perfusion 2005;20:91–99.
47. Shapira OM, Aldea GS, Treanor PR, Chartrand RM, DeAndrade KM, Lazar HL, et al. Reduction of allogenic blood transfusions after open heart operations by lowering CPB prime volume. Ann Thorac Surg 1998;65:724–730.
48. te Velthuis H, Jansen PG, Hack CE, Eijsman L, Wildevuur CR. Specific complement inhibition with heparin-coated extracorporeal circuits. Ann Thorac Surg 1996;61:1153–1157.
49. Keil LB, Jimenez E, Guma M, Reyes MD, Liguori C, DeBari VA. Biphasic response of complement to heparin: fluid-phase generation of neoantigens in human serum and in a reconstituted alternative pathway amplification cycle. Am J Hematol 1995;50:254–262.
50. Khuri SF, Valeri CR, Loscalzo J, et al. Heparin causes platelet dysfunction and induces fibrinolysis before CPB. Ann Thorac Surg 1995;60:1008–1014.
51. Bruins P, te Velthuis H, Eerenberg-Belmer AJ, et al. Heparin-protamine complexes and C-reactive protein induce activation of the classical complement pathway: studies in patients undergoing cardiac surgery and in vitro. Thromb Haemost 2000;84:237–243.
52. Lilly KJ, O'Gara PJ, Treanor PR, et al. Heparin-bonded circuits without a cardiotomy: a description of a minimally invasive technique of CPB. Perfusion 2002;17:95–97.
53. Habib RH, Zacharias A, Schwann TA, Riordan CJ, Durham SJ, Shah A. Adverse effects of low hematocrit during CPB in the adult: should current practice be changed? J Thorac Cardiovasc Surg 2003;125:1438–1450.
54. Hare GMT. Anaemia and the brain. Curr Opin Anaesthesiol 2004;17:363–369.
55. Alexander JC, Kronenfeld MA, Dance GR. Reduced postoperative length of stay may result from using cerebral oximetry monitoring to guide treatment. Ann Thor Surg 2002;73:S373.
56. Yao FSF, Tseng CCA, Ho CYA, Levin SK, Illner P. Cerebral oxygen desaturation is associated with early postoperative neuropsychological dysfunction in patients undergoing cardiac surgery. J Cardiothorac Vasc Anesth 2004;18(5):552–558.
57. van Kempen RAB, Gasiorek JM, Bloemendaal K, Storm van Leeuwen RPH, Bulder ER. Low-prime perfusion circuit and autologous priming in CABG surgery on a Jehovah's Witness: a case report. Perfusion 2002;17:69–72.

58. Sistino JJ, Michler RE, Mongero LB. Laboratory evaluation of a low prime closed-circuit CPB system. J Extra Corporeal Technol 1993;24:116–119.
59. Wiesenack C, Liebold A, Philipp A, et al. Four years' experience with a miniaturized extracorporeal circulation system and its influence on clinical outcome. Artif Organs 2004;28:1082–1088.
60. Calafiore AM, Teodori G, Di Giammarco G, Bosco G, Mezzetti A, Lapenna D, Verna AM. Intermittent antegrade cardioplegia: warm blood vs cold crystalloid. A clinical study. J Cardiovasc Surg 1994; 6 Suppl 1:179–184.
61. Remadi JP, Rakotoarivello Z, Marticho P, et al. Aortic valve replacement with the minimal extracorporeal circulation (Jostra MECC System) versus standard CPB: a randomized prospective trial. J Thorac Cardiovasc Surg. 2004;128:436–441.
62. Norman MJ, Sistino JJ, Acsell JR. The effectiveness of low-prime CPB circuits at removing gaseous emboli. J Extra Corporeal Technol 2004;36:336–342.
63. Morita M, Yozu R, Matayoshi T, Mitsumaru A, Shin H, Kawada S. Closed Circuit CPB with Centrifugal Pump for Open-Heart Surgery: New Trial for Air Removal. Artif Organs 2000;24:442–445.
64. Ojito JW, Hannan RL, Miyaji K, et al. Assisted venous drainage CPB in congenital heart surgery. Ann Thorac Surg 2001;71:1267–1272.
65. Stringer SK, Hultquist KL, Farhangnia M, et al. Integrated blood handling system having active gas removal system and methods of use. US Patent Appl No: 780923, 2001 Feb 9. (Issued as US Patent 6,730,267 assigned to Cardiovention, Inc.)
66. Yamut T. FDA 510(k) Premarket Notification. Cardiovention CORx System, K012325, April 9, 2002.
67. Guidance for CPB Oxygenators 510(k) Submissions; Final Guidance for Industry and FDA Staff Document issued on: November 13, 2000 available from http://www.fda.gov/cdrh/ode/guidance/1361.pdf.
68. Von Segesser LK, Tozzi P, Mallbiabrrena I, Jegger D, Horisberger J, Corno A. Miniaturization in CPB. Perfusion 2003;18:219–224.
69. Rawles TA, Litzie KA, Fallen DM, Stringer SK. Tubing set for blood handling system and methods of use. US Patent Appl No: 134138, 2002 Apr 25. (Issued as US Patent 6,890,316 assigned to Cardiovention, Inc).
70. Lambert E. First, Do No Harm. Forbes Magazine. June 06, 2005;170.
71. Medtronic.com [homepage on the Internet]. [cited 2005 Jun 5]. Available from: http://www.medtronic.com/
72. Huybregts MA, de Vroege R, Christiaans HM, Smith AL, Paulus RC. The use of a mini bypass system (Cobe Synergy) without venous and cardiotomy reservoir in a mitral valve repair: a case report. Perfusion 2005;20:121–124.
73. Litzie KA, Stringer SK, Farhangnia M, Tyebjee M, Afzal TA, Brian BF 3rd. Extracorporeal blood handling system with automatic flow control and methods of use. US Patent Appl No 392441, 2003 Mar 17.
74. Gourlay T, Stefanou DC, Asimakopoulos G, Taylor KM. The effect of circuit surface area on CD11b(mac-1) expression in a rat recirculation model. Artif Organs 2001;25:475–479.
75. Ullmann C. Automated ECC Management. Presented at the Bottlenecks in Cardiac Surgery and Satellite-Symposium on Cardiovascular Perfusion 2005, Heiligendamm, Germany.
76. Wendel HP, Philipp A, Weber N, Birnbaum DE, Ziemer G. Oxygenator thrombosis: worst case after development of an abnormal pressure gradient—incidence and pathway Perfusion 2001;16:271–278.

77. Fisher AR, Baker M, Buffin M, et al. Normal and abnormal trans-oxygenator pressure gradients during CPB. Perfusion 2003;18:25–30.
78. De Somer F, Toubert L, Schacht E, van Nooten G. Nitric oxide donors attenuate increase in pressure drop across membrane oxygenators. Perfusion 1999;14: 331–336.
79. Palanzo D, Zarro D, Montesano R, Manley N, Quinn M, Elmore B, et al. Effect of Trillium™ Biopassive Surface coating of the oxygenator on platelet count drop during CPB. Perfusion 1999;14:473–479.
80. Afzal TA, Dueri JP, Leynov A, Makarewicz A, Piplani A, inventors; Assignee: Cardiovention, Inc. Integrated blood oxygenator and pump system. United States Patent Appl No: 475467, 1999 Dec 30. (Issued as US Patent 6,503,450 assigned to Cardiovention, Inc).
81. Maloney JV Jr, Buckberg GD, inventors. Mass and thermal transfer means for use in heart lung machines, dialyzers, and other applications. US Patent Appl No:940922, 1997 Sept 30. (issued as United States Patent 5,900,142).
82. Reeder GD, Gartner MJ, Borovetz HS, Litwak P, inventors; University of Pittsburgh, assignee. Membrane apparatus with enhanced mass transfer, heat transfer and pumping capabilities via active mixing. United States Patent Appl No; 157815, 1998 Sept 21. (issued as US patent 6,217,826 assigned to University of Pittsburgh).
83. Gartner MJ, Litwak P, Borovetz HS,Griffith BP. Development of a pumping artificial lung. Eng Med Biol 2002;2:1589–1590.
84. Smartcanula.com [homepage on the Internet]. [updated 2002 May 16; cited 2005 Jun 5]. Available from: http://www.smartcanula.com/
85. Jegger D, Corno AF, Mucciolo A, et al. A prototype paediatric venous cannula with shape change in situ. Perfusion 2003;18:61–65.
86. Jegger D, Horisberger J, Boone Y, et al. Vascular access for CPB procedures. Artif Organs 2004;28:649–654.
87. Bird RB, Stewart WE, Lightfoot EN. Transport phenomena. John Wiley & Sons, New York, 1960.
88. Shaaban Ali M, Harmer M, Kirkham F. CPB temperature and brain function. Anaesthesia 2005;60:365–372.
89. Grigore AM, Mathew J, Grocott HP, et al. Prospective randomized trial of normothermic versus hypothermic CPB on cognitive function after coronary artery bypass graft surgery Anesthesiology 2001;95:1110–1119.
90. Cook DJ, Orszulak TA, Zehr KJ, et al. Effectiveness of the Cobra aortic catheter for dual-temperature management during adult cardiac surgery. J Thorac Cardiovasc Surg 2003;125:378–384.
91. Kaukuntla H, Walker A, Harrington D, Jones T, Bonser RS. Differential brain and body temperature during CPB–a randomised clinical study. Eur J Cardiothorac Surg 2004;26:571–579.
92. Paparella D, Brister SJ, Buchanan MR. Coagulation disorders of CPB: a review. Intensive Care Med 2004;30:1873–1881.
93. Stanley TO, Grocott HP, Phillips-Bute B, Mathew JP, Landoflo KP, Newman MF. Preliminary evaluation of the arctic sun temperature controlling system during off-pump coronary artery bypass surgery. Ann Thorac Surg 2003;75: 1140–1144.
94. Doufas AG, Akca O, Barry A, et al. Initial experience with a novel heat-exchanging catheter in neurosurgical patients. Anesth Analg 2002;95:1752–1756.

95. Dixon SR, Whitbourn RJ, Dae MW, et al. Induction of mild systemic hypothermia with endovascular cooling during primary percutaneous coronary intervention for acute myocardial infarction. J Am Coll Cardiol 2002;40:1928–1934.
96. Kaza AK, Cope JT, Fiser SM, et al. Elimination of fat microemboli during CPB. Ann Thorac Surg 2003;75:555–559.
97. Martens S, Dietrich M, Pietrzyk R, Graubitz K, Keller H, Moritz A. Elimination of microbubbles from the extracorporeal circuit: dynamic bubble trap versus arterial filter. Int J Artif Organs 2004;27:55–59.
98. Haemonetics.com [homepage on the Internet]. [cited 2005 Jun 7]. Available from: http://www.haemonetics.com/site/content/km/news_179.asp.
99. Warner C. The use of the orthopaedic perioperative autotransfusion (OrthoPAT) system in total joint replacement surgery. Orthop Nurs 2001;20:29–32.
100. Headley TD, Powers ET. Fluid separation system. US Patent Appl No: 843218, 1997 April 14. (Issued as US Patent 6,099,491 assigned to Transfusion Technologies Corporation).
101. Calafiore AM, Teodori G, Mezzetti A, et al. Intermittent antegrade warm blood cardioplegia. Ann Thorac Surg 1995;59:398–402.
102. Sellke FW, DiMaio JM, Caplan LR, et al. Comparing on-pump and off-pump coronary artery bypass grafting: numerous studies but few conclusions: a scientific statement from the American Heart Association council on cardiovascular surgery and anesthesia in collaboration with the interdisciplinary working group on quality of care and outcomes research. Circulation 2005;111:2858–2864.
103. Harringer W. Capture of particulate emboli during cardiac procedures in which aortic cross-clamp is used. International Council of Emboli Management Study Group. Ann Thorac Surg 2000;70:1119–1123.
104. Chai PJ, Williamson JA, Lodge AJ, et al. Effects of ischemia on pulmonary dysfunction after CPB. Ann Thorac Surg 1999;67:731–735.
105. Alwan K, Falcoz PE, Alwan J, et al. Beating versus arrested heart coronary revascularization: evaluation by cardiac troponin I release. Ann Thorac Surg 2004;77:2051–2055.
106. Fallen D, Komorowski B, Groh M. Perfusion-assisted beating heart CABG with a miniature bypass system is associated with improved outcomes compared to traditional CPB-supported CABG. Abstracts, Outcomes 2003 Meeting. Available from: http://www.outcomeskeywest.com/Pdfs/2003/11-1.pdf.
107. Falk V, Jacobs S, Gummert J, Walther T. Robotic coronary artery bypass grafting (CABG)–the Leipzig experience. Surg Clin North Am 2003;83:1381–1386.
108. Autschbach R, Onnasch JF, Falk V, et al. The Leipzig experience with robotic valve surgery. J Card Surg 2000;15:82–87.

2 Pediatric Perfusion Techniques for Complex Congenital Cardiac Surgery

Kevin A. Charette, BS, CCP,
Ryan R. Davies, MD,
Jonathan M. Chen, MD,
Jan M. Quaegebeur, MD, PhD,
and Ralph S. Mosca, MD

Contents

HISTORICAL CONSIDERATIONS

Motivated by the inadequacy of nonsurgical therapy in ameliorating congenital cardiac disease, surgical pioneers in the 1940s and 1950s began to develop techniques that would allow for the intracardiac repair of congenital heart disease. The first operation on the open human heart under direct vision—closure of an atrial septal defect (ASD) in a 5-year-old girl—was performed at the University of Minnesota by Dr. F. John Lewis on September 2nd, 1952 *(1)*. This

From: *Current Cardiac Surgery: On Bypass: Advanced Perfusion Techniques*
Edited by: L. B. Mongero and J. R. Beck © Humana Press Inc., Totowa, NJ

operation was performed using inflow stasis and moderate total body hypothermia. Within 1 year, Lewis reported closure of 11 ASDs with only 18% mortality *(2)*. This success, however, could not be extended to more complex defects without a system of extracorporeal oxygenation and perfusion. On May 6, 1953, John Gibbon used his extracorporeal oxygenation system to successfully close an ASD in a young woman *(3)*. Despite this success, initial attempts at mechanical cardiopulmonary bypass (CPB) were uniformly dismal; of 18 reported cases between 1951 and 1954, using a variety of methods for total CPB (film oxygenators, bubble oxygenators, and monkey lungs), only those with ASDs survived *(4–10)*. Faced with these results, alternative methods of perfusion were pursued, and on March 26, 1954, C. Walton Lillehei and colleagues successfully closed a ventricular septal defect (VSD) in a 12-month-old infant using controlled cross-circulation with the patient's father functioning as the extracorporeal oxygenator *(11)*. From the late 1950s to well into the 1980s, bubble oxygenators were utilized in most extracorporeal oxygenation circuits. However, the high amount of embolic materials that were released by these devices led to the development of membrane oxygenators, which are now the gold standard for extracorporeal oxygenation *(3)*.

CONGENITAL HEART SURGERY AT NEW YORK PRESBYTERIAN HOSPITAL/COLUMBIA CAMPUS

Pediatric congenital heart surgery has been performed for over 30 years at New York Presbyterian Hospital's Columbia Campus, which is located in upper Manhattan. The Morgan Stanley Children's Hospital of New York (CHONY) is the children's hospital of the Columbia Campus, and is currently the largest congenital heart surgical center in New York State, performing over 500 congenital heart surgeries on CPB per year.

The following chapter outlines general considerations for the pediatric perfusionist, including many of the policies and procedures currently used at CHONY.

CHALLENGES OF CARDIOPULMONARY BYPASS IN THE PEDIATRIC POPULATION

Perfusionists who specialize in pediatric perfusion are challenged to prepare for different sized patients; therefore, they need to employ a variety of oxygenators and circuitry to accommodate children who could be as small as 1 kg or as large as an adult.

Circuits

A current trend in bypass surgery is toward decreasing the overall prime volume that the patient encounters during CPB. Moreover, utilizing the lowest prime possible for neonates and infants is especially important because of their particularly high extracorporeal circuit prime volume/patient blood volume ratio. This ratio can be decreased by employing small diameter, and therefore low prime, tubing (Table 1). Cardiac indices of 2.2–2.5 can be utilized to calculate extracorporeal flow, thereby providing appropriate full flow bypass, while avoiding overcirculation (Table 2). For children less than 5 kg, a circuit that primes with 220 cc is possible; this can be accomplished by utilizing 1/8 in. tubing for the arterial line and 3/16 in. in the venous line. The raceway and sump tubing for this circuit are 3/16 in. and the vent tubing is 1/8 in. Small diameter vent and sump tubing decreases the overall surface area and requires less steal from the total circulating volume when actively filled. An additional 40 cc of prime volume can be saved if the arterial filter is excluded, making the prime 180 cc. This circuit has been successfully used (no arterial filter) to perform a bloodless arterial switch on a 3.4-kg Jehovah's Witness. Even though the necessity of arterial filtration for neonates is debatable, Sorin Group (Mirandola, Italy) has recently developed a low prime arterial line filter (D 130 kids®, 16 cc). Certainly the development of even lower prime arterial filters is merited.

For children who weigh between 5 and 13 kg, a perfusion circuit that primes with 270 cc is available. This system utilizes the standard 3/16 × 1/4 loop and a 1/4 raceway. The use of low prime, high-flow oxygenators, such as the Baby-RX™ by Terumo®, has given the perfusionist the opportunity to offer a bloodless prime to some children who

Table 1
Common Tubing Diameters and Their Associated Prime Volumes Per Inch of Tubing

Tubing Diameter in Inches	*Cc/inch*
1/2	3.5
3/8	1.8
5/16	1.3
1/4	.82
3/16	.45
1/8	.20

Table 2
Appropriate CI Per Patient Temperature

Core temp °C	*Cardiac index M^2*	**Approx DHCA*
37–35	2.2–2.5	5 min
<35–32	2.0–2.2	
<32–28	1.8–2.0	
<28–24	1.6–1.8	20 min
<24–20	1.0–1.5	
<20	0.5–0.8	45 min

*90% probability of absence of structural or functional damage.

(*Source*: Kirklin JW, Barratt-Boyes GB, eds. Cardiac Surgery. Churchill-Livingstone, New York, 1993:61–127.)

would previously have required exogenous packed red blood cells; it can be particularly useful for children in the 10–15-kg range.

The Sorin D 100 Kids oxygenator® primes with 31 cc and is now available for neonates, and hopefully even lower prime devices will be developed.

A 1/4 × 3/8 in. A–V loop and pediatric oxygenator are used for children between 15 and 30 kg (some centers report the use of 5/16 in. venous line tubing in place of 3/8 in. for this patient population). From 30 to 55 kg, a 3/8 × 3/8 in. A–V loop and 3/8 in pump boot are routinely utilized, also with a pediatric oxygenator, and all patients over 55 kg receive an adult setup (Table 3).

Table 3
CHONY Bypass Circuits

Circuit FLOW	*cc/L per min*	*OXYGENATOR*	*LOOP*	*PRIME**	*FILTER*	*BOOT*
A.	<650 cc	**Baby-RX™**	1/8–3/16	220 cc	AF02	3/16-
B.	>650 cc–1.3 L	**Baby-RX™**	3/16–1/4	270 cc	AF02	1/4-
B1.	>1.3 L–1.5 L	**Baby-RX™**	1/4–3/8	375 cc	AF02	1/4-
C.	>1.5–2.5 L	**SX10R®**	1/4–3/8	610 cc	AF02	3/8-
D.	>2.5–3.5 L	**SX10R®**	3/8–3/8	850 cc	AL-8	3/8-
E.	>3.5 L	**SX18R®**	3/8–1/2	1150 cc	AL-8	1/2-

*Represents the minimum dynamic prime at the onset of CPB, excluding the cardioplegia prime.

In addition to constructing extracorporeal circulation systems that are honed to the varying sizes of a pediatric population, other factors must be considered, including degree of hypothermia, acid–base management strategy, cardiopulmonary and cerebral protection, and techniques to manage bypass-induced inflammation.

Hypothermia

In 1950, Bigelow first demonstrated the linear relationship between falling temperature and falling metabolic rate when anesthesia was used to control shivering and the increased muscle tone generated in response to cold *(12)*. These findings were applied by Lewis et al. during their first open intracardiac repair in 1953 *(1)*. After the development of the pump oxygenator, CPB and hypothermia were combined by Sealy, and some degree of hypothermia became common practice in the conduct of cardiac surgery *(13)*.

Use of Hypothermia in Congenital Heart Surgery

The degree of hypothermia used during congenital heart surgery depends primarily on the reduction in flow required to perform an accurate repair. Mild (34–30°C), moderate (<30–25°C) or deep hypothermia (<25°C) may be employed. Mild hypothermia can be used in many simpler procedures, where the period of myocardial ischemia is relatively short. For more complex repairs, moderate hypothermia allows for longer aortic cross-clamp times and temporary periods of lower flow with maintenance of adequate myocardial protection (Table 2). The maintenance of a bloodless operative field in infants and neonates can be particularly challenging for several reasons, including aortopulmonary collaterals, increased pulmonary venous return and anomalous anatomy. Furthermore, the arterial and venous cannula themselves may make adequate exposure difficult. The use of deep hypothermia enables low flow CPB or circulatory arrest, which mitigates all of these problems. CPB may be initiated with a single atrial venous cannula that can be removed (along with the arterial cannula) during the circulatory arrest portion, thereby providing a bloodless and cannula-free operative field. The following chart represents a basic CPB temperature guideline for many congenital heart anomalies. (Table 4).

CO_2 Management: Alpha-Stat Versus pH-Stat

One of the most studied aspects of hypothermia is its effect on the acid–base balance during CPB. In humans, the extracellular fluid pH

Table 4
CHONY Hypothermia Chart

Procedure	*Temperature °C*
ASD secundum	36
ASD Sinus Venosus	34
VSD	32
Sub Aortic Stenosis	32–35
Tetralogy of Fallot	28–32
TAPVR	18
PAPVR	34
Norwood	18
Bidirectional Glenn	32–35
Hemi-Fontan	18
Fontan (lateral tunnel)	18–32
Fontan (extra cardiac)	34
Atrioventricular Septal Defect	28–32
Ross Procedure	28–32
Arterial Switch-VSD	18
Arterial Switch-ASD	18–24
MVR/AVR/TVR	32
Interrupted Aortic Arch	18
Ebstein's Anomaly	28–32
Truncus Arteriosus	18–24
RV-PA conduit	28–32

(pH_e) is maintained within a narrow range between 7.36 and 7.44 at normothermic temperatures. Intracellular pH (pH_i, which is more difficult to measure, but of significantly more importance to optimal intracellular enzymatic functions), is maintained at around 7.1, which is close to the pH of neutrality (pN) of water where the hydroxyl/hydrogen ion ratio approaches unity *(14,15)*. Maintenance of the intracellular environment at a pH close to pN ensures that enzymatic processes occur at an optimal rate *(15)*. As temperature falls, the dissociation constant of water increases, resulting in a decrease of both hydrogen and hydroxyl ions. Thus, maintenance of neutrality requires a rise in pH (decrease in hydrogen concentration).

In ectothermic (i.e., cold-blooded) animals, blood pH increases to maintain intra- and extracellular pH close to the pN of water. To do this, ectotherms allow $PaCO_2$ to fall by maintaining normothermic ventilation despite the decreased CO_2 production that occurs with falling temperature *(16,17)*. This method of pH management is called alpha-stat because the ratio (termed "alpha") of dissociated-to-nondissociated imidazole groups (the primary blood buffer at hypothermic temperatures) remains constant *(16)*. Although a full discussion of the biochemistry of alpha-stat pH management is beyond the scope of this chapter, it appears to offer biochemical stability in the setting of falling temperature *(16)*. The other method of acid-base management is termed pH-stat; in this method, despite the rising pN of water, blood pH is maintained at a constant 7.40 through the addition of CO_2. This method lowers pH_i resulting in loss of intracellular electro-chemical neutrality. Heterothermic (ie. hibernating) animals use a predominantly pH-stat method of acid-base management during hibernation. However, certain active tissues (e.g., heart and liver) actively extrude H^+ across their cell membrane, resulting in the maintenance of pH_i near values predicted by alpha-stat management *(18)*. Furthermore, during awakening, animals begin to hyperventilate, reverting to overall alpha-stat pH management and regaining optimal enzymatic function.

Choice of Acid–Base Management Strategy

The traditional preference for the pH-stat method in the 1960s and 1970s was predicated on two theories: (a) hypercarbia would ameliorate the leftward shift of the oxyhemoglobin dissociation curve which occurs with hypothermia, thereby increasing tissue oxygen availability, and (b) cerebral vasodilation in response to elevated CO_2 would selectively increase cerebral blood flow during the period of CPB *(18,19)*. However, the leftward shift of the dissociation curve is balanced by the increase in oxygen dissolved in plasma during hypothermia, and the dissolved oxygen may be sufficient to fully support cerebral metabolism at hypothermic temperatures *(20,21)*. Although pH-stat management does appear to enhance distribution of extracorporeal perfusate to the brain, and thereby improve the speed and distribution of brain cooling, it is also associated with impaired metabolic recovery after circulatory arrest *(22–24)*.

Most evidence suggests that, in adults, the management strategy does not matter, or there may be benefit to the use of alpha-stat management *(25–27)*. In children, however, the data is more controversial. Although some studies do report improved outcomes using alpha-stat, others have demonstrated shorter recovery of electroencephalographic activity, decreased incidence of electroencephalographic seizures, and improved postoperative developmental scores using pH-stat *(28,29)*. The heterogeneity of results has led some authors to recommend a combined strategy where 10 min of pH-stat management is used to promote brain cooling, followed by alpha-stat management to return the cerebral milieu to electrochemical neutrality *(23,30)*. This crossover method or pH-stat management alone may be the best method in pediatric patients, particularly those in whom large aortopulmonary collaterals impair cerebral cooling *(31–33)*.

The perpetual debate between alpha- and pH-stat blood gas management is ongoing, with many centers reporting good results utilizing either strategy. Therefore, intercenter differences in intraoperative patient management may create a multifactorial milieu that favors one method over another. Therefore, the alpha-stat management strategy has always been utilized at CHONY for all congenital heart surgery. However, current low prime oxygenators are capable of transferring CO_2 over a large range of patients ranging from less than 2 to 15 kg. These units tend to be too efficient for neonates, so low sweep rates are necessary to avoid hypocapnea, especially when cooling to and warming from DHCA and, most importantly, during procedures where aortopulmonary collaterals are present.

A 1995 CHONY study, which used ultrasound to interrogate the middle cerebral artery (MCA) during DHCA and hypothermic low flow bypass, found that patients who underwent deep hypothermia had lower cerebral blood flow velocities after rewarming than those who only experienced moderate hypothermia *(34)*. It was also noted anecdotaly, that middle cerebral artery flow could be used to predict low pCO_2 levels. At a given mean arterial pressure with obvious detectable MCA flow, pCO_2 was above 30 mmHg; in contrast, marked decreases in MCA flow velocity were associated with a pCO_2 that was less than 20 mmHg.

Myocardial Protection

Despite the increased tolerance for hypoxia and ischemia in experimental evaluation of the immature myocardium, in clinical practice, immature myocardium appears to be more susceptible to injury than the adult heart *(35–37)*. Both the hypoxia and the volume and pressure overload common with congenital heart defects result in increased preoperative myocardial stress and susceptibility to perioperative injury *(35)*. Several conditions, including left-to-right shunts, single ventricle with mixed circulation, and atrioventricular valve insufficiency, may lead to volume overload, and then to ventricular hypertrophy and dilatation; similarly, outflow tract obstruction or elevated vascular resistance may result in elevated ventricular pressures and, ultimately, to hypertrophy *(36,38,39)*. Ventricular compensation in both cases leads to myocardium that may be more susceptible to ischemic insult during operative repair *(38,40–42)*.

Proper management of pO_2 is also important for neonatal myocardial protection, especially in the setting of cyanotic lesions *(43)*. To avoid excessive hyperoxygenation, a slightly hyperoxic blood gas strategy can be utilized by maintaining a pO_2 goal in the high 200 s.

Cardioplegia

There are a variety of recipes for cardioplegia solutions and circuit configurations for their delivery. For patients less than 30 kg, a potassium solution of 60 Meq/L with a low prime circuit (75 cc) has proven reliable. This method allows for a quick dose of 15 cc/kg, followed by subsequent doses of 5–7 cc/kg at 20–30-min intervals. The cardioplegia delivery system utilizes a 1:1 blood/clear solution with a 3/16 over 3/16 raceway, the Sorin Vanguard™, and a 1/8-in. delivery line. The cardioplegia solution consists of: 900 cc D5W, 60 Meq KCL, 30 Meq $NaHCO_3$ and 12.5 g of Mannitol. Even lower cardioplegia prime volumes are possible by using 1/8-in tubing in the raceway and smaller conducers. For children over 30 kg, a 4:1 blood cardioplegia system can be used. With this configuration, a high dose of 120 Meq/L is delivered until 7 cc per kg is administered, and then the low dose of 60 Meq/L is given until an additional 8 cc/kg (for a total of 15 cc/kg) is achieved.

There are a variety of cannulae available for pediatric cardioplegia delivery, including Angiocaths®, DLP® aortic root cannulae, and DLP® balloon tip cannulae for individual coronary ostial cardioplegia delivery (Fig. 1). It is possible to perform most pediatric congenital heart surgery without the use of retrograde cardioplegia.

Systemic Responses to CPB

Pulmonary Dysfunction

The lungs are at risk for injury during CPB from two perioperative processes: ischemia/reperfusion and the systemic inflammatory response; these are exacerbated by the frequent coexistence of varying degrees of preoperative pulmonary hypertension. With the onset of total CPB, the lungs become dependent on the bronchial arteries for nutrient and oxygen delivery; where these are not adequate, ischemic injury may occur *(44–47)*. The inflammatory response to CPB contributes to postoperative pulmonary hypertension, leading to increased

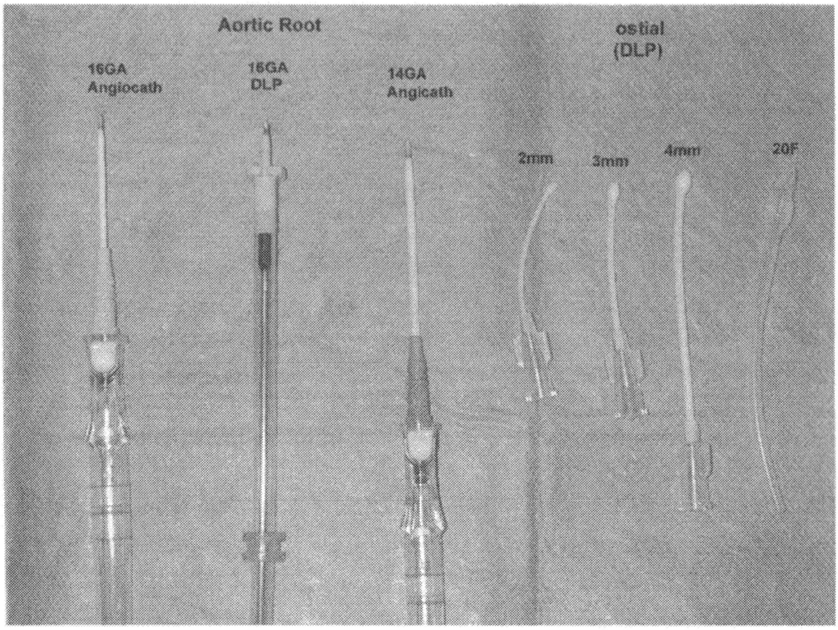

Fig. 1. Cardioplegia Cannulae (Angiocath®, DLP®).

right ventricular work in the postcardiotomy heart and, more importantly, results in pulmonary edema with its attendant decrease in functional residual capacity, compliance, and gas exchange *(48–52)*. The relative impact of and interaction between these processes is complex, as illustrated by the fact that low-flow CPB appears to cause worse lung injury than does circulatory arrest *(53,54)*.

Several strategies have been proposed to limit pulmonary injury during and after CPB. Steroid treatment mitigates the systemic inflammatory response and improves pulmonary compliance and vascular resistance *(55)*. Ultrafiltration also appears to limit post-CPB pulmonary dysfunction *(56–59)*. Experimentally, liquid lung ventilation appears to improve postoperative pulmonary function, but the application of this technique awaits human trials *(60–62)*.

In the post-CPB phase, pulmonary hypertension may be ameliorated through the use of inhaled nitric oxide (NO), and the use of NO may facilitate weaning from CPB, making it an essential tool for pediatric congenital heart surgery *(63)*. The intraoperative administration of NOi can be managed by the respiratory therapists, perfusionists, and/or the anesthesiologists. The respiratory therapists should supply the NO delivery system (INOvent®). After delivery of the system to the operating room, the perfusion or respiratory teams can purge it of nitrogen dioxide, ensure that the system is running smoothly, and then set the requested dose (usually 20 PPM). Anesthesiologists then connect the NOi system in-line with their ventilator tubing.

Neurologic Injury

Mediators of Neurologic Injury. The conduct of CPB in neonates, infants, and children exposes these patients to biological extremes far in excess of those present in most adult operations: deep hypothermia, hemodilution, low perfusion pressures, and wide variations in pump flow rates are common *(64)*. In addition, variability in glucose supplementation, cannula placement, the presence of aortopulmonary collaterals, patient age and predilection for neurologic damage, prior episodes of severe hypoxia, and brain mass may all affect the neurological response to and morbidity from CPB *(64)*. Because of difficulties with neurological and cognitive assessment in infants and children, accurate estimates of the long-term neurological impact of CPB in the pediatric population are difficult to obtain *(65)*. However, estimates of acute neurological morbidity approach 25% *(66)*. Such morbidity may take many forms including stroke, diffuse hypoxic–ischemic lesions, intracranial hemorrhage, delayed choreoathetoid syndrome, spinal cord lesions, cerebral infarction, diffuse cortical atrophy and seizures *(65)*. Several potential mechanisms have been proposed for these injuries *(65)*:

1. Unrecognized preoperative neurological abnormalities;
2. Hypoxic insults;
3. Altered cerebral blood flow and cerebral metabolism with hypothermia;
4. Embolic events; and
5. Low cardiac output states following cardiac surgery.

Unrecognized preoperative neurological abnormalities complicate the analysis of postoperative neurological defects in children. Up to 1/3 of patients may have abnormal preoperative magnetic resonance brain imaging without neurological symptoms or deficits *(67)*. The natural history of such lesions cannot be known for certain, given that many of these patients present with cardiac defects requiring emergent repair. However, clearly many patients have abnormal cerebral blood flow even before being subjected to CPB *(68)*.

With decreasing temperature, cerebral blood flow decreases linearly due to autoregulation, but cerebral metabolism decreases exponentially, resulting in ample cerebral oxygen delivery at low temperature, despite minimal pump flow rates (Table 2) *(69)*. However, even with deep hypothermia, cerebral metabolism continues at a low level, leading to hypoxia and ischemia when the pump is turned off for circulatory arrest. As noted above, hypothermia has additional protective effects on the ischemic brain that help mitigate the resultant damage. Nonetheless, prolonged circulatory arrest time is associated with an increasing risk of neurological injury regardless of the techniques of neuroprotection used *(70)*. Methods that may help limit ischemic injury during DHCA, in addition to hypothermia, include intravenous methylprednisolone *(55)* and the use of aprotinin *(68,71)*. Other methods, including blockade of thromboxane A2 receptors, free radical scavengers, and platelet-activating factor inhibitors, remain experimental at this time.

Although less frequently the cause of neurological morbidity in children than in adults, microembolic events occur commonly and may contribute to end-organ injury. Air embolism may be particularly likely where operative repair necessitates opening the left side of the circulation to the air *(68)*. The use of membrane oxygenators and arterial filters has minimized but not eliminated the risk of air embolism *(72,73)*. When cerebral air embolism does occur, both reestablishment of hypothermic CPB and hyperbaric O_2 therapy may reduce the size of microbubbles, allowing them to pass through capillary beds, and thereby reduce tissue damage *(74)*. Furthermore, the risk of neurological injury does not end with the termination of CPB; in the postoperative period, factors that increase brain metabolic demand (hyperthermia), or decrease substrate and oxygen delivery (low cardiac output or hypoglycemia), may lead to brain injury *(64)*.

Traditionally, DHCA was used for most cardiac repairs in the pediatric population. While its use has enabled technically successful cardiac repairs, DHCA in the format used in the 1980s and early 1990s did not provide adequate protection for the brain *(75)*. Improvements in technology have made it feasible to use bicaval cannulation and continuous low-flow perfusion even in neonates *(75)*. Although neurological outcomes, including stroke rates and long-term developmental outcomes, were improved using continuous low-flow perfusion *(76)*, evidence continues to accumulate that this method may result in increased soft tissue edema, poor pulmonary function, and

Table 5
Common Strategies for Limiting Neurologic Injury with the Use of Deep Hypothermic Circulatory Arrest

Prebypass treatment with steroids and aprotinin *(71,78)*
Adequate duration of cooling (≥20 min) to ensure more uniform and homogeneous brain protection *(79,80)*
Maintenance of higher hematocrits during the cooling phase
**Using pH stat blood gas management strategy during the cooling phase *(23,28,81)*
**Use of intermittent hypothermic cerebral perfusion for 1 to 2 min at 15–20 min intervals *(77,82)*
**Use of MUF after CPB *(83)*
Attention to postoperative cerebral metabolic demand and substrate delivery through limitation of hyperthermia and maintenance of adequate cardiac output I *(64,75)*

DHCA, deep hypothermic circulatory arrest; CPB, cardiopulmonary bypass.
Recommendations based on ref. 75.
**Not used at CHONY.

substantial cerebral edema and neuronal Golgi apparatus damage *(53,54,75,77,78)*. In addition, the inability to remove the cannula during low flow bypass may make a technically accurate repair more difficult. Where DHCA is required, current research suggests a variety of modifications that mitigate the risk of neurological injury (Table 5[23,28,64,71,75,77–83]) *(75)*. Safe and appropriate application of DHCA is essential to ensuring the best cardiac repair, as well as the best neurological outcomes.

Systemic Inflammatory Response

Modern CPB leads to a systemic inflammatory and immunological response through injury of specific blood elements, embolic events, and the activation of complex systems designed to protect the body against bleeding, thrombosis, and invasion by foreign organisms *(84)*. In most patients, these processes are well tolerated; however, they pose an additional risk to patients at the extremes of age where the accompanying morbidity may increase mortality *(84)*.

Antiinflammatory Strategies. Several therapeutic strategies have been promulgated to attenuate the CPB-induced inflammatory process. Corticosteroids have been used for years to moderate the inflammatory cascades. Most of the powerful effects of steroids occur through inhibition of signal transduction and gene transcription in inflammatory cells; because these processes take time, administration of high-dose steroids is most effective when it occurs several hours before CPB *(55)*. Other potential pharmacologic strategies include: serine protease inhibitors (aprotinin) *(85)*, phosphodiesterase inhibitors (milrinone and pentoxifylline), NO donors (sodium nitroprusside), antioxidants (superoxide dismutase and *N*-acetylcysteine), and complement inhibitors *(86)*. Unfortunately, despite encouraging experimental results, most of these strategies have yielded equivocal results in clinical trials *(86)*. Mechanical techniques including hemofiltration, circuit miniaturization to reduce priming volumes and oxygenator exposure, leukocyte filters, the use of DHCA to mitigate postbypass edema and heparin-bonded circuits have generally been more successful, particularly in the pediatric population *(68,86)*.

A successful strategy for reducing postoperative inflammation uses a combination of the aforementioned techniques. The overall conduct of perfusion should be based on the idea that low prime volumes, and therefore diminished surface areas, are essential to mitigating postoperative inflammation. Other strategies employed to reduce excessive postoperative inflammation include: (a) the use of α- and β-antagonist sodium nitroprusside for DHCA procedures at 3–5 mcg/kg/min for vasodilatation during cooling and rewarming, (b) the administration of aprotinin (Trasylol®) during all DHCA procedures, as well as most cases with average bypass times exceeding 1.5 h, and (c) the liberal use of intraoperative hemoconcentration, including postbypass modified ultrafiltration, when indicated (*see* Hemodilution). These techniques may minimize the requirement for delayed postoperative sternal closure.

Concerning the use of aprotinin, a modified half dose protocol that is based on the patient's weight may be efficacious *(87)*. Anecdotaly, using aprotinin on all DHCA procedures has not resulted in clots in the bypass circuit, a disruption in graft flow or any significant renal dysfunction *(88,89)*. The protocol consists of (a) a test dose that is given by the anesthesiologist after heparinization, (b) a loading dose that is also administered by the anesthesiologist, (c) a pump prime dose which the perfusionist adds 5 min after the infusion of the test dose (except when clear prime replacement is utilized, in which case the aprotinin (Trasylol®) pump prime dose is added to the prime after the clear has been removed), and (d) a continuous infusion that is maintained by the anesthesiologist until the patient leaves the operating room (Table 6).

Table 6
Trasylol®

TEST DOSE
Administered by anesthesia after heparinization
<15 Kg = 0.3 cc
15–30 Kg = 0.6 cc
>30 Kg = 1 cc

PATIENT DOSE
LOAD- Administered by anesthesia after heparinization
<51 Kg————20,000 KIU/Kg (2 cc/Kg)
>50 Kg————100 cc
PUMP-Added to the pump prime after the load is started.
<21 Kg————40,000 KIU/Kg (4 cc/Kg)
21–50 Kg———80 cc
>50 Kg————100 cc

MAINTENANCE—RUN BY ANESTHESIA UNTIL THE PATIENT LEAVES THE OR

25% of the Pump Prime dose in cc/h

TECHNIQUE FOR CARDIOPULMONARY BYPASS IN THE PEDIATRIC POPULATION

Prime/Hemodilution

The small size of infants and neonates in comparison to the extracorporeal circuit significantly complicates several aspects of the conduct of CPB. In adults, the priming volume accounts for only 25–33% of the patient's blood volume; in neonates, the priming volume may exceed the blood volume by 200–300% (common pediatric pump circuits have total volume between 500 and 1200 mL). This inevitably leads to significant hemodilution with the onset of extracorporeal circulation (Table 7). Hemodilution reduces plasma proteins and clotting factors (contributing to interstitial edema and coagulopathy), produces electrolyte imbalances, results in a release of stress hormone, and activates inflammatory pathways. The optimal hematocrit will vary from case to case and depends on the diagnosis, degree of functional impairment, and planned surgical procedure; for example, those patients in whom a palliative procedure will result in postoperative mixed circulation with cyanosis will be poorly tolerant of a low hematocrit and may require physiologic normal hematocrit at the termination of the procedure *(90)*.

Table 7
Prime Constituents

Circuit	*Albumin*	*FFP*	*PRBCs*	*Heparin*	*CaCl*	*NaHCO3*	*∧Mannitol∧*	*Total prime*
A <3 kg	coat circuit with 50 cc of 25%	60 cc	125 cc	500 U	75 mg	(10 mEq + 1 mEq/kg)/2	(250 mg/kg)/2	220 cc
A	50 cc of 25%	none	125 cc	500 U	50 mg	(10 mEq + 1 mEq/kg)/2	(250 mg/kg)/2	220 cc
B	50 cc 25%	none	#180 cc	700 U	*75 mg	(10 mEq + 1 mEq/kg)/1.5	(250 mg/kg)1.5	270 cc
B1	75 cc 25%	none	#250 cc	1,000 U	*100 mg	(10 mEq + 1 mEq/kg)/1.5	(250 mg/kg)1.5	375 cc
C	100 cc 25%	none	*350 cc	1,200 U	*100 mg	10 mEq + 1 mEq/kg up to a total of 25 mEq	250 mg/kg	640 cc
D	150 cc 25%	none	*350 cc	1,700 U	*100 mg	25 mEq	250 mg/kg	850 cc
E	200 cc 25%	none	*350 cc	2,200 U	*100 mg	25 mEq	250 mg/kg	1,150 cc

All circuits are initially primed with Plasmalyte®, which is partially chased out by the albumin, blood, or FFP,and then the drugs are added; therefore, the balance of all prime volumes is Plasmalyte®.

#A blood prime is often not necessary; *Calcium is added only if blood is used; ∧An equivalent dose is given at cross clamp removal.

$$V_{blood} = \frac{\left[Hct_d \times \left(V_{pt} + V_{circuit}\right)\right] - \left[Hct_{pt} \times V_{pt}\right]}{Hct_{blood}}$$

V_{blood} = volume of blood needed in prime
Hct_d = desired hematrocit on CPB
Hct_{pt} = patient hematocrit prior to CPB
Hct_{blood} = hematocrit of blood to be added to prime
V_{pt} = patient's circulating blood volume
$V_{circuit}$ = extracorporeal circuit volume

Fig. 2. Estimating blood needed for priming.

The level of hemodilution at the initiation of bypass is determined by the addition of donor blood to the prime solution (otherwise consisting mainly of crystalloids and colloids). Given the risks associated with the use of donor blood (viral particle transmission; complement activation; transfusion reaction; lactate, potassium, citrate-phosphate-dextrose, and glucose infusion) *(91–93)*, attempts have been made to minimize the priming volume required as well as the need for transfusion. Following determination of the desired hematocrit, blood is added to the prime according to the following formula. (Fig. 2). The blood added to the prime may be either packed red blood cells (PRBCs) or whole blood. The use of fresh PRBCs has been advocated, although concerns about using stored blood may be overstated *(94)*. Where PRBCs are used, colloid is also usually added to increase the oncotic pressure of the perfusate and decrease edema formation; maintenance of normal osmotic pressure has been associated with improved survival in infants after CPB *(95)*. Other additives to the prime solution include: variable levels of electrolytes, buffer, calcium (though hypocalcemic primes are generally preferred to mitigate the risk of calcium during ischemic arrest), glucose, and lactate. More controversial is the use of mannitol, both as an osmotic diuretic and free-radical scavenger, and the addition of steroids to reduce the systemic inflammatory response to CPB and ischemia.

Hemodilution

Although previously thought to be safe, bypass strategies employing hemodilution to a hematocrit of less than 25% have been associated with poor perioperative hemodynamics and adverse psychomotor outcomes *(96)*; therefore, an on-bypass hematocrit of 28–35% is a reasonable goal. To achieve this hematocrit goal, small circuits, clear

Table 8
Common Cannulae and Associated Flows

CHONY VENOUS CANNULAE

DLP® single stage straight	*Max Flow cc/min*	*Venous line*	*Biomedicus®*	*Max Flow Cc/min*	*Aug flow*	*Bi-caval Angled DLP® or Angled Edwards®*		*Max Flow cc/min*
14 Fr	300		8 Fr	300		12 Fr	12 Fr	500
16 Fr	450		10 Fr	600		12	14	750
18 Fr	800	3/16	12 Fr	900		12	16	1000
18 Fr	1000	1/4	14 Fr	1200		14	14	1000
20 Fr	1200	1/4	15 Fr	750	2000	14	16	1200
22 Fr	1600	1/4	17 Fr	1100	2600	16	16	1500
22 Fr	1800	3/8	19 Fr	1500	3500	16	18	1800
24 Fr	2200	3/8	21 Fr	2000	4500	18	18	2100
28 Fr	2800	3/8	23 Fr	2500		18	20	2500
30 Fr	3100	3/8	25 Fr	3000		20	20	2800
32 Fr	3500	3/8	27 Fr	3500		20	24	3200
32 Fr	4000	1/2	29 Fr	4500		24	24	4000
34 Fr	4400	1/2				24	28	5000
36 Fr	5000	1/2				28	28	6000
38 Fr	5500	1/2						
40 Fr	6000	1/2						

CHONY ARTERIAL CANNULAE

DLP® wire	*Max Flow Cc/min*	*Biomedicus®*	*Max Flow Cc/min*
6 Fr	400	8 Fr	650
8	650	10	1100
10	1100	12	2200
12	2200	14	2900
14	2900	15	3000
16	4000	17	4000
		19	5500
		21	6500
		23	8000

prime replacement, hemoconcentration, and PRBC transfusions can be utilized. Certain procedures, including short bypass runs, such as during subaortic stenosis resections and ASD closures, may merit lower hematocrits (in the mid 20 s).

If a blood prime is not indicated, then pre-CPB prime replacement can be accomplished (clear prime replacement). First, remove any extra circuit volume over that necessary to make the connection to the arterial cannula. Next, with a clamped arterial line, drain the patient via the venous line into a transfer bag—thereby chasing out the prime. If the connection to the transfer bag is on the venous line, then gravity draining into the bag will suffice (although only the venous volume can be removed). In contrast, if the transfer setup is connected on the arterial line, then all of the volume up to that point may be translocated by running the arterial head and controlling the speed of removal with a venous line clamp. Blood pressure during the exchange can be augmented with α-agonists. However, only the available extra fluid may be removed, so an overaggressive removal strategy is not recommended. Often, much of the fluid that is removed is ultimately transfused back to the patient during the procedure, especially during rewarming. While this would appear to nullify the effect of the replacement procedure, there is evidence that intraoperative fluid shifts can be minimized if a mostly autologous prime is encountered by the patient at the onset of CBP *(97)*.

Hemoconcentration, either conventional or post-bypass, is an important tool for managing excess circuit volume, removing proinflammatory mediators and controlling excess potassium levels. To manage excess circuit volume during pediatric congenital heart surgery, 8 and 27 cc prime hemoconcentrators are available. The 8 cc (Hemocor Junior®) is primarily used on circuits where the prime is 270 cc or less, and the 27 cc (Hemocor 400®) on all others (Fig. 3).

Extended bypass times are associated with increasing expression of proinflammatory mediators *(98)*. Therefore it is helpful to use hemoconcentrators for all cases with expected bypass times exceeding 1.5 h, even in the absence of extra circuit volume requiring removal. This is accomplished by adding a balanced electrolyte solution to the circulating volume and then removing that same amount of volume with the hemoconcentrator. Also, excess potassium levels can be safely managed with aggressive ultrafiltration using normal saline to "wash out" the excess potassium. Normal saline is relatively acidotic, so serial blood gasses are necessary when employing this technique.

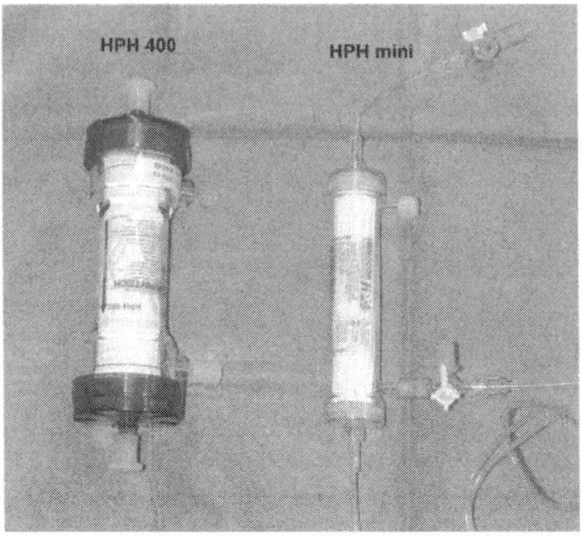

Fig. 3. Hemoconcentrators (HPH 400®, HPH mini®).

Modified Ultrafiltration

At CHONY there are three reasons that we do not routinely use modified ultrafiltration (MUF). First, when using very low prime circuits (180–270 cc), it is difficult to use MUF because there is very little excess circuit volume left in the reservoir after the cessation of CPB. Therefore, flushing the MUF circuit usually requires the addition of volume to the bypass circuit. Second, in larger children (over 25 kg), the amount of time necessary to remove enough volume to effect a significant change reduces the positive effects of MUF. Finally, there is evidence that utilizing conventional hemoconcentration for the removal of pro-inflammatory mediators is as effective as MUF *(99)*. However, children between 14 and 20 kg are subjected to a circuit with a relatively high prime volume compared to their blood volume. Therefore, MUF can effectively increase postbypass hematocrit and remove proinflammatory mediators. For these patients, we utilize a simple arterial-venous MUF circuit. The MUF access line is connected to the arterial manifold sample port, then threaded through a small twin pump and connected to the Hemocor 400® hemoconcentrator. Next, the MUF tubing exits the hemoconcentrator and is connected, via a lucred connection, to the cardioplegia set, ultimately terminating in the right atrium. A stopcock is connected to the lucred site so that flow can be diverted to the venous reservoir for priming and to create a continuous circuit for intraoperative hemoconcentration. A DLP® vessel cannula with a one way valve is placed on the end of the cardioplegia line and, after flushing the system, the right atrium is cannulated via the venous cannula site (the venous cannula has been removed). (Fig. 4). This system is easy to set up, simple to de-air (via the bypass line which runs to the venous reservoir), is protected by a one way valve, and, since it utilizes a vacant twin pump, does not compromise circuit integrity by necessitating the removal of a pump sucker or cardioplegia tubing to attain flow. (Fig. 5)

Prime Solutions

Priming of the bypass circuit is undertaken with a mixture of crystalloid and colloid solutions, as well as PRBCs (when needed) and additives. The crystalloid component is Plasmalyte® and the colloid is 25% albumin. When a child is less than 3 kg, fresh frozen plasma can be included in the prime to avoid excessive fibrinogen and clotting factor dilution.

As a general rule, most patients less than 10 kg require PRBCs in the prime. For neonates and infants, the target hematocrit for the procedure can usually be achieved by utilizing one unit of washed packed red blood cells with part of the unit given in the prime and the remainder transfused while on CPB. All PRBC units should be leukodepleted and, for children under 4 months old, they should also be irradiated and CMV negative. To ensure a physiologic potassium level in the prime, a cell saver is utilized to wash all donor blood with a balanced electrolyte solution.

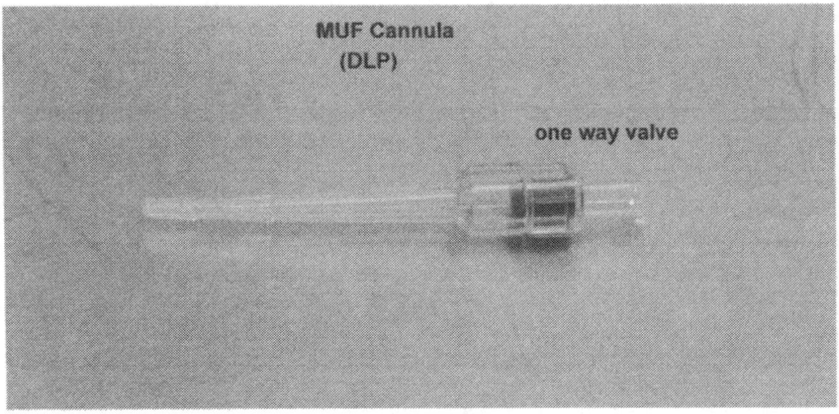

Fig. 4. DLP® MUF cannula.

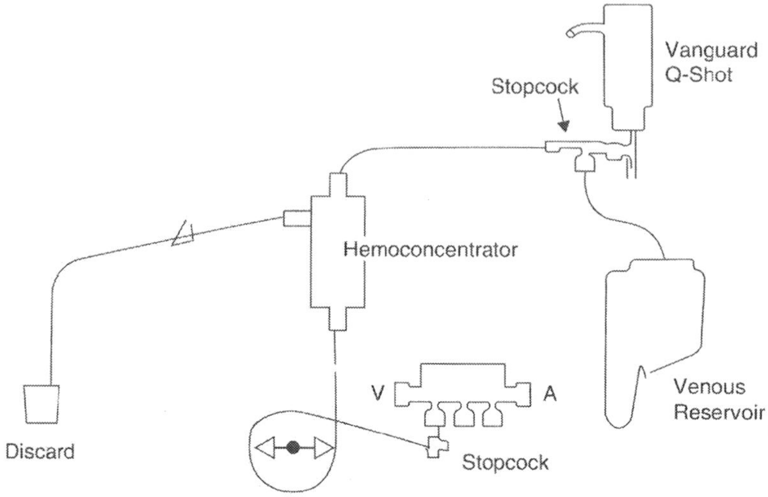

Fig. 5. MUF setup with Sorin Vanguard®.

Mannitol, sodium bicarbonate, heparin, and calcium chloride are also routine pump prime additives. (Table 7. Prime constituents)

Pumps

Both centrifugal and roller pumps have been used for pediatric CPB. The main advantages of using roller pumps for all neonatal and infant bypass procedures are lower prime when 1/4 in. and 3/16 in. tubing are used in the raceway and more accurate low-flow capabilities. However, the priming volume of centrifugal heads has decreased significantly in recent years, making them a viable alternative for larger patients. Centrifugal pumps have several potential advantages, including reduced priming volumes over 3/8 in. and 1/2 in. tubing, diminished damage to formed elements in the blood, and enhanced air removal *(70)*. In addition, these pumps are capable of delivering pulsatile perfusion, which may improve microcirculatory flow *(24)*.

Cannulation

The art of connecting the CPB circuit to the patients' circulation is governed by cannula selection and placement. The goal of cannulation is to use the lowest profile cannula with the best flow dynamics for the patient's calculated blood flow, combined with optimal placement for the prescribed corrective procedure. (Table 8. Cannulae flow) Pediatric bypass procedures are commonly associated with a variety of cannulation schemes. Table 9 gives a general cannulation site guideline,

Table 9
Pediatric Cannulation

Procedure	*Venous Location/Type*	*Venous Location/Type*	*Arterial Location*	*Arterial Location*
ASD secundum	SVC/Rt ang	IVC/Rt ang	Asc Aorta	
ASD Sinus Venosus	SVC/Rt ang	IVC/Rt ang	Asc Aorta	
VSD	SVC/Rt ang	IVC/Rt ang	Asc Aorta	
Sub Aortic Stenosis	RA/Str		Asc Aorta	
Tetralogy of Fallot	SVC/Rt ang	IVC/Rt ang	Asc Aorta	
TAPVR	RA/Str		Asc Aorta	
Norwood	RA/Str		PDA	Neo aorta
Bidirectional Glenn	RA/Str	SVC/Rt ang	Asc Aorta	
Hemi-Fontan	RA/Str		Asc Aorta	
Fontan (lateral tunnel)	RA/Str or SVC/Rt ang	IVC/Rt ang	Asc aorta	
Fontan (extra cardiac)	RA/Str		Asc aorta	
Artrioventricular Septal Defect	SVC/Rt ang	IVC/Rt Ang	Asc aorta	
Ross Procedure	SVC/Rt ang	IVC/Rt Ang	Asc aorta	
Arterial Switch	RA/Str		Asc aorta	
MVR/AVR/TVR	SVC/Rt ang	IVC/Rt ang	Asc aorta	
Interrupted Aortic Arch	RA/Str		Pre interruption	Post interruption
Ebstein's Anomaly	SVC/Rt ang	IVC/Rt ang	Asc aorta	
Truncus Arteriosus	RA/St		Asc aorta	
RV-PA conduit	RA/St		Asc aorta	
Rastelli	SVC/Rt ang	IVC/Rt ang	Asc aorta	
AVR	RA/Str		Asc aorta	

RA, right atrium; SVC, superior vena cava; IVC, inferior vena Cava; Rt ang, right angled; Str, straight.

however, consideration must be given to intercenter differences of bypass technique. For example, whether DHCA will be used for an arterial switch operation (a current trend in pediatric congenital heart surgery is toward the elimination of circulatory arrest) or whether certain procedures will be done off bypass (BDG, Fontan). Moreover, cardiopulmonary bypass may become unnecessary or relegated to a back-up roll for the repair of some congenital heart lesions due to the emergence of hybrid cardiology techniques. (Table 9. cannulation site summary) Vacuum assist has been used to augment venous return in the piglet model, mainly as a means to decrease priming volumes, although this technique is not widely used for neonatal surgery *(100)*.

Cannulation for multiple reoperations can be challenging, especially when immediate bypass is necessary. For larger children, the femoral artery is a common cannulation site; however, in infants it is very difficult to cannulate the femoral artery, so the auxiliary and carotid arteries are possible alternative sites. Venous cannulation can also be achieved in the associated veins of the alternative arterial cannulation sites. It is a safe practice to establish both arterial and venous cannulation before attempting sternotomy when there is a high likelihood of injuring the heart or great arteries. However, it is also common to use the bypass suckers to provide venous drainage until an adequate venous cannula can be inserted into the heart.

CONCLUSION

The use of CPB in congenital heart surgery requires specialized techniques and attention to the specific age-dependent physiologic differences of this diverse patient cohort. Considering the technical and physiologic complexity of conducting successful CPB for these patients, they should ideally be managed by perfusionists who specialize in a primarily congenital heart disease caseload. Delivery of the best possible care is likely to occur when children with congenital heart disease are treated at centers that see large numbers of these patients. Of further interest, approximately 80–85% of these children will survive to become adults with congenital heart disease. This distinct group of patients presents unique challenges to health care providers; therefore, they may be best managed within specialized adult congenital heart disease centers *(101)*.

REFERENCES

1. Lewis FJ, Taufic M. Closure of ASDs with the aid of hypothermia; experimental accomplishments and the report of one successful case. Surgery 1953;33(1):52–59.

2. Lewis FJ, Varco RL, Taufic M. Repair of ASDs in man under direct vision with the aid of hypothermia. Surgery 1954;36(3):538–556.
3. Edmunds LH, Jr. Advances in the heart-lung machine after John and Mary Gibbon. Ann Thorac Surg 2003;76(6):S2220–S2223.
4. Clowes GH, Jr., Neville WE, Hopkins A, Anzola J, Simeone FA. Factors contributing to success or failure in the use of a pump oxygenator for complete by-pass of the heart and lung, experimental and clinical. Surgery 1954;36(3):557–579.
5. Dennis C. Perspective in review. One group's struggle with development of a pump-oxygenator. Trans Am Soc Artif Intern Organs 1985;31:1–11.
6. Dennis C, Spreng DS, Jr., Nelson GE, et al. Development of a pump-oxygenator to replace the heart and lungs; an apparatus applicable to human patients, and application to one case. Ann Surg 1951;134(4):709–721.
7. Dodrill FD, Hill E, Gerisch RA, Johnson A. Pulmonary valvuloplasty under direct vision using the mechanical heart for a complete by-pass of the right heart in a patient with congenital pulmonary stenosis. J Thorac Surg 1953;26(6):584–594; discussion 195–197.
8. Gibbon JH, Jr. Application of a mechanical heart and lung apparatus to cardiac surgery. Minn Med 1954;37(3):171–185.
9. Mustard WT, Thomson JA. Clinical experience with the artificial heart lung preparation. Can Med Assoc J 1957;76(4):265–269.
10. Kirklin JW. Open-heart surgery at the Mayo Clinic. The 25th anniversary. Mayo Clin Proc 1980;55(5):339–341.
11. Warden HE, Cohen M, Read RC, Lillehei CW. Controlled cross circulation for open intracardiac surgery: physiologic studies and results of creation and closure of ventricular septal defects. J Thorac Surg 1954;28(3):331–341.
12. Bigelow WG, Lindsay WK, Greenwood WF. Hypothermia; its possible role in cardiac surgery: an investigation of factors governing survival in dogs at low body temperatures. Ann Surg 1950;132(5):849–866.
13. Sealy WC, Brown IW, Jr., Young WG, Jr. A report on the use of both extracorporeal circulation and hypothermia for open heart surgery. Ann Surg 1958;147 (5):603–613.
14. Swan H. The hydroxyl-hydrogen ion concentration ratio during hypothermia. Surg Gynecol Obstet 1982;155(6):897–912.
15. White FN, Somero G. Acid-base regulation and phospholipid adaptations to temperature: time courses and physiological significance of modifying the milieu for protein function. Physiol Rev 1982;62(1):40–90.
16. Lloyd-Thomas A. Acid base balance. In: Jonas RA, Elliott MJ, eds. Cardiopulmonary Bypass in Neonates, infants and Young Children. Oxford, UK: Butterworth-Heinemann, Ltd.; 1994:100–109.
17. Swan H. The importance of acid-base management for cardiac and cerebral preservation during open heart operations. Surg Gynecol Obstet 1984;158(4): 391–414.
18. Swain JA, McDonald TJ, Jr., Robbins RC, Balaban RS. Relationship of cerebral and myocardial intracellular pH to blood pH during hypothermia. American Journal of Physiology 1991;260(5 Pt 2):H1640–H1644.
19. Belsey RH, Dowlatshahi K, Keen G, Skinner DB. Profound hypothermia in cardiac surgery. J Thorac Cardiovasc Surg 1968;56(4):497–509.
20. Davies LK. Hypothermia. In: Gravlee GP, Davis RF, Kurusz M, Utley JR, eds. Cardiopulmonary Bypass: Principles and Practice. 2nd ed. Lippincott, Williams & Wilkins: Philadelphia, PA; 2000:197–213.

21. Dexter F, Kern FH, Hindman BJ, Greeley WJ. The brain uses mostly dissolved oxygen during profoundly hypothermic cardiopulmonary bypass. Ann Thorac Surg 1997;63(6):1725–1729.
22. Sakamoto T, Kurosawa H, Shin'oka T, Aoki M, Isomatsu Y. The influence of pH strategy on cerebral and collateral circulation during hypothermic cardiopulmonary bypass in cyanotic patients with heart disease: results of a randomized trial and real-time monitoring. J Thorac Cardiovasc Surg 2004;127(1):12–19.
23. Skaryak LA, Chai PJ, Kern FH, Greeley WJ, Ungerleider RM. Blood gas management and degree of cooling: effects on cerebral metabolism before and after circulatory arrest. J Thorac Cardiovasc Surg 1995;110(6):1649–1657.
24. Watanabe T, Miura M, Orita H, Kobayasi M, Washio M. Brain tissue pH, oxygen tension, and carbon dioxide tension in profoundly hypothermic cardiopulmonary bypass. Pulsatile assistance for circulatory arrest, low-flow perfusion, and moderate-flow perfusion. J Thorac Cardiovasc Surg 1990;100(2):274–280.
25. Patel RL, Turtle MR, Chambers DJ, James DN, Newman S, Venn GE. Alpha-stat acid-base regulation during cardiopulmonary bypass improves neuropsychologic outcome in patients undergoing coronary artery bypass grafting. J Thorac Cardiovasc Surg 1996;111(6):1267–1279.
26. Murkin JM, Martzke JS, Buchan AM, Bentley C, Wong CJ. A randomized study of the influence of perfusion technique and pH management strategy in 316 patients undergoing coronary artery bypass surgery. I. Mortality and cardiovascular morbidity. [see comment]. J Thorac Cardiovasc Surg 1995;110(2):340–348.
27. Stephan H, Weyland A, Kazmaier S, Henze T, Menck S, Sonntag H. Acid-base management during hypothermic cardiopulmonary bypass does not affect cerebral metabolism but does affect blood flow and neurological outcome. British Journal of Anaesthesia 1992;69(1):51–57.
28. Jonas RA, Bellinger DC, Rappaport LA, et al. Relation of pH strategy and developmental outcome after hypothermic circulatory arrest. J Thorac Cardiovasc Surg 1993;106(2):362–368.
29. du Plessis AJ, Jonas RA, Wypij D, et al. Perioperative effects of alpha-stat versus pH-stat strategies for deep hypothermic cardiopulmonary bypass in infants. J Thorac Cardiovasc Surg 1997;114(6):991–1000.
30. Kern FH, Greeley WJ. Pro: pH-stat management of blood gases is not preferable to alpha-stat in patients undergoing brain cooling for cardiac surgery. J Cardiothorac Vasc Anesth 1995;9(2):215–218.
31. Kirshbom PM, Skaryak LR, DiBernardo LR, et al. pH-stat cooling improves cerebral metabolic recovery after circulatory arrest in a piglet model of aortopulmonary collaterals. J Thorac Cardiovasc Surg 1996;111(1):147–155; discussion 156–157.
32. Jonas RA. Deep hypothermic circulatory arrest: current status and indications. Seminars in Thoracic & Cardiovascular Surgery Pediatric Cardiac Surgery Annual 2002;5:76–88.
33. Laussen PC. Optimal blood gas management during deep hypothermic paediatric cardiac surgery: alpha-stat is easy, but pH-stat may be preferable. Paediatr Anaesth 2002;12(3):199–204.
34. Jonassen AE, Quaegebeur JM, Young WL. Cerebral blood flow velocity in pediatric patients is reduced after cardiopulmonary bypass with profound hypothermia. J Thorac Cardiovasc Surg 1995;110(4 Pt 1):934–943.
35. Allen BS, Barth MJ, Ilbawi MN. Pediatric myocardial protection: an overview. Seminars in Thoracic & Cardiovascular Surgery 2001;13(1):56–72.

36. Hammon JW, Jr. Myocardial protection in the immature heart. Ann Thorac Surg 1995;60(3):839–842.
37. Yee ES, Ebert PA. Effect of ischemia on ventricular function, compliance, and edema in immature and adult canine hearts. Surg Forum 1979;30:250–252.
38. Allen BS. Pediatric myocardial protection: a cardioplegic strategy is the "solution". Seminars in Thoracic & Cardiovascular Surgery Pediatric Cardiac Surgery Annual 2004;7:141–154.
39. Friedman WF. The intrinsic physiologic properties of the developing heart. Prog Cardiovasc Dis 1972;15(1):87–111.
40. Nienaber CA, Gambhir SS, Mody FV, et al. Regional myocardial blood flow and glucose utilization in symptomatic patients with hypertrophic cardiomyopathy. Circulation 1993;87(5):1580–1590.
41. Peyton RB, Jones RN, Attarian D, et al. Depressed high-energy phosphate content in hypertrophied ventricles of animal and man: the biologic basis for increased sensitivity to ischemic injury. Ann Surg 1982;196(3):278–284.
42. Sink JD, Pellom GL, Currie WD, et al. Response of hypertrophied myocardium to ischemia: correlation with biochemical and physiological parameters. J Thorac Cardiovasc Surg 1981;81(6):865–872.
43. Bandali KS, Belanger MP, Wittnich C. Hyperoxia causes oxygen free radical-mediated membrane injury and alters myocardial function and hemodynamics in the newborn. Am J Physiol Heart Circ Physiol 2004;287(2): H553–H559.
44. Serraf A, Robotin M, Bonnet N, et al. Alteration of the neonatal pulmonary physiology after total cardiopulmonary bypass. J Thorac Cardiovasc Surg 1997;114(6):1061–1069.
45. Friedman M, Sellke FW, Wang SY, Weintraub RM, Johnson RG. Parameters of pulmonary injury after total or partial cardiopulmonary bypass. Circulation 1994; 90(5 Pt 2):II262–II268.
46. Friedman M, Wang SY, Sellke FW, Franklin A, Weintraub RM, Johnson RG. Pulmonary injury after total or partial cardiopulmonary bypass with thromboxane synthesis inhibition. Ann Thorac Surg 1995;59(3):598–603.
47. Kuratani T, Matsuda H, Sawa Y, Kaneko M, Nakano S, Kawashima Y. Experimental study in a rabbit model of ischemia-reperfusion lung injury during cardiopulmonary bypass. J Thorac Cardiovasc Surg 1992;103(3):564–568.
48. Komai H, Adatia IT, Elliott MJ, de Leval MR, Haworth SG. Increased plasma levels of endothelin-1 after cardiopulmonary bypass in patients with pulmonary hypertension and congenital heart disease. J Thorac Cardiovasc Surg 1993;106 (3):473–478.
49. Komai H, Haworth SG. Effect of cardiopulmonary bypass on the circulating level of soluble GMP-140. Ann Thorac Surg 1994;58(2):478–482.
50. Kirshbom PM, Jacobs MT, Tsui SS, et al. Effects of cardiopulmonary bypass and circulatory arrest on endothelium-dependent vasodilation in the lung. J Thorac Cardiovasc Surg 1996;111(6):1248–1256.
51. Kirshbom PM, Page SO, Jacobs MT, et al. Cardiopulmonary bypass and circulatory arrest increase endothelin-1 production and receptor expression in the lung. J Thorac Cardiovasc Surg 1997;113(4):777–783.
52. Kirklin JK, Westaby S, Blackstone EH, Kirklin JW, Chenoweth DE, Pacifico AD. Complement and the damaging effects of cardiopulmonary bypass. J Thorac Cardiovasc Surg 1983;86(6):845–857.

53. Skaryak LA, Lodge AJ, Kirshbom PM, et al. Low-flow cardiopulmonary bypass produces greater pulmonary dysfunction than circulatory arrest. Ann Thorac Surg 1996;62(5):1284–1288.
54. Wernovsky G, Wypij D, Jonas RA, et al. Postoperative course and hemodynamic profile after the arterial switch operation in neonates and infants. A comparison of low-flow cardiopulmonary bypass and circulatory arrest. Circulation 1995; 92(8):2226–2235.
55. Lodge AJ, Chai PJ, Daggett CW, Ungerleider RM, Jaggers J. Methylprednisolone reduces the inflammatory response to cardiopulmonary bypass in neonatal piglets: timing of dose is important. J Thorac Cardiovasc Surg 1999;117(3): 515–522.
56. Bando K, Vijay P, Turrentine MW, et al. Dilutional and modified ultrafiltration reduces pulmonary hypertension after operations for congenital heart disease: a prospective randomized study. J Thorac Cardiovasc Surg 1998;115(3):517–525; discussion 525–527.
57. Elliott MJ. Ultrafiltration and modified ultrafiltration in pediatric open heart operations. Ann Thorac Surg 1993;56(6):1518–1522.
58. Koutlas TC, Gaynor JW, Nicolson SC, Steven JM, Wernovsky G, Spray TL. Modified ultrafiltration reduces postoperative morbidity after cavopulmonary connection. Ann Thorac Surg 1997;64(1):37–42.
59. Ungerleider RM. Effects of cardiopulmonary bypass and use of modified ultrafiltration. Ann Thorac Surg 1998;65(6 Suppl):S35–S38; discussion S9, S74–S76.
60. Williams EA, Welty SE, Geske RS, et al. Liquid lung ventilation reduces neutrophil sequestration in a neonatal swine model of cardiopulmonary bypass. Crit Care Med 2001;29(4):789–795.
61. Cannon ML, Cheifetz IM, Craig DM, et al. Optimizing liquid ventilation as a lung protection strategy for neonatal cardiopulmonary bypass: full functional residual capacity dosing is more effective than half functional residual capacity dosing. Crit Care Med 1999;27(6):1140–1146.
62. Cheifetz IM, Cannon ML, Craig DM, et al. Liquid ventilation improves pulmonary function and cardiac output in a neonatal swine model of cardiopulmonary bypass. J Thorac Cardiovasc Surg 1998;115(3):528–535.
63. Miller OI, Tang SF, Keech A, Pigott NB, Beller E, Celermajer DS. Inhaled nitric oxide and prevention of pulmonary hypertension after congenital heart surgery: a randomised double-blind study. Lancet 2000;356(9240):1464–1469.
64. Kern FH, Hickey PR. The effects of cardiopulmonary bypass on the brain. In: Jonas RA, Elliott MJ, eds. Cardiopulmonary bypass in neonates, infants and young children. Oxford, UK: Butterworth-Heinemann, Ltd.; 1994:263–281.
65. Pua HL, Bissonnette B. Cerebral physiology in paediatric cardiopulmonary bypass. Canadian Journal of Anaesthesia 1998;45(10):960–978.
66. Ferry PC. Neurologic sequelae of open-heart surgery in children. An 'irritating question'. Am J Dis Child 1990;144(3):369–373.
67. McConnell JR, Fleming WH, Chu WK, et al. Magnetic resonance imaging of the brain in infants and children before and after cardiac surgery. A prospective study. Am J Dis Child 1990;144(3):374–378.
68. Jaggers J, Shearer IR, Ungerleider RM. Cardiopulmonary bypass in infants and children. In: Gravlee GP, Davis RF, Kurusz M, Utley JR, eds. Cardiopulmonary Bypass: Principles and Practice. 2nd ed. Phiadelphia, PA: Lippincott, Williams & Wilkins; 2000:633–661.

69. Kern FH, Greeley WJ, Ungerleider R. The effects of bypass on the developing brain. Perfusion 1993;8(1):49–54.
70. Kirklin JW, Barratt-Boyes BG. Cardiac Surgery. 1st ed. New York: John Wiley & Sons; 1986.
71. Aoki M, Jonas RA, Nomura F, et al. Effects of aprotinin on acute recovery of cerebral metabolism in piglets after hypothermic circulatory arrest. Ann Thorac Surg 1994;58(1):146–153.
72. Blauth C, Smith P, Newman S, et al. Retinal microembolism and neuropsychological deficit following clinical cardiopulmonary bypass: comparison of a membrane and a bubble oxygenator. A preliminary communication. Eur J Cardiothorac Surg 1989;3(2):135–138; discussion 9.
73. Semb BK, Pedersen T, Hatteland K, Storstein L, Lilleaasen P. Doppler ultrasound estimation of bubble removal by various arterial line filters during extracorporeal circulation. Scand J Thorac Cardiovasc Surg 1982;16(1):55–62.
74. Armon C, Deschamps C, Adkinson C, Fealey RD, Orszulak TA. Hyperbaric treatment of cerebral air embolism sustained during an open-heart surgical procedure. Mayo Clin Proc 1991;66(6):565–571.
75. Shen I, Giacomuzzi C, Ungerleider RM. Current strategies for optimizing the use of cardiopulmonary bypass in neonates and infants. Ann Thorac Surg 2003;75(2): S729–S734.
76. Bellinger DC, Jonas RA, Rappaport LA, et al. Developmental and neurologic status of children after heart surgery with hypothermic circulatory arrest or low-flow cardiopulmonary bypass. N Engl J Med 1995;332(9):549–555.
77. Langley SM, Chai PJ, Miller SE, et al. Intermittent perfusion protects the brain during deep hypothermic circulatory arrest. Ann Thorac Surg 1999;68 (1):4–12.
78. Langley SM, Chai PJ, Jaggers JJ, Ungerleider RM. Preoperative high dose methylprednisolone attenuates the cerebral response to deep hypothermic circulatory arrest. Eur J Cardiothorac Surg 2000;17(3):279–286.
79. Hindman BJ, Dexter F, Cutkomp J, Smith T, Todd MM, Tinker JH. Brain blood flow and metabolism do not decrease at stable brain temperature during cardiopulmonary bypass in rabbits. Anesthesiology 1992;77(2):342–350.
80. Greeley WJ, Kern FH, Ungerleider RM, et al. The effect of hypothermic cardiopulmonary bypass and total circulatory arrest on cerebral metabolism in neonates, infants, and children. J Thorac Cardiovasc Surg 1991;101(5):783–794.
81. Aoki M, Nomura F, Stromski ME, et al. Effects of pH on brain energetics after hypothermic circulatory arrest. Ann Thorac Surg 1993;55(5):1093–1103.
82. Schultz S, Creed J, Schears G, et al. Comparison of low-flow cardiopulmonary bypass and circulatory arrest on brain oxygen and metabolism. Ann Thorac Surg 2004;77(6):2138–2143.
83. Skaryak LA, Kirshbom PM, DiBernardo LR, et al. Modified ultrafiltration improves cerebral metabolic recovery after circulatory arrest. J Thorac Cardiovasc Surg 1995;109(4):744–751; discussion 51–52.
84. Edmunds LH, Jr. Inflammatory and immunogical response to cardiopulmonary bypass. In: Jonas RA, Elliott MJ, eds. Cardiopulmonary bypass in neonates, infants, and young children. Oxford, UK: Butterworth-Heinemann; 1994: 225–241.
85. Jansen PG, Baufreton C, Le Besnerais P, Loisance DY, Wildevuur CR. Heparin-coated circuits and aprotinin prime for coronary artery bypass grafting. Ann Thorac Surg 1996;61(5):1363–1366.

86. Pintar T, Collard CD. The systemic inflammatory response to cardiopulmonary bypass. Anesthesiol Clin North America 2003;21(3):453–464.
87. Nuttall GA, Fass DN, Oyen LJ, Oliver WC, Jr., Ereth MH. A study of a weight-adjusted aprotinin dosing schedule during cardiac surgery. Anesth Analg 2002; 94(2):283–289.
88. Mangano DT, Tudor IC, Dietzel C. The risk associated with aprotinin in cardiac surgery. N Engl J Med 2006;354(4):353–365.
89. Heindel SW, Mill MR, Freid EB, Valley RD, White GC, 2nd, Norfleet EA. Fatal thrombosis associated with a hemi-fontan procedure, heparin-protamine reversal, and aprotinin. Anesthesiology 2001;94(2):369–371.
90. Bailey JM, Daly WL. Pediatric cardiopulmonary bypass. In: Mora CT, ed. Cardiopulmonary bypass : principles and techniques of extracorporeal circulation. New York: Springer-Verlag; 1995:312–328.
91. Ratcliffe JM, Elliott MJ, Wyse RK, Hunter S, Alberti KG. The metabolic load of stored blood. Implications for major transfusions in infants. Arch Dis Child 1986;61(12):1208–1214.
92. Salama A, Mueller-Eckhardt C. Delayed hemolytic transfusion reactions. Evidence for complement activation involving allogeneic and autologous red cells. Transfusion 1984;24(3):188–193.
93. Hall TL, Barnes A, Miller JR, Bethencourt DM, Nestor L. Neonatal mortality following transfusion of red cells with high plasma potassium levels. Transfusion 1993;33(7):606–609.
94. Keidan I, Amir G, Mandel M, Mishali D. The metabolic effects of fresh versus old stored blood in the priming of cardiopulmonary bypass solution for pediatric patients. J Thorac Cardiovasc Surg 2004;127(4):949–952.
95. Marelli D, Paul A, Samson R, Edgell D, Angood P, Chiu RC. Does the addition of albumin to the prime solution in cardiopulmonary bypass affect clinical outcome? A prospective randomized study. J Thorac Cardiovasc Surg 1989;98(5 Pt 1):751–756.
96. Jonas RA, Wypij D, Roth SJ, et al. The influence of hemodilution on outcome after hypothermic cardiopulmonary bypass: results of a randomized trial in infants. J Thorac Cardiovasc Surg 2003;126(6):1765–1774.
97. Rosengart TK, DeBois W, O'Hara M, et al. Retrograde autologous priming for cardiopulmonary bypass: a safe and effective means of decreasing hemodilution and transfusion requirements. J Thorac Cardiovasc Surg 1998;115(2):426–438; discussion 38–39.
98. Huang H, Yao T, Wang W, et al. Continuous ultrafiltration attenuates the pulmonary injury that follows open heart surgery with cardiopulmonary bypass. Ann Thorac Surg 2003;76(1):136–140.
99. Thompson LD, McElhinney DB, Findlay P, et al. A prospective randomized study comparing volume-standardized modified and conventional ultrafiltration in pediatric cardiac surgery. J Thorac Cardiovasc Surg 2001;122(2):220–228.
100. Ahlberg K, Sistino JJ, Nemoto S. Hematological effects of a low-prime neonatal cardiopulmonary bypass circuit utilizing vacuum-assisted venous return in the porcine model. J Extra Corpor Technol 1999;31(4):195–201.
101. Grown-up congenital heart (GUCH) disease: current needs and provision of service for adolescents and adults with congenital heart disease in the UK. Heart 2002;88 Suppl 1:i1–i14.

3 Separation from Cardiopulmonary Bypass: Hemodynamic Considerations

Marc L. Dickstein, MD

Contents

INTRODUCTION

The successful transition from full circulatory support to the normal circulatory physiology requires careful attention to a number of parameters that are often perturbed while on cardiopulmonary bypass (CPB). Many of these parameters, such as temperature, extracellular glucose and potassium concentrations, hematocrit, and acid-base status, are relatively easy to restore. However, the re-establishment of many aspects of normal cardiovascular function, such as peripheral vascular resistance, blood pressure, and cardiac function, are not as straightforward, due in part to the unusual physiologic conditions imposed. The purpose of this chapter is to elaborate the cardiovascular physiology relevant to the transition from full circulatory assist, and to describe a model that will allow for a better understanding of the unique consequences that occur.

From: *Current Cardiac Surgery: On Bypass: Advanced Perfusion Techniques*
Edited by: L. B. Mongero and J. R. Beck © Humana Press Inc., Totowa, NJ

THE DETERMINANTS OF VENTRICULAR FUNCTION

The fundamental determinants of ventricular function are classically separated into heart rate, preload, afterload, and contractility. It is particularly important to review these concepts in the context of external circulatory support, as the conditions under which the heart operates are far from classical. For example, consider that while on CPB the heart is performing no external work, despite the fact that it may have normal electrical activity, normal excitation—contraction coupling, and normal myocyte function. In other words, despite the fact that the heart may have normal function on the cellular level, the heart is not participating in generating pressure or flow in the vasculature. Although this point may seems obvious, it is important to understand these conditions to appreciate the types of physiologic changes that occur during the transition to the normal circulatory state.

Preload

Preload represents the stretch on the muscle just prior to its contraction. The Frank-Starling relationship, arguably the most important observation in cardiovascular physiology, describes the increased strength of contraction associated with increased preload (Fig. 1). While preload is most simply represented by a weight hanging from a muscle strip just prior to contraction, preload in the intact heart is quite a bit more complicated and is influenced by a number of factors that impact on ventricular filling (and hence end-diastolic stretch). These factors include blood volume, venous capacitance, ventricular compliance, atrial function, valvular function, and heart rate. As intravascular volume increases, so too increases venous pressure, and hence, the driving force for ventricular filling. Constriction or dilation of the venous capacitance vessels will alter the venous pressure associated with a given intravascular volume; sudden changes in venous capacitance may be associated with considerable hemodynamic instability, which are predominantly caused by changes in the driving force for ventricular filling. Although the filling pressure provides the energy for ventricular distention, the ventricular volume that results is also determined by the compliance of the ventricle. Ventricular compliance may be thought of as the passive mechanical properties of the chamber; a noncompliant ventricle will require higher filling pressures to achieve a given ventricular volume. The majority of ventricular filling occurs early in diastole, and it is manifest on the transmitral flow tracing as the "e" wave (Fig. 2). The pressure gradient between the atrium and ventricle is rapidly dissipated by the rapid movement of blood out of

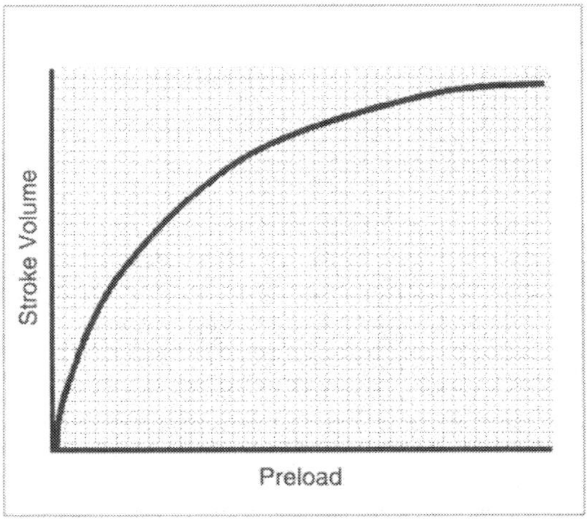

Fig. 1. The Frank-Starling relationship demonstrates increasing stroke volume with increasing preload. Notice that stroke volume is more sensitive to changes in preload at low values compared to high values.

the atria (hence, lowering atrial pressure) and into the ventricle (hence, raising ventricular pressure), and a period of diastasis occurs wherein there is little flow into the ventricle. Moderate increases in heart rate decrease the time period of diastasis, and therefore do not impact greatly on ventricular filling; more significant increases in heart rate

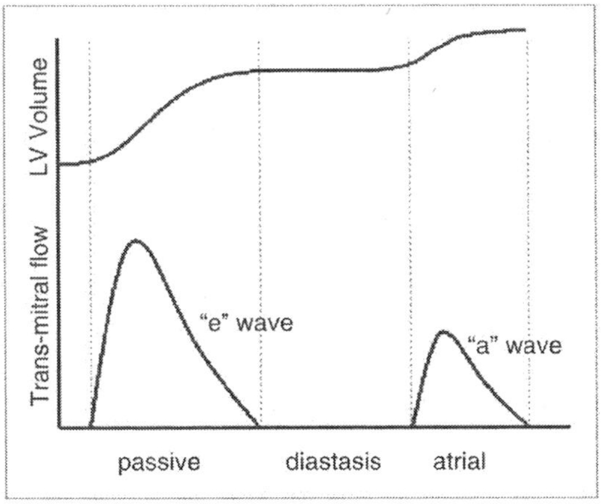

Fig. 2. There are normally two bursts of transmitral flow (bottom tracings) that contribute to ventricular filling (top tracing): The first occurs immediately after ventricular relaxation ("e" wave) and the second occurs with atrial contraction ("a" wave).

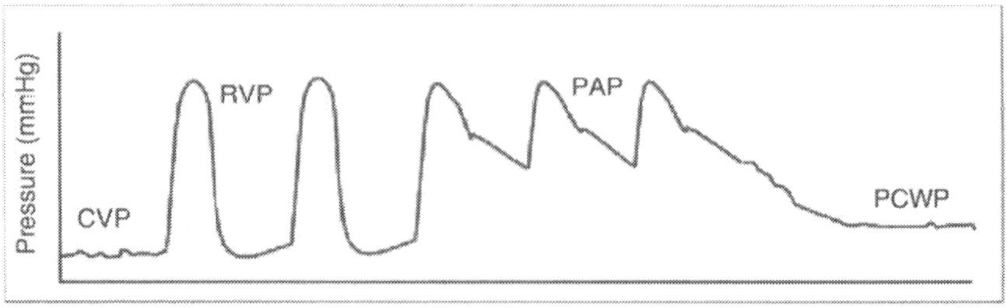

Fig. 3. This tracing represents the progression of waveform morphology that occurs as the pulmonary arterial catheter is advanced from the right atrial [central venous pressure (CVP)], across the tricuspid valve into the right ventricle (RVP), across the pulmonic valve into the pulmonary artery (PAP), and into the "wedged position whereby the balloon tip occludes arterial flow [pulmonary capillary wedge pressure (PCWP)].

may impact on the early filling phase, and thereby reduce ventricular preload. Mitral stenosis decreases the flow rate into the ventricle for a given pressure gradient; hence, mitral stenosis causes hemodynamic instability, which is predominantly caused by reductions in ventricular preload. Atrial contraction reestablishes a pressure gradient between the atrium and ventricle, and thereby accounts for additional ventricular filling ("a" wave). In normal patients, atrial contraction accounts for 20–30% of the total flow across the atrioventricular valves. The loss of normal sinus rhythm may be associated with a significant reduction in ventricular preload, especially in patients with noncompliant ventricles or mitral stenosis; often A-V sequential pacing is necessary to restore ventricular preload.

How do we estimate preload clinically? With the widespread use of transesophageal echocardiography (TEE), it is possible to get a reasonable estimate of chamber size and, hence, preload. In the absence of TEE, we substitute the pressure at end-diastole with the assumption that the higher the pressure, the greater the size and the greater the stretch on the contractile elements. EDP can be assessed clinically by measuring the pulmonary capillary wedge pressure (PCWP) using a Swan-Ganz catheter that is placed through the right ventricle (RV) into the pulmonary artery (PA) (Fig. 3). When the balloon at the tip of the catheter is inflated, it occludes flow in that small branch of the PA; the pressure distal to the balloon quickly equilibrates with the pressure in the pulmonary venous system. As the risk of pulmonary rupture and hemorrhage is increased with anticoagulation, the pulmonary arterial diastolic pressure is often used instead of the PCWP. In the absence of a PA catheter, central venous pressure is used to assess volume status with the assumption that there is a positive association between changes in central venous pressure and LV size.

Afterload

Afterload is the hydraulic *load* imposed on the ventricle during ejection, usually by the arterial system and the interaction of the heart with the vasculature into which it ejects. The most important parameter that confers this afterload stress to the heart is the aortic blood pressure; hypertension is associated with greater opposition to ventricular ejection. However, because aortic pressure normally varies throughout the ventricular ejection phase, no single value of aortic pressure accurately measures ventricular afterload. Moreover, the pressure in the aortic root is determined by the interplay of ventricular output (which determines the volume of blood in the aortic tree), arterial compliance (which determines the pressure associated with a particular volume in the arterial tree), and systemic vascular resistance (SVR) (which determines the rate that the blood volume leaves the aortic tree). Under pathologic conditions, when either the mitral valve is incompetent (i.e., leaky) or the aortic valve is stenotic, *afterload* is determined by factors other than the properties of the arterial system.

Similar to the pump function curves for centrifugal pumps, ventricular stroke volume decreases as afterload increases (Fig. 4). Weaker hearts tend to be more sensitive to changes in afterload (hence, the importance of pharmacologic afterload reduction for treatment of heart failure), and stronger hearts tend to be less sensitive. Systemic vasodilation is associated with decreased aortic pressure and lower ventricular afterload. Importantly, the performance of the ventricle plays a large role in determining its own afterload. For example, if cardiac function is suddenly depressed, the decreased ejection into the vascular tree would be associated with a lower arterial pressure, and hence a lower afterload, thus promoting ejection. However, this important homeostatic mechanism is derailed while on CPB when the arterial pressure is governed independently of ventricular performance.

Contractility

Contractility is an ill-defined concept that refers to the intrinsic strength of the ventricle or cardiac muscle. By intrinsic strength, we mean those features of the cardiac contraction process that are intrinsic to the ventricle (and cardiac muscle) and are independent of external conditions imposed by either the preload or the afterload. During the cardiac cycle, as calcium is released from internal cellular stores and becomes available to facilitate the interaction of the contractile elements actin and myosin, the physical properties of the muscle change and the ventricular chamber become more stiff. The consequence of this change in chamber stiffness is that, for a given volume, there will be a greater chamber pressure. Positive inotropic agents (i.e., lead to an increase in contractility) all work by increasing the amount of available calcium during systole and result in a stiffer ventricle at the end of systole (i.e., increased end-systolic elastance), and hence a greater pressure generation.

Changes in contractility may occur chronically (cardiomyopathy decreases maximal elastance, whereas left ventricular hypertrophy increases maximal elastance) or acutely by pharmacologic therapy (such as beta-adrenergic agonists, phosphodiesterase inhibitors, and calcium, which increase contractility, and beta-adrenergic and calcium channel antagonists, which decrease contractility), myocardial ischemia, reperfusion injury, acute overdistension, etc. A change in contractility results in a shift in the Frank—Starling relationship (Fig. 5); reductions in contractile strength lead to a decreased stroke volume at a given preload.

How do we measure contractility clinically? Although ventricular stiffness and contractility may be assessed by analyses of pressure—

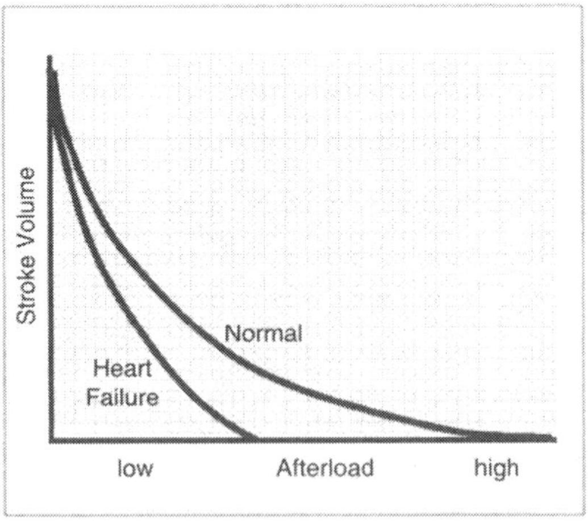

Fig. 4. In all cases, stroke volume decreases as afterload increases. This relationship is shifted leftward in patients with heart failure; the less contractile heart is more sensitive to changes in afterload, and thus there is a greater reduction in stroke volume as afterload is increased.

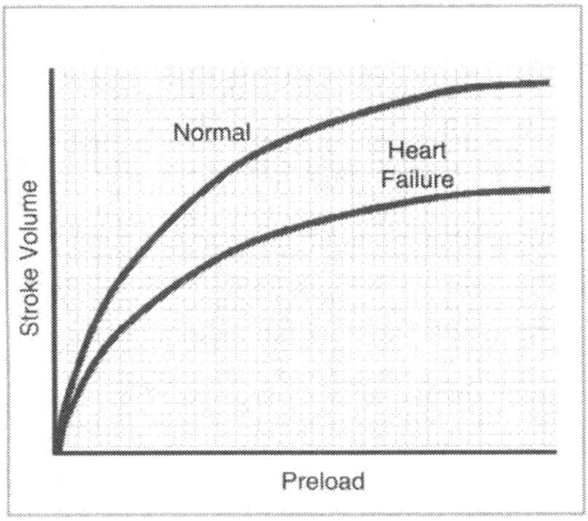

Fig. 5. These two tracings both represent Frank-Starling relationships. Notice that decreased contractility (heart failure) shifts the relationship down and to the right. To achieve the same stroke volume, preload must be increased. Furthermore, there is less sensitivity to preload in the failing heart.

volume loops, the most common clinical method for assessment of contractility is the TEE-derived ejection fraction (end-diastolic chamber area—end-systolic chamber area/end-diastolic chamber area). However, it is important to appreciate that ejection fraction is also sensitive to changes in afterload. Moreover, contractility cannot be assessed by this method while on CPB; cardiac output and ejection fraction may be zero, despite the fact that the ventricle may have normal contractility!

VASCULAR FUNCTION

Blood flows because of pressure gradients in the vascular tree. Normally, the heart ejects blood intermittently; hence, both pressure and flow in the vascular tree are pulsatile. However, understanding the determinants of pulsatile flow as opposed to steady flow requires acquisition of instantaneous measurements and complex calculations. Consider that we calculate vascular resistance in the intact circulation by relating mean pressure and mean flow, as if flow was laminar and steady, and pressure was nonpulsatile. In fact, a more complete representation of the pressure and flow relations in the arterial tree is provided by an analysis of aortic impedance that relates pressure and flow ratios in a frequency domain; these types of analyses are generally confined to research labs and are not used clinically because of the inherent difficulties of measuring instantaneous flow. Hence, the clinical assessment of blood flow in the vasculature is typically limited to the consideration of mean pressures and mean flows in the system, as if the flow of blood occurred at a steady rate and laminar fashion in the arterial tree. Principles gleaned from Poiseuille's Law are used to understand the factors governing vascular resistance, and Ohm's law is applied to aid in understanding the relationship of pressure, resistance, and flow. However, as will be described in the following sections, the transition off of CPB represents a time during which many of the assumptions are invalid.

Steady-State Versus Non—Steady-State Relationships

While on full CPB, flow is simply governed by the rate of the CPB pump. Pressure is typically measured in the radial or femoral artery, and SVR is calculated as a ratio of pressure and flow (assuming venous pressure is quite low relative to arterial pressure). Consequently, the treatment of hypotension on CPB simply requires one to increase flow (increase the pump speed) or increase resistance (administer a vasoconstrictor or raise viscosity via transfusion or hemoconcentration). However, it is important to appreciate that the term flow in Ohm's law specifically refers to the flow across the resistance vessels (i.e., across the systemic arterioles and capillaries). During periods of steady state, the flow into the aorta is the same as the flow across the capillaries, and we may thus use the flow rate into the aorta to calculate SVR. In contrast, these two flow rates may be quite different during non—steady state events, and thus the use of aortic flow would be misleading if used to estimate vascular resistance.

Rapid Change in Blood Volume as an Example of A Non—Steady State

Let's look at an example of emergently initiating CPB immediately after a patient exsanguinates during sternotomy. Despite valiant attempts to support the blood pressure with potent vasoconstrictors before "crashing on," the blood pressure will undoubtedly be quite low upon initiation of normal flow into the aortic root. What is the reason for low blood pressure in the face of presumably high SVR and normal flow? In this situation, despite the fact that the flow into the aortic tree may be normal, the flow across the arterioles and capillaries initially will be much lower than the flow into the aortic tree. If one could measure flow across the capillaries, the relationship $P = F \cdot SVR$ would still hold. However, an estimation of SVR based on aortic flow would result in an erroneous conclusion that SVR was inappropriately low. If one waited a brief period, the volume in the aortic tree would continue to increase (as volume into the aortic tree continues to exceed volume out across the capillary bed) until the pressure in the aortic tree becomes quite high. At this point, the pressure in the aortic tree is sufficient to drive blood across the high SVR at the same rate that volume is entering via the aortic cannula. Now, in steady state, the calculation of SVR would properly reflect the fact that it is quite high because of the vasoconstrictors administered before the initiation of CBP. However, during non—steady state, a better understanding of the determination of blood pressure comes from an appreciation of the simple relationship of pressure and volume within a compartment, rather than pressure and flow out of the compartment.

THE VOLUME COMPARTMENT MODEL

The cardiovascular system may be thought of as a series of compartments that contain the totality of a patient's blood volume (Fig. 6). Blood flows from one compartment to the next based on the pressure gradient between the two compartments and the resistance to flow

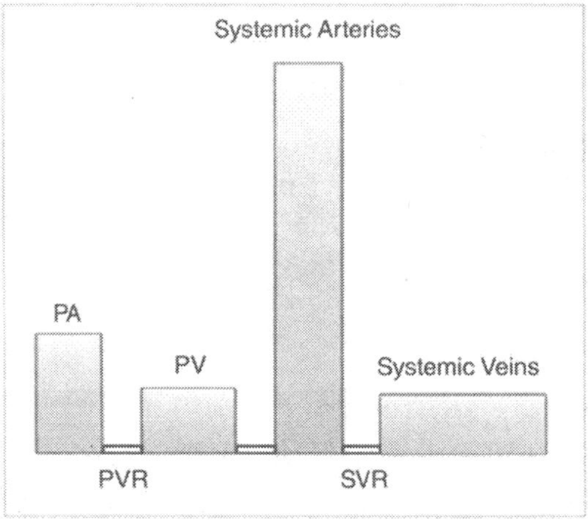

Fig. 6. This figure illustrates the pressures and volumes in the four main volume compartments of the circulation. The heights of the bar represent the mean pressure; the pressure drop from the pulmonary artery (PA) to the pulmonary vein (PV) provides the energy for forward flow across the pulmonary capillary bed. Similarly, the pressure drop from the system arteries systemic veins provides the energy for forward flow across the systemic capillary bed. The area of the compartments illustrates the distribution of blood volume.

between the two compartments. The pressure in a given compartment depends on the volume contained in that compartment and the compliance of the compartment. Changes in the volume of a compartment occur when there is a difference between the flow rate into the compartment compared with the flow rate out of the compartment. In normal circulation, one can consider four compartments: systemic veins, PAs, pulmonary veins (PVs), and systemic arteries. Importantly, at any given moment the total blood volume is accounted for as the sum of the volumes contained in the individual compartments. While on CPB, one considers a fifth compartment placed in parallel with the PAs and PVs. In this case, the reservoir chamber in the CPB circuit provides a unique opportunity to directly observe changes in the distribution of blood volume into the various compartments. This point will be elaborated in the following three examples.

Sudden Systemic Vasodilation

If the resistance of flow between the systemic arterial and systemic venous compartments suddenly decreased, there would be increased flow out of the systemic arterial compartment. If the inflow (the CPB rate) remained constant, then there would no longer be a steady state, in that flow out of the arterial tree would exceed flow in, and volume in the compartment would decrease. It should be no surprise then that arterial pressure is reduced. Where is the blood volume? The flow rate into the systemic venous circulation is increased; because of the high compliance of this system, the consequent pressure rise in the venous systemic compartment is quite small. Hence, venous return to the venous reservoir is only slightly increased. Moreover, the response to a decrease in pressure in the systemic circulation is to increase flow in an attempt to restore systemic arterial compartment volume. This would further reduce reservoir volume.

Temporary Discontinuation of CPB with Aortic Cross-Clamp in Place

Occasionally, to reduce arterial wall stress while repairing a defect in the aorta, the surgeon may request that flow be temporarily halted. If aortic flow were suddenly reduced to zero, then arterial pressure would exponentially decrease as blood continued to leave the arterial compartment into the systemic veins. As long as a pressure gradient exists between the systemic arteries and veins, then blood will continue to flow proportional to the pressure gradient and inversely related to the peripheral vascular resistance. The volume in the reservoir chamber would continue to increase as the volume in (from the systemic veins) exceeds the volume out (pump flow rate). Upon resumption of CPB, the flow into the arterial compartment will exceed the flow out, and the compartment will continue to increase its volume, and hence, its pressure. Steady state is achieved when the pressure in the arterial compartment is sufficient to drive the same flow rate out of the compartment as the flow rate into the compartment. From this example, it is clear that substitution of CPB rate for flow across the resistance vessels for the estimation of PVR is only valid during steady state.

"Giving 100"

After discontinuation of CPB, a volume bolus is frequently administered via the arterial cannula in response to hypotension and the diagnosis of inadequate preload. The 100 ml of volume is administered directly into the systemic arterial compartment with a resultant increase in systemic blood pressure. However, the increase in blood pressure does not indicate the preload sensitivity of the heart; rather, the resultant increase in pressure is a function of the compliance of the vasculature at that particular pressure. The two sources of volume input to the systemic arterial compartment are the heart and the aortic cannula; the flow rate from the CPB pump transiently adds to the cardiac output. In addition, the "extra" increase in volume, and hence pressure, in the aortic root increases afterload; a weak heart will decrease its output in response to this, thus blunting the pressure increase one normally sees when "giving 100."

THE PHYSIOLOGY OF PARTIAL BYPASS

The transition off of full CPB includes a variable period of time during which the heart is ejecting volume while the flow rate is reduced. Typically, this is accomplished by imposing graded resistance on the venous cannula and adjusting the pump speed to match inflow and outflow rates; in other words, at each level of partial bypass, the goal is to reestablish steady state in respect to the venous reservoir compartment. With that goal in mind, let's look at the implications of these maneuvers for the cardiovascular system.

Coincident with and proportional to increasing venous cannula resistance, blood returning in the vena cava is redirected to the right heart, thus increasing preload. Initially, blood volume in the pulmonary circulation is extremely low, and thus the RV initially does not face a significant afterload challenge; therefore RV ejection occurs early in this process and at low pressures. Conversely, the left ventricle (LV) finds itself in quite a different situation. Left ventricular preload increases as a consequence of the restoration of pulmonary venous blood volume; for some patients, such as those with pulmonary hypertension or congestive heart failure, the amount of volume the RV must eject to restore LV preload to the normal range is much greater, and thus may take a longer period of time. In addition, this period is most notable for the increase in LV afterload that results from persistent aortic flow; the volume and pressure in the aorta is maintained by energy derived from the bypass pump rather than the LV; hence, the LV must pump against an artificially high afterload during a period of time that LV preload is low. It should be no surprise that LV ejection fraction is often significantly reduced during partial bypass. The common echocardiographic finding of impaired ejection fraction while on partial bypass, followed by improvement after separation from bypass, should now be expected and understood as an obligatory consequence of the change in LV loading conditions; the sensitivity of the LV to the artificially high afterload imposed by partial bypass is, however, related to LV contractility.

CONCLUSION

The smooth transition from CPB to the unassisted circulation is an obvious goal. The unique challenges of non—steady state physiology often complicate interpretation of the hemodynamic changes associated with this transition. An understanding of the relationships between pressures, volumes, and flows into the vascular compartments, as well as the recognition of the alterations in loading conditions that occur during this transition, will allow for more timely and more appropriate interventions.

4 Prime Solutions for Extracorporeal Circulation

Robert J. Frumento, MS, MPH, *and*
Elliott Bennett-Guerrero, MD

CONTENTS

Summary

Various crystalloid and colloidal solutions, as well as various volumes of these solutions, are used to prime the cardiopulmonary bypass (CPB) circuit. Several institutions have developed "standard" priming solutions and volumes for all adult patients, whereas other institutions base their primes on body weight and body surface area. The significant variability in both CPB prime content and volume is primarily caused by the lack of data from well-designed trials evaluating differences in patient outcomes. Several studies have been performed examining intermediate outcomes, such as biochemical markers, and special concerns, including transfusion requirements; however, much of the available data are inconsistent and inconclusive.

The aim of this chapter is to review the specific components of the CPB prime, focusing on the constituents of the priming solution and the priming volume. Although the adult cardiac surgical patient is the primary patient population to be reviewed, a section on pediatric CPB prime is also included.

From: *Current Cardiac Surgery: On Bypass: Advanced Perfusion Techniques*
Edited by: L. B. Mongero and J. R. Beck

CARDIOPULMONARY BYPASS PRIME SOLUTIONS

There is significant interinstitutional variability regarding the specific components of priming solutions. In general, priming solutions have osmolality and electrolyte content that is similar to human plasma. The optimal priming fluid, as well as specific additives in cardiac surgery, is a topic of continuing debate.

FLUID

Crystalloid

Crystalloid solutions are composed of electrolytes and water. Because of their composition, crystalloid solutions will move across the vascular membrane and pass into the interstitial space, which results in only 10–25% of the crystalloid solution remaining within the vascular space.

There are three types of crystalloid solutions: isotonic (the solute concentration equals the solute concentration of plasma), hypotonic (the solute concentration is less than the solute concentration of plasma), and hypertonic (the solute concentration is greater than the solute concentration of plasma). Various available crystalloid solutions and their respective compositions are shown in Table 1.

Colloid

Colloids refer to large molecules that do not pass readily across capillary walls. These compounds exert an oncotic (i.e., they attract fluid) load and are usually administered to restore intravascular volume and improve tissue perfusion. Various colloid solutions available in the United States, and their respective compositions, are shown in Table 2.

Hetastarch (HES), which is a synthetic colloid, is a derivative of amylopectin, which is a highly branched starch. Amylopectin is rapidly hydrolyzed and renally excreted. To slow down this degradation, anhydroglucose residues are substituted with the hydroxyethyl groups of amylopectin. Hetastarch preparations have historically been characterized by their mean molecular weight (Mw), molar substitution (MS; mol of hydroxyethyl residues per mol of glucose subunits), and the C2/C6 ratio (pattern of substitution at the glucose subunit carbon atoms) *(1,2)*. In the United States, there are currently two available hydroxyethyl starch preparations; however, in Europe several preparations are available (Table 3). Both preparations available in the United States contain the identical starch, 6% with a Mw of 450 kD, and differ only

Table 1
Crystalloid Solutions

Solution	*Osmolarity mOsmol L^{-1}*	*PH*	*Na^+ mEq L^{-1}*	*CL^- mEq L^{-1}*	*K^+ mEq L^{-1}*	*Ca^{2+} mEq L^{-1}*	*Mg^- mEq L^{-1}*	*Acetate Mg L-1*	*Lactate mEq L^{-1}*
0.9% NaCl	308	5	154	154	—	—	—	—	—
Ringer's Lactate	273	6.5	130	109	4	2.7	—	—	28
Plasmalyte-A	294	7.4	140	98	5	—	3	27	—
Normasol-R	295	7.4	140	98	5	—	3	27	—
0.9% NaCl (Saline) and Glucose*	264	5.5	31	31	—	—	—	—	—

*40 mg/L glucose, Normasol contains 23 mmol/L gluconate.

Table 2
Colloid Solutions Available in the United States

Solution	*Osmolarity mOsmol L^{-1}*	*Molecular Weight kD*	*pH*	*COP mmHg*	*Na^+ mEq L^{-1}*	*CL^- mEq L^{-1}*	*K^+ mEq L^{-1}*	*Ca^{2+} mEq L^{-1}*	*Glucose Mg/L*	*Lactate mEq L^{-1}*
Albumin (5%)	300	66	6.9	20	145	160	—	—	—	—
6% HES in 0.9% Saline	308	450	5	30	154	154	—	—	—	
6% HES in Balanced Salt	307	450	6.0	30	143	124	3	5	99	28
Albumin (25%)	1,500	66	6.9	100	145	160				—

Table 3
Colloid Solutions Available Outside the United States

Solution	*Degree of Substitution*	*Mw kD*	*pH*	*Na^+ mEq L^{-1}*	*CL^- mEq L^{-1}*	*K^+ mEq L^{-1}*	*Ca^{2+} mEq L^{-1}*	*Glucose mEq L^{-1}*	*Lactate mEq L^{-1}*
Albumin (5%)	—	66	6.9	145	160	—	—	—	—
Albumin (25%)	—	66	6.9	154	154	—	—	—	—
6% HES in 0.9% NaCl	0.7	450	5	143	124	3	5	—	28
6% XES in 0.9% NaCl	0.6	200	5	154	154	—	—	—	—
6% TES in 0.9% NaCl	0.4	130	5	154	154	—	—	—	—
10% PES in 0.9% NaCl	0.5	200	5	154	154	—	—	—	—
Gelofusine (succinylated gelatin)	—	30	5.9	154	125	—	—	—	—
Haemaccel (polygeline)	—	35	6	145	145	5.1	6.25	—	—

HES, Hetastarch; XES, hexastarch; PES, pentastarch; TES, tetrastarch.

in the solution they are prepared in. They are 6% hetastarch in normal saline (Abbott Laboratories; Chicago, Ill.; Hespan®, DuPont Pharm) and 6% hetastarch in a balanced salt solution (Hextend™; BioTime, Berkeley, CA).

Albumin was the first natural colloid for clinical use as a volume expander, and it is the standard colloidal agent for comparison with other colloid products. Albumin for commercial use is obtained from source blood, plasma, or serum of healthy human donors by fractionation according to the Cohn cold ethanol process *(3)*. Albumin is pasteurized for 10h at 60°C to inactivate human immunodeficiency virus (HIV) and hepatitis viruses. Sodium caprylate and sodium acetyltryptophanate are added to prevent denaturation during pasteurization. Currently, there are three commercially available forms of albumin (5% albumin, 25% albumin, and plasma protein fraction).

Crystalloid Versus Colloid

Proponents of colloid-based prime emphasize the importance of avoiding a colloid osmotic pressure (COP) decline and concomitant edema that can compromise organ function. Crystalloid advocates note the lack of clear evidence that more expensive colloidal priming fluids quantifiably improve patient outcomes.

The use of pure crystalloid CPB priming solutions results in a rapid fall of COP at the onset of CPB, and it has been associated with postoperative organ dysfunction *(4)*. The sudden hemodilution and decrease in COP increases macro- and microvascular filtration pressure, causing a rise in extravascular lung water *(5)* and myocardial edema *(6,7)* upon weaning from CPB.

There are no controlled randomized trials assessing the effects of different crystalloid solutions (Table 1) on avoiding a decline in COP and concomitant edema. The rationale for adding colloidal solutions to CPB prime is preservation of COP and, hence, less fluid retention. Hydroxyethyl starch (HES) is as effective as albumin as an intravascular volume expander *(8)*. Hydroxyethyl starch may also be a less expensive alternative to albumin as a colloidal solution. However, concerns remain about the adverse effects of HES on blood coagulation, especially when it is used in patients undergoing CPB. In these patients, the deleterious effects of the extracorporeal circulation, by itself, already compromise effective hemostasis *(9,10)*. The use of albumin may not affect blood coagulation to the same degree as HES *(11)*. Albumin may even be advantageous when used in patients undergoing CPB, because preexposure of the synthetic surfaces of the

CPB circuit to albumin has been shown to decrease the affinity of platelets to these surfaces *(8)*.

The addition of colloid to the priming solution has been shown to result in a reduction in the amount of fluid accumulation and organ edema *(12)*. Several studies using a variety of colloidal priming solutions have been performed, but only four have been performed using priming solutions that are currently available in the United States. Two of these studies were prospective, randomized studies that were limited by small sample size, and reported no differences between groups in terms of patient outcomes *(13,14)*. Canver et al. *(15)* reported a large retrospective study showing no differences in bleeding-related outcomes between those patients with a HES-primed CPB circuit and those with albumin- or crystalloid-primed circuits. However, Herwaldt et al. *(16)* performed a case control study on the use of HES as a CPB priming solution and reported an increased risk for blood/blood product use and higher chest tube drainage in those patients who received HES in the CPB priming solution.

Acting on the recommendation of its Blood Products Advisory Committee (BPAC), the U.S. FDA has recently (2004) approved the following new warning in the labeling of all 6% hetastarch products formulated in 0.9% sodium chloride:

> *[6% hetastarch] is not recommended for use as a cardiac bypass pump prime, while the patient is on cardiopulmonary bypass, or in the immediate period after the pump has been discontinued because of the risk of increasing coagulation abnormalities and bleeding in patients whose coagulation status is already impaired.*

The FDA did not recommend this labeling change for 6% hetastarch in a balanced salt solution.

Albumin avidly binds calcium and reduces the fraction of ionized calcium. The reduction in ionized calcium can cause myocardial depression *(17)*. When compared with crystalloid prime, albumin-treated patients required more intravascular fluid replacement, produced less urine output, and had decreased renal function *(18,19)*. Furthermore, studies have examined the effect of albumin on glomerular filtration rate (GFR), particularly in burn patients, and found a 40% increase in plasma volume and a paradoxical decrease in GFR and urine output *(20,21)*. The mechanism of albumin-induced reduction in GFR is unknown; however, studies show that albumin increases the oncotic pressure within the peritubular vessels, causing a decrease in sodium and water excretion *(21)*.

Inclusion of albumin in the prime may help avoid oxygenator thrombosis (1 in every 20,000 cases), which is the leading cause of emergency oxygenator replacement *(22)*. Furthermore, inclusion of albumin in the prime has been shown to reduce extravascular lung water accumulation and pulmonary shunt fraction *(22)*.

Evidence from trials comparing albumin with crystalloid as the priming fluid has recently been systematically reviewed *(23)*. The authors conducted a metaanalysis of such trials to test the hypothesis that an albumin prime better maintains platelet count and COP and lessens on-bypass and postoperative fluid imbalance. They also assessed whether the choice of priming fluid significantly affects postoperative colloid usage, time to extubation, allogeneic blood transfused, and length of stay. They found that albumin exerts significant favorable effects during bypass on platelet count, COP, and positive fluid balance, as well as on postoperative COP, weight gain, and colloid usage in patients undergoing CPB. The authors also found no significant differences in markers of hemorrhagic complications. Unfortunately, thrombotic complications, such as stroke and myocardial infarction, as well as other outcome data, were not reported.

ADDITIVES TO CARDIOPULMONARY BYPASS PRIME SOLUTION

Glucose

The use of glucose has received some recent attention due to observed adverse neurologic outcomes associated with hyperglycemia in noncardiac surgery *(24)*. A theoretical advantage of adding glucose to priming solutions is that the osmotic pressure of the prime is increased; thus, perioperative fluid requirements and the use of albumin may be reduced. Glucose also provides a substrate for energy production during myocardial ischemia *(25)*. A clinical audit by Newland et al. *(26)* evaluating the removal of glucose from the CPB prime reported a 66% reduction in the incidence of hyperglycemia during CPB when glucose was removed from the CPB prime; however, a significant reduction in osmolality was also observed, and there were no differences in terms of overall patient outcomes. The clinical relevance of glucose in the CPB prime is still unclear.

Mannitol

The use of mannitol in the CPB priming solution has been advocated for several years. Animal models have demonstrated the use of mannitol to attenuate tissue edema, promote diuresis, and protect the kidneys from ischemia/reperfusion injury. However, human studies have been unable to duplicate these findings *(27,28)*. Indeed, several human studies have indicated that the use of mannitol in the CPB prime may be detrimental to renal function after cardiac surgery, regardless of its ability to increase urinary output *(28,29)*.

Aprotinin

Aprotinin, a serine protease inhibitor, has both antifibrinolytic and platelet-preserving activity *(30–32)*, and it reduces blood loss and transfusion requirements in cardiac surgical patients. The use of aprotinin as an additive to the CPB prime has been specifically studied. Schonberger et al. *(33)* demonstrated that addition of aprotinin to the CPB prime resulted in reduced blood transfusion, although no difference was found in perioperative blood loss. A large multicenter trial *(31)* evaluating the effectiveness of aprotinin in cardiac surgical reoperations demonstrated that an aprotinin dosing regimen that included a loading dose and a continuous infusion, in addition to the CPB prime dose, significantly reduced blood loss and transfusion requirements compared with the CPB prime dose alone. Although a multicenter study in primary coronary artery bypass grafting demonstrated similar efficacy between the infusion group and the CPB prime only dose group, significantly more perioperative myocardial infarction occurred in the CPB prime dose only group. Therefore, it is currently recommended that aprotinin be administered as a loading dose and infusion in addition to the priming dose.

CARDIOPULMONARY BYPASS PRIME VOLUME

Differences in priming volumes can vary significantly due to differences in oxygenators, arterial filters, and connective tubing. Potential advantages and disadvantages of different priming volumes include anemia and dilution of clotting factors when larger priming volumes are used and the potential for increased blood viscosity with subsequent alterations in microcirculatory blood flow when smaller priming volumes are used.

The lower safe limit of the hematocrit on CPB is not known, although there is probably little benefit and some risk in maintaining a hematocrit below 15% *(34)*. This is especially true during the period of separation from bypass, when maldistribution of coronary blood flow away from the subendocardium and the risk of dilutional coagulopathy mitigate against maintaining an excessively low hematocrit. In general, however, because hemodilution has a beneficial effect on perfusion and there is a theoretical decrease in microcirculatory flow with high hematocrits above 30%, it is generally acceptable to maintain a hematocrit below 30% while on CPB *(35)*.

Priming volumes between 1,400 and 2,000 mL are generally used by perfusionists during CPB. Therefore, a certain degree of hemodilution is inevitable, and this magnitude depends on the volume of the solution used for priming, the patient's preoperative hematocrit, and baseline blood volume. Low preoperative hematocrit, small body surface area (BSA), and low red blood cell mass have been shown to be independent predictors of allogeneic blood transfusion, and these values are exacerbated by the hemodilution induced by a large nonsanguinous prime. Shapira et al. randomized 114 patients to either full prime volume (1,400 mL) or reduced prime volume (600–800 mL) and found that patients receiving the reduced prime volume received statistically significantly fewer allogeneic blood products, had higher hematocrit values on CPB, and had equivalent 24-h chest tube drainage between groups *(36)*. These results suggest that the use of a reduced prime volume may reduce allogeneic blood product use.

There are several techniques that can be used to reduce pump prime volume, such as retrograde autologous priming (RAP). Several small European studies have demonstrated that by reducing the rapid crystalloid administration, which occurs at the commencement of CPB by using the RAP technique, the number of allogeneic red cell transfusions can be reduced *(37)*. Retrograde autologous priming may also be a promising technique to reduce the rapid hemodilution-associated fall in COP and metabolic acidosis *(38)*. Furthermore, Eising et al. demonstrated that RAP can also reduce the amount of extravascular lung water and myocardial edema upon weaning from CPB, compared with crystalloid priming *(39)*. However, their use is not widespread, and popularity varies among perfusionists because safety may be compromised. Antegrade autologous priming is a good alternative, also known as clear prime replacement. Reducing the clear fluid by replacing the circuit volume with the patient's blood volume in the routine direction of bypass flow, thereby minimizing possible air entrainment and accidents associated with RAP procedures.

PEDIATRIC PATIENTS

Crystalloids and Colloids

The priming of the extracorporeal circuit is of particular importance in pediatric cardiac surgery, as the priming volume of the circuit often equals or exceeds the patient's total blood volume. Hence, when CPB is instituted in the pediatric patient, the composition and volume of the priming solution determines the composition of the circulating fluid to a far greater degree than in the adult patient. There is also a great degree of variability in the *volume* of the priming solutions used, related mainly to the variety of oxygenators, connecting tubing, and arterial filters that are employed in different size pediatric patients.

Although variation exists, the use of priming solution composed of a crystalloid base to which blood and albumin are added is generally favored in children. The crystalloid base is similar in electrolyte content and osmolarity to plasma, with Plasmalyte, Normosol, and lactated Ringer's solution being commonly used base-priming solutions.

The use of colloids in pediatric patients may be beneficial for several reasons. There is some evidence to suggest that the addition of colloid to the priming solution may counteract the increased permeability of capillaries and the decline in oncotic pressure that has been shown to occur with purely crystalloid priming solutions *(40)*. The clinical relevance of this, however, has not been adequately studied. Although the addition of colloid to the prime solution has been shown to prevent excessive edema formation in long-duration CPB, the differences in lung water or total body water are not significant for very long postoperatively *(40)*.

The most commonly used colloid added to the extracorporeal circuit is albumin, although many others have been used, including 6% hydroxyethyl starch and human plasma. The relative importance of colloids in short-term CPB remains a matter of speculation. The addition of albumin to achieve a 5% solution probably has some advantages at minimal risk, but may not be benign *(41)*. The largest randomized controlled trial to date randomized 86 children, ranging in age from 3 days to 4 years, to receive either 5% albumin or crystalloid prime. Although patients in the albumin group had a higher COP and gained less weight postoperatively, those receiving the albumin prime required significantly more transfusions *(41)*. Therefore, the risk/benefit ratio of albumin prime in this patient population requires further investigation.

Blood-Based Priming Solutions

Due to the relatively high ratio of the extracorporeal circuit volume to the patient's total blood volume in neonates and small children, an unacceptable degree of hemodilution may occur if a purely crystalloid/colloid solution is used as the sole priming solution. Thus, packed red blood cells (PRBCs) are often added to the priming circuit to avoid an unacceptable degree of hemodilution. The degree of hemodilution may be predicted by knowing the weight of the patient, the hematocrit, the amount of intravenous fluids administered before CPB, and the oxygenator's/circuits's priming volume.

Several centers advocate the use of fresh whole blood (i.e., collected within 48 hours of surgery) when priming the CPB circuitry in infants and children, in an attempt to diminish the inflammatory response and abnormal coagulation that often occurs in these patients *(42,43)*. However, the majority of evidence to support this technique has come from adult trauma and transplantation studies where patients often receive complete exchange transfusion, as is often the case in neonates and infants undergoing cardiac surgery with CPB *(44–46)*. Mou et al. recently reported the largest randomized trial to date, in which children less than 1 year of age were randomized to receive either fresh whole blood or reconstituted blood (a combination of PRBCs and fresh frozen plasma) for CPB circuit priming *(47)*. These authors found that the use of whole blood had no advantage over the use of reconstituted blood, and that the use of whole blood was associated with longer hospital and intensive care unit stays and an increase in perioperative fluid overload *(47)*. Therefore, as the authors from this trial have stated, it seems that the use of fresh whole blood in this patient population is not justified.

CONCLUSIONS

Theoretical evidence, case reports, and anecdotal evidence demonstrating the hazards associated with each kind of priming solutions available in the United States must be interpreted with caution. The choice of priming solutions is one of many factors that can influence bleeding, acid-base balance, edema, and patient outcomes in the complex arena of cardiac surgery. Hence, to better define the specific impact of priming solutions, randomized blinded clinical trials need to be conducted.

Based on the existing literature, no single best CPB fluid, volume, or additives can be singled out as being most beneficial in the cardiac surgical patient. There is little peer-reviewed data from adequately powered randomized blinded clinical trials to suggest that the administration of any particular priming solution to cardiac surgical patients is associated with an improvement in clinically relevant outcomes.

REFERENCES

1. Prien T, Thulig B, Wusten R, Schoofs J, Weyand M, Lawin P. [Hypertonic-hyperoncotic volume replacement (7.5% NaCl/10% hydroxyethyl starch 200.000/0.5) in patients with coronary artery stenoses]. Zentralbl Chir 1993;118:257–263; discussion 264–266.
2. Prien T, Backhaus N, Pelster F, Pircher W, Bunte H, Lawin P. Effect of intraoperative fluid administration and colloid osmotic pressure on the formation of intestinal edema during gastrointestinal surgery. J Clin Anesth 1990;2:317–323.
3. Tollofsrud S, Svennevig JL, Breivik H, et al. Fluid balance and pulmonary functions during and after coronary artery bypass surgery: Ringer's acetate compared with dextran, polygeline, or albumin. Acta Anaesthesiol Scand 1995;39:671–677.
4. Foglia RP, Lazar HL, Steed DL, et al. Iatrogenic myocardial edema with crystalloid primes: effects on left ventricular compliance, performance, and perfusion. Surg Forum 1978;29:312–315.
5. Hoeft A, Korb H, Mehlhorn U, Stephan H, Sonntag H. Priming of cardiopulmonary bypass with human albumin or Ringer lactate: effect on colloid osmotic pressure and extravascular lung water. Br J Anaesth 1991;66:73–80.
6. Mehlhorn U, Allen SJ, Davis KL, Geissler HJ, Warters RD, Rainer de Vivie E. Increasing the colloid osmotic pressure of cardiopulmonary bypass prime and normothermic blood cardioplegia minimizes myocardial oedema and prevents cardiac dysfunction. Cardiovasc Surg 1998;6:274–281.
7. Geissler HJ, Allen SJ. Myocardial fluid balance: pathophysiology and clinical implications. Thorac Cardiovasc Surg 1998;46 Suppl 2:242–245; discussion 246–247.
8. Boldt J, Zickmann B, Ballesteros BM, Stertmann F, Hempelmann G. Influence of five different priming solutions on platelet function in patients undergoing cardiac surgery. Anesth Analg 1992;74:219–225.
9. Kuitunen A, Hynynen M, Salmenpera M, et al. Hydroxyethyl starch as a prime for cardiopulmonary bypass: effects of two different solutions on haemostasis. Acta Anaesthesiol Scand 1993;37:652–658.
10. Cope JT, Banks D, Mauney MC, et al. Intraoperative hetastarch infusion impairs hemostasis after cardiac operations. Ann Thorac Surg 1997;63:78–82; discussion 82–83.
11. Kuitunen AH, Hynynen MJ, Vahtera E, Salmenpera MT. Hydroxyethyl starch as a priming solution for cardiopulmonary bypass impairs hemostasis after cardiac surgery. Anesth Analg 2004;98:291–297.
12. Gravlee D, Kurusz, Utley. Cardiopulmonar Bypass: Principles and Practice. Second Edition. Lippincott Williams, Philadelphia, 2000.
13. Sade RM, Stroud MR, Crawford FA, Jr., Kratz JM, Dearing JP, Bartles DM. A prospective randomized study of hydroxyethyl starch, albumin, and lactated Ringer's solution as priming fluid for cardiopulmonary bypass. J Thorac Cardiovasc Surg 1985;89:713–722.
14. Lumb PD. A comparison between 25% albumin and 6% hydroxyethyl starch solutions on lung water accumulation during and immediately after cardiopulmonary bypass. Ann Surg 1987;206:210–213
15. Canver CC, Nichols RD. Use of intraoperative hetastarch priming during coronary bypass. Chest 2000;118:1616–1620.

16. Herwaldt LA, Swartzendruber SK, Edmond MB, et al. The epidemiology of hemorrhage related to cardiothoracic operations. Infect Control Hosp Epidemiol 1998;19:9–16.
17. Kovalik SG, Ledgerwood AM, Lucas CE, Higgins RF. The cardiac effect of altered calcium homeostasis after albumin resuscitation. J Trauma 1981;21: 275–279.
18. Scott DA, Hore PJ, Cannata J, Masson K, Treagus B, Mullaly J. A comparison of albumin, polygeline and crystalloid priming solutions for cardiopulmonary bypass in patients having coronary artery bypass graft surgery. Perfusion 1995;10:415–424.
19. Bennett-Guerrero E, Frumento RJ, Mets B, Manspeizer H, Hirsh A. Impact of normal saline based versus balanced salt intravenous fluid replacement on clinical outcomes: a randomized blinded clinical trial. Anesthesiology 2001;92:A106.
20. Gore DC, Dalton JM, Gehr TW. Colloid infusions reduce glomerular filtration in resuscitated burn victims. J Trauma 1996;40:356–360.
21. Lucas CE. Renal considerations in the injured patient. Surg Clin North Am 1982;62:133–148.
22. Fisher AR. The incidence and cause of emergency oxygenator changeovers. Perfusion 1999;14:207–212.
23. Russell JA, Navickis RJ, Wilkes MM. Albumin versus crystalloid for pump priming in cardiac surgery: meta-analysis of controlled trials. J Cardiothorac Vasc Anesth 2004;18:429–437.
24. Pulsinelli WA, Levy DE, Sigsbee B, Scherer P, Plum F. Increased damage after ischemic stroke in patients with hyperglycemia with or without established diabetes mellitus. Am J Med 1983;74:540–544.
25. Metz S, Keats AS. Benefits of a glucose-containing priming solution for cardiopulmonary bypass. Anesth Analg 1991;72:428–434.
26. Newland RF, Baker RA, Mazzone AL, Ottens J, Sanderson AJ, Moubarak JR. Removal of glucose from the cardiopulmonary bypass prime: a prospective clinical audit. J Extra Corpor Technol 2004;36:240–244.
27. Stanic M, Sindjelic R, Neskovic V, Davidovic L, Lotina S. [Renal protection during surgical procedures on the infrarenal aorta]. Srp Arh Celok Lek 2002; 130:168–172.
28. Carcoana OV, Mathew JP, Davis E, et al. Mannitol and dopamine in patients undergoing cardiopulmonary bypass: a randomized clinical trial. Anesth Analg 2003;97:1222–1229.
29. Ip-Yam PC, Murphy S, Baines M, Fox MA, Desmond MJ, Innes PA. Renal function and proteinuria after cardiopulmonary bypass: the effects of temperature and mannitol. Anesth Analg 1994;78:842–847.
30. Maquelin KN, Nieuwland R, Lentjes EG, Boing AN, Mochtar B, Eijsman L, Sturk A: Aprotinin administration in the pericardial cavity does not prevent platelet activation. J Thorac Cardiovasc Surg 2000;120:552–557.
31. Levy JH, Pifarre R, Schaff HV, et al. A multicenter, double-blind, placebo-controlled trial of aprotinin for reducing blood loss and the requirement for donor-blood transfusion in patients undergoing repeat coronary artery bypass grafting. Circulation 1995;92:2236–2244.
32. Poullis M, Manning R, Laffan M, Haskard DO, Taylor KM, Landis RC. The antithrombotic effect of aprotinin: actions mediated via the proteaseactivated receptor 1. J Thorac Cardiovasc Surg 2000;120:370–378.

33. Schonberger JP, Everts PA, Ercan H, et al. Low-dose aprotinin in internal mammary artery bypass operations contributes to important blood saving. Ann Thorac Surg 1992;54:1172–1176.
34. Liam BL, Plochl W, Cook DJ, Orszulak TA, Daly RC. Hemodilution and whole body oxygen balance during normothermic cardiopulmonary bypass in dogs. J Thorac Cardiovasc Surg 1998;115:1203–1208.
35. Osawa H, Yoshii S, Abraham SJ, et al. Critical values of hematocrit and mixed venous oxygen saturation as parameters for a safe cardiopulmonary bypass. Jpn J Thorac Cardiovasc Surg 2004;52:49–56.
36. Shapira OM, Aldea GS, Treanor PR, et al. Reduction of allogeneic blood transfusions after open heart operations by lowering cardiopulmonary bypass prime volume. Ann Thorac Surg 1998;65:724–730.
37. Rosengart TK, DeBois W, O'Hara M, et al. Retrograde autologous priming for cardiopulmonary bypass: a safe and effective means of decreasing hemodilution and transfusion requirements. J Thorac Cardiovasc Surg 1998;115:426–438; discussion 438–439.
38. Liskaser FJ, Bellomo R, Hayhoe M, et al. Role of pump prime in the etiology and pathogenesis of cardiopulmonary bypass-associated acidosis. Anesthesiology 2000;93:1170–1173.
39. Eising GP, Pfauder M, Niemeyer M, et al. Retrograde autologous priming: is it useful in elective on-pump coronary artery bypass surgery? Ann Thorac Surg 2003;75:23–27.
40. Groom RC, Akl BF, Albus R, Lefrak EA. Pediatric cardiopulmonary bypass: a review of current practice. Int Anesthesiol Clin 1996;34:141–163.
41. Riegger LQ, Voepel-Lewis T, Kulik TJ, et al. Albumin versus crystalloid prime solution for cardiopulmonary bypass in young children. Crit Care Med 2002; 30:2649–2654.
42. Kern FH, Morana NJ, Sears JJ, Hickey PR. Coagulation defects in neonates during cardiopulmonary bypass. Ann Thorac Surg 1992;54:541–546.
43. Kirklin JK, Westaby S, Blackstone EH, Kirklin JW, Chenoweth DE, Pacifico AD. Complement and the damaging effects of cardiopulmonary bypass. J Thorac Cardiovasc Surg 1983;86:845–857.
44. Petaja J, Lundstrom U, Leijala M, Peltola K, Siimes MA. Bleeding and use of blood products after heart operations in infants. J Thorac Cardiovasc Surg 1995;109:524–529.
45. Shoemaker WC, Wo CC. Circulatory effects of whole blood, packed red cells, albumin, starch, and crystalloids in resuscitation of shock and acute critical illness. Vox Sang 1998;74 Suppl 2:69–74.
46. Ramsey G, Sherman LA. Transfusion therapy in solid organ transplantation. Hematol Oncol Clin North Am 1994;8:1117–1129.
47. Mou SS, Giroir BP, Molitor-Kirsch EA, et al. Fresh whole blood versus reconstituted blood for pump priming in heart surgery in infants. N Engl J Med 2004; 351:1635–1644.

5 Blood Flow During Cardiopulmonary Bypass

Terence Gourlay, PhD
and Tipo Qureshi, MD

CONTENTS

SUMMARY

Clinical cardiopulmonary bypass (CPB) has been with us now for over 50 years, and in that time it has evolved technologically and practically, embracing all of the major scientific and clinical innovations of the later half of the last century in the fields of material development, electronics, and computer technology. However, despite the adsorption of all of these emerging technologies, materials, and techniques, the CPB system used today would be largely recognizable to the early CPB pioneers. Without a doubt, the materials and devices have improved over the evolution of CPB, but the basic techniques and fundamental principles remain largely unchanged. Despite the continued improvement in devices and better understanding of the mechanisms underlying CPB pathophysiology, which have led to generally

From: *Current Cardiac Surgery: On Bypass: Advanced Perfusion Techniques*
Edited by: L. B. Mongero and J. R. Beck © Humana Press Inc., Totowa, NJ

improved patient outcome, several aspects of CPB remain controversial. Amongst these controversial issues are the mechanism and nature of blood flow delivery to the patient. That the patient requires artificial provision of blood flow during the procedure is essential and is, in itself, not at all controversial. However, there are issues relating to blood flow which remain controversial, e.g., whether to use pulsatile or nonpulsatile blood flow, which is the most appropriate blood flow index for a particular environment, and which pumping mechanism is most suitable. In this chapter, we will explore these issues, and endeavor to answer some of these fundamental questions relating to blood flow by referring to the medical literature and clinical evidence.

THE PHYSIOLOGY OF BLOOD FLOW

It is reasonable to assume that the blood flow delivered by the native heart, which evolved over millions of years for the purpose, is the ideal flow modality for CPB. Therefore, in considering our ideal CPB blood flow delivery system, the mechanisms underlying normal physiological blood flow should be the point of reference. The fundamental requirement of blood flow delivery to organs and tissues, which is that of delivering nutrients and enhancing the removal of waste matter, is well understood. However, the system is far more complex than this insofar as blood flow plays a very important role in the maintenance of homeostasis. This maintenance of a constant internal environment, despite a changing external environment, requires constant control and monitoring of many factors, often reduced to six basic control levels: CO_2, urea, ionic concentration, water content, blood sugar, and temperature *(1)*. This is perhaps an overly simplistic view of homeostasis, which we know to be extremely complex and to involve many receptors, communicators, effectors, and both positive- and negative-feedback systems. However, in principal, blood flow is central to the control of all of these parameters. A good example of the complexity of these mechanisms is the physiological response to temperature. When the body is exposed to low temperatures, the hypothalamus will initiate a sequence of events that have evolved to maintain the "core" temperature at a near normal level. This response involves muscular and secretory responses, such as vasoconstriction, to minimize blood flow to the effected region, reducing heat loss. This peripheral vasoconstriction in response to low temperature, results in shunting of blood flow to the vital organs and the maintenance of a physiologically acceptable core temperature. This is an important response in the context of blood flow distribution during CPB, as we shall discuss later.

The distribution of blood flow within the body varies greatly under a broad spectrum of stress conditions. For example, during exercise, blood flow increases most significantly to the muscles. However, the brain, which has a powerful autoregulatory mechanism, maintains a relatively stable blood flow independent of systemic conditions. Clearly, the homeostatic control mechanisms are complex and a full discussion of the various central, regional, and local aspects involved in these systems is beyond the scope of this chapter, but the important parameters can be summarized as follows.

LOCAL CONTROL OF BLOOD FLOW

By the Tissues: Metabolic Control of Blood Flow

Blood flow is necessary for the delivery of oxygen and nutrients to tissues, the removal of carbon dioxide, and the maintenance of ionic balance. However, the delivery requirements vary, depending on the function of the organ or tissue, and in response to local and systemic need. The variation in tissue blood flow delivery, as a measure per gram of tissue, is reflective of both metabolic requirement and the specific function of the tissue in maintaining homeostasis (Fig. 1). Some organ systems, such as the skin or kidneys, have specific blood flow requirements in order for them to perform their specialized functions, and this may be considerably higher than other tissues.

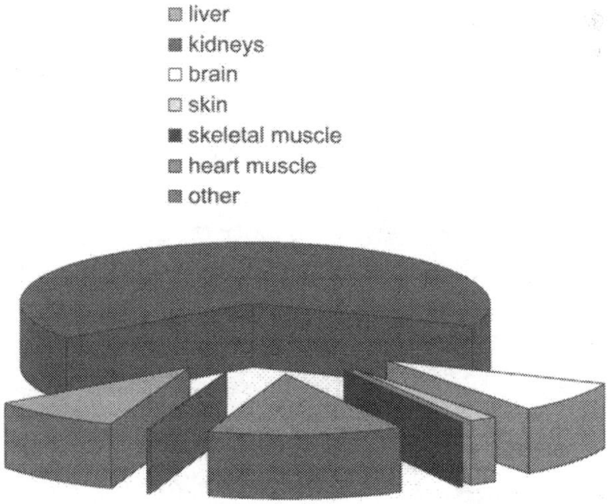

Fig. 1. The distribution of blood flow in milliliters per gram of tissue to the vital tissues in the human body. This illustrates quite clearly the varying metabolic demand of these tissues under physiological conditions.

In general however, in all tissues, the blood flow increases proportionally depending on its metabolic requirements, but is usually regulated at the minimal level that will supply the tissue's demand to minimize the workload of the heart. Local control of blood flow can be characterized in two phases:

1. Short-term control is achieved within seconds to minutes, with rapid local control of tissue blood flow through changes in local vasoconstriction and vasodilatation of the arterioles, met arterioles, and precapillary sphincters. As these are poorly innervated, contraction is controlled by local metabolites.
2. Long-term control is a much slower process that occurs over days or weeks and results in changes in the numbers or physical sizes of the blood vessels supplying the tissues. In the context of CPB, which is of relatively short duration, these long-term control and response mechanisms are of lesser importance.

The metabolic changes that produce vasodilatation by relaxation of the arterioles and precapillary sphincters include, in most tissues, decreases in O_2 tension and pH and an increase in CO_2 tension and osmolality, with the direct dilator action of CO_2 being most pronounced in the skin and brain. K^+ and lactate are other dilator substances that accumulate locally, especially in skeletal muscle. The vasodilator effect of these metabolites is graphically demonstrated during exercise. A rise in temperature, especially in metabolically active tissues, also exerts a direct vasodilator effect. In injured tissues such as one might encounter in the post-CPB patient, histamine released from damaged cells increases capillary permeability, thereby contributing to the inflammatory response.

Local blood flow decreases during injury as injured arteries and arterioles constrict strongly due to local liberation of serotonin from platelets. A drop in tissue temperature also causes vasoconstriction, and this local response to cold plays a major part in temperature regulation. In terms of general blood flow distribution, it is important to note that the blood flow rate/gram of tissue is very high in the liver, brain, and kidneys. This reflects the high metabolic demands of these tissues, even in the resting state.

The Role of Oxygen and Other Nutrients in Local Control of Blood Flow

One of the most important and vital nutrients to all tissues is oxygen. A reduction in the availability of oxygen to tissues or a rise in the rate of metabolism markedly increases the blood flow to the tissue under normal conditions. This is caused, in part, by oxygen and other nutrient deficiencies, resulting in the greater rate of formation of vasodilator substances. Some of the different vasodilator substances released under these conditions include: adenosine, carbon dioxide, adenosine phosphate, histamine, potassium ions, and hydrogen ions. Of these, adenosine is believed to be the most important of the local vasodilators in terms of its influence on the local environment. In addition to its effect on the release of vasodilatory substances, a lack of an adequate supply of oxygen and other nutrients required to maintain vascular smooth muscle contraction directly results in relaxation and consequent dilatation *(2)*. The number of open precapillary sphincters at any given time has been shown to be proportional to the oxygen and nutrient requirements of the tissue, with their relaxation occurring below a critical oxygen or nutrient level and vice versa *(3)*.

Other nutrients besides oxygen that have been shown to exert an effect in the local control of blood flow include glucose, amino acids, fatty acids, and certain vitamins, all of which cause vasodilatation if deficient. These vascular responses in response to local metabolic changes are also responsible for the auto regulation that occurs in tissues in response to changes in arterial pressure.

Two additional special instances of metabolic control of local blood flow, which are of significant interest in the field of CPB, are reactive hyperemia and active hyperemia. Reactive hyperemia occurs after blockage of blood flow to a tissue. Once flow is reestablished it increases several fold and continues at this rate for seconds to hours, depending on the duration of the original blockage and the oxygen deficit that has accrued during the period of occlusion. In effect, the lack of flow sets into motion all the factors that cause vasodilatation. Active hyperemia occurs when any tissue becomes highly active with the increase in local metabolism resulting in the release of vasodilator substances increasing blood flow through the tissue. In the case of skeletal muscle, this can be an up to 20-fold increase in local blood flow during exercise *(4)*.

In addition to the general mechanisms for local control of blood flow that have been described, certain organs have specific blood flow requirements to allow them to perform their specialized functions. Blood flow to the kidney remains fairly constant, despite changes in arterial pressure caused by the action of the juxtaglomerular apparatus operating via the sodium concentration within the tubule through a mechanism called tubuloglomerular feedback. In the brain, in addition to the control of blood flow by tissue oxygen concentration, the local regulation of blood flow is based on the concentrations of carbon dioxide and hydrogen ions. An increase in either of these dilates the cerebral vessels and increases local blood flow, resulting in the rapid washout of the excess carbon dioxide or hydrogen ions. Exact control of the concentrations of these two ions and pH is of importance, as neuronal activity and the level of brain excitability is very sensitive to changes in their concentrations. These functions are readily influenced during CPB, where the ionic balance is disturbed and oxygen delivery is highly variable. Recent studies have demonstrated the interruption of normal cerebral arterial vasomotion function during CPB, which could lead to a loss of some of the autoregulatory function of the brain and subsequent neurological injury *(5)*.

Systemic Control of Blood Flow by the Autonomic Nervous System and Humoral Control

The nervous system can function extremely rapidly and provides a means of controlling large parts of the circulation simultaneously, allowing blood flow redistribution and rapid control of blood pressure, often overriding local blood flow mechanisms. The nervous system controls the circulation almost entirely through autonomic mechanisms, with the sympathetic nervous system playing the dominant role and the parasympathetic nervous system contributing specifically to the regulation of heart function. The sympathetic nerves innervate vascular smooth muscle causing vasoconstriction in all segments of the circulation except the capillaries and venules. In general terms, sympathetic innervation of the small arteries and arterioles allows vasoconstriction, thereby increasing resistance to blood flow, whereas innervation of the large arteries and veins decreases the volume in these vessels, resulting in the redistribution of blood volume. In addition, almost all blood vessels of the body innervated by peripheral sympathetic nerves are maintained in a partial state of contraction referred to as resting vasomotor tone originating from the vasomotor center in the reticular substance of the medulla. This center transmits signals continuously to the sympathetic vascular vasoconstrictor nerve fibers, causing continuous slow firing of these fibers resulting in partial contraction. Humoral control of blood flow relies on substances such as hormones or ions, which are secreted or absorbed into body fluids. They are produced either locally and cause local effects or at distant sites and then transported throughout the body. They can be divided into vasoconstrictor or vasodilator agents. The name and effect of the most important of these agents can be seen in Table 1.

The main vasoconstrictor agents include adrenalin, noradrenalin, angiotensin, and vasopressin. Noradrenaline, which is an extremely potent vasoconstrictor agent, is released from sympathetic nerve endings in almost all parts of the body in response to stress or exercise. In addition the sympathetic nerves to the adrenal medullae cause these glands to secrete both noradrenaline and adrenaline. These hormones then cause the same excitatory effects as sympathetic stimulation. Adrenalin also has a mild vasodilatory action in skeletal and cardiac muscle. The octapeptide angiotensin II has a generalized arteriolar vasoconstrictor action resulting in an increase in arterial pressure. It is formed from angiotensin I liberated by the action of renin from the kidney on circulating angiotensinogen. Renin secretion is increased in response to a fall in blood pressure or reduction in extracellular fluid volume, and has been shown to be effected by the presence or absence of a pulse during CPB *(6)*. Vasopressin is produced within the hypothalamus and

Table 1
Humoral Vasoactive Agents

Agent	*Action*	*Source*
Adrenaline	VC	Adrenals
Noradrenaline	VD	Sympathetic NS / Adrenals
Angiotensin II	VC	Action of renin on circulating angiotensin I
Vasopressin	VC	Hypothalamus
Endothelin	VC	Endothelial cells
Ca^{2+} increase	VC	Body and tissue fluids
CO_2 decrease	VC	Body and tissue fluids
H^+ decrease	VC	Body and tissue fluids
Bradykinin	VC	Body and tissue fluids
Serotonin	VD	Platelets/ GIT
Histamine	VD/VC	Any tissue esp. Mast cells / Basophils/
Prostaglandins	VD/VC	Eosinophils
K^+	VD	Body and tissue fluids
Mg^{2+}	VD	Body and tissue fluids
H^+ increase	VD	Body and tissue fluids
Glucose	VD	Body and tissue fluids
CO_2 increase	VD esp. brain	Body and tissue fluids
		Body and tissue fluids

transported to the posterior pituitary, where it is secreted into the blood. Normally secreted in only small amounts, the concentration of this hormone rises after severe hemorrhage and circulatory shock and is important in raising arterial pressure. Endothelin is another vasoconstrictor substance present within endothelial cells and is released after trauma. An increase in calcium ion concentration also causes vasoconstriction, as calcium has a general effect to stimulate smooth muscle contraction. Carbon dioxide acting on the brain vasomotor center has a powerful indirect effect that is transmitted through the sympathetic nervous vasoconstrictor system to cause widespread vasoconstriction throughout the body. Finally, it is also well known that a slight decrease in hydrogen ion concentration causes arteriolar constriction.

The main vasodilator agents include bradykinin, serotonin, and histamine. Bradykinin is a short half-life small polypeptide derived from alpha-globulins activated by blood trauma, dilution, and contact with foreign substances. It causes both powerful arteriolar dilatation and increased capillary permeability. Serotonin, found in high concentrations in platelets and certain tissues of the gastrointestinal tract, can also exert a vasoconstrictor effect depending on the area of the circulation. Histamine is released mainly from mast cells and basophils in response to damage or inflammation, and from eosinophils during an allergic reaction. Histamine has a powerful vasodilator effect on arterioles and can also significantly increase capillary permeability. Prostaglandins are produced from an arachidonic acid precursor via the cyclooxygenase pathway and are released by all tissues producing vasodilatation or vasoconstriction. Various ions can also promote vasodilatation, including a rise in potassium, magnesium, and hydrogen ion concentration. The increase in osmolality resulting from a rise in hydrogen ion or glucose concentration also results in arteriolar dilatation. Finally, an increase in carbon dioxide concentration causes moderate vasodilatation in most tissues by a local effect, but marked vasodilatation in the brain. This is central to the question of whether to employ alpha-stat or pH-stat control during hypothermic CPB. These strategies will be discussed in more detail elsewhere in this volume, but briefly, Alpha-stat results in a lower pCO_2, which may have an adverse effect on cerebral blood flow, especially in cyanotic congenital heart conditions caused by pulmonary vasodilatation and cerebral vasoconstriction redistributing blood flow. With pH-stat, respiratory acidosis and hypercarbia results in an increase in cerebral blood flow, which may be advantageous in some but may also expose the brain to greater microembolic complications. pH-stat has also been shown to result in more homogenous cooling, greater reduction of oxygen consumption, and increased tissue oxygen availability. However, regional distribution of blood flow has been shown in a canine model to be similar in normothermic and hypothermic full flow CPB with alpha-stat and pH-stat strategies. The alpha-stat pH Stat debate very clearly demonstrates the importance of local blood flow control and the potential for tissue/organ function influence by the clinician responsible for CPB control. Furthermore it highlights the complex nature of the feedback and control mechanisms involved in organ blood flow maintenance and response.

As we have seen, it is clear that the control systems for maintaining and regulating blood flow at the systemic, regional and local level are very complex indeed, and the influence of the heart as the main provider of blood flow to the tissues plays a central role, both in controlling systemic blood flow, and hence nutrient delivery, and in responding to systemic and local demands. The heart, as part of an integrated control system, can respond to the demand and changing conditions incredibly well, being able to increase blood flow from a resting 4–6 L/min^{-1} to more than 20 L/min^{-1} *(7)*. Such changes in systemic output are rarely required under CPB conditions, but highlight the potential supply/demand requirement under normal physiological conditions. Critically, during CPB, the heart is replaced by a mechanical pump, which is not normally sensitive to the changing requirements of the challenged tissues. Such control is in the hands of the surgical team who act upon a different set of indicators for the status of blood flow demand for any given set of circumstances. These markers tend to be at the systemic level and are barometric in nature, including PO_2, PCO_2, and arterial and venous blood pressures, because under normal clinical conditions, clinicians operate in an information vacuum, in regard to more sensitive local tissues, which are indicators of both the adequacy of supply, the demand for blood, and the changing local environment. The maintenance of adequate perfusion during CPB has been one of the most intensively studied aspects of perfusion practice, and has resulted in the development of both new technologies designed to generate more physiological flow, and new techniques aimed at minimizing the pathophysiological consequences of delivering blood flow extracorporeally.

What is clear is that physiological blood flow delivery is complex and goes far beyond simply pumping blood around the circulation. It is pulsatile in nature, and is sensitive to global and local demand for nutrients and interaction with the external environment. In short, even with our present advanced knowledge of physiology and technology, it would be very difficult to produce a system that approaches the human homeostatic system. To date, those involved with CPB have had to accept a compromise situation, which meets only the very basic clinical demands.

BLOOD FLOW DURING CARDIOPULMONARY BYPASS

The physiological control of local and systemic blood flow is extremely complex, and although these control mechanisms persist during CPB, the feedback mechanisms present in the physiological setting, resulting in changes to systemic regional and local blood flow, are largely overridden during clinical CPB. Therefore, clinical CPB tends to be unreactive to developing local changes, and only reactive to the systemic consequences of these. Blood flow delivery by mechanical means, combined with artificial oxygenation and the many other parameters altered during CPB, e.g., the introduction of hemodilution and changes in body temperature, render even the best approach to clinical CPB, at the very most, a compromise solution. Clinical CPB, despite the use of the best technology and technique, is an entirely nonphysiological event, and, given the presence of highly evolved sensor and feedback mechanisms within the body, it is not surprising that the reaction to the initiation and conduct of CPB on the part of this complex physiological system is both complicated and dynamic.

There are several main events that effect local, regional, and systemic responses to the initiation of CPB; the introduction of hemodilution, changes in cardiac index, the introduction of nonpulsatile blood flow, and a drift downward in core body temperature, possible hyper- or hypooxygenation, and the chemistry of the priming fluid employed. The chemical effects associated with the presence of priming fluids are complex and have been described earlier in this chapter. These primarily revolve around the pH effects, and have largely been eliminated by the introduction of more controlled and buffered priming solutions. Additionally, the introduction of largely primeless minibypass systems, which are in some instances autologously primed with the patient's own blood, further diminish the priming solution chemistry effect *(8)*. Similarly, the known clinical effect of priming solution on viscosity, and hence peripheral vascular resistance, which is seen particularly at the onset of CPB (Fig. 2), has been largely diminished by the utilization of lower priming volumes and autologous prime *(9)*. However, several questions still remain to be answered in terms of the ideal blood flow regime for clinical CPB. Principal among these are questions relating

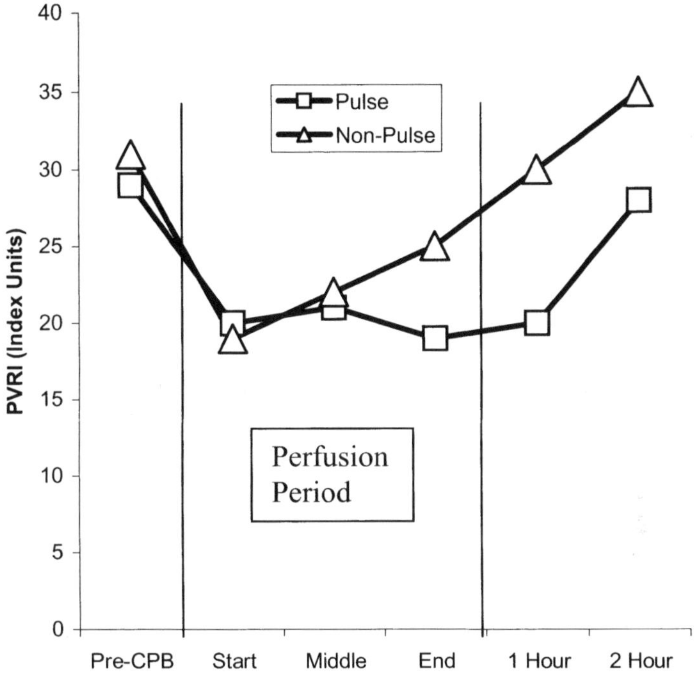

Fig. 2. Peripheral vascular resistance (Index Units) associated with pulsatile and nonpulsatile perfusion. These are data taken from two groups of 10 patients undergoing routine elective CABG procedures; the data demonstrate the commonly observed effect of a rapid drop in PVRI associated with the initiation of CPB (thought to be caused by hemodilution), followed by a rising level throughout the perfusion period in the nonpulsatile group that is not present in the pulsatile group. The difference in PVRI in the immediate postbypass phase is considered to be clinically significant insofar as the nonpulsatile group exhibits a higher PVRI that may effect a strain on the already insulted myocardium that is often countered by using vasodilator therapy. This is not the case with pulsatile perfusion.

to the ideal bulk flow rate employed and the modality of perfusion, whether pulsatile or nonpulsatile.

Determination of Systemic Blood Flow Rate During Cardiopulmonary Bypass

The systemic blood flow rate delivered during CPB varies, depending on the size of the patient and the clinical protocol. This is one of the basic tenets of CPB, and several tools have evolved over the years to help predict the blood flow rate for patients of varying sizes under various clinical protocol conditions. Generally, the predicted blood flow rate is obtained by calculation, using both measured and derived parameters, conventionally involving the Body Surface Area (BSA) and Flow Index, in the manner described in equation 1:

$$\text{Calculated Blood Flow Rate } (\text{l}\,\text{min}^{-1}) = \text{BSA } (\text{m}^2) \times \text{FI } (\text{l}\,\text{min}^{-1}\,\text{m}^{-2}) \quad (1)$$

The BSA is a calculated parameter derived from patient height and weight using a nomogram tool (Fig. 3). The nomogram permits the calculation of body surface area from two these two input factors, and simplifies the calculation shown below and first described by Boyde in 1935 *(10)*

$$\text{BSA } (\text{m}^2) = \text{Weight}^{0.425} (\text{kg}) \times \text{Height}^{0.725} (\text{m}) \times 0.007184^3 \quad (2)$$

Flow index is generally a preset constant that may vary according to temperature and preferred protocol conditions. In modern adult clinical practice, where profound cooling is utilized less frequently, the Flow Index normally ranges from $2–2.8\,\text{l}\,\text{m}^{-2}\,\text{min}^{-1}$ *(11)*. This is a simplistic approach to estimating blood flow during CPB, and although it has been shown to be generally adequate over almost half a century of clinical practice, it does not take into consideration many important factors, such as the differential in metabolic requirements of various tissues, and tissue distribution *(12)*. It is interesting to note that the Flow Index levels commonly employed in clinical CPB practice do not truly reflect those encountered in the normal physiological state. The normal range for cardiac index in adult humans is $2.3–4.2\,\text{l}\,\text{m}^{-2}\,\text{min}^{-1}$, which would suggest that the values employed in clinical perfusion practice are potentially rather low. Indeed, a cardiac index of between 1.8 and 2.2, which is very close to clinical CPB levels, is considered to be indicative of clinical hypoperfusion in normal medical practice, and levels of less than 1.8 are indicative of cardiogenic shock. Clearly, under routine CPB conditions, where cardiac index (Flow Index) levels of between 2 and 2.8 are common, patients are being perfused at the very edge of acceptable physiological levels.

Perhaps in this modern era another method for calculating systemic blood flow during CPB should be considered. Such a proposition may very well be timely, as over its evolution it is not only the technologies and techniques of CPB that have changed, but the patients themselves may be quite different in relation to some very important parameters. Patients presenting for CPB in the western world in particular tend to be considerably more obese than those in the early days of CPB, and perhaps the method for predicting the systemic blood flow rate for these patients should take this into consideration. The contribution of fat

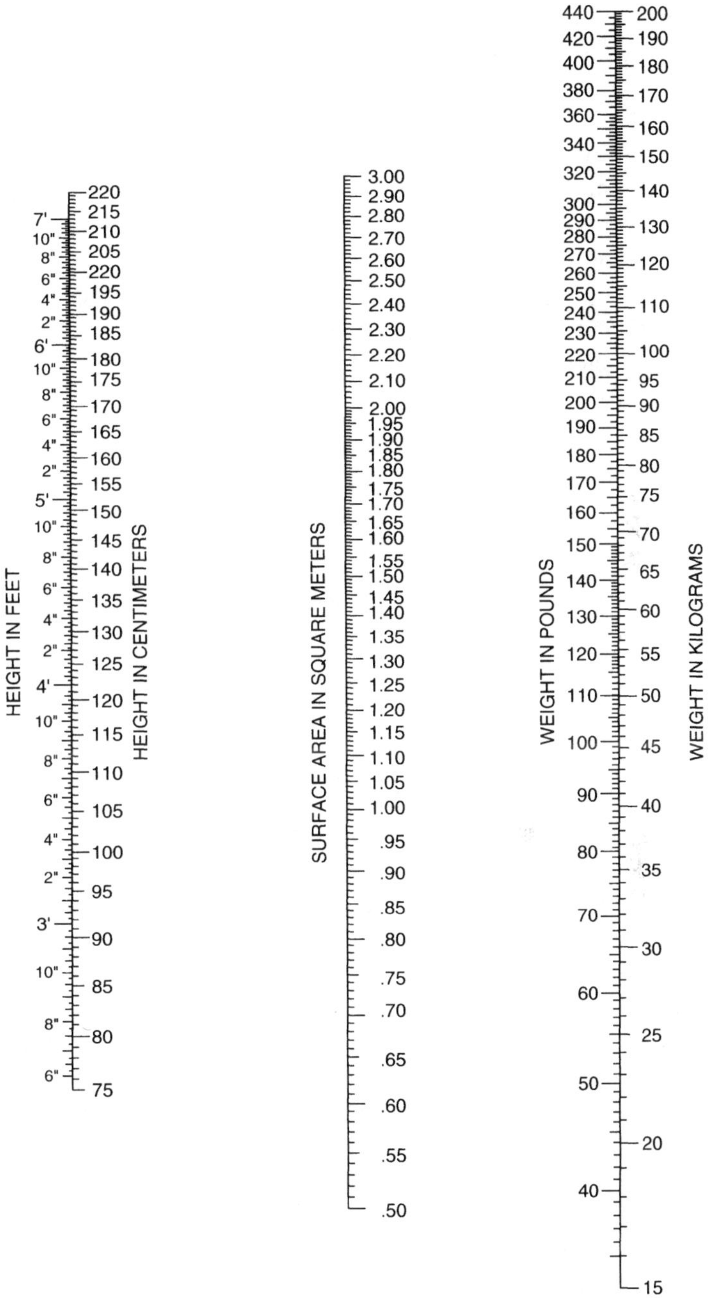

Fig. 3. The nomogram generally used to calculate BSA, which is employed to calculate the systemic blood flow rate in patients undergoing CPB.

content to the overall body mass in these patients, and hence to the BSA, has increased disproportionately. Muscle is the major contributor to basal metabolic requirements, but when excess fat is present, the calculated blood flow rate, which is derived through body surface area calculation, may exceed the actual required level, when only those tissues that contribute to the metabolic rate are considered. Recently, Alston and co-workers *(13)* suggested that a more appropriate and accurate method for predicting blood flow during CPB might involve estimation of Lean Body Mass (equation 3), and confirmed that this is positively correlated with SVO^2 during clinical CPB, whereas BSA and BMI do not when blood flow is maintained at the clinically normal fixed rate of $2.4\,lm^{-2}\,min^{-1}$.

$$\text{Lean body mass (\%)} = 100 - \text{Fat\%} \tag{3}$$

$$\text{Total fat (\%)} = (4.95/\text{density} - 4.5) \times 100 \tag{4}$$

$$\text{Density} = c - m \times \log(\text{biceps} + \text{triceps} + \text{superailiac} + \text{subcapsularis}), \tag{5}$$

where c and m are regression coefficients taken from age- and sex-specific tables.

Studies by this group suggest that BSA and BMI, commonly employed to predict flow rate during CPB, may no longer be appropriate. These studies represent a patient-focused concept in blood flow estimation, and may significantly influence future clinical practice.

Flow, or flow index, has been intensively studied in the context of CPB for over 50 years; however, whatever flow index is employed, and this will vary depending on the hemodynamic and temperature conditions required by the operating team, the basic rule for clinical perfusion is simply that one can only deliver to the patient as much blood flow as one receives from the patient. This balance clearly does not apply during initiation and cessation of CPB, but during the maintenance period of CPB this is an important rule, and changes in the blood flow output from the patient can be a good diagnostic indicator of the hemodynamic status of the patient and the adequacy of cannulation, among other important factors. The pump undoubtedly is the major circulatory driving force, but many other nonpump-related factors influence blood flow delivery, both systemically and at the tissue level, as we have already discussed. Despite the most sensitive and accurate predictive methodology in estimating systemic blood flow rate before the operative period, one must always remember that this is no more than a guideline and that the actual flow rate is an extremely dynamic factor.

Blood Pumps for Cardiopulmonary Bypass

During CPB, blood flow is delivered by a mechanical pump, which fulfills the role of the heart in maintaining systemic circulation. Several different pumping mechanisms are available to clinicians, and these have been the focus of considerable research effort since the very early days of CPB. Indeed, the pumps we know today owe much to pioneers in other branches of medical and engineering practice *(14)*. Some of the earliest systems were exotic in the extreme, and included, amongst other variations, modified motorcar engines *(15)*. However, emerging from this complex, and in some instances exotic, past has been the two principal mechanisms, which are employed in clinical practice today, the roller pump and the centrifugal pump. Both systems have several advantages and disadvantages in terms of their efficiency in delivering blood flow without compromising clinical safety. The roller pump has been in clinical use since the very early days of CPB and in many ways is a very elegant yet simple solution to the blood flow delivery issue. The simplicity of the roller pump, which is neither preload nor afterload dependent, has led to its widespread use in modern clinical practice. However, this independence of inlet or outlet conditions remains both its most commonly criticized characteristic and its greatest perceived advantage *(16)*. The ability of the roller pump to continue to pump against excessive outlet resistance has led to some concern with regard to potential for circuitry rupture in the event of outlet-side occlusion. This remains a concern despite the common practice of monitoring outlet-side pressure during clinical use. Similarly, the independence of the roller pump to its inlet conditions gives rise to concern in some quarters relating to its ability to effectively empty inlet reservoirs and, as a consequence, pump air to the patient. This remains one of the most common and injurious accident scenarios in clinical CPB practice *(17)*. Over the years, several safety devices have been developed to address these concerns, including level sensors placed on inlet reservoirs that will both warn the user of low level conditions and simultaneously deactivate the pump, and air sensors that deactivate the pumping system if gross amounts of air are detected. Although these safety devices have improved the safe application of roller pump technology, they do add complexity to the system and there is a genuine fear of an inappropriate "reliance" on this technology overriding conventional personal vigilance.

The most commonly used alternative to the roller pump for arterial or systemic pumping is the centrifugal pump. A full description of the science underlying this technology is beyond the scope of this chapter, but in general these systems function by imparting kinetic energy to the patient's blood by spinning either a veined or smooth impeller very rapidly in the fluid path, resulting in positive displacement of blood. Such pumps, being nonocclusive and lacking a "direct-drive" mechanism with respect to propelling blood, are load dependent, in terms of both pre- and afterload. This load dependence has both benefits and disadvantages. It is beneficial insofar as such pumps cannot overpressure in the presence of an obstruction, avoiding the danger of circuit rupture associated with the roller pump under similar circumstances. In the presence of a blockage, the kinetic pump will simply continue to rotate harmlessly without any further positive displacement of blood or dangerous increase in line pressure. Another advantage of such systems is their inherent inability to pump gross amounts of air *(18)*. In the presence of gross air, particularly volumes of air approaching the priming volume of the pump head, kinetic pumps will simply deprime, and will rotate relatively harmlessly. These important safety features, together with the ability to locate the pump head anywhere within the perfusion circuit, have led to widespread use of kinetic pumps in routine clinical practice, and in the artificial heart/ventricular support arenas. However, these advantages of the kinetic mechanism also carry with them disadvantages. In particular, it is not always possible to determine the exact output of such a system due to the relationship between afterload and pump speed. As the afterload increases, for example, in circumstances of increasing patient peripheral vascular resistance or tubing obstruction, the rotational speed of the pump, and hence the kinetic energy delivered to overcome increasing resistance to flow, requires an increase to compensate, otherwise blood flow delivery rate will decay. Although, at first sight, this is a simple relationship, in practice, successful compensation is entirely dependent on data obtained from a flow sensor positioned in the arterial line of the perfusion circuitry, and hence on the accuracy of this device. Technologies have evolved, in the form of laser electromagnetic and ultrasonic sensors, which are capable of delivering fairly accurate assessment of blood flow, and such systems can now be employed safely in clinical practice, but always with considerable vigilance on the part of the operator to ensure that an adequate blood flow rate is being delivered to the patient.

Over the past few years attempts have been made to produce hybrid pumping systems, which have the advantages of both primary pumping systems. These pumps, although not in regular routine clinical practice at present, employ roller technology with a flexible ventricle in the pump raceway. Such pumps are dependent on a head of pressure at the inlet side to effectively fill the ventricle behind the roller, and in this regard function rather like a centrifugal pump. The drive for positive displacement is derived from the roller itself; in this regard, such systems function like a roller pump. This combination of characteristics eliminates the unpredictability of preload dependence while eliminating the ability of the ventricle to pump air. If the inlet reservoir supplying the pump were to empty, the system ventricle would simply "suck flat." This seems to be an ideal compromise system, combining the desirable characteristics of both roller and centrifugal mechanisms; however, clinical application of such systems has been slow.

WHAT IS THE IDEAL FLOW MODALITY FOR CARDIOPULMONARY BYPASS?

As already described in this chapter, the blood flow requirements of the tissues and organs are very dynamic, and the controlled delivery of blood flow is dependent upon local, regional, and systemic conditions. It is also clear that several chemical agents are involved in the control of blood flow delivery, and that the release of these agents is promoted by the enduring conditions either locally or systemically. The body will respond to changes in these conditions very rapidly, leading to short and/or long term changes to local or systemic conditions. Under the circumstances encountered during CPB, clinicians are normally dealing with short-term changes in blood flow requirements to the tissues; however, in the absence of real-time indicators of local chemistry, control of regional conditions is beyond the scope of clinical perfusion practitioners. Therefore, clinical perfusion can at best be only a compromise situation where the clinician is responsive to the systemic indicators of regional and local events, indicated by changes in pressure, electrolytes, and oxygen consumption, etc. In accepting that clinical perfusion is indeed a compromise that falls far short of physiological blood delivery and feedback systems, it is important that the very best pumping parameters are employed, but what are these and what control parameters are available? The primary aim, as in all perfusion practice, should be to be biomimetic in terms of the flow generated. This of course means delivering pump flow architecture that is as near to the physiological state as possible. In short, the flow should be pulsatile and have pulse architecture, which is similar to that of the native heart. The human organism has evolved over millions of years with the result that we have a blood flow system that most appropriately matches our living environment. It is therefore reasonable to assume that a flow modality that most closely matches our normal physiological state is the one that is most suitable for any circumstances, including circulatory support.

The pulsatile nature of blood flow has been the focus of considerable research effort for millennia. Aristotle noted that "The blood in animals throbs within their veins" and that "the veins pulsate as a whole synchronously and successively inasmuch as they depend on the heart. It keeps moving and so do they." This reference to throbbing pulses is one of the first that hints at the pulsatile nature of blood flow. Its importance to the maintenance of normal organ and tissue function was, however, beyond the abilities of these very early academics to investigate or understand. It was not until much later that the critical importance of the pulse element of blood flow in maintaining organ and tissue function was investigated and confirmed. That a pulsatile flow regime may be better for extracorporeal circulation applications certainly makes sense intuitively; however, the mechanisms underlying the pulsatile nature of blood flow as the best option for tissue perfusion in the mammalian organism have been investigated, and a scientific foundation for the pulse in these circumstances confirmed.

Why Use Pulsatile Flow During Cardiopulmonary Bypass?

In addition to the intuitive view that a pulsatile flow regime is a more physiological option for circulatory support, there is evidence that supports the role of the pulse, per se, in the maintenance of more normal circulatory architecture than is the case with nonpulsatile flow. Burton et al. suggested that arterial pressure decay after systole results in a critical closing pressure being reached within the microcirculation, at which point flow within the capillaries ceases *(19)*. They demonstrated that the pulse prolongs the period of capillary opening and hence blood flow. This is critical in the context of CPB, where the circulation is supported by artificial means, and may suggest that in the presence of inadequate nonpulsatile flow regimes, capillary fallout may occur, and hence reduced peripheral perfusion. Subsequent studies have confirmed this. Ogata et al. *(20)* demonstrated that the presence of a pulse has a direct effect on capillary blood flow and diameter irrespective of the total blood flow and mean pressure. This finding correlates closely with the clinical finding of increased peripheral vascular resistance with nonpulsatile flow. In a series of animal experiments, Takeda et al. *(21)* demonstrated that nonpulsatile flow caused a general collapse of capillary structure, a reduction in blood flow, and an increase in capillary shunting, irrespective of the mean blood flow and arterial pressure.

Baba et al. *(22)* confirmed this in a series of studies involving the physical observation of the microcirculation using a high-definition microscope. They observed a drop during nonpulsatile flow in erythrocyte velocity within the capillaries, as well as a reduction in the number of perused capillaries with reversal of these changes on resuming pulsatile flow. He proposed that the basal and flow stimulated endothelium-derived nitric oxide release in the microvessels decreased with the loss of pulsatility, and that this induced the constriction of arterioles after the flow pattern was changed to the nonpulsatile mode.

The critical closing pressure argument was taken a step further by Shepard et al., who postulated that it was the additional energy delivered to the tissues with pulsatile flow, as opposed to nonpulsatile flow, that was responsible for keeping the peripheral circulation open *(23)*. Interestingly, he determined by mathematical modeling that pulsatile flow delivered 2.4 times as much energy at the same mean pressure than nonpulsatile perfusion, a finding confirmed in principle by other researchers *(24)*. The energy generation issue is an important factor when comparing pulsatile with nonpulsatile flow. However, it is not a factor that is easily measured during clinical perfusion. Recently, Undar *(25)* proposed that because pulsatile flow depends on an energy gradient and this directly effects its physiological outcome, investigators need to specify the difference in hemodynamic energy produced between the flow modalities by use of an energy equivalent formula, commonly known as energy equivalent pressure (EEP), which was first described by Shepard et al., for meaningful comparisons to be made. He also stressed the importance of suitable patient selection criteria, continuous use of pulsatile flow during the period of CPB, and appropriate selection of extracorporeal circuit components, all of which can have an effect on the quality of pulsatile blood flow delivered. Undar has also recently generated a surplus hemodynamic energy formula as a novel method to precisely quantify different levels of pulsatility and nonpulsatility for direct and meaningful comparisons *(26)*. Shepard et al. *(23)* had previously suggested that this increase in energy delivery with pulsatile flow was responsible for maintaining capillary patency, and that the pulse itself was responsible for extracellular fluid exchange. As early as 1938, McMaster and Parsons had demonstrated that lymph flow is greatly reduced with nonpulsatile blood flow *(27)*. By using an isolated ear preparation from a rabbit model, they noted that edema only developed with the use of nonpulsatile flow, and that clearance of dye from the rabbit ear was more rapid with pulsatile flow, suggesting that fluid exchange and clearance is improved with pulsatile flow. Prior et al. *(28)* proposed that the pulse is responsible for fluid exchange at the capillary level, whereas the mean pressure is responsible for maintenance of fluid balance. He suggested that the pulse pressure profile at the capillary level, along with the mean blood pressure and extracellular osmotic pressures, were the main factors responsible for the maintenance of fluid balance and exchange of nutrients at the cellular level. This concept is the focus of further research, and is gaining general acceptance.

The critical factor supporting the use of pulsatile flow revolves around the enhanced energy delivery associated with its use when compared to nonpulsatile flow. This has been demonstrated in both clinical and nonclinical studies *(29,30)*; however, the most important factor to the clinician is the clinical evidence of the differences between pulsatile and nonpulsatile modalities. These are not always apparent in normal clinical practice, as the adequacy of the pulse delivered can be hampered by several factors, including the anesthesia, the use of vasoactive agents, temperature, and the configuration of the perfusion circuit. Despite these confounding factors, there is a body of evidence from those involved in the investigation of blood flow that suggests the benefits of pulsatile flow might be considered in terms of two factors: hemodynamic effects and metabolic effects.

Hemodynamic Effects of Pulsatile Flow

The most commonly observed consequence of nonpulsatile blood flow is a progressive systemic arterial vasoconstriction *(31–33)*, ultimately leading to a general reduction in visceral perfusion. This has important clinical consequences because upon separation from CPB, the left ventricle is already functionally compromised from the insult of the operative procedure. Any increase in afterload during this critical period predisposes to low cardiac output syndrome and potential organ damage that, with the use of nonpulsatile CPB, is usually successfully prevented in the immediate postperfusion period by vasodilator and inotropic intervention. Several studies have shown improved myocardial performance with vasodilator drugs, such as sodium nitroprusside, used to control this increased systemic vascular resistance *(34,35)*. However, Taylor and colleagues demonstrated that the use of pulsatile flow during the period of perfusion prevented the initiation of this vasoconstriction during the operative period *(36)*. This led to the potential use of pulsatile blood flow as a physiological tool to prevent systemic arterial vasoconstriction, and hence, reduce or eliminate the need for pharmacological intervention in the early postperfusion period. Clinical studies have demonstrated that pulsatile CPB reduces the requirements for inotropic agents and intraaortic balloon pump support after CPB, suggesting the maintenance of a more normal hemodynamic state even in the postperfusion phase *(37,38)*.

The mechanisms underlying the hemodynamic effects of the different flow modalities during CPB remain the subject of investigation and are not yet fully understood. Various theories have been proposed to explain the progressive systemic arterial vasoconstriction that occurs with nonpulsatile CPB, most of which focus on humoral deregulation, including activation of the rennin–angiotensin system and the release of catecholamines, vasopressin, and other local tissue vasoconstrictors. In a series of animal experiments, Many et al. found increased renin levels with nonpulsatile blood flow, a finding that was confirmed by other investigators *(33,39–42)*. Taylor et al. *(43)* addressed the concomitant rise in levels of the potent vasoconstrictor angiotensin II, which is responsible for the systemic arterial vasoconstriction, with the use of angiotensin I and II inhibitors during CPB; they found a highly significant and rapid reduction in vascular resistance during CPB and a rise in cardiac index immediately after CPB. Plasma catecholamines have also been shown to be elevated during nonpulsatile CPB, and further studies have shown that these can be attenuated by utilizing a pulsatile blood flow regime *(44–46)*. It is a similar picture with vasopressin levels, again with attenuation associated with pulsatile blood flow *(47)*. In a recent clinical study comparing a range of biochemical indices and their effects on pulmonary and renal functions during pulsatile and nonpulsatile flow, Sezai et al. found lower levels of inflammatory mediator interleukin-8 and catecholamines in the pulsatile group after CPB. He concluded that the inhibitory effects on cytokine activity, endothelial damage, and pulmonary alveoli edema were additional favorable effects to those on catecholamine levels, renal function, and peripheral circulation already documented *(48)*.

Pulsatile CPB would therefore seem to offer advantages over nonpulsatile flow in terms of preventing unwanted physiological postoperative sequelae that require pharmacological and other intervention, and this has been demonstrated in some studies that have confirmed a reduction in hemodynamically related mortality in patients receiving pulsatile CPB as opposed to nonpulsatile perfusion *(37,38)*. However, despite this body of evidence opinion still seems to be divided as to the importance of pulsatile flow in clinical practice from the hemodynamic standpoint *(49)*. Perhaps the origins of this controversy lie with the numerous and varied anesthetic and perfusion protocols and regimes employed throughout the clinical world. However, studies continue in this field with particular emphasis on metabolic issues.

Metabolic Effects of Pulsatile Blood Flow

The metabolic effects of pulsatile and nonpulsatile CPB have been investigated at the cellular and vital organ level. At the cellular level, nonpulsatile CPB has been associated with metabolic acidosis and reduced tissue oxygen consumption *(50–53)*, whereas the opposite has been found with pulsatile blood flow *(41)*. In general, the reason suggested by researchers for this difference is the additional energy delivered by pulsatile flow improving the delivery of nutrients *(28,54)*.

The effect of pulsatile CPB on organ function has been the focus of many studies over the years, and, indeed, predates the clinical application of CPB by many years. Many of the effects of pulsatile blood flow on major organ function have now been well documented and described. Herreros et al. assessed organ injury provoked by pulsatile and nonpulsatile perfusion by conducting a morphological study on animal heart, liver, lung, and kidney tissue harvested after CPB. His results suggested a better peripheral perfusion in the pulsatile group for all tissue types *(55)*. However, research groups have focused on the effect of pulsatile perfusion on individual organs and organ systems, and their findings have been generally supportive of pulsatile blood flow as the perfusion modality of choice in terms of the preservation of vital organ function.

Pulsatile Blood Flow and the Kidney

The importance of pulsatile flow on renal function was established long before the clinical application of CPB. In 1889, Hamel *(56)* demonstrated the effect of the pulse on renal function using an isolated renal preparation. Studies subsequently carried out by Gesell in 1913 *(57)* supported these findings and suggested that the improved kidney function with pulsatile flow is the result of better gas exchange at the capillary level and the maintenance of improved lymph flow. In a later series of experiments, Kohlstaedt and Page *(58)* subjected isolated kidneys to depulsed and pulsed flow at the same mean pressure and found an elevation in renin secretion and a reduction in urine flow in the group exposed to nonpulsatile flow. After the development and application of CPB, researchers had the opportunity to investigate the effect of pulsatile flow on renal function under controlled clinical conditions. In a clinical study of infants, Williams et al. found that urine output in patients subjected to pulsatile flow was double that of patients who underwent a nonpulsatile regime *(59)*. These clinical findings were supported by Taylor et al. *(38)* who found that pulsatile flow resulted in an increase in urine production and a decrease in plasma angiotensin II levels during adult cardiac surgery *(8)*.

Because of these fairly early studies, the effect of flow modality on renal blood flow and function has been extensively investigated in both clinical and animal models. The findings have been almost entirely supportive of the use of pulsatile blood flow in the preservation of renal function. These studies suggest that pulsatile flow is associated with better renal function and the preservation of renal microcirculatory architecture compared with nonpulsatile flow *(60–67)*.

At a cellular metabolic level, studies of renal function in patients exposed to CPB have shown that nonpulsatile blood flow is associated with a more rapid onset of renal hypoxia and acidosis than pulsatile flow *(68–70)* and confirmed these findings by demonstrating decreased tissue oxygen pressure in the renal medulla, increased local lactate levels, and decreased oxygen uptake with nonpulsatile blood flow.

The investigation of the effects of pulsatile flow on renal function has not been universally supported. Although with one exception, that of Ritter et al. *(71)* who concluded that pulsatile CPB was associated with reduced urine output and reduced creatinine clearance postoperatively, there are no reports in the literature of pulsatile flow resulting in an inhibition of renal function. Several studies have resolved that pulsatile flow has relatively no effect, and suggested that the maintenance of normal physiological mean pressure levels is of more importance *(71–74)*. However, it must be stressed that, as stated by Mavroudis in his excellent review of the subject, the pulse architecture employed in these studies was by no means physiological, or common to all studies *(75)*.

The real benefit of pulsatile blood flow over depulsed perfusion may be in patients with preexisting renal dysfunction. Several clinical studies have focused on patients with preoperative renal insufficiency requiring cardiac surgery. Matsuda et al. *(76)* established that renal function is best preserved in these patients by the use of pulsatile CBP and on the basis of a substantial clinical trial recommended that pulsatile flow be employed in this group. Kocakulak et al. *(77)* investigated the effects of pulsatile perfusion on microcirculation and renal function in high-risk patients either having chronically obstructive pulmonary disease or chronic renal failure. He observed that pulsatile perfusion improved microcirculation and renal function in the high-risk patients.

Pulsatile Blood Flow and the Brain

Despite the protective mechanisms in place to protect the brain from disturbances in blood flow, it is still susceptible to injury during CPB.

Factors shown to affect the brain during cardiac surgery include temperature, pattern of blood flow, viscosity, oxygen tension, carbon dioxide tension, and pharmacological agents. But pulsatile blood flow employed during CPB has been shown to preserve cerebral function and moderate cerebral injury. Early studies by Sanderson et al. *(78)* and Taylor et al. *(79)*, using creatine kinase isoenzyme in cerebrospinal fluid as a marker for cerebral injury in a canine model found significantly lower levels with the use of pulsatile blood flow, indicating significantly less diffuse brain injury in this group. In keeping with the general effects of nonpulsatile flow, DePaepe et al. *(80)* found a reduction in cerebral capillary diameter, and therefore cerebral blood flow, potentially resulting in diffuse cerebral injury under nonpulsatile conditions.

A significant effect on the physiological response of the brain by flow modality has also been demonstrated in several studies. Taylor et al. *(19,81)* found markedly different hypothalamic—pituitary responses to surgical stress between the two flow modalities, and that pulsatile flow was associated with the preservation of more normal function.

The influence of pulsatile flow on regional cerebral blood flow was demonstrated by DePaepe et al. *(80)* and Simpson et al. *(82)* who found disruption of regional flow with nonpulsatile flow, but not pulsatile perfusion. In contrast to nonpulsatile CPB, pulsatile flow also seems to prevent the cerebral acidosis normally encountered during the early phase of CPB *(83)*. Collectively, these findings may help to explain the reduced lactate production reported by Mori et al. *(84)*, who suggested that pulsatile blood flow maintains regional blood flow and suppresses anaerobic metabolism, especially during the critical cooling and rewarming phases of the operation.

Once again, there is little or no evidence suggesting that pulsatile blood flow is injurious when the brain is considered. However, there are some authors who contest the benefits of pulsatile flow in this regard. Hindman et al. *(85)*, Grubhofer et al. *(86)*, and Kawahara et al. *(87)* focused on cerebral blood flow and cerebral oxygen consumption and found no difference between pulsatile and nonpulsatile flow regimes. Chow et al. *(88)* also found no difference in several cerebral metabolic markers. Clinically, two studies *(89,90)* found no differences in neurological or neuropsychological outcomes between the two flow modalities. However, it is not clear from these studies how the hemodynamics of pulsatile flow were controlled; this is one very important factor, which we will return to later in this chapter.

Pulsatile Blood Flow and the Liver and Pancreas

The adverse effects of CPB on the liver and pancreas have been well documented after early sporadic findings of raised levels of plasma amylase during clinical CPB. Feiner *(91)* reported a 16% incidence of ischemic pancreatitis in patients subjected to CPB. However, Baca et al. *(92)*, using a canine model, demonstrated that pancreatic function was attenuated with pulsatile blood flow. Saggau et al. *(93)* in animal and human studies examined plasma levels of insulin, glucose, glucagons, and growth hormone and found disruption of pancreatic function with nonpulsatile CPB and normal function of the pancreatic B cells under pulsatile conditions. Mori et al. *(64)* confirmed these findings by demonstrating that in dogs perfused under both hypothermia and normothermia, pancreatic function was preserved only in the presence of pulsatile blood flow and reduced with nonpulsatile flow.

Several researchers have investigated the effect of flow modality on hepatic function by employing serum markers as indicators of hepatic injury. Pappas et al. *(94)*, using serum glutamic oxaloacetic transaminase as an indicator of hepatic injury, concluded that pulsatile blood flow was associated with the preservation of hepatic function. These findings were confirmed by Chiu et al. *(95)*, who reported on clinical studies focusing on postoperative serum glutamic oxaloacetic transaminase levels, and concluded that hepatic function was preserved with pulsatile blood flow during CPB. Critically, Mathie et al. *(96)* found that pulsatile CPB in a canine model preserved hepatic blood flow and function. He also demonstrated that nonpulsatile flow resulted in vasoconstriction of hepatic blood flow, coupled with a reduction in hepatic oxygen consumption. More recently, Kamiyashiki et al. confirmed these findings in a clinical model *(97)* and concluded that pulsatile normothermic CPB, in this case generated by using an IABP, provided better liver perfusion and resulted in better hepatic metabolism than nonpulsatile CPB.

Pulsatile Blood Flow and the Gut

The seriousness of abdominal complications resulting from CPB has long been recognized as a significant factor in operative morbidity and mortality. Gauss et al. *(98)* reported an abdominal complication in 1.8% of 500 patients who underwent cardiac surgery, with a mortality of 44% in this group. Similarly, in a large series of 5,924 patients, Baue *(99)* observed postoperative gastrointestinal morbidity in 0.29–2% of patients undergoing CPB, with a mortality rate of 23.5–44%. He attributed this complication to mesenteric hypoperfusion leading to bowel ischemia occurring as part of the generalized hypoperfusion seen with nonpulsatile perfusion. Bowles et al. *(100)* suggested that mesenteric ischemia leading to increased gut permeability might be an important factor contributing to the endotoxemia seen as a result of CPB in some patients. This theory was also postulated by Andersen and Baek *(101)* investigating post-CPB endotoxemia in children. Earlier studies by Andersen et al. *(102)* added weight to this theory, as they demonstrated that preoperative infection was not associated with endotoxemia seen during and after bypass. Tao et al. *(103)* demonstrated that pig gut mucosa becomes ischaemic during CPB as a result of blood flow distribution and shifting tissue oxygen demand. These findings were confirmed in a clinical setting by Riddington et al. *(104)* that showed that patients undergoing CPB exhibited increased gut mucosal ischemia and permeability, with endotoxin detectable in 42% of the patients. They also found that any elevation in intestinal pH did not return to normal until the nonpulsatile flow was terminated and pulsatile flow was resumed by the beating heart. This effect was later reported by Hamulu et al. *(105)* and Quigley et al. *(106)*, and it established the importance of perfusion pressure in preventing endotoxemia in both pulsatile and nonpulsatile perfusion, as a perfusion pressure maintained above 60 mmHg prevented endotoxemia in both groups.

The potential beneficial effect of pulsatile flow in preventing gut-related complications by reducing mucosal ischemia and increasing oxygen delivery was proposed by Fiddian-Green *(107)*, who also suggested the application of preoperative gut lavage and prophylactive antibiotics to reduce the incidence of endotoxemia. Reilly and Bulkey *(108)* proposed that the vasoactive gut response to circulatory shock is mediated by the activation of the renin-angiotensin system, which increases gut permeability. More recent studies by Gu et al. *(109)* examined the effect of a pulsatile catheter pump applied in the descending aorta on abdominal organ perfusion in a pig model. He found that compared to the nonpulsatile group during the ischemic phase of CPB, the pulsatile group had higher flow to the superior mesenteric artery, greater delivery of haemodynamic energy as indicated by the energy equivalent pressure, and higher organ perfusion status.

Overall, the medical literature is quite clear, pulsatile blood flow maintains organ function during CPB and prevents the onset of significantly increased vascular resistance in CPB patients. These findings are particularly evident in studies carried out on the kidneys and gut, where the maintenance of normal function and structure is of great importance to recovery and prevention of postoperative complications. Several authors have highlighted the beneficial effects of reducing the activation of, for example, the renin-angiotensin system to the prevention of postoperative vasoconstriction, which has been highlighted as one of the most common, but challenging, complications in the post-CPB patient. This, together with the complications associated with increased gut permeability and endotoxemia, which carries a very high mortality (up to 44%), can be largely prevented by applying pulsatile perfusion during the operative period. This proactive technique avoids the need to be reactive in the postoperative period.

However, it must be recognized that many of the studies carried out on pulsatile flow have been performed on nonclinical models, where there are no limitations on the technology employed to generate the pulse. Although clinical studies are largely supportive of pulsatile flow, it is important to look at the types of pumps available, the ability of these pumps to generate pulsatile flow of physiological proportions, and the limitations of such systems in clinical practice.

PUMPING SYSTEMS FOR PULSATILE PERFUSION

A variety of pumping options are available to clinicians to provide cardiopulmonary support to patients during cardiac surgery. Bregman et al. *(*110*)* conveniently divided these pumps into two categories, namely positive displacement pumps and the kinetic or centrifugal pumps. In general these are the pumping options, which are available for providing both nonpulsatile flow *(*as discussed earlier in this chapter*)* and pulsatile flow. The kinetic pumps are, as we have already discussed, load-sensitive pumps in which the generation of positive displacement of blood flow is achieved by increasing the velocity of blood at the inlet of the pump by rotating an impeller resulting in an increase in the kinetic energy of blood at the outlet. Kinetic pumps are the only true nonpulsatile pumps, as the output pulse architecture bears no resemblance to physiological pulsatile flow. Attempts to generate some degree of pulsatility with such systems have met with only limited success, with conflicting views by several researchers on the degree of hemolysis and pulsatility *(111,112)*. Clinical acceptance of pulsatile centrifugal pumps has been slow, with some researchers encountering difficulties in generating acceptable pulsatile flow *(113)* and others not finding any clinical benefit in the pulsatile flow generated by these devices *(114)* in contrast to roller pumps. However, recent studies focusing on the new Jostra centrifugal pump have been more encouraging *(115,116)*.

The positive-displacement pumping systems, particularly the roller pump systems, have been more successfully integrated into clinical practice in the pulsatile mode. The roller pump offers the capability to generate a pulse by accelerating the pump head without fear of significant backflow at the termination of the pulse cycle. Additionally, the roller pump mechanism as we know it today offers some degree of control of pulse architecture, in terms of frequency, delay time, ejection time (run-time), and after-run, which permits some degree of control of the "systolic" aspect of pulse architecture. If triggered by an electrocardiograph, the roller pump, if properly timed, can function in rather the same manner as a balloon assist pump (IABP), by ejecting at the appropriate time in the cardiac cycle. Overall, the roller mechanism has been very useful in the investigation of pulsatile flow, but its uptake in the clinical world has been slow. This may be due to several factors, but certainly early attempts at achieving pulsatile flow met with limited success *(117–119)* and there were, and in some quarters there still exists, a fear of excess generation of hemolysis. Clinical and animal studies suggest this fear of damage to formed blood elements *(120–123)*. However, there persist some conflicting views on the efficiency of roller pumps in generating pulsatile flow in the physiological sense *(124)*. It has been suggested that it is capable of, at best, only generating a nonphysiological "ripple" flow pattern Fig. 4. As we have

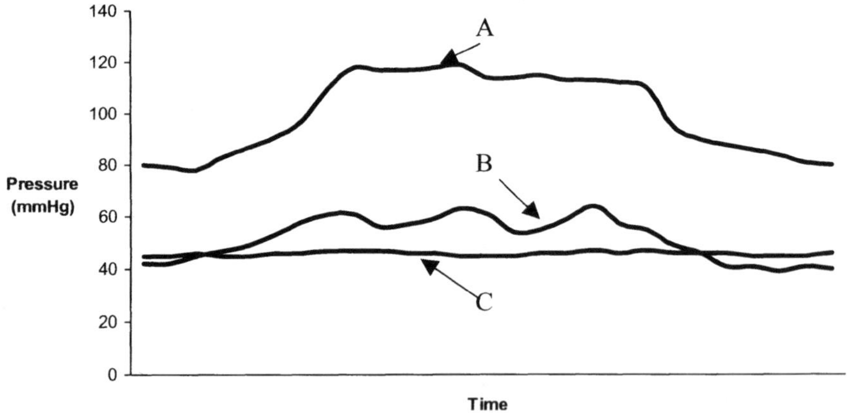

Fig. 4. Comparison of the pressure profiles generated in the radial artery by the native heart (A), a pulsatile roller pump (B) and a centrifugal pump (C). Neither pumping mechanism is capable of producing a pressure profile that is in any way mimetic of the native heart. The frequently referred to "ripple flow" pattern associated with the roller mechanism is quite clear in this illustration, and it is thought to be caused by the effect of the rollers making and breaking contact with the pump tubing.

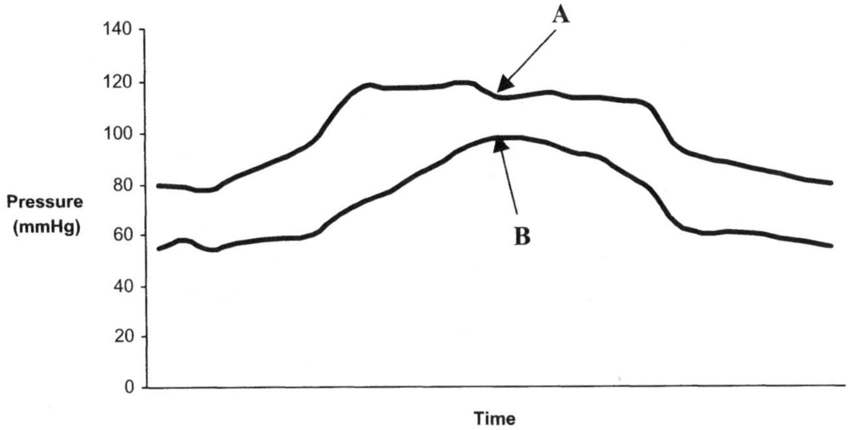

Fig. 5. Comparison of the radial artery pressure profiles generated by the native heart (A) and a ventricular pulsatile pump (B). The ventricular mechanism generates a profile that more closely resembles the native heart, but remains suboptimal in many ways.

already discussed in this chapter, there remains clear evidence that despite the suboptimal output of such systems in the physiological sense, there are still considerable clinical benefits associated with its use, and such systems remain the main pulsatile option for clinical practice.

There are other pumping systems available to the research and clinical fields that are capable of generating pulsatile flow; these include ventricular pumps and pulsatile assist pumps. The ventricular mechanisms function in a similar manner to native heart insofar as blood flows in and out of the system, with the direction of flow restricted and governed by inlet and outlet valves. The power for positive displacement of blood is provided by mechanical, hydraulic, or pneumatic compression of a flexible ventricle. Insofar as the operating mechanics of such systems closely resembles the native heart, the outlet architecture also closely resembles the physiological architecture (Fig. 5). These systems have been extensively studied in both the research and laboratory settings with considerable success *(125–128)*. However, widespread use of these systems has been limited by cost and complexity.

The pulsatile assist device (PAD), which employs an intermittent occlusive device such as an intraaortic balloon pump positioned in the arterial line of the CPB, is another device that has been employed to generate pulsatile flow during CPB. The versatility and degree of control offered by this method has impressed some researchers

(129,130), but uptake of this system has been hampered by fears on the part of users of balloon rupture *(131)*, haemolysis *(132)*, and the added complexity of the system.

FACTORS LIMITING BLOOD FLOW DURING CARDIOPULMONARY BYPASS

The provision of blood flow is one of the two main functions of CPB, the other being the provision of gas exchange. On the surface it would appear to be the simplest function, to simply provide blood flow to the patient during the operative procedure. However, as we have seen, blood flow delivery and requirement are very complex issues, requiring consideration of local, regional, and systemic issues. Acceptance of the inability of the clinician to adequately monitor the changing local and regional issues makes the blood flow provision to the patient a simple matter of following systemic markers of the adequacy of blood flow. A range of factors have evolved to aid the clinician in this task, including blood pressure (venous and arterial), line pressure, local temperatures, level sensors, and online blood gas analysis (particularly venous saturation), amongst others. However, even if one accepts that provision of blood flow with either nonpulsatile or pulsatile characteristics, which matches the inlet blood flow, is the only requirement of the clinician, several additional limitations must be borne in mind. For example, there is the thorny matter of damage and activation of formed blood elements associated with excessive sheer stress within the perfusion circuitry. That high sheer activates blood cells and results in excessive hemolysis has been well described *(133)*, and it is clear that this is a blood flow issue. It is therefore important that the clinician vectors this factor into his rational when configuring the CPB system. Minimizing velocity and directional changes within the circuitry, minimizing the number of devices in the arterial line of the circuit, and optimizing the diameter of the arterial cannula will help with this, together with optimizing the occlusive setting of the roller pump mechanism. These are all blood flow issues, which are even further complicated when pulsatile blood flow is employed. Pulsatile flow accentuates the deleterious effects of all of the above, if proper steps are not taken to minimize these factors. For example, the primary aim of pulsatile flow generation is, in the context of pulse generation, to be as biomimetic as possible; in other words, to generate pulsatile blood flow architecture that is similar to the physiological state. We have already seen that there are considerable technological hindrances to this objective in the normal clinical environment. Routine clinical technology is currently not able to generate physiological pulsatile flow. However, it is also clear that the best current compromise solution, the roller pump, although suboptimal in terms of output profile, is associated with considerable clinical advantages. It is therefore necessary to ensure that the pumping system employed is given the very best environment in which to generate pulsatile flow. As already discussed in this chapter, the benefits of pulsatile flow are generally attributed to enhanced energy delivery to the tissues. It is therefore necessary that the pump be employed in an environment in which the energy delivered by the pump to the patient is optimized and not adsorbed by inline circuitry components and cannulae. The energy adsorption associated with various circuitry components has been the subject of considerable study *(134–136)* (Fig. 6). The blood oxygenator, the arterial line tubing, and the arterial filter were found to adsorb some energy, but by far the most limiting factor is the arterial cannula *(137–139)*. This will remain a limitation of CPB unless surgeons are prepared to employ cannulae of the same

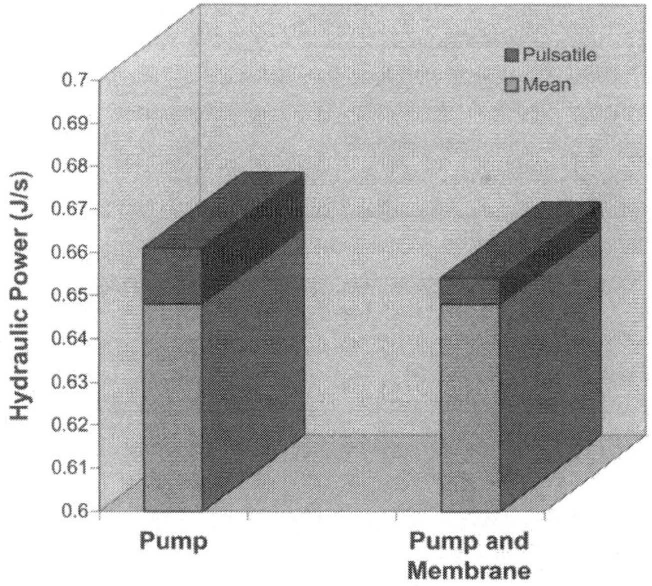

Fig. 6. The hydraulic power output of a pulsatile pump used in a mock circulation model in which an oxygenator is alternately included and removed from the system. The presence of the oxygenator in the arterial line results in a reduction in the total hydraulic power, but not in the mean domain. The oxygenator effects the power delivery primarily to the pulsatile domain.

dimensions as the arterial line itself; reassuringly, this is a most unlikely event.

CONCLUSION

At the beginning of this chapter we referred to several controversies associated with blood flow during CPB, including the most appropriate blood flow rate, pulsatile versus nonpulsatile flow, and the best delivery system for clinical applications. We have tried to deliver a balanced view on these issues with reference to the appropriate medical literature. However, these matters remain unresolved. There are clear advantages of pulsatile flow, demonstrated in both the clinical and research environments. Yet, clinical adoption of pulsatile flow has been sparse and slow. Perhaps this is because of several matters, largely unrelated to the physiological nature of pulsatile flow. The technology generally employed to deliver blood flow during CPB is not suitable for delivering pulsatile flow of physiological proportions, and this coupled with the clinical trend of employing flow rates that are analogous to clinically inappropriate hemodynamic states may explain the reports both literal and anecdotal that suggest that pulsatile flow is of little clinical benefit. So, the controversy persists, in relation to all of the issues surrounding blood flow delivery, and it appears that using current methods for calculating systemic blood flow, our patients may not be receiving blood flow rates that are entirely suitable. The overly obese may be receiving excessive blood flow, and hence face the risk of vascular hemorrhage, whereas those of a more petite stature may be underperfused in terms of satisfying the demands of those tissues and structures which contribute to the metabolic demand. One major benefit of these continued controversies and debates is that research in this field continues. At the moment, perhaps those who persevere with the old perfusionist's rule of thumb, that one can only pump to the patient that which one receives from him/her, are as close to offering optimal blood flow to the clinical cardiac patient as are those who employ the very best technology and physiological data. However, it is clear that with evolving technology we can take the blood flow delivery aspect of CPB a little closer to the physiological state, at which point it becomes a more practical science.

REFERENCES

1. Schulkin J. Allostasis, Homeostasis, and the Costs of Physiological Adaptation. Cambridge University Press, London, 2004.

2. Granger HJ, Goodman AH, Cook BH. Metabolic models of microcirculatory regulation. Fed Proc 1975;34(11):2025–2030.
3. Kessler M. Oxygen Supply: Theoretical and Practical Aspects of Oxygen Supply and Microcirculation of Tissue. University Park Press, Baltimore, 1973.
4. Tortora GD. Principles of Anatomy and Physiology. John Wiley & Sons, Inc., Hoboken, NJ, 2005.
5. Modine T, Azzaoui R, Ouk T, et al. Changes in cerebral vascular reactivity occur early during cardiopulmonary bypass in the rat. Ann Thorac Surg 2006;82(2): 672–678.
6. Canivet JL, Larbuisson R, Damas P, et al. Plasma renin activity and urine beta 2-microglobulin during and after cardiopulmonary bypass: pulsatile vs non-pulsatile perfusion. Eur Heart J 1990; 11(12):1079–1082.
7. Nicols WW, O'Rourke MF. McDonald's Blood Flow in Arteries. Hodder Arnold, London, 2005.
8. Lau CL, Posther KE, Stephenson GR, et al. Mini-circuit cardiopulmonary bypass with vacuum assisted venous drainage: feasibility of an asanguineous prime in the neonate. Perfusion 1999;14(5):389–396.
9. Gourlay T, Samartzis I, Taylor KM. The effect of haemodilution on blood-biomaterial contact-mediated CD11b expression on neutrophils: ex vivo studies. Perfusion 2003;18(2):87–93.
10. Boyd E. The Growth of the Surface Area of the Human Body. University of Minnesota Press, Minneapolis, 1935.
11. Johnson JM, Robins S, Hyde JAH. Monitoring and safety in cardiopulmonary bypass. In: Techniques in Extracorporeal Circulation. Kay and Munsch, editors. Arnold Hodder, London, 2004.
12. Alston RP, Anderson A, Sanger K. Is body surface area still the best way to determine pump flow rate during cardiopulmonary bypass? Perfusion 2006;21(3): 139–147.
13. Bayliss WM, Muller EA. A simple high speed rotary pump. J Sci Instrum 1928; 5:278–279.
14 DeBakey ME. A simple continuous blood flow instrument. New Orleans Med Surgical J 1934;87:387–389.
15. Daly Ide B. A seven horse power Austin engine adapted as a blood pump. J Physiol 1933;77:199–217.
16. Gourlay T. Perfusion Pumps in Cardiopulmonary Bypass in Neonates, Infants and Young Children. Richard Jonas and Martin Elliott, editors. Butterworth Heinemann Press, Oxford, 1994.
17. Palanzo DA. Perfusion safety: defining the problem. Perfusion 2005;20(4):195–203.
18. Kolff J, Ankney RN, Wurzel D, Devineni R. Centrifugal pump failures. J Extra Corpor Technol 1996;28(3):118–122.
19. Burton AC. Relationship of structure to function of the tissues of the wall of blood vessels. Physiol Rev 1954;34:618
20. Ogata T, Ida Y, Takeda J. Experimental studies on the extracorporeal circulation by use of our pulsatile arterial pump. Lung 1959;6:381.
21. Takeda J. Experimental study on peripheral circulation during peripheral circulation, with special reference to a comparison of pulsatile flow with non-pulsatile flow. Arch Japan Chir 1960;29:1407–1430.
22. Baba A, Dobsak P, Saito I. Microcirculation of the bulbar conjunctiva in the goat implanted with a total artificial heart: effects of pulsatile and nonpulsatile flow. ASAIO J 2004;50(4):321–327.

23. Shepard RB, Simpson DS, Sharp JF. Energy equivalent pressure. Arch Surg 1966;93:730–740.
24. Wilcox BR, Coulter NA, Peters RM, Stacey RW. Power dissipation in the systemic and pulmonary vasculature of dogs. Surgery 1967;62:25–29.
25. Undar A. Energy equivalent pressure formula is for precise quantification of different perfusion modes. Ann Thorac Surg 2003;76(5):1777–1778.
26. Undar A. Pulsatile versus nonpulsatile cardiopulmonary bypass procedures in neonates and infants: from bench to clinical practice. ASAIO J 2005;51(5): vi–x.
27. McMaster PD, Parsons RJ. The effect of the pulse on the spread of substances through tissues. J Exp Med 1938;68:377–400.
28. Prior FGR, Moorcroft V, Gourlay T, Taylor KM. Further testing of pulse reverse osmosis. A new theory of the maintenance and control of blood pressure. Int J Artif Organs 1995;18:469.
29. Undar A, Eichstaedt HC, Masai T, Bigley JE, Kunselman AR. Precise quantification of pulsatility is a necessity for direct comparisons of six different paediatric heart-lung machines in a neonatal CPB model. ASAIO J 2005; 51(5):600–603.
30. Wright G. Hydraulic power outputs of pulsatile and non-pulsatile cardiopulmonary bypass pumps. Perfusion 1988;3:251–262.
31. Hornick P, Taylor KM. Pulsatile and Nonpulsatile Perfusion: The Continuing Controversy. J. Cardiovasc and Vasc Anaesth, Vol 1997;11(3):310–315.
32. Videcoq M, Desmonts JM, Marty J, Hazebroucq J, Langlois J. Effects of droperidol on peripheral vasculature: use of cardiopulmonary bypass as a study model. Acta Anaesthesiol Scand 1987;31:370–374.
33. Taylor KM. Effect of pulsatile flow and arterial line filtration on cerebral cellular damage during open heart surgery. Proceedings of Second International Symposium on Psychopathological and Neurological Dysfunction following Open-Heart Surgery. 1980.
34. Stinson EB, Holloway EL, Derby GC, et al. Control of myocardial performance early after open heart operations by vasodilator treatment. J Thorac Cardiovasc Surg 1977;73:523.
35. Taylor KM, Bain WH, Russell M, Brannan JJ, Morton IJ. Peripheral vascular resistance and angiotensin II levels during pulsatile and no-pulsatile cardiopulmonary bypass. Thorax 1979;34(5):594–598.
36. Taylor KM, Bain WH, Morton JJ. The role of angiotensin II in the development of peripheral vasoconstriction during open heart surgery. Am Heart J 1980; 100:935–937.
37. Gourlay T, Taylor KM, Russell M, Wheatley D. Comparative retrospective study of pulsatile and non-pulsatile flow in 380 consecutive cardiac patients. Proc. First World Congress on Extracorporeal Circulation. Brighton, England, 1983.
38. Taylor KM, Bain WH, Davidson KG, Turner MA. Comparative clinical study of pulsatile and non-pulsatile perfusion in 350 consecutive patients. Thorax 1982; 37(5):324–330.
39. Many M, Soroff HS, Birtwell WC, Giron F, Wise H, Deterling RA Jr. The physiologic role of pulsatile and nonpulsatile blood flow. II. Effects on renal function. Arch Surg 1968;95(5):762–767.
40. Kohlstaedt LA, Page IH. The liberation of renin by perfusion of kidneys following reduction of pulse pressure. J Exp Med 1940;72:201–211.

41. Taylor KM, Bain WH, Russell M, Brannan JJ, Morton I.J. Peripheral vascular resistance and angiotensin II levels during pulsatile and non-pulsatile cardiopulmonary bypass. Thorax 1979a;34:594–598.
42. Townsend GE, Wynands JE, Whalley DG, Wong P, Bevan DR. Role of renin-angiotensin system in cardiopulmonary bypass hypertension. Can Anaesth Soc J 1984;31:160–165.
43. Taylor KM, Casals J, Morton JJ. The haemodynamic effect of angiotensin blockage after cardiopulmonary bypass. Br Heart J 1979;41:380.
44. Minami K, Korner M, Vyska K. Effects of pulsatile perfusion on plasma catecholamine levels and haemodynamics during and after cardiac operations with cardiopulmonary bypass. J Thorac Cardiovasc Surg 1990;99:82–91.
45. Taylor KM. Pulsatile Perfusion. In Cardiopulmonary Bypass-Principles and management (KM Taylor ed). Chapman and Hall, London, 1986.
46. Hutcheson IR, Griffith TM. Release of endothelium-derived relaxing factor is modulated both by frequency and amplitude of pulsatile flow. Am J Physiol 1991;261:H257–H262.
47. Levine FH, Philbin DM, Kono K, Coggins, et al. Plasma vasopressin levels and urinary sodium excretion during cardiopulmonary bypass with and without pulsatile flow. Ann Thorac Surg 1981;32:63–67.
48. Sezai A, Shiono M, Nakata K, Effects of pulsatile CPB on interleukin-8 and endothelin-1 levels. Artif Organs. 2005;29(9):708–713.
49 Weinstein GS, Zabetakis PM, Clavel A, et al. The renin angiotensin system is not responsible for hypertension following coronary artery bypass grafting. Ann Thorac Surg 1987;43:74–77.
50. Jacobs LA, Klopp EH, Seamone W, Topaz SR, Gott VL. Improved organ function during cardiac bypass with a roller pump modified to deliver pulsatile flow. J Thorac Cardiovasc Surg 1969;58(5):703–712.
51. Dunn J, Kirsh MM, Hrness J, Carroll M, Straker J, Sloan H. Hemodynamic, metabolic and hematologic effects of pulsatile cardiopulmonary bypass J Thorac Cardiovasc Surg 1974;68(1):138–147.
52. Steed D, Follette D, Foglia R. Effetcs of pulsatile and nonpulsatile flow on subendocardial perfusion during cardiopulmonary bypass. Ann Thorac Surg 1978; 26:133–141.
53. Shepard RB, Kirklin JW. Relation of pulsatile flow to oxygen consumption and other variables during cardiopulmonary bypass. J Thorac Cardiovasc Surg 1969; 58(5):694–702.
54. Prior FGR, Moorecroft V, Gourlay T, Taylor KM. The therapeutic significance of pulse reverse osmosis. Int J Artif Organs 1996;19(8):487–492.
55. Herreros J, Berjano EJ, Sola J. Injury in organs after cardiopulmonary bypass: a comparative experimental morphological study between a centrifugal and a new pulsatile pump. Artif Organs 2004;28(8):738–742.
56. Hamel G. Dei Bedeutung des pulses fur den blutstrom. Ztschr Biol NSF 1889; 474–497.
57. Gesell RA. On relation of pulse pressure to renal function. Am J Physiol 1913;32:70.
58. Kohlstaedt LA, Page IH. The liberation of renin by perfusion of kidneys following reduction of pulse pressure. J Exp Med 1940;72:201–211.
59. Williams GD, Seifen AB, Lawson NW, et al. Pulsatile perfusion versus conventional high flow non-pulsatile perfusion for rapid core cooling and rewarming of

infants for circulatory arrest in cardiac operation. J Thorac Carciovasc Surg 1979;78:667–677.
60. Fintersbuch W, Long DM, Sellers RD. Renal arteriography during extracorporeal circulation in dogs with preliminary report upon effects of low molecular weight dextran. J Thorac Cardiovasc Surg 1961;41:252–260.
61. Nakayama K, Tamiya T, Yamamoto K, et al. High amplitude pulsatile pump in extracorporeal circulation with particular reference to hemodynamics. Surgery 1963a;54:798.
62. Barger AC, Herd JA. Study of renal circulation in the un-anaesthetized dog with inert gases (proceedings of the Third International Congress of Nephrology). Nephrology 1966;1:174.
63. Boucher JK, Rudy LW, Edmunds LH. Organ blood flow during pulsatile cardiopulmonary bypass. J Appl Physiol 1974;36:86–90.
64. Mori A, Watanabe K, Onoe M, et al. Regional blood flow in the liver, pancreas and kidney during pulsatile and nonpulsatile perfusion under profound hypothermia. Jpn Circ J 1988;52:219–227.
65. Nakamura K, Koga Y, Sekiya R, et al. The effects of pulsatile and non-pulsatile cardiopulmonary bypass on renal bloodflow and function. Jpn J Surg 1989;19:334–345.
66. Undar A, Masai T, Beyer EA. Pediatric physiologic pulsatile pump enhances cerebral and renal blood flow during and after cardiopulmonary bypass. Artif Organs 2002;26(11):919–923.
67. Nakamura K, Harasaki H, Fukumura F, et al. Comparison of pulsatile and non-pulsatile cardiopulmonary bypass on regional renal blood flow in sheep. Scand Cardiovasc J 2004;38(1):59–63.
68. Kim HK, Son HS, Fang YH. The effects of pulsatile flow upon renal tissue perfusion during cardiopulmonary bypass: a comparative study of pulsatile and non-pulsatile flow. ASAIO J 2005;51(1):30–36.
69. German JC, Chalmers GS, Hirai J, Mukherjee ND, Wakabayashi A, Connolly JE. Comparison of nonpulsatile and pulsatile extracorporeal circulation on renal tissue perfusion. Chest 1972;61(1):65–69.
70. Mukherjee ND, Beran AV, Hirai J. In vivo determination of renal tissue oxygenation during pulsatile and non-pulsatile left heart bypass. Ann Thorac Surg 1973;15:334.
71. Ritter ER. Pressure-flow relations in kidney: alleged effects of pulse pressure. Am J Physiol 1952;168:480–489.
72. Goodyer AVN, Glenn WL. Relation of arterial pulse pressure to renal function. Am J Physiol 1951;167:689–697.
73. Oelert H, Eufe R. Dog kidney function during total left heart bypass with pulsatile and non-pulsatile flow. J Cardiovasc Surg (Torino) 1974;15:674.
74. Selkurt EE. Effects of pulse pressure and mean arterial pressure modification on renal haemodynamics and electrolyte and water excretion. Circulation 1951;4:541.
75. Mavroudis C. To pulse or not to pulse. Ann Thorac Surg 1978:25:259–271.
76. Matsuda H, Hirose H, Nakano S, et al. Results of open heart surgery in patients with impaired renal function as creatinine clearance below 30 ml/min. The effects of pulsatile perfusion. J Cardiovasc Surg (Torino) 1986;27(5):595–599.
77. Kocakulak M, Askin G, Kucukaksu S. Pulsatile flow improves renal function in high-risk cardiac operations. Blood Purif 2005;23(4):263–267.

78. Sanderson JM, Wright G, Sims FW. Brain damage in dogs immediately following pulsatile and non-pulsatile blood flows in extracorporeal circulation. Thorax 1972;27(3):275–286.
79. Taylor KM, Devlin BJ, Mittra S, Gillan JG, Brannan JJ, McKenna JM. Assessment of cerebral damage during open heart surgery. A new experimental model. Scand J Thorac Cardiovasc Surg 1980;14:197–203.
80. DePaepe J, Pomerantzeff PMA, Nakiri K, Armelin E, Verginalli G, Zerbini EJ. Observations of the microcirculation of the cerebral cortex of dogs subjected to pulsatile and non-pulsatile flow during extracorporeal circulation. In: A Propos Du Debit Pulse. Cobe Laboratories, Inc., Belgium, 1979.
81. Taylor KM, Wright GS, Reid JS, et al. Comparative studies of pulsatile and non-pulsatile flow during cardiopulmonary bypass. II The effects on adrenal secretion of cortisol. J Thorac Cardiovasc Surg 1978;75:574.
82. Simpson JC. Cerebral perfusion during cardiac surgery using cardiac bypass. In: Towards Safer Cardiac Surgery. Longmore D, editor. MTP, Lancaster, 1981.
83. Briceno JC, Runge TM. Monitoring of blood gasses during prolonged cardiopulmonary bypass and their relationship to brain pH, PO2 and PCO2. ASAIO J 1994;40:M344–M350.
84. Mori A, Sono J, Nakashima M, Minami K, Okada Y. Application of pulsatile cardiopulmonary bypass for profound hypothermia in cardiac surgery. Jpn Circ J 1981;45:315–322.
85. Hindman BJ, Dexter F, Smith T, Cutkomp J. Pulsatile versus nonpulsatile flow. No difference in cerebral blood flow or metabolism during normothermic cardiopulmonary bypass in rabbits. Anaesthesiology 1995;82(1):241–250.
86. Grubhofer G, Mares P, Rajek A, et al. Pulsatility does not change cerebral oxygenation during cardiopulmonary bypass. Acta Anaesthesiol Scand 2000;44: 586–591.
87. Kawahara F, Kadoi Y, Saito S, Yoshikawa D, Goto F, Fujita N. Balloon pump induced pulsatile perfusion during cardiopulmonary bypass does not improve brain oxygenation. J Thorac Cardiovasc Surg 1999;118:361–366.
88. Chow G, Roberts IG, Harris D, et al. Stockert roller pump generated pulsatile flow: cerbral metabolic changes in adult cardiopulmonary bypass. Perfusion 1997;12(2):113–119.
89. Henze T, Stephen H, Sonntag H. Cerebral dysfunction following extracorporeal circulation for aortocoronary bypass surgery: no differences in neuropsychological outcome after pulsatile versus nonpulsatile flow. Thorac Cardiovasc Surg 1990;38:65–68.
90. Murkin JM, Martzke JS, Buchan AM, et al. A randomized study of the influence of perfusion technique and pH management strategy in 316 patients undergoing coronary artery bypass surgery: II. Neurological and cognitive outcomes. J Thorac Cardiovasc Surg 1995;110:349–362.
91. Feiner H. Pancreatitis after cardiac surgery. Am J Surg 1976;131:684. Baca I, Beiger W, Mittmann U, Saggau W, Schmidt-Gayk H, Storch HH. Comparative studies of pulsatile and continuous flow during extracorporeal circulation. Effects on liver function and endocrine pancreas secretion. Chir Forum Exp Klin Forsch 1979;49–53.
92. Baca I, Beiger W, Mittmann U, Saggau W, Schmidt-Gayk H, Storch HH. Comparative studies of pulsatile and continuous flow during extracorporeal circulation. Effects on lver function and endocrine pancreas secretion. Chir Forum Exp Klin Forsch 1979;49–53.

93. Saggau W, Baca I, Ros E, Storch HH, Schmitz W. Clinical and experimental studies on pulsatile and continuous flow during extracorporeal circulation. Herz 1980;5:42–50.
94. Pappas G, Winter SD, Kopriva CJ, Steele PP. Improvement of myocardial and other vital organ functions and metabolism with a simple method of pulsatile flow (IAPB) during clinical cardiopulmonary bypass. Surgery 1975;77:34–44.
95. Chiu IS, Chu SH, Hung CR. Pulsatile flow during routine cardiopulmonary bypass. J Cardiovasc Surg (Torino) 1984;25(6):530–536.
96. Mathie R, Desai J, Taylor KM. Hepatic blood flow and metabolism during pulsatile and non-pulsatile cardiopulmonary bypass. Life Support Sys 1984;2:303–305.
97. Kamiyashiki S, Hashimoto K. Superior results of ketone body ratio in pulsatile normothermic cardiopulmonary bypass; comparison with non-pulsatile cardiopulmonary bypass. Kyobu Geka. 2003;56(5):365–370.
98. Gauss A, Druck A, Hemmer W, Georieff M. Abdominal complications following heart surgery. Anaesthesiol Intensivmed Notfallmed Schmerzther 1994;29:23–29.
99. Baue AE. The role of the gut in the development of multiple organ dysfunction in cardiothoracic patients. Ann Thorac Surg 1993;55:822–829.
100. Bowles CT, Ohri SK, Nongchana K, Keogh BE, Yacoub MH, Taylor KM. Endotoxaemia detected during cardiopulmonary bypass with a modified Limulus amoebocyte lysate asay. Perfusion 1995;10:219–228.
101. Andersen LW, Baek L. Transient endotoxaemia during cardiac surgery. Perfusion 1992;7:53–58.
102. Andersen LW, Baek L, Degen H, Lehd J, Krasnik M, Rasmussen JP. Presence of circulating endotoxins during cardiac operations. J Thorac Cardiovasc Surg 1987;93:115–119.
103. Tao W, Zwischenberger JB, Nguyen TT, et al. Gut mucosal ischaemia during normothermic cardiopulmonary bypass results from blood flow redistribution and increased oxygen demand. J Thorac Cardiovasc Surg 1995;110:819–828.
104. Riddington DW, Venkatesh B, Boivin CM, et al. Intestinal permeability, gastric intramucosal pH, and systemic endotoxemia in patients undergoing cardiopulmonary bypass. JAMA 1996;275:1007–1012.
105. Hamulu A, Atay Y, Yagdi T, et al. Effects of flow types in cardiopulmonary bypass on gastric intramucosal pH. Perfusion 1998;13:129–135.
106. Quigley RL, Caplain MS, Perkins JA, et al. Cardiopulmonary bypass with adequate flow and perfusion pressure prevents endotoxaemia and pathologic cytokine production. Perfusion 1995;10:27–33.
107. Fiddian-Green RG. Gut mucosal ischaemia during cardiac surgery. Semin Thorac. Cardiovasc Surg 1990;4:389–399.
108. Reilly PM, Bulkey GB. Vasoactive mediators and splanchnic perfusion. Crit Care Med 1993;21:S55–S68.
109. Gu YJ, De Kroon TL, Elstrodt JM, et al. Augmentation of abdominal organ perfusion during cardiopulmonary bypass with a novel intra-aortic pulsatile catheter pump. Int J Artif Organs 2005;28(1):35–43.
110. Bregman D, Kesselbrenner M, Sack JB. Pulsatile flow during cardiopulmonary bypass. In: Techniques in extracorporeal circulation. Kay P, editor. Butterworth-Heinemann, London, 1991.
111. Takami Y, Makinouchi K, Nakazawa T, et al. Hemolytic characteristics of a pivot bearing supported Gyro centrifugal pump (C1E3) simulating various clinical applications. Artif Organs 1996;20:1042.

112. Tayama E, Nakazawa T, Takami Y, et al. The hemolysis test of the Gyro C1E3 pump in pulsatile mode. Artif Organs 1997;21:675–679.
113. Nishida H, Uesugi H, Nishinaka T, et al. Clinical evaluation of pulsatile flow mode of Terumo Capiox centrifugal pump. Artif Organs 1997;21(7): 816–821.
114. Komada T, Maet H, Imawaki S, Shiriashi Y, Tanaka S. Haematologic and endocrinologic effects of pulsatile cardiopulmonary bypass using a centrifugal pump. Nipon Kyobu. Geka.Zashii 1992;40:901–911.
115. Orime Y, Shiono M, Hata H, et al. Cytokine and endothelial damage in pulsatile and nonpulsatile cardiopulmonary bypass. Artif Organs 1999;23:508–512.
116. Hata M, Shiono M, Orime Y, et al. Clinical use of Jostra Rota Flow centrifugal pump: the first case report in Japan. Ann Thorac Cardiovasc Surg 1999;5:230–223.
117. Ogata T, Ida Y, Takeda J. Experimental studies on the extracorporeal circulation by use of our pulsatile arterial pump. Lung 1959;6:381.
118. Nonoyama A. Haemodynamic studies on extracorporeal circulation with pulsatile and non-pulsatile blood flows. Arch Jpn Chirurgie 1960;29:381–406.
119. Nakayama K, Tamiya T, Yamamoto K, et al. High amplitude pulsatile pump in extracorporeal circulation with particular reference to hemodynamics. Surgery 1963;54:798.
120. Wright G. Blood cell trauma. In: Cardiopulmonary Bypass. Taylor KM, editor. Chapman and Hall, London, 1986:249–276.
121. Gourlay T, Taylor KM. Pulsatile flow and membrane oxygenators. Perfusion 1994(a);9:189–196.
122. Taylor KM, Bain WH, Maxted KJ, Hutton MM, McNab WY, Caves PK. Comparative studies of pulsatile and nonpulsatile flow during cardiopulmonary bypass. I. Pulsatile system employed and its hematologic effects. J Thorac Cardiovasc Surg 1978;75(4):569–573.
123. Adams S, Fleming J, Gourlay T, Taylor KM. Clinical experience with the Sarns pulsatile pump during open heart surgery. Perfusion 1986;1:53–56.
124. Wright G. The hydraulic power outputs of pulsatile and nonpulsatile cardiopulmonary bypass pumps. Perfusion 1988;3:251–262.
125. Runge TM, Grover FL, Cohen DJ, Bohls FO, Ottmers SE. Preload-responsive, pulsatile flow, externally valved pump: cardiovascular bypass. J Invest Surg 1989;2(3):269–279.
126. Rottenberg D, Sondak E, Rahats S, Borman JB, Dviri E, Uretzky G. Early experience with a true pulsatile pump for heart surgery. Perfusion 1995;10(3):171–175.
127. Mutch WA, Lefevre GR, Theissen DB, Girling LG, Warrian RK. Computer controlled cardiopulmonary bypass increases jugular venous oxygen saturation during rewarming. Ann. Thorac. Surg. 1998;65(1):59–65.
128. Waldenberger FR, Vandezande E, Janssens P, et al. A new pneumatic pump for extracorporeal circulation: TPP (true pulsatile pump). Experimental and first clinical results. Int J Artif Organs 1997;20:447–454.
129. Maddoux G, Pappas G, Jenkins M, Battock D, Trow R, Smith SC Jr, Steele P. Effect of pulsatile and nonpulsatile flow during cardiopulmonary bypass on left ventricular ejection fraction early after aortocoronary bypass surgery. Am J Cardiol 1976;37(7):1000–1006.
130. Philbin DM, Levine FH, Emerson CW, Coggins CH, Buckley MJ, Austen WG. Plasma vasopressin levels and urinary flow during cardiopulmonary bypass in

patients with valvular heart disease: effects of pulsatile flow. J Thorac Cardiovasc Surg 1979;78(5):779–783.
131. Tomatis L, Nemiroff M, Raihi M, et al. Massive atrerial air embolism due to rupture of pulsatile assist device. Successful treatment in the hyperbaric chamber. Ann Thorac Surg 1981;32(6):604–608.
132. Zumbro GL, Shearer G, Fishback ME, Galloway RF. A prospective evaluation of the pulsatile assist device. Ann Thorac Surg 1978;28:269.
133. Wright G. Blood cell trauma. In: Cardiopulmonary Bypass. Taylor KM, editor. Chapman and Hall, London, 1986:249–276.
134. Gourlay T, Taylor KM. Pulsatile flow and membrane oxygenators. Perfusion 1994(a);9:189–196.
135. Gourlay T. Controlled Pulsatile Architecture in Cardiopulmonary Bypass: In-vitro and Clinical Studies. PhD thesis 1997; Strathclyde University.
136. Wright, G. Factors affecting the pulsatile hydraulic power output of the Stockert roller pump. Perfusion 1989;4:187–195.
137. Runge TM, Cohen DJ, Hantler CB, Bohls FO, Ottmers Se, Briceno JC. Achievement of physiologic pulsatile flow on cardiopulmonary bypass with a 24 French cannula. ASAIO 1992;38:M726–M729.
138. Kayser KL. Pulsatile perfusion problems. Ann Thorac Surg 1979;27:284–285.
139. Taylor KM. Pulsatile Perfusion. In: Cardiopulmonary Bypass: Principles and Management. Taylor KM, editor. Chapman and Hall, London, 1986.

6 The Inflammatory Response to Cardiopulmonary Bypass

Roman M. Sniecinski, MD, and Jerrold H. Levy, MD

CONTENTS

INTRODUCTION

Inflammation is a protective response of vascular tissue. Under normal circumstances, it functions as part of a surveillance system designed to quarantine and destroy harmful agents. The system is complex, with redundant cascades and amplification built into it. Because of this, inflammation is often exaggerated out of proportion to the inciting stimulus, and results in pathologic injury to the host. Certain types of clinical injury, such as severe trauma, burns, pancreatitis, and major surgery, can provoke such a profound response that it results in respiratory failure, coagulopathy, and multiorgan system dysfunction. These phenomena are often summarized under the term "systemic inflammatory response syndrome (SIRS)."

INFLAMMATORY CELLS

Neutrophils

Multiple cells are involved in the inflammatory response, but perhaps the best-characterized effector cell is the neutrophil. These

From: *Current Cardiac Surgery: On Bypass: Advanced Perfusion Techniques*
Edited by: L. B. Mongero and J. R. Beck © Humana Press Inc., Totowa, NJ

polymorphonuclear leukocytes (PMNs) are involved in the phagocytosis of pathogens and damaged tissue. They belong to the family of immune cells known as granulocytes, which are named for their abundant cytoplasmic granules. These granules contain proteolytic enzymes, precursors to oxygen radicals, and proinflammatory mediators. These toxic substances are released from the activated neutrophil in a process known, quite appropriately, as degranulation. The result is endothelial cell injury, production of cytolytic oxygen species, and further recruitment of leukocytes.

Although they circulate in the blood, neutrophils exert their effects by migrating into the interstitium. This is accomplished in a three-step process involving margination, adherence, and extravasation. First, the expression of adhesion molecules known as selectins on the neutrophil (L-selectin) and the endothelial cell (E- or P-selectin) slows the neutrophil and causes it to "roll" along the microvasculature. Next, the interaction of integrins located on the neutrophil with adhesion molecules on endothelial cells causes the leukocyte to adhere to the endothelium. The leukocyte integrins thought to play an important role are CD11a/18 and CD11b/18, whereas the adhesion molecules on the endothelium are ICAM-1 and VCAM-1 *(1)*. Once fully arrested, extravasation of the neutrophil is mediated by chemoattractants from the interstitial space. After moving through the endothelial junctions, neutrophils degranulate, leading to the release of their toxic substances. However, because the attack is nonspecific, neutrophils have been implicated in producing the clinical manifestations of acute lung injury, reperfusion injury, and transfusion reactions *(2,3)*.

Basophils and Mast Cells

Like neutrophils, basophils also have cytoplasmic granules that contain inflammatory mediators. Among them, histamine is perhaps the best characterized. Through interaction with H1 receptors, histamine causes an increase in vascular permeability, bronchoconstriction, vasodilatation, and chemotaxis of neutrophils. Although the basophil's granules are chiefly released in response to the binding of immunoglobulin (Ig) E antibodies, complement represents another pathway to activation. This has an important implication in cardiac surgical patients, in that institution of cardiopulmonary bypass (CPB) is associated with massive complement activation *(4)*.

Mast cells are another inflammatory cell important in the inflammatory response, and they share many similarities with basophils. Unlike basophils, however, they do not circulate in the blood. Instead, they are fixed in various perivascular spaces, including the heart, lungs, and skin. When activated, these cells release a wide variety of proteases, interleukins (ILs), and other inflammatory mediators. In addition to IgE and compliment, mast cells can also be activated by thrombin. Thus, they play a role in linking the inflammatory and coagulation systems.

Monocytes

Monocytes are incompletely differentiated phagocytes that travel in the blood stream. Once they are activated and mature, they settle into tissue and are termed macrophages. They are best known for phagocytosing pathogens and presenting the antigens to lymphocytes. Their role in the inflammatory response to CPB, however, is becoming increasingly recognized *(5)*. Monocytes can be activated via the complement system, endothelial cells, or endotoxin. In response, they release a host of proinflammatory factors, including ILs and tumor necrosis factor (TNF)-α (*see* following sections). It seems likely that inflammatory damage to organs is preceded by the accumulation of macrophages in the respective tissue.

INFLAMMATORY MEDIATORS

Complement

The complement system represents one of the most primitive, yet most powerful, defenses against microbial invasion. It can be found throughout the evolutionary chain, from mammals down to sea urchins *(6)*. It was first described over 100 years ago as a serum protein that "complemented" antibodies in killing bacteria. It is now known that the complement system consists of 30 or more plasma and membrane proteins that assist in opsonization, cytolysis, and amplification of inflammation.

The complement system can be activated via one of three independent pathways. There is, however, "cross-talk" between complement and other serum proteases, so activation can also occur at different steps in the cascade (Fig. 1). The convergence point of all pathways is the cleaving of factor C3 into C3a and C3b. C3a is an anaphylatoxin that diffuses into the circulation and causes smooth muscle contraction, increased vascular permeability, and release of mediators from mast cells. C3b binds to bacteria, tagging them for phagocytosis, and cleaves factor C5 into C5a and C5b. Like C3a, C5a is an anaphylotoxin, but also a powerful attractant and activator of neutrophils. C5b is the first component of the membrane attack complex (MAC) formed from factors C5–C9. In prokaryotes, the MAC creates transmembrane pores, causing intracellular swelling and, ultimately, cell death.

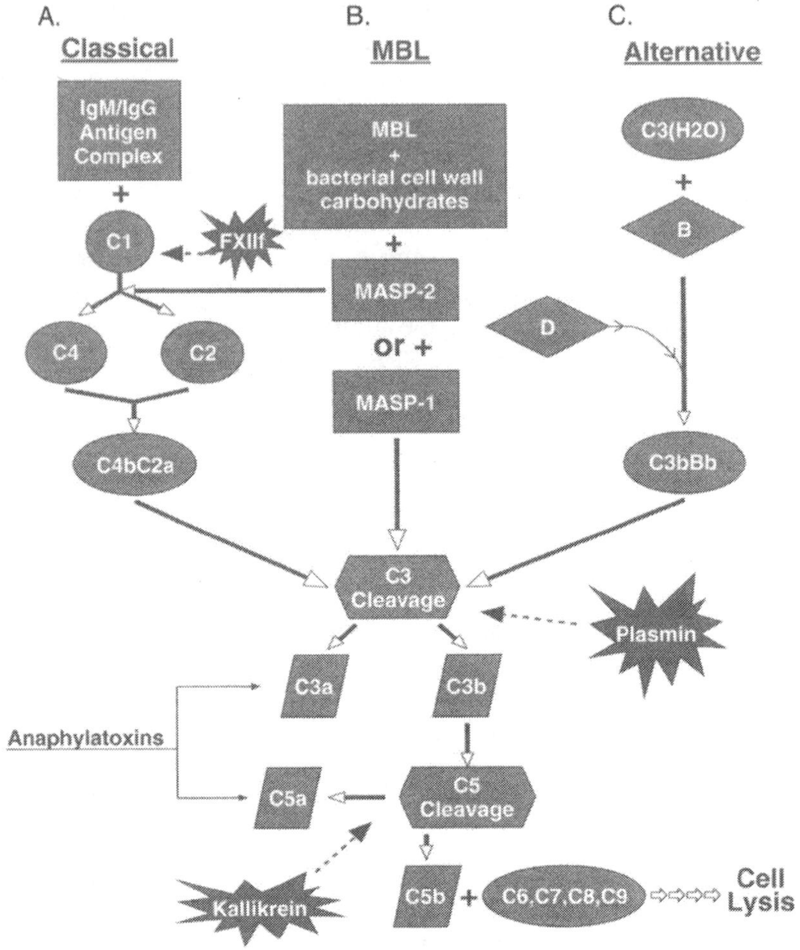

Fig. 1. Activation of the complement system can occur via three different pathways: (A) The classical pathway is initiated when IgM or IgG antigen/antibody complexes bind to C1. This results in a complex that cleaves C2 and C4, resulting in C4bC2a, which cleaves C3. (B) The mannose binding lectin (MBL) pathway starts by the binding of MBL to specific carbohydrates on the bacterial cell wall. In conjunction with MBL associated serine proteases (MASPs), the complex either cleaves C4 and C2 (MASP-2) or C3 directly (MASP-1). (C) The alternative pathway is initiated by the hydrolysis of C3 (C3-H2O), which binds to factor B. Factor B is activated by factor D and the complex of C3bBb can cleave C3. Dashed lines indicate crosstalk from other protease systems. (Adapted from Mojcik CF, and Levy JH: Aprotinin and the systemic inflammatory response after cardiopulmonary bypass. Ann Thorac Surg 71:745, 2001.)

Cytokines

Cytokines are polypeptides that allow communication between cells. They initiate actions by binding to specific targets on nearby cells, or, by traveling through the circulation, act as hormones to influence distant cells. The expression of cytokine receptors on target cells is highly regulated, and often under the influence of more than one cytokine. The actions that cytokines influence usually involve the transcription of new proteins, stimulation of cell growth, and regulation of cell differentiation.

Tumor necrosis factor α is one of the principal mediators of the inflammatory response to gram-negative bacteria. In response to lipopolysaccharide (LPS), also called endotoxin, which is derived from the bacterial cell wall, monocytes, mast cells, and T-cells secrete TNF-α. This results in expression of endothelial adhesion molecules, activation of neutrophils and phagocytes, and other aspects of a local inflammatory response. In high systemic levels, however, TNF-α causes the lethal symptoms of sepsis. Myocardial contractility is depressed, blood vessels become dilated and permeable, and intravascular thrombosis can lead to severely reduced tissue perfusion.

Interleukins are cytokines primarily synthesized by leukocytes that act on other leukocytes. Important ILs involved in the inflammatory response to cardiac surgery are IL-1, -6, and -8 *(7)*. Interleukin-1 is secreted by activated monocytes in response to TNF-α or anaphylatoxins. It plays a central role in inflammation by stimulating the production of IL-6 and -8 in target cells, such as lymphocytes, macrophages, and endothelial cells. Interleukin-6 helps mediate the "acute phase response" to tissue injury by inducing the liver to produce peptides, such as C-reactive protein, α1-antitrypsin, and fibrinogen. Some of the phenomena associated with the acute phase response include fever, leukocytosis, and gluconeogenesis. Plasma levels of adrenocorticotropic hormone, cortisol, and catecholamines also become elevated. Interleukin-8 is a potent attractor of neutrophils, and it is considered the primary mediator of lung neutrophilia. It up-regulates PMN adhesion molecules and causes increased degranulation.

Not all ILs promote inflammation, however. Interleukin-10 is considered antiinflammatory, and it actually antagonizes some of the actions of IL-6, -8, and TNF-α. It is produced by T-cells and monocytes in response to IL-6 and TNF-α, respectively, and likely acts as negative feedback on the inflammatory response. It inhibits the synthesis of proinflammatory cytokines, including IL-1, -6, -8, and TNFα, by macrophages. It also reduces the production of superoxide ions by neutrophils and macrophages, playing an important role in the suppression of chronic inflammatory states such as arthritis. Interestingly, just like IL-1, -6, and -8, levels of IL-10 are also elevated during CPB.

Kallikrein–Kinin System

The kinins are a group of serum proteins involved in the regulation of vascular tone, patency, and repair *(8)*. They are synthesized in the liver and circulate in bodily fluids as an inactive form known as kininogens. Two forms of kininogens exist in humans: high molecular weight kininogen (HMWK) and low molecular weight kininogen (LMWK). Although the two differ in their pharmacologic properties, they are both activated by proteases called kallikreins.

Tissue kallikrein is synthesized in cells from the heart and kidney, as well as other organs. Once activated, tissue kallikrein acts on LMWK to release kallidin, which is further converted to bradykinin. Bradykinin acts on specific receptors to cause the release of nitric oxide and prostacyclin from endothelial cells, resulting in vasodilation and increased vascular permeability. In addition, bradykinin participates in inflammation by releasing TNF and ILs from macrophages.

Plasma kallikrein exists in the circulation in an inactive form known as prekallikrein. It travels with HMWK and is activated by factor XIIa, or Hageman factor, from the contact system (*see* Contact Activation). Once activated, plasma kallikrein releases bradykinin from HMWK and activates additional factor XII in a positive-feedback loop. Proinflammatory actions of the two proteins are promoting neutrophil aggregation and up-regulating their elastase release. One of the ultimate results of kallikrein and factor XIIa interactions is the generation of thrombin in parallel with kinins, thus providing a link between inflammation and coagulation.

Thrombin, Plasmin, and Platelets

From a teleological perspective, it makes sense that the immune system and the coagulation system are activated at the same time. When breaks in the skin occur, not only must blood loss be stopped, but foreign invaders must be neutralized as well. Unfortunately, in the postoperative setting, this cross-talk can create overload in one system, and cause problems in the other. The coagulation cascade is reviewed elsewhere, but it is important to note that several key components also function as mediators of inflammation *(9)*.

Thrombin has a variety of effects that augment the inflammatory response. By itself, it is a powerful attractant for PMNs. On endothelial cells, it causes the up-regulation of selectins and the secretion of platelet-activating factor (PAF). Thrombin also causes the release of IL-6 and -8 from monocytes, macrophages, and endothelial cells. On the fibrinolytic side of coagulation, plasmin can directly cleave complement factor C3, leading to the formation of the C3 convertase via the classical pathway (Fig. 1). Additionally, fibrin split products, which are formed by plasmin's degradation of fibrin, are inherently proinflammatory, and they stimulate further complement activation.

Platelets have long been recognized as a key component of coagulation. However, evidence for their contribution to the inflammatory response is accumulating *(10)*. Once activated, platelets bound to the endothelium release IL-8 and express P-selectin, which is important in the rolling phase of neutrophils (Fig. 1). Named for its actions of aggregation and activation of platelets, PAF is also a potent attractor and activator of neutrophils. It is released by mast cells, along with leukotriene C4 and prostaglandin D2, as part of the acute phase hypersensitivity immune response.

CARDIOPULMONARY BYPASS-INDUCED INFLAMMATION

Cardiopulmonary bypass incites a systemic inflammatory response. The severity of SIRS can range from being barely detectable to severe multiple organ dysfunction. Other than the actual operative trauma, the factors thought responsible for CPB-induced inflammation are blood contact with the extracorporeal circuit, ischemia/reperfusion injury, and endotoxemia. These processes are briefly described below, and Table 1 summarizes some of the inflammatory factors activated by CPB.

Contact Activation

Factor XII, factor XI, HMWK, and prekallikrein are associated proteins that travel together and are collectively known as the "contact system." In the setting of CPB, the name is particularly appropriate because it is the touching of blood with the artificial surface of the bypass circuit that activates the system (Fig. 2). When factor XII contacts the negatively charged surface, a conformational change occurs and the protein is autoactivated. This produces factors XIIa and XIIf.

Table 1
Levels of Humoral Inflammatory Mediators During CPB and Their Role in Inflammation

Mediator	*Levels during/after CPB*	*Comments*
TNF-α	• Rapid rate of rise during cannulation process • Peaks about 2 h after CPB onset, often reaching 10 times the baseline level • May have a second peak 18–24 h post-op	• Initiates the production of other humoral inflammatory mediators, including IL-1, -6, and leukotrienes • Direct cardiac depressant
IL-1	• Level increases after onset of CPB, reaching peak 24 h later	• Plays a central role by increasing PMN adhesion and stimulating production of IL-6 and -8
IL-6	• Increased level 2 h after CPB onset, peaking about 4 h after onset • May remain elevated for up to 24 h	• Peak levels correlate with RWMA and post-op ischemic episodes • Induces hepatic synthesis of acute phase proteins
IL-8	• Begin rising during rewarming stage and peak 1–3 h later	• Powerful chemotaxis for PMNs
C3a	• Level rises after onset of CPB, peaking at the end of CPB	• Binds to mast cells and basophils, causing histamine release
C5a	• Plasma level difficult to for measure because it is rapidly taken up and internalized by neutrophils	• Powerful chemotaxis PMNs • Stimulates PMN respiratory burst, leading to O_2 free radicals
Bradykinin	• Level rises after onset of CPB, peaking at the end of CPB	• Potent vasodilator that increases vascular permeability

This table shows levels of important humoral mediators during CPB and their role in inflammation.

In addition to activating factor XI and starting the coagulation cascade (*see* Chapter 1), XIIa cleaves prekallikrein to its active form. Kallikrein then cleaves HMWK, releasing bradykinin. Factor XIIf, also known as Hageman fragment, is derived from XIIa. Both kallikrein and XIIf can activate complement. Complement is also

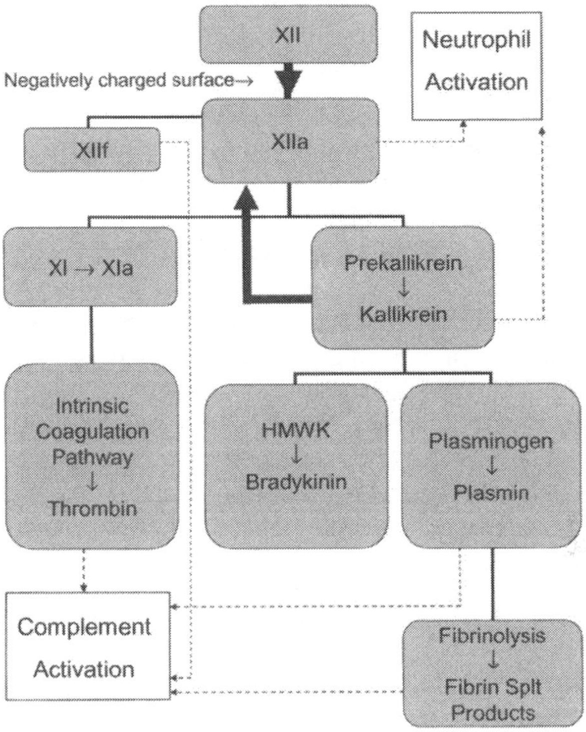

Fig. 2. The contact system cascade initiates interactions with coagulation, inflammation, and fibrinolysis. Note that kallikrein and XIIa form a positive-feedback loop. Dashed lines indicate cross-talk with inflammation. XIIa, activated factor; XII XIIf, Hageman fragments; Xia, activated factor XI; HMWK, high molecular weight kininogen.

activated via the alternative pathway during CPB. This is because the extracorporeal circuit lacks the endothelial cell surface inhibitors that normally limit that pathway. The end result of blood passing though the CPB apparatus is the production of multiple inflammatory factors and their circulation throughout the body.

Ischemia/Reperfusion

The use of an aortic cross-clamp excludes portions of the arterial tree from perfusion by the CPB circuit. It provides the advantage of a bloodless surgical field at the expense of inducing ischemia in the excluded organs, most notably the heart. Strategies for myocardial protection, such as cooling and cardioplegia, have evolved over the years, but the initial insult still exists. Upon removal of the cross-clamp, ischemic tissue is reperfused and, perhaps paradoxically, further damage is done.

Under normal circumstances, 95% of myocardial O_2 is reduced to H_2O in the mitochondria. The remaining 5% produces oxygen free radicals, which are quickly scavenged by various defense enzymes, such as superoxide dismutase. During ischemia, however, these natural antioxidants become depleted. Then, when reperfusion occurs, the cells can no longer handle the overload of reactive oxygen species. The number of free radicals formed on reperfusion is related to the duration of the preceding ischemic event. Thus, during persistent ischemia, cell damage may be slow and progressive, but explosive damage can occur at the onset of reperfusion. Myocardial stunning may occur secondary to free radical disruption of cell membranes and the disturbance of calcium homeostasis.

Although reactive oxygen species are directly toxic to myocytes, their existence is transient. Further damage takes place because of the inflammatory response they incite *(11)*. Disrupted cell membranes become vulnerable to attack by the complement system, resulting in the release of anaphylatoxins. Oxygen-derived free radicals have also been shown to activate transcription factors in endothelial cells, specifically the DNA-binding protein NF-κB. This transcription factor induces the rapid expression of TNF-α, and several ILs, including IL-6 and -8. Activation of NF-κB also up-regulates endothelial adhesion molecules, such as the selectins and ICAM-1. So, the damage initially done by free radicals is compounded by the production of proinflammatory mediators.

Endotoxemia

Lipopolysaccharide molecules are components of the gram-negative bacterial cell wall, and are collectively known as endotoxin. When combined with the LPS-binding protein found in plasma, it activates macrophages and enhances their production of TNF-α. LPS also stimulates endothelial cells to produce IL-6, setting up the inflammatory response.

Increased levels of LPS are associated with CPB and aortic cross clamping. Over 40% of these patients experience intermittent levels of significant endotoxemia *(12)*. The most likely source is the intestines, as CPB is known to increase gut permeability *(13)*. Whether this is caused by intestinal ischemia, nonpulsatile flow, or hypooncotic conditions remains an area of considerable debate. Failure of the liver to clear the portal circulation, or even contaminants in the bypass circuit itself, may also play a role in this phenomenon.

ANTIINFLAMMATORY STRATEGIES

Off-Pump Cardiac Surgery

Perhaps the most direct way to avoid SIRS, secondary to CPB use, is to avoid CPB itself. Although the operative trauma of median sternotomy is similar in off-pump coronary artery bypass surgery (OPCAB), there is no artificial surface present for contact activation and there is less of a global ischemia/reperfusion injury response. There have been many small trials comparing levels of inflammatory mediators in patients undergoing CABG with or without the use of CPB. In general, patients undergoing OPCAB have less production of TNF-α and IL-8, and an overall limitation of the inflammatory response *(14)*.

Removal of CPB does not completely eliminate SIRS, however. Levels of IL-6 during OPCAB are consistent with those during CPB, and conflicting data exists regarding complement activation *(15,16)*. Also, activation of the hemostatic system and the generation of thrombin occur secondary to surgical trauma alone. This suggests that modulation of the inflammatory response may be justified during all cardiac surgery, both with and without the use of CPB.

Heparin-Coated Cardiopulmonary Bypass Circuits

Endothelial cells have heparin sulphate glycosaminoglycans attached to their surface, which can mediate cellular interactions. Other than an anticoagulant effect (*see* Chapter 1), heparin may also have an antiinflammatory role *(17)*. It has been shown to block L- and P-selectin interactions in vitro, thereby inhibiting neutrophil adhesion *(18)*. Heparin inhibits IL-1, -6, and TNF-α gene expression in endotoxin-stimulated monocytes, and can interfere with IL-8–induced neutrophil chemotaxis.

Efforts to make CPB more biocompatible have focused on bonding a layer of heparin molecules to the circuit. In theory, this should somewhat emulate the endothelium and reduce blood cell contact with foreign material. Indeed, some clinical studies have shown decreased complement activation and cytokine release with the use of heparin-coated circuits *(19,20)*. Despite a reduction in inflammatory markers, significant clinical benefits, in terms of hemodynamics, transfusion requirements, or length of intensive care unit stay, have been difficult to demonstrate.

Leukocyte Filtration

With neutrophils playing such a prominent role in the damage inflicted by the inflammatory response, it seems logical that reducing their numbers would decrease the severity of SIRS. When connected in series with either the arterial or venous lines of the CPB circuit, leukocyte-depleting filters moderately decrease the patient's total leukocyte count. The potential benefit would seem to be highest for postoperative respiratory function because the lungs are a major source of sequestered PMNs after CPB. Unfortunately, despite some small studies showing minor improvements in postoperative respiratory index, the prevailing notion is that leukocyte depletion does not prevent lung dysfunction *(21)*. This is likely because the inflammatory response is complex and has many more mediators than just neutrophils. Systemic levels of complement activation, ILs, and TNF-α have not been shown to be affected by leukocyte depletion.

Corticosteroids

Corticosteroids, or more specifically glucocorticoids, have been used as antiinflammatory agents for more than 50 years. Although they actually increase the number of PMNs released from the bone marrow into the circulation, glucocorticoids exert their effects by interfering with the recruitment and activation of inflammatory cells. Increases in IL-1, -6, -8, and TNF-α have all been shown to be attenuated with corticosteroid use. Also, levels of the antiinflammatory cytokine IL-10 are increased. More recently, glucocorticoids have been shown to suppress the transcription factor NF-κB (*see* Ischemia/Reperfusion). Given the potential of CPB to cause SIRS, it is not surprising that the prophylactic use of corticosteroids has been widely investigated in cardiac surgery since the 1970s.

Despite several randomized, blinded, placebo-controlled investigations, the exact role for corticosteroids is still being defined. Traditionally, one or two prophylactic doses of 30 mg/kg of hydrocortisone have been given intraoperatively to patients undergoing CPB. Although most studies have shown a decrease in proinflammatory mediators, as well as an increased cardiac index, clinical endpoints, such as time to extubation, have failed to show improvement. One of the problems may be that glucocorticoids have little, if any, effect on complement levels. They also promote hyperglycemia, which possibly increases patient morbidity. In a recent review of over 30 years worth of studies in the field *(22)*, Chaney concluded that the prophylactic use of glucocorticoids in patients undergoing cardiac surgery with CPB "does not appear to offer any clinical benefits and may be detrimental."

On the other hand, smaller "stress doses" of hydrocortisone, rather than the massive 1–2 g traditionally given, may have potential benefits in a select group of patients. Much like septic shock, SIRS can be associated with low cardiac output and profound vasodilation. Kilger et al. *(23)* postulated that certain subgroups of patients, mainly those undergoing prolonged bypass runs or those having a preoperative ejection fraction of less than 40%, suffer from a relative adrenocortical insufficiency. By administering a stress dose regimen over 4 d (100 mg load, followed by 10 mg/h at 24°C, 5 mg/hr at 24°, 20 mg TID for 1 d, and 10 mg TID for 1 d), they found a reduced need for vasopressor use and a shorter length of stay both in the ICU and total hospitalization. Larger clinical trials are still needed to define specific doses and patient populations that may benefit from corticosteroid use.

Aprotinin

Aprotinin is a nonspecific serine protease inhibitor, or serpin, best known for its antifibrinolytic effect by blocking plasmin (*see* Chapter 1). Because it is nonspecific, it also inhibits other components of coagulation and inflammation, including kallikrein, trypsin, and elastase. However, these antiinflammatory actions appear to be dose dependent. The "full Hammersmith" dose of aprotinin (280 mg load, 280 mg in CPB prime, and 70 mg/h infusion), which targets the inhibition of kallikrein production and function, appears to be necessary to suppress SIRS amplification *(24)*.

Although the exact antiinflammatory mechanism of aprotinin is not fully understood, levels of IL-6 after CPB are significantly reduced. At the same time, levels of IL-10 are significantly increased, thus shifting the balance toward antiinflammatory mediators *(25)*. Neutrophils also appear to be affected by aprotinin. Their extravasation may be impeded by decreased expression of the CD11b/CD18 integrin and the inhibition of ICAM-1 on endothelial cells *(26)*. Clinical evidence supporting a neutrophil effect includes brochoalveolar lavage fluid from patients undergoing CPB. When collected from patients given high-dose aprotinin, it has a lower concentration of IL-8 and less PMN accumulation *(27)*.

Complement Inhibitors

Given the key role complement plays in initiating and propagating inflammation, it is not surprising that it is a target for pharmacological intervention. Efforts to decrease the damage it does in myocardial reperfusion injury have been ongoing for the past 20 years. C1 esterase inhibitor (C1-Inh) is an endogenous serpin that acts on complement factors C1s and C1r, thus blocking the classical pathway of activation *(28)*. Concentrates of C1-Inh have been shown to decrease myocardial damage after thrombolytic therapy for acute myocardial infarction *(29)*. Its use has also lead to lower levels of C3a in septic shock patients *(30)*. Enthusiasm for its use during CPB has been tempered, however, by the report of fatal thromboembolic events with high doses *(31)*. This is likely caused by the fact that C1-Inh also inhibits other serine proteases, including those of the fibrinolytic system, which may cause it to have procoagulant effects. It also fails to have a significant effect on the alternative pathway of complement activation, which may play the major role during CPB.

A more specific inhibition of complement can be achieved using monoclonal antibodies. Pexelizumab is a recombinant antibody fragment that targets and binds C5. By doing so, it blocks the formation of the anaphylatoxin C5a, as well as the MAC. In a recent multicenter trial, pexelizumab was associated with a risk reduction of myocardial infarction and 30-d mortality in patients undergoing CABG surgery on CPB *(32)*. While promising, routine use of complement inhibitors is still under investigation.

In summary, CPB incites a systemic inflammatory response that varies widely in its clinical severity. Multiple strategies are being developed to attenuate this response. Due to the complexity and redundancy of the inflammatory cascade, however, there will probably not be one magic bullet. Instead, a combination of pharmacology and surgical techniques will likely be needed to further improve patient outcomes.

REFERENCES

1. Asimakopoulos G, Taylor KM. Effects of cardiopulmonary bypass on leukocyte and endothelial adhesion molecules. Ann Thorac Surg 1998;66:2135–2144.
2. Nishimura M, Ishikawa Y, Satke M. Activation of polymorphonuclear neutrophils by immune complex: possible involvement in development of transfusion-related acute lung injury. Transfus Med 2004;14:359–367.
3. Park JL, Lucchesi BR. Mechanisms of myocardial reperfusion injury. Ann Thorac Surg 1999;68:1905–1912.
4. Chenoweth DE, Cooper SW, Hugli TE, et al. Complement activation during cardiopulmonary bypass: evidence for generation of C3a and C5a anaphylatoxins. NEJM 1981;304:497–503.
5. Ernofsson M, Thelin S, Siegbahn A. Monocyte tissue factor expression, cell activation, and thrombin formation during cardiopulmonary bypass: a clinical study. J Thorac Cardiovasc Surg 1997:113:576–584.
6. Fujita T, Endo Y, Nonaka M. Primitive complement system—recognition and activation. Mol Immun 2004;41:103–111.

7. Tonnesen E, Christensen VB, Toft P. The role of cytokines in cardiac surgery. Int J Cardiol 1996;53(supplement):S1.
8. Campbell DJ. The kallikrein-kinin system in humans. Clin Exp Pharm Physiol 2001;28:1060.
9. Levy JH, Tanaka KA. Inflammatory response to cardiopulmonary bypass. Ann Thorac Surg 2003;75:S715–S720.
10. Weerasinghe A, Taylor KM. The platelet in cardiopulmonary bypass. Ann Thorac Surg 1998;66:2145–2152.
11. Anaya-Prado R, Toledo-Pereyra LH, Lentsch AB, Ward PA. Research Review: Ischemia/reperfusion injury. J Surg Res 2002;105:248–258.
12. Riddington DW, Venkatesh B, Boivin CM, et al. Intestinal permeability, gastric intramucosal pH, and systemic endotoxemia in patients undergoing cardiopulmonary bypass. JAMA 1996;275:1007–1012.
13. Ohri SK, Desai JB, Gaer JAR, et al. Intraabdominal complications following cardiopulmonary bypass. Ann Thorac Surg 1991;52:826–831.
14. Asimakopoulos G. Systemic inflammation and cardiac surgery: an update. Perfusion 2001;16:353–360.
15. Gu YJ, Mariana MA, Boonstra PW, et al. Complement activation in coronary artery bypass grafting patients without cardiopulmonary bypass: the role of tissue injury by surgical incision. Chest 1999;116:892–898.
16. Tarnok A, Hambsch J, Emmrich F, et al. Complement activation, cytokines, and adhesion molecules in children undergoing surgery with and without cardiopulmonary bypass. Ped Cardiol 1999;20:113–125.
17. Tyrrell DJ, Horne AP, Holme KR, et al. Heparin in inflammation: potential therapeutic applications beyond anticoagulation. Adv Pharmacol 1999;46:151–206.
18. Nelson RM, Cecconi O, Roberts GW, et al. Heparin oligosaccharides bind L- and P-selectin and inhibit acute inflammation. Blood 1993;82:3253–3258.
19. Fosse E, Moen O, Johnsson E, et al. Reduced complement and granulocyte activation with heparin coated cardiopulmonary bypass. Ann Thorac Surg 1994;58:472–477.
20. Steinberg BM, Grossi EA, Schmartz DS, et al. Heparin bonding of bypass circuits reduces cytokine release during cardiopulmonary bypass. Ann Thorac Surg 1995;60:525–529.
21. Asimakopoulos G. The inflammatory response to CPB: the role of leukocyte filtration. Perfusion 2002;17:7–10.
22. Chaney MA. Corticosteroids and cardiopulmonary bypass: a review of clinical investigations. Chest 2002;121:921–931.
23. Kilger E, Weis F, Briegel J, et al. Stress doses of hydrocortisone reduce severe systemic inflammatory response syndrome and improve early outcome in a risk group of patients after cardiac surgery. Crit Care Med 2003;31:1068–1074.
24. Englberger L, Kipfer B, Berdat PA, et al. Aprotinin in coronary operation with cardiopulmonary bypass: Does "low dose" aprotinin inhibit the inflammatory response? Ann Thorac Surg 2002;73:1897–1904.
25. Tassani P, Augustin N, Barankay A, et al. High dose aprotinin modulates the balance between proinflammatory and anti-inflammatory responses during coronary artery bypass graft surgery. J Cardiothor Vasc Anes 2000;14:682–686.
26. Asimakopoulos G, Thompson R, Nourshargh S, et al. An anti-inflammatory property of aprotinin detected at the level of leukocyte extravasation. J Thorac Cardiovasc Surg 2000;120:361–369.

27. Hill GE, Pohorecki R, Alonso A, et al. Aprotinin reduces interleukin-8 production and lung neuttrophil accumulation after cardiopulmonary bypass. Aneth Analg 1996;83:696–700.
28. Caliezi C, Wuillemin WA, Zeerleder S, et al. C1-esterase inhibitor: An anti-inflammatory agent and its potential use in the treatment of diseases other than hereditary angioedema. Pharmacol Rev 2000;52:91–112.
29. Zwaan C, Kleine AH, Diris JHC, et al. Continuous 48-h C1-inhibitor treatment, following reperfusion therapy, in patients with acute myocardial infarction. Eur Heart J 2002;23:1670–1677.
30. Hack CE, Ogilvie AC, Eisele B, et al. C1-inhibitor substitution therapy is septic shock and in vascular leak syndrome induced by high doses of IL-2. Intensive Care Med 1993;86:S19–S28.
31. Horstick G, Berg, O, Heimann, A, et al. Application of C1-esterase inhibitor during reperfusion of ischemic myocardium: Dose related beneficial versus detrimental effects. Circulation 2001;104:3125–3131.
32. Verrier ED, Shernan, SK, Taylor KM, et al. Terminal complement blockade with pexelizumab during coronary artery bypass graft surgery requiring cardiopulmonary bypass: A randomized trial. JAMA 2004;291:164.

7 Minimally Invasive Perfusion Techniques

Sandhya K. Balaram, MD, PhD,
John Markham, MS, MBA, CCP,
and Joseph J. DeRose, Jr., MD

Contents

WHAT IS MINIMALLY INVASIVE CARDIAC SURGERY?

The "invasiveness" of most surgical and interventional procedures relies heavily on the physician's access to the operative field. In the majority of surgical specialties, a procedure is deemed less "invasive" when it is performed with limited or no incisions. In cardiac surgery, the invasiveness of an operation has at least two components: the incision and the presence of the cardiopulmonary bypass machine.

The primary operative incision in cardiac surgery is the median sternotomy. The median sternotomy affords unlimited exposure to all

From: *Current Cardiac Surgery: On Bypass: Advanced Perfusion Techniques*
Edited by: L. B. Mongero and J. R. Beck

surfaces of the heart, as well as to all internal chambers of the heart. However, this incision is hampered by the potential side effects and complications of wound infection, brachial plexus palsies, postoperative pain, pulmonary dysfunction, and poor cosmesis. Alternative incisions and totally endoscopic approaches to the heart have been devised for a select group of cardiac procedures to minimize some of these untoward effects of median sternotomy. Such cardiac procedures at times require novel approaches to both the institution of cardiopulmonary bypass and the delivery of cardioplegia.

However, the cardiopulmonary bypass circuit itself can be the most invasive component of any cardiac procedure. The inflammatory response elicited by the bypass circuit may result in end-organ manifestations, particularly in high-risk patients. The coagulopathy and hemodilution of cardiopulmonary bypass can result in increased bleeding and necessitate blood transfusion, which is another potentially invasive therapy. Furthermore, manipulation of the aorta with cannulation and cross-clamping increases the potential risk for arterial embolization and stroke. Interventions to ameliorate all of these potential side effects of cardiopulmonary bypass can be included under the umbrella of minimally invasive cardiac surgery.

Minimally invasive cardiac surgical procedures, then, can include operations that eliminate or minimize cardiopulmonary bypass, as well as those operations that are performed endoscopically or through limited, alternative incisions. Similarly, the most minimally invasive of all cardiac surgical operations are performed endoscopically on the beating heart. However, the degree of invasiveness of each component of a cardiac operation can only be interpreted when it is evaluated for each particular patient. For some patients, the most morbid component of cardiac surgery might be cardiopulmonary bypass, while for other, lower risk patients, the sternotomy might hold the highest potential for postoperative morbidity.

There are numerous minimally invasive perfusion techniques for each minimally invasive operation. It is incumbent upon the minimally invasive cardiac surgeon and the perfusion team to be familiar with all such approaches and select the most appropriate approach for each patient about to undergo heart surgery. The following chapter will outline the full range of perfusion circuits and cannulation schemes that are at the disposal of the minimally invasive cardiac surgical team. Specific minimally invasive approaches to each operation will then be outlined.

OVERVIEW OF MINIMALLY INVASIVE PERFUSION

Throughout the history of cardiac surgery, there have been many instrumental highlights and milestones. One of these is the innovation of minimally invasive surgical techniques. When discussing minimally invasive cardiac surgery, it is imperative to both recognize and understand the rationale for this technological surge. Perfusion has a traceable extension in theory and practice to the surgical procedure itself. One should envision perfusion as an extension of all operative support systems.

The basic principles of heart–lung bypass allow effective and logical circuit choices. During the period of cardiopulmonary bypass, there are essentially two circuits involved: the patient's circuit and the perfusion circuit. If the patient's circulating blood volume added to the perfusion circuit, the prime volume, is not sufficient to accommodate both circuits during cardiopulmonary bypass, then both the chosen circuit and the size of the circuit will be ineffective. The underlying principle of circuit design is to use the smallest circuit possible while maintaining adequacy of perfusion.

Conceptual knowledge may be the perfusionist's most important attribute in regard to minimally invasive perfusion techniques. The perfusionist is an extension of the surgical procedure itself. Minimally invasive surgery does not necessarily require a complex array of perfusion and circuitry alterations. However, circuitry considerations are imperative for successful delivery of circulatory support.

Surgical philosophy and preference often dictate the perfusionist's approach to the procedure at hand. We prefer to keep circuitry simple and to change isolated parameters only when appropriate. The segmentation of specific surgical procedures can be useful in classifying these procedures according to perfusion requirements. At our institution, we classify our perfusion selections according to clinical drivers. In other words, specific surgical alterations dictate a different course of action from a perfusion viewpoint. Our number one clinical driver is surgical choice of access. In addition, several team-related factors define the effective application of such techniques and should not be overlooked. These include accurate assessment of the perfusion team's comfort level, competence, and support.

The process flow that is helpful in determining a set course of action can be radically altered during the operating procedure. The illustration (Fig. 1) contains the exact parameters and stages in

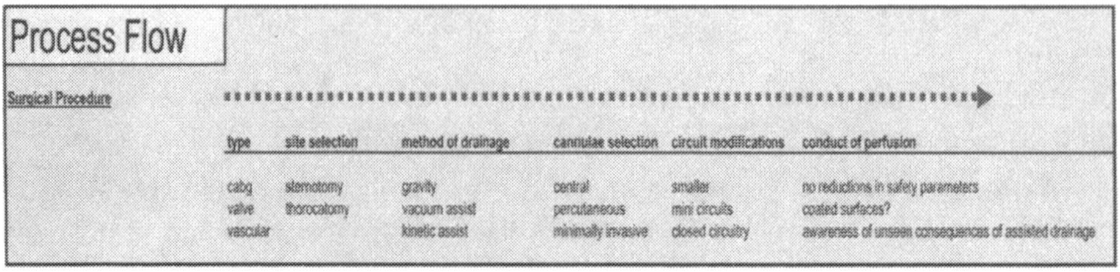

Fig. 1. Parameters and stages in protocol development.

protocol development. During the minimally invasive procedure, however, these are all interrelated, and a change in one parameter may affect any or all of the others. This supports the idea that conceptual knowledge and competency remain vital to quality perfusion. The competency and experience threshold to confidently use minimally invasive systems is undetermined at this time. However, it is well accepted that all individuals learn as a result of absolute experience and the collective learning process *(1)*. Any cardiac team faced with the development of a minimally invasive program will certainly have to consider an appropriate time frame for staff competency, comfort, and skill development.

The movement towards less invasive cardiac procedures has altered the clinical approach to perfusion. Our industry has long been accommodating to demands of reduced surface area and reduction of hemodilution. Concerns about surface activation, complement activation, platelet dysfunction, and postoperative edema have been partially offset by the use of smaller circuits and more biocompatible surfaces. These issues, while some of the most heavily researched perfusion topics for several decades, do not necessarily correspond with minimally invasive techniques. Minimally invasive perfusion is primarily concerned with the alteration of the physics of perfusion. This can be broken down into two main components: size and construction.

CIRCUIT CONSIDERATIONS

Size

The reduction of the perfusion surface area is considered essential to minimally invasive perfusion. However, it is more appropriate to consider circuit reduction and decreased priming volume as a standard approach to everyday perfusion techniques. The choices of incision and access will dictate the use of smaller cannulae at the surgical field. However, in many instances, the ability of the surgeon to have optimal visualization will not affect the gross size of the perfusion circuit. Parallel motivations to reduce circuit size and alter technique will overlap. In respect to size, smaller circuits require less prime and result in less hemodilution of the patient. The reduction of homologous blood requirements through smaller circuit surface area has been well documented *(2)*.

Configuration

The configuration of the circuit is important in providing necessary elements for the planned surgical procedure. Regardless of the possible circuit changes and the intent behind them, standard principles and parameters should be upheld.

When designing a circuit, it is imperative to continually ask two essential questions:

1. Are the changes I am making necessary to the implementation and flow of the surgery?
2. Am I compromising any standards of perfusion?

Circuitry considerations and changes in the perfusionist's mindset are imperative aspects to the successful delivery of circulatory support. Fig. 2 provides an example of a perfusion strategic process flow to aid in the implementation of minimally invasive perfusion protocols. The use of such a tool can be helpful, and we routinely use it in the development of specific perfusion accommodations.

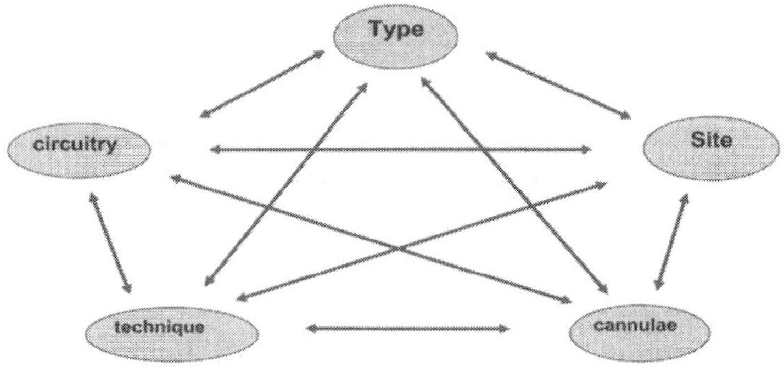

Fig. 2. Interdependency of related parameters.

COMPONENT SELECTION IN MINIMALLY INVASIVE PERFUSION

Assisted Venous Drainage

As discussed earlier, the surgical procedure and cannulation technique dictate the perfusion circuitry and techniques necessary during the perioperative period. Gravity siphon (venous reservoir 40–70 cm below the surface of the heart) is determined by the central venous pressure; this, in turn, is dependent on intravascular volume and venous compliance. Venous compliance is regulated and manipulated by the usage of anesthesia, medications, and changes in sympathetic tone *(3)*. The gravity siphon utilized in a traditional sternotomy approach will, under most circumstances, be unable to provide adequate venous drainage. Small incisions require that the perfusionist maintain ability to drain and perfuse the patient from alternative sites, thereby adding increased resistance to flow in the venous portion of the bypass circuit. This change in resistance often requires active emptying of the patient's blood volume to augment venous drainage. Some indications for augmented venous return are:

- Percutaneous cannulation
- Robotic and/or endoscopic procedures requiring CPB
- Minimally invasive cardiac surgery where surgical visualization is a concern
- Altered surgical approaches, such as hemisternotomy or thoracotomy
- Prime reduction and minimizing hemodilution *(4)*

Currently, there are three methods to assist venous drainage and facilitate the surgical process: kinetic assist, vacuum assist, and roller-pump assist. Each method, although significantly different in technique, will accomplish the same result and facilitate the surgical process. Each method of drainage has its specific requirements, as well as its advantages and disadvantages (Fig. 3). It is up to the perfusionist, in consultation with the surgeon, to decide which method better suits the capabilities of the team and allows the **safest** and most **reproducible** result. We believe that vacuum assist and kinetic assist fit these criteria and suggest their usage for routine perfusion protocol.

Vacuum-Assisted Venous Drainage

Vacuum-assisted venous drainage (VAVD) entails the application of a **regulated** amount of negative pressure to a closed and nonvented venous reservoir/perfusion circuit. The negative pressure exerted on the

METHOD OF ASSIST	ADVANTAGES	DISADVANTAGES
VACUUM	• EASE OF SETUP • INEXPENSIVE • EASE OF CONVERSION	• INVOLVES CHANGING THE DYNAMICS OF THE VENOUS RESERVOIR • POSSIBLE AIR ENTRAINMENT • POSSIBLE PRESSURIZATION OF RESERVOIR
KINETIC	• MISMATCH OF DRAINAGE / ARTERIAL FLOW EASILY RECOGNIZED • EASILY REGULATED	• MOST EXPENSIVE • HAVE TO TERMINATE CPB TO CONVERT TO KINETIC
ROLLER	• LEAST EXPENSIVE OF THE THREE	• DIFFICULT TO REGULATE AND MONITOR NEGATIVE PRESSURE • HAVE TO TERMINATE CPB TO CONVERT TO ROLLER ASSIST

Fig. 3. Method of drainage.

venous reservoir is transferred to the blood pathway of the perfusion tubing and, subsequently, to the patient's venous system. The use of negative pressure to augment return has been well documented for its efficiency, and is often questioned for its potential negative affects. Some of these negative effects include the potential to introduce microbubbles into the systemic circulation and physical changes to the pressure dynamics in the venous reservoir *(5)*. The application of vacuum has been speculated to increase the amount of air introduced into the circuit, as well as change the behavior of the gaseous emboli in the circuit *(6)*.

Vacuum-assisted venous drainage needs to be carefully planned and discussed among the surgical team. Primary problems and initial troubleshooting can be ineffective and potentially dangerous. The surgical team, particularly the perfusionists, should have the sense and presence of mind to cope with the common and uncommon possibilities presented with VAVD. Several safety measures will have to be employed if a perfusion team is to effectively attempt to perform this minimally invasive technique.

Table 1
Key Components to VAVD

Components
Minimally invasive venous cannulae selection
Approved vacuum assist venous reservoir
Vacuum regulator
Pressure monitor to measure the venous reservoir pressure(Inlet)
Reservoir positive and negative pressure alert
Positive pressure relief (10 mmHg or less)
One-way valve in arterial line (if centrifugal pump is used)
Arterial line pressure monitoring
Flow meter post filter (optional)
Reduced visual noise whenever possible

Tables 1 and 2 display the key components and required processes for the safe implementation and management of vacuum-assisted venous return. Table 1 focuses on the physical application, and Table 2 addresses the mental component of preparation. We recommend their consideration in protocol development, and discourage ignorance as to their importance. The perfusionist should be familiarized with their individual value, as well as their limitations. In analyzing the key components, it is best to start at the incision site and work backwards; this seems to be an appropriate way to handle any proactive or reactive concerns regarding the procedure.

Kinetic-Assist Venous Drainage

Kinetic assist involves the introduction of a constrained vortex (centrifugal) pump into the venous line immediately proximal to the inlet

Table 2
Preparation for VAVD

Review
Literature
Manufacturer's recommendations and suggestions
Current demand and surgical needs
Discuss
Surgeon
Anesthesia
Other perfusionists with experiences
Perfusion team members

of the venous reservoir. The generation of sufficient RPMs and negative pressure facilitates the venous drainage. Logistically speaking, actively pumping into the venous reservoir poses additional challenges to the perfusionist. These challenges include the necessity to operate and concentrate on two pumps (as a primary perfusionist) as opposed to a single arterial pump. The main constraint of this type of system is that it needs to be set up and primed before bypass. The main advantage to kinetic-assist is in its associated (and potential) use with a closed, soft-shell venous reservoir, thus offsetting the effects of air–blood interface and potentially diminishing the inflammatory response.

Kinetic-assist drainage, similar to VAVD, may be responsible for the introduction of air into the venous line. In general, it has been suggested that the entrainment of venous air, which is exacerbated through the use of such augmenting techniques, may in fact lead to an increase in postoperative neurocognitive deficits *(7)*. It is clear that the addition of negative pressure to the venous system of the heart–lung circuit will indeed alter the behavior of gaseous emboli. Wilcox et al., have demonstrated that downstream embolic counts and rate of air entrainment were significantly greater with VAVD as opposed to kinetic-assisted drainage *(8)*. The authors claim that there is nearly a 10-fold increase in the arterial line emboli count, with the main determinants of this increased count being the rate of entrainment *(8)*.

In addition to the potential increase in harmful microembolic counts, increasing negative pressure has been postulated to have a damaging effect on the blood cells, mainly through the increased turbulence generated throughout the bypass circuit and at the smaller minimally invasive cannula tip *(9)*. Lactate dehydrogenase (LDH) and plasma hemoglobin are hemolytic parameters associated with increased sheer stress and cellular damage. Mueller et al. found that in regard to these parameters, VAVD did not cause any significant increase over gravity drainage *(10)*. The same was noted for thrombocyte and white blood cell counts *(10)*. Future analysis regarding outcome-related effects of these systems and continued comparisons between vacuum and kinetic drainage will be helpful in guiding our protocols and judgment.

Clearly, the same principles that guide us in our daily preparation should remain prevalent in the various decisions that we make in our minimally invasive approaches. These principles include the reduction of venous air and reduction of blood cell trauma. Augmented venous return is the basis of minimally invasive perfusion. The choice as to which method of drainage is suitable depends on surgeon's requirements, the perfusion team, and the overall strengths and weaknesses of the operative team. We reiterate the notion that if a technique is not safe and reproducible, then it is the wrong choice. To illustrate, our team performs approximately 30% of all cases with some form of minimally invasive approach (of which approximately 10% are learned near the time of the surgery). In addition, we are asked to augment our drainage another 10% of the time for routine sternotomy. We use vacuum with a hard-shell venous reservoir because of the uncertainty of the demand, the limited number of perfusion staff, the desire for standardization, and the safety and effectiveness of routine.

Specific Circuit Alterations

Minimally invasive surgery may require assembly of a bypass circuit using an FDA-approved vacuum-assist venous reservoir. The surgical access and desired cannulation will dictate the necessity to split the venous line and add a Y connector to the venous line of the bypass circuit. Minimally invasive atrial septal defects, minimally invasive mitral valve repairs, and robotically-assisted procedures will usually require some manipulation to accommodate bicaval drainage.

At our institution, if the internal jugular vein is required for venous drainage, then the perfusionist will prepare the heparin flush for the percutaneous cannula insertion. A Biomedicus (Medtronic) 15-Fr arterial cannula is used for the right internal jugular vein. A 1-L normal saline bag (0.9% sodium chloride), three 60-ml syringes, one 10 ml syringe, one IV infusion set, porcine heparin, 3/8 inch tubing, and tubing clamps are required for the setup. 2,000 U of heparin are added to the liter of normal saline. The 60-ml syringes are drawn from this solution and ready for flush. 5,000 U heparin are drawn up in a 10-ml syringe, and an additional 5 ml are drawn from the liter of normal saline. The cannula is handed to the table and a pig tail is attached. The cannula is flushed, inserted, and advanced to the SVC–RA junction and confirmed by TEE. After the cannula is deaired and flushed with heparinized saline, the 3/8-inch line will be connected and the patient clamped out with double tubing clamps. The 3/8-inch line will then be primed with either the IV infusion or the 60-ml syringes. After the line is primed, it is double clamped. The heparin flush is then connected to the three-way stop cock, and the infusion to the patient through the cannula is begun. Note that taking the baseline ACT after the infusion of heparin will inflate the baseline ACT. One should consider taking this sample after the Swan–Ganz insertion but before the internal jugular cannulation. The cannula and lines are then sutured and secured for later connection to the bypass circuit.

The venous line should be prepared with alcohol and cut with sterile tubing scissors. The Y-connector can be placed in several places in the venous line. We prefer to cut it in about 12–18 inches from the inlet of the cardiotomy. The 3/8-inch portion of the connector can be capped and remain as such until it is time to connect to the patient. Connection of the circuit to the patient *should be delayed* until ready to initiate bypass, or at least until the administration of heparin. Early connection of the lines may increase the risk of accidental decannulation of the internal jugular vein.

CANNULATION SCHEMES

Planning of access for cannulation for cardiopulmonary bypass is integral to minimally invasive cardiac surgery. Unlike routine cardiac operations in which cannulation is often standardized, these new techniques require complex, and sometimes creative, planning. Often, it is the chosen surgical incision that limits and necessitates preoperative decisions regarding access. The minimum size of cannulas required must be discussed with the perfusion team to ensure adequate drainage and flows for each patient. The requirements for cardioplegia delivery and monitoring should be determined. Current technology has resulted in specialized cannulas that may be placed directly into the operating field or in a more remote location. Techniques such as percutaneous cannulation are considered a safe option for cardiopulmonary bypass. A specific cannulation scheme must be created for each operation that takes into consideration all options for access, cannulas, and perfusion circuits.

ARTERIAL ACCESS

The placement of arterial cannulas is almost entirely dependent on the choice of incision for a given minimally invasive surgery. Any surgery requiring sternotomy or upper hemisternotomy may utilize standard aortic cannulation of the ascending aorta. The site of access with this incision is the upper portion of the ascending aorta, just inferior to the innominate artery. The presence of any palpable or echocardiographic calcifications at this site may necessitate, as in a standard procedure, insertion of the cannula, either along the inferior aortic arch or into a peripheral site.

Femoral arterial cannulation may be performed using an open or percutaneous technique. Complete percutaneous femoral artery cannulation may be performed using progressive dilatation and a basic

Seldinger technique over a guidewire. In obese patients or elderly patients with diseased vessels, this access may be technically difficult. If significant atherosclerotic disease is suspected, the open technique is considered safer. A 3-cm horizontal incision is made over the femoral arterial pulse and dissected through the femoral sheath to expose the femoral artery. Vessel loops are placed around the artery and a 6-0 purse-string suture is placed on the anterior surface of the vessel. An 18-gauge needle is used to access the artery directly, and a guidewire is passed into the ascending aorta and checked using echocardiographic guidance. An arterial cannula may then be inserted over the guidewire without the need for extra manipulation or additional dilations. The arteriotomy is directly opened to accommodate the size of the cannula. The cannula is secured, deaired, and connected to the bypass circuit.

Another option for arterial access is the right subclavian artery. This access site is best utilized when the ascending aorta and arch are to be replaced or antegrade cerebral perfusion is required as an adjunct to hypothermic circulatory arrest. The exposure of the subclavian artery requires a 3-cm horizontal incision made just inferior and parallel to the clavicle. Dissection into the deltopectoral groove exposes the subclavian vein, which is gently retracted to expose the subclavian artery. Once intravenous heparin is delivered, the artery may be cannulated directly or through an interposition graft. Our group prefers to use an 8-mm Gore-Tex® graft anastamosed to the artery in an end-to-side fashion, with a partial occluding clamp placed on the artery *(11)*. A 20-Fr straight arterial cannula is secured into the graft and the cannula is deaired in a standard fashion before connection to the bypass circuit. This facilitates decannulation at the completion of the procedure with simple oversewing of the graft stump, thereby preventing unnecessary manipulation of the subclavian artery.

Venous Access

If the right atrium is accessible, as in a hemisternotomy, venous drainage may be obtained through an open technique using a standard two-stage oval cannula placed directly into the right atrium. Placement of this cannula is facilitated through this minimally invasive incision with gentle retraction of the atrial appendage toward the patient's left side. Placement of the cannula into the inferior vena cava (IVC) from this site should be confirmed with echocardiography.

Femoral cannulation is another good option for drainage. A two-stage femoral venous cannula may be placed into the femoral vein and directed into the IVC using echo guidance. Similar to arterial cannulation, this catheter may be placed using an open technique with initial placement of a wire followed by progressive dilators and, finally, placement of a venous cannula. Alternatively, when femoral venous cannulation is used without concomitant arterial cannulation, a routine percutaneous Seldinger technique can be used.

Bicaval cannulation is often required for mitral valve or right heart procedures. A percutaneous right internal jugular vein line may be placed using the Seldinger technique before patient positioning. It is critical that this cannula is filled with 5,000 U of heparin and that the patient is placed on a continuous low-dose heparin drip through this cannula to prevent clot formation before the institution of cardiopulmonary bypass. The tip of the cannula should be placed just into the superior vena cava to prevent an injury during retraction of the atria. After the patient is positioned and prepped, an inferior venous cannula may be placed either in the femoral vein or directly into the lower right atria through the working incision. Alternatively, a small venous cannula may be placed just inferior to the wound, through the skin, and brought into the IVC for drainage.

Arterial Cannulas

Cannulas specifically designed for minimally invasive cardiac surgery are all unique in size, material, pliability, and methods of insertion. One system is considered the most "minimally invasive" in that its placement of the arterial, venous, and cardioplegia systems is entirely percutaneous. Completely endoscopic systems include the Heartport Endovascular catheter system (Endo Cardiopulmonary Bypass System; Heartport, Inc., Redwood City, CA) and the Estech Remote Access Perfusion System (ESTECH, Inc., Danville, CA). These include a specialized arterial cannula that is placed percutaneously through the femoral artery into the ascending aorta. This cannula is a thin-walled, wire-wound 21- or 23-Fr cannula that includes an endoaortic balloon that inflates to occlude the aorta and allow delivery of antegrade cardioplegia through the tip of the catheter. The corresponding 28-Fr venous drainage cannula contains multiple side holes and is placed into the right atrium or IVC using a percutaneous femoral technique with either fluoroscopic or transesophageal echocardiographic (TEE) guidance. The endoaortic balloon position must be carefully confirmed using TEE guidance. Careful monitoring of pressures and flow into both the endoaortic and endocoronary cannulas is required to prevent and recognize any potential dislodgement.

Direct arterial cannulas are also specifically made for minimally invasive surgeries. These cannulas are made of pliable materials that allow for ease of insertion.

The Gem-Flex II arterial cannulas (Edwards Lifesciences, Midvale, CA) are available in 16-, 18-, and 20-Fr (5.3–6 mm) at a length of 15 cm. These may be placed in the femoral, axillary, or ascending aorta positions, as previously described. Adequate flows are expected with each of these cannulas.

Our preferred technique of cannulation in minimal access surgery involves the use of direct arterial cannulation, aortic cross-clamping through a small percutaneous incision site, and direct cardioplegia delivery. This method decreases the potential risk of endovascular balloons. Although it does require direct access to the arterial system, it ensures adequate delivery of cardioplegia and complete aortic occlusion.

Venous Cannulas

The venous cannula used in percutaneous techniques must be thin-walled and flexible to enhance blood flow and allow the possibility of kinetic or VAVD. Constructed with polyurethane to prevent kinking, the Edwards VFEM venous cannula (Edwards Lifesciences, Irvine, CA) is available in 18–31-Fr sizes with lengths of 55–65 cm. Guide-wires and dilator kits are available for percutaneous positioning of these cannulas. In addition, the RMI Avid Cannulas (Edwards Lifesciences) are 22-Fr, thin-walled, curved, and composed of a triple-hole design that is useful in many procedures in which the IVC is directly accessible. These cannulas may be placed through the wound or through a small skin incision into the lower right atrium/IVC. Exposure is often limited in these procedures, and these small, easily maneuverable cannulas are useful for drainage. Medtronic venous cannulas (Biomedicus 15-, 17-, 19-, and 21-Fr) are also used in the femoral position.

During some procedures, additional venous drainage may be helpful to decompress the heart and improve visualization. Peripheral cannulation systems using gravity may drain only 75–80% of the venous return to the heart. Assisted drainage using either kinetic pump or vacuum assist offers complete support of the circulation and prevents heart filling and ejection. In our program, we use a carefully regulated suction to apply vacuum to an open venous system. Flow rates are given from the manufacturer and should become familiar as part of the selection process. As a general guide, you can expect to augment return by approximately 30% with assisted venous drainage. Depressed venous flow rates can be affected by surgical positioning, cannula position, volemic state, and degree of negative pressure exerted on the circuit.

Cardioplegia Cannulas

Delivery of cardioplegia antegrade through the aorta or retrograde through the coronary sinus must also be planned. With the Heartport® system, antegrade cardioplegia is delivered directly into the aorta through the aortic cannula after balloon inflation. A specialized 9-Fr endocoronary sinus catheter (Endo CPB system; Heartport, Inc.; Redwood City, CA) may be placed into the coronary sinus via the right internal jugular vein using TEE guidance. Its balloon is inflated, and cardioplegia is delivered into the coronary sinus at a line pressure of approximately 250–350 mmHg, and a coronary sinus pressure not to exceed the manufacturer's recommendation of 40–50 mmHg. Alternatively, antegrade cardioplegia may be delivered directly into the aorta using an 18-Fr-long angiocatheter placed through the anterior chest wall into the aorta. Another option is to place an aortic root needle (Medtronic Inc., Minneapolis, MN) through the small hemisternotomy or thoracotomy incision for delivery of cardioplegia and deairing of the heart. Appropriate line pressures should be insured for all cardioplegia delivery techniques. A myocardial temperature probe may be used to check adequate delivery. Exposure to any portion of the right heart through a hemisternotomy or small right thoracotomy allows for placement of a direct retrograde cannula with gentle retraction of the right atrium towards the patient's left side and TEE-directed positioning of the cannula itself.

COMPLICATIONS OF CANNULATION

Care should be taken with placement of these cannulas, and patient selection is a critical aspect of these cases. This may often be a laborious and time-intensive portion of the procedure. Older patients may have significant atherosclerotic disease of their peripheral arterial vessels, making cannulation at these sites more morbid. Some female patients may have small femoral vessels that make it difficult to pass the appropriately sized cannulas required for bypass. Several complications have been linked to the use of remote access systems. Femoral artery dissections and occlusions have been reported *(12)*. Limb ischemia and plaque dislodgement have also been described *(12)*. Overall, the incidence of these complications is reported as less than 1% *(12,13)*. The risk of femoral artery injury with cannulation has been shown to be higher in women *(12)*. There may also be problems specific to certain specialized intraarterial cannula, such as balloon migration, inadequate cardioplegia delivery, or balloon rupture *(13)*. Any intrinsic aortic disease may put the patient at risk from femoral cannulation *(14)*. The possibility of these complications should be considered during decision-making for access for each specific patient. Good patient selection will help avoid significant complications.

MINIMALLY INVASIVE MITRAL VALVE SURGERY

Currently existing minimally invasive approaches to the repair and replacement of the mitral valve are directed at the size and location of the incision for access to the surgical field. Although percutaneous procedures are being developed for mitral valve repair, present techniques do not allow for both the elimination of cardiopulmonary bypass and the application of alternative incisions. As such, the various cannulation schemes and perfusions techniques previously outlined become paramount to the successful completion of a minimally invasive mitral valve operation. The various approaches to mitral valve surgery range from direct surgery through small incisions to completely endoscopic operations.

Hemisternotomy

Minimally invasive approaches to both the mitral and aortic valve were first described in the mid 1990s through a variety of both upper and lower hemisternotomy incisions *(15–18)*. Although parasternal and "j" type incisions have been reported, complications with wound dehiscence, lung herniation, and postoperative pain limited their universal application *(19)*.

An upper hemisternotomy incision with a division of the sternum into the left fourth interspace is the approach popularized by the Cleveland Clinic group *(15,18,20,21)*. The mitral valve is exposed through a transseptal incision that is extended onto the dome of the left atrium. In most cases, the aorta can be cannulated directly. Similarly, direct bicaval cannulation can be accomplished through the wound. The use of either VAVD or kinetic-assisted drainage allows for the use of small, wire-reinforced, angled venous cannulae (18–24-Fr), resulting in less obstruction of the operative field. Femoral arterial and venous cannulation can also be used, but is rarely necessary for increased exposure. The aorta is cross-clamped directly, and cardioplegia is delivered in a conventional manner with standard antegrade and retrograde catheters.

This approach has been described in over 400 patients at the Cleveland Clinic, with conversion necessary in less than 1% of patients and a hospital mortality of 0.3% *(20,21)*.

A lower hemisternotomy incision can also be used with division of the sternum into the right second intercostal space. Cannulation can typically be performed centrally; however, femoral arterial or venous cannulation can also be performed to increase operating space if needed. Assisted venous drainage is, again, critical for minimizing cannulation size and decreasing priming volume. Aortic cross clamping is done directly through the wound with either a traditional clamp or a flexible clamp, and cardioplegia is given in a conventional fashion. The mitral valve can be approached with either a transseptal incision through the right atrium or with a conventional left atrial incision through the interatrial groove. The Brigham and Women's group has championed this approach, and it has reported excellent results in over 400 patients *(19,22)*. The preferred cannulation scheme used by this group includes direct aortic cannulation with a flexible cannula and direct SVC cannulation with a 24-Fr vacuum-assisted, thin-walled wire-reinforced cannula. The IVC is cannulated percutaneously from the femoral vein with a long 21-Fr cannula. When comparing patients undergoing minimally invasive mitral valve surgery to those undergoing full sternotomy, Mihaljevic et al. demonstrated decreases in the length of stay, cardiopulmonary bypass time, and cross-clamp time among those patients undergoing minimally invasive surgery *(22)*.

Right Thoracotomy

Several different minimally invasive approaches can be used when approaching the mitral valve through the right chest. Understanding the specific surgical approach will allow both surgeon and perfusionist to select the appropriate cannulation scheme and cardioplegia delivery system for each circumstance. Potential advantages to the right chest approach include preserved integrity of the chest wall, rapid recovery to full activity, and improved cosmesis. For all right-chested approaches, double lumen intubation with selective left lung ventilation is necessary. The patient is then typically positioned in the anterolateral thoracotomy position, with the hips left at 45 degrees for femoral vessel access if needed. The use of a beanbag is typically helpful for patient positioning, and care needs to be taken to ensure appropriate padding of potential pressure points. The right arm can be positioned either tucked back at the side or supported over the head. Our group has found that placing the arm comfortably over the head on a pillow, as is used for a posterolateral thoracotomy, to be the safest and most effective way to position the patient.

The simplest right chested approach involves making a 6-cm "mini" thoracotomy incision in the fourth or fifth interspace. A small retractor is used for rib spreading, and direct cannulation of the aorta is possible with a cannula brought either through the wound or through a separate stab incision. Although small, wire-reinforced cannulae can be used for direct SVC and IVC cannulation, working space can be limited with such an approach. Our group prefers to cannulate the SVC percutaneously through an internal jugular vein puncture before positioning and draping of the patient. A 15- or 17-Fr percutaneous arterial perfusion cannula is used for venous drainage in this circumstance. The cannula is flushed with heparin and maintained with a heparin/saline drip until full heparinization is instituted. If it is elected to cannulate the IVC directly, a 22- or 24-Fr vacuum assist cannula can be brought through a future chest tube site to improve operating space. Alternatively, the femoral vein can be percutaneously cannulated with a 19- or 21-Fr-long vacuum assist cannula, which is advanced to the IVC–RA junction under echo guidance. Likewise, if working space is limited, the femoral artery can be cannulated as described previously.

Any of three techniques of aortic cross clamping can be used when a rib-spreading thoracotomy is used: transaxillary cross clamping, direct cross clamping with a flexible cross-clamp, and endoaortic balloon clamping. Our group favors the transaxillary clamp as an excellent space-saving technique for direct aortic occlusion. When a minithoracotomy is used, antegrade and retrograde cardioplegia cannula can be inserted directly through the wound. Our group favors repeated doses of antegrade cardioplegia for the minithoracotomy approach. It is critical to monitor and maintain aortic root pressure during the delivery of antegrade cardioplegia, as the anterior retraction of the left atrium during mitral valve exposure can render the aortic valve insufficient. We favor release of the minimally invasive retractor during each cardioplegia dose to ensure adequate antegrade delivery.

Surgery is then performed under direct vision with special long instruments for better access to the operative field. Although knots can occasionally be tied conventionally, it is typically less traumatic to the surgical tissues to use a knot pusher for all knot tying. Video assistance can also be used for this procedure by introducing a small camera through a port posterior to the incision. Multiple groups have reported excellent short- and medium-term results with the minithoracotomy approach, using both central and peripheral cannulation techniques *(23,24)*.

The minithoracotomy approach can also be performed with completely peripheral cannulation. The use of an endoaortic balloon clamp for antegrade cardioplegia delivery can also be used, allowing for a completely free operative field. Although this technique adds significantly to the complexity of the operation and may not be warranted in the setting of a rib-spreading thoracotomy, it does lend itself to a non–rib-spreading thoracotomy or completely endoscopic approach. For totally endoscopic approaches to the mitral valve, our group favors internal jugular and femoral venous cannulation, as well as standard femoral arterial cannulation. Transthoracic aortic clamping can be performed, and an antegrade aortic cardioplegia needle can be delivered through the non–rib-spreading incision. Alternatively, a long 14-gauge angiocath can be introduced through a separate chest wall puncture and placed in the ascending aorta.

When a non–rib-spreading incision is used, surgery is performed with video assistance and special long instruments. Although this approach requires a significantly longer learning curve, several groups have reported excellent results with totally endoscopic mitral valve surgery *(25)*.

Robotic Mitral Valve Surgery

To improve the learning curve and visualization of minimally invasive mitral valve surgery, robotic technology was applied to this procedure in 1999. The da Vinci robotic system (Intuitive Surgical Incorporated, Sunnyvale, CA) is composed of a surgeon control console and a surgical arm unit that positions and directs the microinstruments. Unlike standard thoracoscopic instruments, these specialized "EndoWrist" instruments have a full 7 degrees of freedom, simulating the motion of a human wrist at the operative site. Insertion of the instruments into the chest cavity is performed through two 8-mm ports. A third 12-mm port is used to insert the endoscope. The instruments are controlled by a surgeon who sits at the operating console away from the operative field. Computer interfacing allows for scaled motion, thereby eliminating tremor and providing for incredibly accurate surgical precision through these small ports. The surgeon views the surgery through the eyepiece in the surgical console, which provides high-definition, magnified, real three-dimensional vision. The potential advantages of robotics when applied to minimally invasive mitral valve surgery are twofold: a) The learning curve of operating with endoscopic instruments and knot pushers is significantly decreased, and b) totally endoscopic operations are much more easily learned and performed.

The surgical and perfusion setup for robotic mitral valve surgery can be identical to that used for a standard "mini" mitral performed through a small rib-spreading right thoracotomy. The East Carolina group has the most experience with robotic mitral valve surgery *(26,27)*. They favor the use of an internal jugular catheter and femoral venous and arterial cannulation. Although direct aortic cannulation can be performed in a similar manner to that used during nonrobotic direct minimitral surgery, eliminating the operative field of extraneous cannulas is helpful during robotic surgery. Aortic occlusion is performed with a transaxillary clamp, and intermittent antegrade cardioplegia is given through an antegrade cardioplegia needle, which is inserted directly through the wound. The camera for the robot is inserted at the medial aspect of the thoracotomy wound, and the robotic arms are positioned through separate 8-mm ports. Sutures and different prostheses are passed through the thoracotomy wound. Other surgeons favor the use of peripheral cannulation with endoaortic balloon occlusion. Good results have been obtained with this perfusion setup amongst groups with extensive endoaortic experience *(24)*.

The robotic "mini" mitral operation, as described most extensively by the East Carolina group, has recently been modified to be performed totally endoscopically. Peripheral cannulation is used, and aortic occlusion can be performed with either a transaxillary clamp or an endoaortic balloon. The camera is placed through a separate port and a 2–4-cm, non–rib-spreading working port is used for the passage of sutures and prostheses. The results of this procedure have yet to be widely reported and await further study. However, early results appear to be equivalent to an open, direct minimitral through a right thoracotomy.

Miniaortic Valve Replacement

Minimally invasive approaches to the aortic valve make use of smaller incisions to access the upper portion of the mediastinum essential in performing the operation. The patient is first positioned supine with a shoulder roll to elevate the upper torso and facilitate exposure of the aortic valve. We use a small oscillating saw to perform an upper hemisternotomy with careful division of the sternum into the right third interspace. Access to the arterial system is performed directly into the upper portion of the aorta, across from the innominate artery, using a Medtronic® standard 20-Fr aortic cannula. A standard 36–46-Fr two-stage, oval, wire-enforced venous cannula (Medtronic, Inc.) is placed through the right atrial appendage and secured laterally to the chest wall to increase the working space. If additional space is required, percutaneous internal jugular and femoral venous lines, as previously described, could also supply ample drainage.

Left ventricular venting is performed in a standard fashion through the right superior pulmonary vein using a small angled metal vent that is secured laterally in the incision. The antegrade cannula is placed in the mid portion of the aorta, and a retrograde cannula may be inserted directly into the right atrium by retracting the right heart and placing the catheter under TEE guidance. The cross-clamp is placed under direct vision, and the aorta is opened transversely in a standard fashion. It is helpful to position the bed in the reverse trendelenberg position for this portion of the procedure.

The upper hemisternotomy, as popularized by Cosgrove and colleagues, continues to show similar perioperative results to conventional sternotomy and is performed in multiple centers *(28,29)*. In addition, the hemisternotomy approach has shown cosmetic advantages and improved sternal stability, as well as decreased blood loss and transfusion *(30)*. Advantages of the sternal-sparing incision include decreased pain, morbidity, and hospital stay *(31)*. Use of the third intercostal space has resulted in decreased pulmonary complications *(32)*. There is some evidence that this approach decreases the systemic inflammatory response as well *(33)*.

Miniaortic Aneurysm Repair

This same sternal-sparing approach may also be used be for an ascending aortic aneurysm or aortic root repair. The patient is positioned again in the supine position with a transverse roll placed behind the shoulder blades to open up the upper torso. An upper hemisternotomy incision with division of the sternum into the left fourth interspace is preferred, as it allows for maximal exposure. The aorta may be cannulated directly at this point if a simple tube graft is planned. However, if circulatory arrest is necessary, cannulation of the arterial system is best obtained with right axillary cannulation through a short interposition graft, as previously described. The benefits of the interposition graft are that it provides unobstructed flow and allows easy removal at case completion with graft ligation, rather than an arterial repair with occasionally difficult exposure. Flow through the axillary cannula proceeds at 300–500 cc/min during the circulatory arrest time, thereby continuously providing cerebral perfusion. Use of cerebral venous saturation monitoring may be helpful in determining the adequacy of cerebral flow. A standard 36–46 oval venous cannula is placed into the atrium. A metal angle vent and retrograde catheter are placed as previously described.

This approach has been used for repair of aneurysm, dissections, reoperations, and root repairs with good results. It has demonstrated significant improvements in transfusion requirements, ICU stay, and length of hospital stay *(34,35)*. Repair of the aortic root through an upper hemisternotomy has also been described, although the increased time of procedure demands careful attention to myocardial protection *(36)*. Mean operating time, as expected, was longer than for control groups, but the patients had similar bypass and cross clamp times. Postop transfusion and ICU length of stay were both decreased, but did not reach statistical significance *(37)*.

Right Thoracotomy for Atrial Septal Defect (ASD)

Repair of ASD is a procedure that shows significant benefits when performed through minimally invasive incisions. Although many of these are closed percutaneously, those patients with a large ASD or with a significant atrial septal aneurysm often require surgical closure. Due to its relative simplicity, ASD closure was one of the earliest performed minimally invasive surgeries, and techniques have continued to be refined over the past several years, with results demonstrating that the procedure is safe, with good long-term outcomes *(38,39)*.

In providing an alternative to median sternotomy, one option is a small right minithoracotomy *(39)*. The patient is placed into a modified left lateral decubitus position with the right arm suspended above the head or tucked underneath the right side. The pelvis must remain flat to allow ease of femoral cannulation with the right chest slightly elevated. A superior vena caval cannula, #18 arterial (Medtronic, Inc.) is placed into the right internal jugular vein and positioned with TEE guidance into the SVC above the right atrium. This is important in preventing any torquing forces on the cannula when the atrium is opened. The IVC is drained by a femoral venous cannula (Edwards Lifesciences; 17- or 19-Fr) placed percutaneously in the femoral vein to increase the working space of the thoracotomy. A cardioplegia needle and cross clamp may be placed directly through the wound. Alternatively, an endoaortic balloon 17- or 21-Fr Remote Access Perfusion cannula (ESTECH, Inc.) may be placed into the ascending aorta using echocardiographic guidance. After selective left lung ventilation, a 4-cm incision is made over the fourth intercostal space, and a soft tissue retractor ring (Cardiovations, Inc.) is placed between the ribs. The pericardium is opened to expose the aorta and right atrium. Caval snares are placed to isolate the right atrium. The procedure is then performed through this small incision using long instruments to close the ASD either primarily or with a small pericardial patch.

Totally Endoscopic/Robotic ASD Repair

With the push for more percutaneous treatments, transitions were soon made to a totally endoscopic procedure *(40)*. Complete endoscopic repair may be performed through four small port incisions with the use of robotic assistance. This helps avoid potential problems of thoracotomy, such as pain caused by spreading of the ribs and division of the intercostal muscles. This method of closure has improved postoperative recovery time and has demonstrated excellent quality of life scores with avoidance of sternotomy or thoracotomy *(41,42)*.

This repair also requires the use of single-lung ventilation, and patients are positioned in the same modified left lateral decubitus position. The right chest is brought forward, but the pelvis again remains flat for adequate exposure of the groin for femoral cannulation. A superior vena cava venous line cannula (Edwards Lifesciences; 17-Fr) is placed into the right internal jugular vein and positioned above the right atrium. The IVC is drained by a femoral venous cannula placed percutaneously in the femoral vein. Direct cannulation of the femoral artery with a 17- or 19-Fr cannula increases the working space of the thoracotomy. Alternatively, using an endoaortic balloon, a 17- or 21-Fr Remote Access Perfusion cannula may be placed into the ascending aorta using echocardiographic guidance. A 1.5-cm port site is created in the right chest for insertion of the camera through a 12-mm incision, and two smaller 8-mm port sites are placed on either side for the arm insertion. One assistant port site is placed just posterior to the site of the camera. The surgical cart is brought to the bedside, and the robotic arms and camera are inserted. Using robotic assistance, the pericardium is opened, and stay sutures are placed, followed by caval snares, initiation of cardiopulmonary bypass, and cooling. Cardioplegia may be delivered directly through a 14-gauge angiocatheter, placed through the anterior chest wall directly into the aorta, or may be delivered using the endoaortic balloon system.

Minimally Invasive Coronary Artery Bypass Grafting (CABG)

OpCAB

Less invasive approaches to CABG surgery may include elimination of cardiopulmonary bypass, elimination of the median sternotomy incision, or both. The most common minimally invasive technique for coronary artery bypass grafting is off-pump CABG (OpCAB). OpCAB allows for grafting of all coronary territories through a conventional median sternotomy. Despite the fact that a conventional incision is used, the procedure's minimally invasive nature arises from the elimination of cardiopulmonary bypass and the deleterious inflammatory response associated with on-pump procedures. Randomized studies have demonstrated decreased blood loss *(43–47)* and early improvements in cognitive function *(43,47–49)* in most patients undergoing OpCAB. Despite the fact that improvements in end organ function and stroke have been documented with OpCAB in high-risk patients *(43,46,50–52)*, these benefits have not been clearly shown over on-pump CABG in lower risk patient populations *(45,53)*.

Procedures regarding pump priming and standby for OpCAB vary between different institutions. It is generally recommended that a perfusionist be in the room with a primed pump for all off-pump cases. Preoperative consultation with the operating surgeon is important for the entire team to be aware of specific time points in each case during which conversion might be necessary. Conversion of OpCAB to an on-pump case has been shown to be associated with poor patient outcomes *(54)*. Good patient selection is critical for avoiding emergency conversion of an OpCAB to an on-pump CABG.

Robotic CABG

Robotic CABG can be divided into three general procedures: robotically assisted CABG (RACAB), totally endoscopic arrested-heart CABG (TECAB), and totally endoscopic beating heart CABG.

RACAB

Robotically assisted CABG employs the robot in the mobilization of one or both internal thoracic arteries, the pericardotomy, and the identification of target vessels *(55,56)*. A small anterior thoracotomy is performed, and the anastomoses are performed on the beating heart by hand. A non–rib-spreading incision can be used, in which the intercostal muscles are divided and the target vessel exposed with a soft tissue retractor. Although multivessel revascularization can be performed with the use of a rib-spreading incision *(57,58)*, this procedure is typically reserved for revascularization of the left anterior descending artery (LAD) and the diagonal vessels. A similar operation can be performed with thoracoscopic mobilization of the left internal thoracic artery (LITA) in lieu of the robot *(59)*. However, widespread adoption of this procedure has been slow, secondary to technical demands and a long learning curve.

RACAB has been shown to have excellent short- and mid-term results with markedly improved recovery times when compared to conventional CABG *(55–58)*. The procedure is minimally invasive in its avoidance of CPB, together with the use of a sternal sparing incision. It is limited by the ability to revascularize only anteriorly located coronary vessels. The combination of RACB and stenting as a "hybrid" revascularization has shown promise in certain high-risk patient populations *(60,61)*.

Because RACAB is performed through limited access, a strategy needs to be in place for the rare case of emergency conversion. The left groin should be available for emergency cannulation. Extended thoracotomy and conventional cannulation of the aorta and right atrium are also possible. Appropriate patient selection and the judicious use of coronary shunting should avoid most instances of conversion to an on-pump operation. Nonetheless, close communication with the perfusion team remains essential.

ARRESTED-HEART TECAB

The robot can also be used for all parts of the operation, including the anastomosis. This can be performed in both on-pump on the arrested heart *(62,63)* and off-pump on the beating heart *(64,65)*.

With arrested heart TECAB, the internal thoracic artery is mobilized with the robot and the pericardotomy is performed. The target vessels are identified, and the LITA is prepared for anastomosis. CPB is then typically instituted through the right femoral vessels, and cardioplegic arrest is achieved with endoaortic balloon clamping. The LAD is then opened with the robot and the anastomosis is performed robotically. Because the heart is decompressed, there is a considerable amount of working space without chest insufflation, and the table surgeon can assist the console surgeon through a working port.

This procedure is minimally invasive in that it is performed through 4 or 5 ports. However, it retains the invasiveness of CPB, aortic cross clamping, and cardioplegic arrest. Some surgeons have performed TECAB on the beating heart while on partial CPB through femoral access. This allows for a decompressed and supported heart, but does not require special endoaortic balloon clamping.

Although arrested heart TECAB has been performed with some success, its minimally invasive nature when compared to RACAB is in question. Nonetheless, as facilitating technology improves, the role of arrested heart TECAB in complete myocardial revascularization remains to be seen.

Beating Heart TECAB

Beating heart TECAB is a procedure in which the robot is used for LITA mobilization, pericardotomy, vessel identification, vessel snaring, and anastomosis, all through four endoscopic ports. When the heart is beating, the anterior working space required for this operation is dependent on good chest insufflation, and tableside assistance is difficult. Several investigators have reported good short-term results for this procedure *(64,65)*. However, the learning curve for this procedure is long, and rapid surgeon adoption requires intensive preprocedure training.

Beating heart TECAB is the ultimate in minimally invasive revascularization, in that it is performed without CPB and with no incisions. Presently, beating heart TECAB can only be used to graft anteriorly located coronary vessels. The learning curve for this procedure has resulted in adoption by only a handful of surgeons, with most surgeons opting for RACAB as an off-pump, minimally invasive approach to LAD revascularization.

As with RACAB, beating heart TECAB requires close communication with the perfusion team. A perfusionist should be in the room with a primed pump, and the left groin should be prepped and accessible. Conversion would typically be performed with femoral bypass and limited thoracotomy.

CONCLUSION

Minimally invasive perfusion techniques involve many choices. These include choices of positioning, access, cannulation, and circuitry. Seemingly small decisions may have a much larger impact on the overall success of a given operation. Thus, all members of a minimally invasive team must understand the basic steps of these cardiac operations. The flow of the surgery and the quality of perfusion should remain constant. Proper attention to detail and careful patient selection are mandatory in the prevention of complications.

As technology moves forward in support of minimally invasive techniques, it is important to remember the basics of surgical success. Diligence in planning and a patient-specific strategy will improve the operational stresses that may present themselves during a minimally invasive procedure. With experience and training, the competence and confidence of the surgeon will grow. Quality assurance in the form of skills assessments, staff meetings, and free discussions of the implications of minimally invasive techniques will add to the basic training of all the team members. Building this strong framework of preparation and communication ultimately leads to successful outcomes.

REFERENCES

1. Pisano GP, Bohmer RM, Edmondson AC. Organizational Differences in Rates of Learning: Evidence from the Adoption of Minimally Invasive Cardiac Surgery. Management Sci 2001;47:752–768.
2. Banbury MK, White JA, Blackstone EH, Cosgrove DM. Vacuum-assisted venous return reduces blood usage. J Thorac Cardiovasc Surg 2003;126:680–687.
3. Hessel EA, II, Edmunds LH, Jr. Extracorporeal Circulation: Perfusion Systems. In Cardiac Surgery in the Adult. Cohn LH, Edmunds LH, Jr, editors. McGraw-Hill, New York. 2003:317–338.
4. Nelson DA, Lich BV. The Ultimate Guide to Assisted Venous Drainage. Available from: http://www.perfusion.com. Accessed.
5. Lapietra A, Grossi EA, Pua BB, Esposito RA, Galloway AC, Deriveux CC, et al. Assisted venous drainage presents the risk of undetected air microembolism. J Thorac Cardiovasc Surg 2000;120:856–862.
6. Barak M, Katz Y. Microbubbles: pathophysiology and clinical implications. Chest. 2005;128:2918–2932.
7. Likosky DS, Groom RC, Cantwell C, Forest RJ, et al. A method for identifying mechanisms of neurologic injury from cardiac surgery. Heart Surg Forum 2004; 7(6):348–352.
8. Wilcox TW, Mitchell MB, Gorman DF. Venous air in the bypass circuit: a source of arterial line emboli exacerbated by vacuum-assisted drainage. Ann Thorac Surg 1999;(68):1285–1289.
9. Cirri S, Negri L, Babbini M, Khlat B, et al. Haemolysis due to active venous drainage during cardiopulmonary bypass: comparison of two different techniques. Perfusion 2000;16(4):313–318.
10. Mueller XM, Tevaerai HT, Horisberger J, Augstburger M, Burke M, von Segesser LK. Vacuum assisted venous drainage does not increase trauma to blood cells. ASAIO J 2001;47(6):651–654.
11. Strauch JT, Spielvogel D, Lauten A, Galla JD, Lansman SL, McMurtry K, Griepp RB. Technical advances in total aortic arch replacement. Ann Thorac Surg 2004; 77(2):581–589; discussion 589–590.
12. Muhs BE, Galloway AC, Lombino M, et al. Arterial injuries from femoralartery cannulation with port access cardiac surgery. Vasc Endovascular Surg 2005:39(2): 153–158.
13. Schachner T, Bonaros N, Feuchtner G, et al. How to handle remote access perfusion for endoscopic cardiac surgery. Heart Surg Forum 2005;8(4):E232–E235.
14. Orihashi K, Sueda T, Okada K, Imai K. Newly developed aortic dissection in the abdominal aorta after femoral arterial perfusion. Ann Thorac Surg 2005;79: 1945–1949.
15. Navia JL, Cosgrove DM III. Minimally invasive mitral valve operations. Ann Thorac Surg 1996;62:1542–1544.

16. Cohn LH, Adams DH, Couper GS, et al. Minimally invasive cardiac valve surgery improves patient satisfaction while reducing costs of cardiac valve replacement and repair. Ann Surg 1997;226:421–426.
17. Gundry SR, Shattuck OH, Razzouk, AJ, et al. Facile minimally invasive cardiac surgery via ministernotomy. Ann Thorac Surg 1998;65:1100–1104.
18. Cosgrove DM, Sabik JF, Navia J. Minimally invasive valve surgery. Ann Thorac Surg 1998;65:1535–1539.
19. Cohn L. Operative incisions for minimally invasive cardiac surgery. Op Tech Thorac Cardiovasc Surg 2000;5:146–155.
20. Gillinov AM, Banbury MK, Cosgrove DM. hemisternotomy approach for aortic and mitral valve surgery. J Cardiac Surgery 2000;15:15–20.
21. Gillinov AM, Cosgrove DM. Minimally invasive mitral valve surgery: ministernotomy with extended transseptal approach. Sem Thorac Cardiovasc Surg 1999; 11:206–211.
22. Mihaljevic T, Cohn LH, Unic D, Aranki SF, Couper GS, Byrne JG. One thousand minimally invasive valve operations: early and late results. Ann Surg 2004;240: 529–534.
23. Grossi EA, Galloway AC, LaPietra A, et al. Minimally invasive mitral valve surgery: a 6 year experience with 714 patients. Ann Thorac Surg 2002;74: 660–663.
24. Vanermen H, Farhat F, Wellens F, et al. Minimally invasive video-assisted mitral valve surgery: from Port-Access towards a totally endoscopic procedure. J Cardiac Surg 2000;15:51–60.
25. Dogan S, Aybek T, Risteski PS, et al. Minimally invasive port access versus conventional mitral valve surgery: prospective randomized study. Ann Thorac Surg 2005;79:492–498.
26. Nifong LW, Chitwood WR, Pappas PS, et al. Robotic mitral valve surgery: A United States multicenter trial. J Thorac Cardiovasc Surg 2005;129:1395–1404.
27. Kypson AP, Chitwood WR, Jr. Robotic mitral valve surgery. Am J Surg 2004; 188(4A suppl):83S–88S.
28. Gillinov AM, Banbury MK, Cosgrove DM. Hemisternotomy approach for aortic and mitral valve surgery. J Card Surg 2000;15(1):15–20.
29. Bouchard D, Perrault LP, Carrier M, Menasche P, Bel A, Pelletier LC. Ministernotomy for aortic valve replacement: a study of the preliminary experience. Can J Surg 2000;43(1):39–42.
30. Bonacchi M, Prifti E, Giunti G, Frati G, Sani G. Does ministernotomy improve postoperative outcome in aortic valve operation? A prospective randomized study. Ann Thorac Surg. 2002;73(2):460–465; discussion 465–466.
31. Liu J, Sidiropoulos A, Konertz W. Minimally invasive aortic valve replacement (AVR) compared to standard AVR. Eur J Cardiothorac Surg 1999;16:280–283.
32. Dias AR, Dias RR, Gaiotto F, et al. Mini-sternotomy for treatment of aortic valve lesions. Arq Bras Cardiol 2001:7:221–228.
33. Hayashi Y, Sawa Y, Nishimura M, Sathoh H, Ohtake S, Matsuda H. Avoidance of full-sternotomy: effect on inflammatory cytokine production during cardiopulmonary bypass in rats. J Card Surg 2003;18(5):390–395.
34. Svensson LG. Progress in ascending and aortic arch surgery: minimally invasive surgery, blood conservation, and neurological deficit prevention. Ann Thorac Surg 2002;74(5):S1786–S1788; discussion S1792–S1799.
35. Svensson LG, Nadolny EM, Kimmel WA. Minimal access aortic surgery including re-operations. Eur J Cardiothorac Surg 2001;19(1):30–33.

36. Byrne JG, Adams DH, Couper GS, Rizzo RJ, Cohn LH, Aranki SF. Minimally-invasive aortic root replacement. Heart Surg Forum 1999;2(4):326–329.
37. Sun L, Zheng J, Chang Q, Tang Y, Feng J, Sun X, Zhu X. Aortic root replacement by ministernotomy: technique and potential benefit. Ann Thorac Surg 2000; 70(6):1958–1961.
38. Demirsoy E, Arbatli H, Unal M, Yagan N, Tukenmez F, Sonmez B. Atrial septal defect repair with minithoracotomy using two stage single venouscannula. J Cardiovasc Surg 2004 Feb;45(1):21–25.
39. Doll N, Walther T, Falk V, et al. Secundum ASD closure using a right lateral minithoracotomy: five-year experience in 122 patients. Ann Thorac Surg 2003; 75(5):1527–1530; discussion 1530–1531.
40. Bonaros N, Schachner T, Oehlinger A, et al. Experience on the way to totally endoscopic atrial septal defect repair. Heart Surg Forum 2004;7(5): E440–E445.
41. Morgan JA, Peacock JC, Kohmoto T, et al. Robotic techniques improve quality of life in patients undergoing atrial septaldefect repair. Ann Thorac Surg 2004 Apr;77(4):1328–1333.
42. Argenziano M, Oz MC, Kohmoto T, et al. Totally endoscopic atrial septal defect repair with robotic assistance. Circulation 2003;108:II191–II194.
43. Puskas J, Cheng D, Knight J, et al. Off-pump versus conventional coronary artery bypass grafting: A meta-analysis and consensus statement from the 2004 ISMICS consensus. Innovations 2005;1:3–27.
44. Cheng DC, Bainbridge D, Martin JA, Novick RJ. Does off-pump coronary artery bypass reduce mortality, morbidity and resource utilization when compared to conventional coronary artery bypass? A meta-analysis of randomized trials. Anesthesiology 2005;102:188–203.
45. Khan NE, De Souza A, Mister R, et al. A randomized comparison of off-pump and on-pump multivessel coronary-artery bypass surgery. N Engl J Med 2004; 350:21–28.
46. Puskas JD, Williams WH, Duke PG, et al. Off-pump coronary artery bypass grafting provides complete revascularization with reduced myocardial injury, transfusion requirements and length of stay: A prospective randomized comparison of two hundred unselected patients undergoing off-pump versus conventional coronary artery bypass grafting. J Thorac Cardiovasc Surg 2003;125:797–808.
47. Zamvar V, Williams D, Hall J, et al. Assessment of neurocognitive impairment after off-pump and on-pump techniques for coronary artery bypass graft surgery: prospective randomized controlled trial. BMJ 2002;325:1268.
48. van Dijk D, Jansen EWL, Hijman R, et al. for the Octopus Study Group. Cognitive outcome after off-pump and on-pump coronary artery bypass graft surgery. A randomized trial. JAMA 2002;287:1405–1412.
49. Lund C, Hol PK, Lundbland R, et al. Comparison of cerebral embolization during off-pump and on-pump coronary artery bypass surgery. Ann Thorac Surg 2003; 76:765–770.
50. Al-Ruzzeh S, Nakamura K, Athanasiou T, et al. Does off-pump coronary artery bypass (OPCAB) surgery improve the outcome in high risk patients?: A comparative study of 1398 high-risk patients. Eur J Cardiothorac Surg 2003;23: 50–55.
51. Boyd WD, Desai ND, Del Rizzo DF, et al. Off-pump surgery decreases postoperative complications and resource utilization in the elderly. Ann Thorac Surg 1999;68:1490–1493.

52. Martinovic I, Farah I, Mair R, et al. Reduced mortality and cerebrovascular morbidity with off-pump coronary artery bypass grafting surgery in octogenarians. Heart Surg Forum 2003;6:S13.
53. Nanthoe HM, van Dijk D, Jansen EWL, et al. A comparison of on-pump and off-pump coronary bypass surgery in low-risk patients. N Engl J Med 2003;348: 394–402.
54. Edgerton JR, Dewey TM, Magee MJ, et al. Conversion in off-pump coronary artery bypass grafting: An analysis of predictors and outcomes. Ann Thorac Surg 2003;76:1138–1143.
55. DeRose JJ, Jr., Balaram SK, Ro C, et al. Mid-term results and patient perceptions of robotically-assisted coronary artery bypass grafting. Interactive Cardiovasc Thorac Surg 2005;4:406–411.
56. Mohr FW, Falk V, Diegeler A, et al. Computer-enhanced robotic cardiac surgery—Experience in 148 patients. J Thorac Cardiovasc Surg 2001;121:842–853.
57. Srivastava S, Gadasalli S, Agusala M, et al. Use of bilateral internal thoracic arteries in CABG through lateral thoracotomy with robotic assistance in 150 patients. Ann Thorac Surg 2006;81:800–806.
58. Subramanian S, Patel NU, Patel NC, Loulmet DF. Robotic assisted multivessel minimally invasive direct coronary artery bypass with port-access stabilization and cardiac positioning: paving the way for outpatient coronary surgery? Ann Thorac Surg 2005;79:1590–1596.
59. Vassiliades. Atraumatic coronary artery bypass: technique and outcomes. Heart Surg Forum 2001;4:331–334.
60. Lee MS, Wilentz JR, Raj R, et al. Hybrid revascularization using percutaneous coronary intervention and robotically-assisted minimally invasive direct coronary artery bypass surgery. J Invasive Cardiol 2004;16:419–425.
61. Riess FC, Bader R, Kremer P, et al. Coronary hybrid revascularization from January 1997 to January 2001: a clinical follow-up. Ann Thorac Surg 2002;73: 1849–1855.
62. Dogan S, Aybek T, Andressen E, et al. Totally endoscopic coronary artery bypass grafting on cardiopulmonary bypass with robotically enhanced telemanipulation: report of forty-five cases. J Thorac Cardiovasc Surg 2002;123:1125–1131.
63. Kappert U, Schneider J, Cichon R, et al. Closed chest totally endoscopic coronary artery bypass surgery: fantasy or reality? Current Card Rep 2000;2:558–563.
64. Mohr FW, Falk V, Diegeler A, et al. Computer-enhanced robotic cardiac surgery—Experience in 148 patients. J Thorac Cardiovasc Surg 2001;121:842–853.
65. Falk V, Diegeler A, Walther T, et al. Endoscopic coronary artery bypass grafting on the beating heart using a computer enhanced telemanipulation system. Heart Surg Forum 1999;2:199–205.

8 Cannulation and Clinical Concerns for Cardiopulmonary Bypass Access

James R. Beck, BS, CCP,
David Y. Park, BS, CCP, and
Linda B. Mongero, BS, CCP

CONTENTS

CANNULATION AND CLINICAL CONCERNS FOR CARDIOPULMONARY BYPASS ACCESS

Diversion of blood into an extracorporeal circuit for facilitation of cardiopulmonary bypass (CPB) and return to the patient is commonplace in today's cardiothoracic theater. However, of late, many new cannula options are allowing remote or noncentral cannulation for specialized procedures, as well as innovative technology to improve existing techniques. The purpose of this chapter is to explore the principles, concepts, and possibilities for various cannulation sites and techniques, coupled with an understanding of flow dynamics necessary for successful implementation of CPB.

From: *Current Cardiac Surgery: On Bypass: Advanced Perfusion Techniques*
Edited by: L. B. Mongero and J. R. Beck © Humana Press Inc., Totowa, NJ

VENOUS CANNULATION

Basics of Venous Return

Facilitation of venous return from the patient to the extracorporeal circuitry may be accomplished via a host of cannula options, as well as cannulation sites *(1–5)*. Before we explore the options of cannula selection and cannulation sites, we must first understand the basics of venous drainage. Blood flows within the extracorporeal circuit because of pressure difference; i.e., blood flows from an area of higher pressure to an area of lower pressure *(6)*. Within the venous limb of the circuit, this area of lower pressure may be created by various techniques. These include gravity siphoning by locating the venous reservoir below the level of the patient or by augmenting venous return by applying negative pressure to the venous line. The latter may be accomplished utilizing vacuum assistance or kinetic assistance by using a pump to actively drain (or create an area of lower pressure within) the extracorporeal circuit. As described by Poiseuille's law, flow within a tube (Q) is equal to pressure (P) divided by resistance (R) ($Q = P/R$), and resistance within a tube may be described by viscosity times length divided by the radius to the forth power ($R = VxL/r^4$) *(6)*. Understanding the forces that determine blood flow is important as we examine the various contributors to venous return.

The amount of venous return will be affected by many factors, including the patient's blood volume, table height and amount of negative pressure, cannula placement, resistance in the venous cannula, CPB tubing, connectors, and circuit configuration *(4,5,7–9,10)*. As clinicians, we devote a great deal of attention to troubleshooting and optimizing various CPB parameters. Often, the most variable of these parameters will be the adequacy of venous return. We could not discuss venous cannulation for CPB without examining each of the factors that play a role in determining the amount of venous return in greater detail.

DETERMINANTS OF VENOUS RETURN

Cannula Selection

Let us begin by looking at cannula selection. For the clinician to choose the proper cannula size and shape, one must first gather some crucial information. First, we need to determine the patient's flow requirements. We should not be fooled by simply calculating flow based solely on body surface area (BSA). We should also consider extenuating circumstances that may necessitate flow requirements above or below those calculated on BSA. These patient conditions may include profound dilatation, volume-overload states, high-output disorders, pregnancy, and any other conditions that may require flow rates in excess of those calculated on BSA. Next, we should consider the surgical plan in respect to cannulation sites. For example, central cannulation may be accomplished with an appropriately sized single venous cannula placed within the right atrium, or via bicaval, i.e., superior vena cava (SVC) and inferior vena cava (IVC) cannulae, depending on the surgical approach. Remote, or noncentral, venous access may include adequately sized and shaped cannulae for groin access (femoral vein), neck access (jugular vein), or less common access sites for CPB drainage *(10–18)*. Once we have gathered the necessary information to determine desired flow rates and cannula shape (based on surgical access and surgeon preference), we must determine cannula size. Cannula size selection is best accomplished by referencing individual cannula flow characteristics established by the manufacturer or by bench-top testing *(3,5)*. Most manufactures provide cannula flow charts that rate pressure drop (or negative pressure) versus flow rates for a particular size and shape cannula, usually rated using water in liters per minute. Using this reference is important, but should not be the sole source for cannula size selection. As clinicians, we must also assess individual patient and surgical parameters that may affect our choice of cannula size. For instance, what will we anticipate for negative pressure during a particular procedure? Negative pressure for gravity siphoning can be estimated (in centimeters of water) as the height difference between the patient and the top of the level in your venous reservoir. During augmented venous return (vacuum or kinetic), additional negative pressure can be added to the height difference to allow greater venous return with smaller sized cannulae *(19–22)*. Patient parameters must also play a role in cannula size selection. For instance, a 27-French femoral vein cannula will provide greater flow than a similar 21-French cannula, but vessel size may prohibit use of such cannulae. Site selection may also play a role in cannula size selection. For example, when cannulating the internal jugular vein for minimally invasive procedures, the smallest sized percutaneous cannula for a given pressure drop and flow may help prevent blocking side branch vessels, thus avoiding cerebral venous congestion and its subsequent sequelae. In another example, choosing too small a cannula can also be problematic. Not only may venous return be inadequate, but undersized cannulae may also produce problematic positioning issues, such as cannula tip occlusion during myocardial retraction or cannulae that may flip or become dislodged during cardiac manipulation. Preoperative discussion of cannula size, shape, composition, and design, as well as the planned surgical procedure, may aid in avoiding venous return issues after initiation of CPB.

Site Selection and Surgical Techniques

As previously discussed, site selection will play a role in determining cannula selection. Equally important is the placement of the venous cannula at a given surgical site, as well as the physical correlation between cannula drainage holes, tissue proximity, available volume, and a host of additional factors. We can get a better understanding of how many of these factors come into play as we look at various cannulation sites. Also, keep in mind that many of these factors may be realized at multiple cannulation sites, and that the clinician should be prudent when troubleshooting venous return issues.

Typically, central venous cannulation is accomplished via insertion of cannulae into the right atrium. This may be facilitated with a single-stage venous cannula, a dual stage cavoatrial cannula, or bicaval cannulation into the SVC and IVC *(1–3,5)*. Although these common approaches to venous return usually provide adequate flow, they are not entirely without limitation. When using a single two-stage (cavoatrial) cannula, it is important to assess venous return shortly after commencement of CPB and before myocardial retraction. The two-stage venous cannula is generally placed in the right atrial (RA) appendage, with the smaller tip positioned in the inferior vena cava. Occasionally, the tip of this cannula can become occluded by the Eustachian valve at the IVC–RA junction, or by improper placement or advancing the cannula into a side branch of the IVC. Likewise, any venous cannula can be partially or totally occluded by entrapment of tissue in cannula drainage holes. Assessing this entrapment can be difficult, and we will discuss the clinical indicators for this situation in greater detail shortly. Bicaval cannulation is often used when right heart access is needed or if myocardial retraction is expected to impede RA venous return. Caval tapes or snares are often placed around the cavae and through small tourniquets, which are cinched down to capture all venous return and prevent air from entering the venous circuit when opening the right heart *(23)*. This can also be problematic if cannulae are malpositioned, or if caval snares occlude the cannula tip. Clinicians should pay careful attention to central venous pressure (CVP) and venous return when these caval tapes or snares are being cinched down and during periods of myocardial positioning and retraction. Changes in venous return should be promptly discussed with the surgical team so adjustments can be made to avoid prolonged periods of poor venous return, venous congestion, and low flow states.

With the advent of minimally invasive surgery, as well as advances in complex cardiac and vascular repair, the need for remote or non-central venous cannulation has continued to grow. As new surgical techniques arise, the perfusion and surgical community will continue to be challenged with new, and sometimes problematic, cannulation issues. For example, new hybrid cannulation techniques are emerging, such as groin and neck cannulation for minimally invasive mitral valve (MV) and robotic surgery, central cannulation with oval, and various innovative cannulae to optimize visualization and use of smaller cannulae with augmented (vacuum and kinetic) venous return. Each of these techniques embraces distinct advantages and, sometimes, new concerns over older, standard cannulation techniques *(24–27)*.

Neck or internal jugular cannulation has proven useful in minimally invasive techniques, as well as some reoperations when sternotomy or thoracotomy is risky. However, clinicians must be prudent when using this technique. Cannula placement should be with the tip of the percutaneous cannula at the SVC–RA junction for MV repairs or just proximal to the SVC–RA junction for procedures requiring caval snares *(14)*. Whenever possible, flow from the neck cannula should be monitored independently from inferior cannula drainage. Cerebral venous congestion can be problematic when using this technique, and adequate cerebral drainage must be monitored. To facilitate drainage with smaller percutaneous neck cannulae, augmented venous return is usually needed. Clinicians should use extreme caution when employing these techniques, and they should become familiar with the many problems and pitfalls that can accompany use of vacuum- or kinetic-assisted venous return *(28,29)*. New pump and circuit technology coupled with various alarms, safety features, and regulator technology has greatly improved the safety of assisted venous return.

Groin or femoral vein access has been used successfully for remote venous access for many years. New, thin-wall, wire-wound, multistage cannula technology coupled with augmented venous return has allowed greater flow rates with smaller percutaneous cannulae. However, these cannulae and percutaneous insertion techniques are not without risk. Injuries to the femoral artery and dissections or lacerations of the femoral vein, iliac, and IVC have been reported *(30)*. Careful placement of these cannulae is necessary to prevent side- and end-hole occlusion or cannula kinking upon retraction, especially when used in conjunction with augmented venous return *(20,21,31)*. Each of these cannulation techniques may play an important role as cardiac surgery leaps into the next century. Careful cannula placement, site selection, and surgical technique will be successful only in the presence of adequate patient blood volume.

Volume Status

Once anticoagulation, cannula choice, site selection, and surgical placement are complete, we turn to assessment of clinical parameters for determination of venous return. It seems painfully obvious that without sufficient patient blood volume, adequate venous return cannot be accomplished. However, venous access and volume assessment are often not clear-cut. So, where do we begin with the assessment of volume available for venous return?

The amount of volume available for venous return is determined by the pressure in the central veins (CVP). This pressure is influenced by several factors, including the intravascular volume, the venous compliance, and the arterial flow rate versus venous drainage relationship on CPB and the inclusion or exclusion of venous compartments during various surgical techniques using caval or vascular snares. Because venous return may vary during manipulation and retraction of the heart, it is important to obtain and assess venous return parameters early during CPB and before cardiac retraction. CVP is a good indicator of venous volume and should be monitored continuously during CPB.

The most commonly used measurement for CVP is obtained via the right atrial port of the Swan–Ganz catheter. It is important to understand the relationship between CVP monitoring from this port, the location or height of the transducer (preferably at the level of the RA), and the surgical approach or technique to be utilized for a given procedure. When a single RA cannula or dual-stage RA cannula is used, CVP monitoring from the RA port of the Swan–Ganz catheter usually provides an adequate assessment of venous volume throughout the cardiac procedure. Early assessment of CVP while on bypass will help the clinician troubleshoot later venous return issues related to positioning and cannula entrapment if cardiac manipulation causes a sharp rise in CVP coupled with acute decreases in venous return. This situation is relatively common and may be rectified by cardiac repositioning or brief periods of lower flow to facilitate surgical repair.

When remote, noncentral, or bicaval cannulation is used, CVP monitoring and assessment may be more tricky *(32)*. If bicaval cannulation is used in conjunction with caval snares, the RA port of the Swan–Ganz catheter may be isolated from the circulation. Relying on the CVP from the RA port of the Swan–Ganz catheter may be erroneous in this situation. It is important to understand this concept because cannula entrapment and loss of venous return may not be reflected by changes in the CVP value. Alternative sources of CVP monitoring may be useful whenever bicaval or noncentral venous cannulation is used and exclusion or isolation of the right atrium is expected. Often, a combination of techniques may be useful in determining venous volume. For example, monitoring the side port of the Swan introducer (usually located proximal to venous cannulae) during procedures requiring RA isolation will allow the clinician to assess volume of the head and neck to ensure adequate cerebral perfusion and avoid cerebral venous congestion. However, this does not offer any indication of IVC or lower body venous return, which may be assessed solely by changes in returning volume or other sites of venous pressure monitoring. Changes and complications associated with venous return may not be limited to subtle variations in the central venous pressure.

Troubleshooting

Troubleshooting poor or suboptimal venous return may include assessment of cannula and surgical site selection, surgical technique, and volume status, as previously discussed, as well as a host of mechanical and clinical issues *(33,34)*. Mechanical opposition to adequate venous return may range from simple occurrences such as kinked venous lines, inadequate patient height for gravity return, airlock, or cannula obstruction, to tricky, less common causes such as partial or total vessel laceration and situations of venous reservoir pressurization.

A no-nonsense approach to troubleshooting mechanical impedance to venous return should begin at the cannula tip and extend to the reservoir outlet. Is the cannula positioned with the tip inserted into the azygous, innominate, or hepatic veins? Has the cannula tip flipped or turned to allow partial or total occlusion of the drainage holes? Have caval snares or myocardial retraction or positioning occluded drainage holes? Has vacuum or assisted drainage caused atria or vessel collapse or tissue entrapment of venous drainage holes? Is the venous line kinked or clamped, and can you visually follow the course of that line from cannula to reservoir? Is an airlock present? Can it be removed, and where is the air originating? Is the table height sufficient? Is the reservoir vented appropriately, and, if augmenting venous return, is the vacuum source on or is the kinetic assist pump on? After assessing the more common causes of mechanical obstruction to venous return, one might consider more unusual occurrences, such as venous dissection and extraluminal or transeptal placement of the venous return catheter into the left atrium. Other unusual mechanical obstructions may include use of augmented or VAVR with improper reservoir venting, and possible venous reservoir pressurization or malfunctioning regulating equipment. Causes of low venous return may also be assessed by evaluating clinical issues *(35)*.

Clinical observation may be helpful in troubleshooting venous return issues. As discussed previously, volume status plays an important role in determining the adequacy of venous return. However, volume assessment should not be based solely on measurements of CVP. Clinicians may begin by asking, "Where is the venous volume? Has the volume moved to an extravascular space?" This condition may be caused by several factors, including bleeding, translocation to extravascular spaces, and urine output. Reduced venous pressure may also be a result of venodilatation with various drug therapies, patient positioning with legs down allowing a large venous capacitance pooling, or pathological conditions of circulating hypovolemia. In addition, intermittent collapse and release of intimal walls around cannula openings (often called venous line chatter) may impede normal flow patterns and cause reduced venous return. This condition may be ameliorated by partially clamping the venous line or slightly raising the venous reservoir to reduce the negative pressure in the venous line to restore normal flow patterns and increase venous return volume. One should exercise care when using these techniques because retarding venous return too much may allow blood to flow around venous cannulae, causing possible premature warming of the myocardium, distention, or obstruction of surgical view.

AUGMENTED VENOUS RETURN

Early CPB circuits used a variety of suction-type pumps to control venous return. Many of these applications were difficult to control and were rapidly abandoned for simpler techniques, such as gravity drainage. Of late, there has been renewed interest in augmented venous return techniques to allow use of miniaturized circuitry and smaller cannulae and tubing for minimally invasive surgical procedures. By increasing the amount of negative pressure applied to the venous line, smaller cannulae and tubing are capable of providing greater flow rates over gravity siphonage alone. The application of negative pressure to the venous line may be facilitated by several methods. These include applying regulated vacuum to a closed hard-shell venous reservoir or a modified soft-shell venous reservoir enclosed within a rigid housing, or by use of a centrifugal or roller pump for kinetically assisted venous drainage (KAVD).

Although each of these techniques is capable of augmenting venous return, each of them carries certain risks, benefits, and possible pitfalls. Using a roller pump in the venous line between the cannula and venous reservoir is one method. Historically, this method carries the risk of generating extremely high negative pressure in the venous line with increased hemolysis; however, newer pump technology may allow automated pressure regulation of these pumps *(36)*. This technique may also be more labor intensive because it requires constant adjustment of pump flow rates based on available venous volume. Also, in the event of cannula entrapment, high negative pressure may injure intimal walls and make cannula release difficult. Another technique allowing kinetic-assisted venous return incorporates a centrifugal pump into the venous line between the cannula and venous reservoir *(20,32)*. Although this method can require less attention to flow rate adjustment than the roller pump technique, it is not without fault. Centrifugal pumps add a component of cost, and if air is entrapped in the venous line, most centrifugal pumps will break the air up into many smaller bubbles, which may readily pass through the extracorporeal circuit and into the patient's systemic circulation.

A third method of augmenting venous return utilizes a vacuum applied to a hard-shell, nonvented venous reservoir or, more recently, applying vacuum to the exterior of a soft-shell venous reservoir enclosed within a rigid sealed housing *(22,37,39)*. When using this method the vacuum source must be regulated to maintain negative pressures below 100 mmHg.

Challenges and Risks

Augmented venous return carries several potential risks over conventional gravity drainage techniques, and clinicians should become familiar with problematic areas associated with these techniques *(38)*. As mentioned, negative pressure should be maintained below 100 mmHg to avoid increased sheer stress on red blood cells and resultant hemolysis. Augmenting negative pressure on the venous line may also increase the risk of cannula tip and side-hole entrapment, as well as increase the risk of air aspiration from RA holes or around cannula purse-string sutures or snares. In addition to clinical concerns, clinicians must be attentive to pump and mechanical functions of augmented venous return to avoid possible catastrophic events. One of the primary pitfalls of augmented and vacuum assisted venous return is air embolization *(28,40,41)*. The possibility of gaseous embolization exists in several different scenarios of augmented venous return. As mentioned, increasing or augmenting the negative pressure in the venous line may increase the amount of air being pulled into the extracorporeal circuit from cardiac and vascular holes, as well as cannula insertion sites. Some degree of venous air may be passed into the systemic circulation *(42)*.

When using VAVR, extreme caution should be observed. Obstruction of the vent or vacuum port could result in pressurization of the reservoir, loss of venous return, and rapid gaseous embolization of the patient. Pressure in the reservoir can quickly exceed relatively low CVP, obstruct venous drainage, and force air retrograde up the venous line causing massive air embolization. A pressurized venous reservoir may also cause the reservoir to empty, allowing air to enter the blood path of the oxygenator. If a vapor trap is used, it should not be allowed to completely fill during use because this condition could obstruct the reservoir vent, causing reservoir pressurization. Clinicians should exercise caution during periods of low flow or when coming off of CPB in cases using VAVR. The vacuum should be released and the reservoir vented to atmosphere before even brief periods of termination of CPB or very low flow states. During these periods, use of a vacuum can lead to negative pressure in the oxygenator and potential air embolization by pulling air across the oxygenator fibers and into the blood path. The sample system, the arterial purge line, a hemoconcentrator, a nonocclusive roller pump, a centrifugal pump, or any other connection between the patient arterial line and the reservoir may provide a conduit for the vacuum to be applied to the arterial side of the oxygenator, thereby facilitating inadvertent air embolization.

Of late, several safety features and techniques have allowed safer conduct of CPB while using VAVR. All reservoirs used in conjunction with VAVR should be equipped with positive pressure-relief valves. In addition, negative pressure should be regulated with a reliable vacuum controller equipped with a negative pressure pop off, preventing excessive negative pressure from being applied to the reservoir *(1,43)*. When using VAVR in conjunction with centrifugal arterial pumps, it is helpful to use a one-way duckbill valve between the centrifugal pump and oxygenator to prevent accidental retrograde flow and to help prevent negative pressurization of the oxygenator with subsequent air embolization. In addition to protected, regulated vacuum sources, positive and negative pressure relief devices, and one-way valves, it is also advisable to monitor reservoir and arterial pressures at all times while employing VAVR. Many newer pumps have both positive and negative pressure-monitoring capabilities, along with audible alarms. Using these features is very helpful in avoiding catastrophic air embolization. For instance, setting an arterial line pressure alarm at –1 mmHg is helpful because you never want negative pressure in your oxygenator or arterial limb of the CPB circuit. Likewise, setting a pressure alarm on your reservoir of 1 or 2 mmHg is helpful because you never want to pressurize your venous reservoir. Clinicians using older pump technology may benefit from simpler indicators. For example, having an empty bag on an open prime line will yield a visual alert to a pressurized reservoir as the bag begins to blow up like a balloon. Another example of simple tricks to avoid mistakes involves vacuum regulation and atmospheric venting of venous reservoirs. Because most centers use tubing with a connection for VAVR (i.e., one end of a "y" open to atmosphere and the other end connected to the vacuum source), placing tape targets on each of these limbs allows the perfusionist to easily identify where to place a single clamp for either VAVR or atmospheric venting, thus reducing the risk of a misplaced clamp and accidental reservoir pressurization (Fig. 1). Early recognition of these conditions may allow the clinician to avoid catastrophic

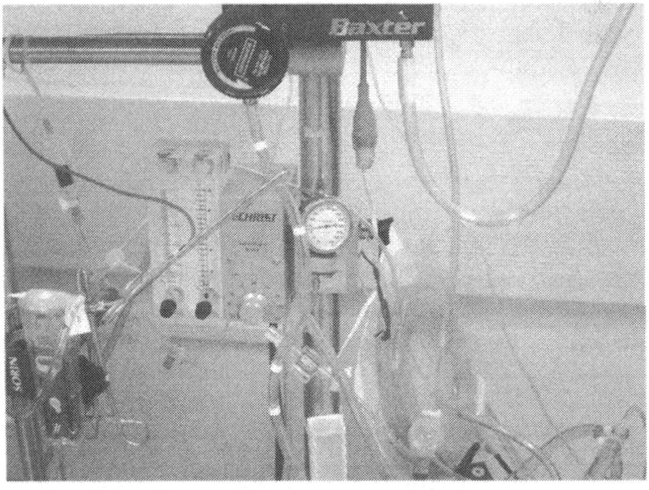

Fig. 1. VAVR line with white tape targets to prevent clamp placement errors.

adverse events. As we advance into a new era of cardiac care, many new techniques and technologies may emerge. We must evaluate these techniques with cautious optimism and sound scientific judgment to ensure safe and improved care for the outpatient population.

ARTERIAL CANNULATION

Basics of Arterial Cannulae

There are a host of various cannula shapes, sizes, and features, each designed to aid in insertion or ameliorate deleterious effects of returning extracorporeal blood flow. For example, the most basic cannula design is an extruded piece of plastic tubing narrowed at one end, usually with a beveled or tapered tip. This cannula type is often referred to as the "Bardic type." Early use of these stiff, relatively thick, plastic-walled cannulae allowed the surgeon to gain arterial access for extracorporeal blood return in an inexpensive, single-use, disposable product. Although some of these cannulae are still in use today, engineers and surgeons quickly began to explore variations to improve on this most basic design. A flange was added to aid in fixation and to prevent too much cannula length from being inserted into the vessel. Further exploration of cannula qualities such as pressure drop, realized that high flow rates through these narrow, thick-walled cannulae led to higher pressure gradients, high flow jets, turbulence, and, ultimately, greater sheer stress with damage to blood components *(44)*. The need for easier cannula insertion coupled with scientific evaluation of cannula flow patterns led to improved cannula design. These improvements included thin-walled plastic and metal-tipped cannulae with lower pressure drop, angled cannulae for improved positioning within the vessel, molded flanges or feet for ease of securing, and integral barbed and luered connectors for quick hookup and deairing, as well as diffusion-tipped cannulae to alleviate the adverse effects of jetting return against intimal vessel walls *(45)*. Today many different cannula shapes, sizes, materials, and features offer the clinician a range of choices based on necessary flow dynamics, surgical site selection, operative plan, and surgeon preference. With the extensive choice of cannula options, it may be difficult to discern which arterial cannula is best suited for any given patient.

Cannula Choice

Cannula choice is easy. Just calculate the flow rate and pick the size. Correct? Well, not so fast! There are multiple factors dictating proper cannula selection, and choosing poorly may end in complications ranging from mild morbidity to catastrophic mortality. As previously discussed, a host of cannula features exist, each of which may offer benefit or risk to a particular surgical approach. Weighing the risk/benefit ratio is essential, and recognizing how each of these features may impact the surgical procedure will allow the perfusion, surgical, and anesthesia teams to discuss the best cannula option for every case. Because it would be impossible to review every arterial cannula, we will discuss various cannula features (i.e., pros and cons) coupled with surgical site selection and operative techniques in greater detail. Keep in mind that basic cannula features may apply to a number of different cannulae used at various insertion sites.

Central Aortic Cannulation

As discussed earlier, any cannula selection should begin by determining patient flow requirements. Remember, simply calculating flow based on BSA may not be sufficient. Consider all patient parameters, including current cardiac output, unusual situations, and pathological states. Next, we must consider the surgical plan in respect to the insertion site for arterial cannulation. Finally, we narrow down our choice based on desired flow rate, cannula shape, size, surgical access, and surgeon preference.

The most common site for arterial cannulation is the ascending aorta or arch. Using the aorta avoids additional surgical site access and possible additional complications. However, where to physically place the arterial cannula within the aorta raises additional concerns *(46,47)*. For instance, the condition or quality of the aortic wall, presence of atherosclerotic disease, or visualization concerns may play a role in aortic cannula site placement and cannula choice. First, we must determine the cannula shape best suited for aortic cannulation. Surgeon preference, belief, and technique often play a major role in selection of the aortic cannula shape. Various angled and straight-tipped cannulae offer a host of benefits in respect to tip positioning within the aorta, length of cannula within the vessel, and lie, or position outside the vessel without impeding surgical access or obstructing surgical view. Next, the desired cannula features, such as material, securing flanges, tip design, and connection options, must be assessed. Cannula materials may play an important role in determining cannula function. These can include choice of metal tip versus plastic, stiff versus soft, and wire-wound versus nonreinforced. Metal tips may provide the best in internal-to-outside diameter ratio (or lowest pressure gradient for a given outer size); however, that same very thin wall may also be somewhat sharp, possibly dislodging atheroemboli or damaging intimal walls. Conversely, plastic tips may yield higher pressure gradients, but may be gentler upon insertion. Stiffer arterial cannulae may offer both risks and benefits as well. Stiffer cannulae may be easier to insert, but can cause vessel injury or possible malpositioning during periods of cardiac manipulation or retraction. Softer bodied cannulae may be more challenging to insert, but may provide free movement for cardiac retraction and cannula positioning within the pericardial well, facilitating improved surgical view. Fixed flanges may provide the most secure placement of aortic cannulae; however, these features may dictate where surgeons must place cannula restraint sutures and may not allow surgeons to determine how far to advance the cannula tip based on a particular surgical procedure or pathological finding. Tip design may play a role in reducing morbidity associated with aortic cannulation. A single end-hole may allow a steady flow centrally directed with less turbulence; however, if poorly positioned, this same feature may cause intimal damage. Multiple side holes may reduce the jetting effect of single end-hole cannulae, allowing pressure relief if poorly positioned, but when in close proximity to vessel walls this may dislodge atheroemboli or even cause intimal wall damage from continuous flow directed toward intimal tissue. Diffusion-tipped cannulae may yield softer or gentler flow, reducing the jetting effects of single end-hole or end-/side-hole combination aortic cannulae. However, these cannulae may cause more turbulent blood flow, possibly disrupting atheroemboli, and may increase pressure gradients over other designs. Connection features like barber connectors make it easier to hook up extracorporeal tubing, but may add cost, and luer connections may facilitate de-airing, but may also be a potential source of blood leakage or air entry if not properly secured.

Various techniques may be employed to reduce the adverse effects associated with arterial cannulation of the ascending aorta and aortic arch *(48–53)*. Atherosclerosis frequently involves the ascending aorta and may pose a challenge during aortic cannulation. Physical disruption of calcifications and atheromatous material during cannula insertion, aortic cross-clamping, aortic manipulation, and cannula flow patterns may lead to increased postoperative morbidity *(54,55)*. Techniques to avoid manipulation of susceptible areas of the aorta include manual palpation, palpation with inflow occlusion, epiaortic scanning, and use of transesophageal echocardiography (TEE) *(48,56)*. Although TEE is convenient and often readily available in the operating suite, its use in selecting cannulation sites is not optimal because of limited views of the ascending aorta. In cases of severe atheroma, some advocate use of noncentral, alternate cannulation sites, such as the femoral or axillary arteries or use of elongated arterial cannulae, which can be advanced past atheromatous areas into the arch or proximal descending aorta. Once aortic cannulation is complete, confirmation of location within the central lumen of the aorta should be made. This may include a combination of techniques, including rapid back bleeding of the cannula, checking for pulsatility within the arterial limb of the extracorporeal circuit, comparing radial pressure to central arterial pressure measured off the aortic cannula, as well as a small "test dose" of forward flow from the extracorporeal circuit while monitoring appropriate line pressure coupled with surgical observation of the aorta and cannulation site. Intraoperative observation of arterial line pressure may often be helpful. Tracking changes in arterial (CPB circuit) line pressure may help avoid complications like cannula tip malposition, arterial tubing, or cannula kink, cannula occlusion by placement of the aortic cross clamp, poor cannula size choice, and aortic dissection. The clinician should be suspect of the latter when accompanied by sudden decrease in venous return volume, decrease in arterial pressure, loss of circulating perfusate, increase in arterial line pressure, bleeding from around the cannulation site, and possible hematoma surrounding the aortic cannula. In addition to injuries of the aorta, alternate cannulation sites may be used when dictated by surgical approach, operative techniques, and pathological findings.

Femoral Artery

Cannulation of the femoral or iliac arteries may be indicated for operative procedures of the ascending arch and descending aorta, reoperations where surgical access may be risky or problematic, and, of late, minimally invasive surgical procedures. Due to limitation of the femoral artery lumen, smaller-sized arterial cannulae are often required. These cannulae may increase the "jetting" effect associated with small end-hole openings at greater flow rates, and may also have higher sheer rates, as is expected with larger pressure gradients. Surgical complications of femoral artery cannulation have also been reported *(57–59)*. The most common complication is trauma to the cannulated vessel, including tears, dissections, bleeding, thrombosis, infection, and limb ischemia distal to cannula insertion sites. The most serious complication of femoral artery cannulation is retrograde arterial dissection, which may extend to the aortic root *(57,60)*. The clinical picture may resemble the antegrade dissection described earlier with sudden decrease in venous return, loss of arterial blood pressure, increased line pressure, excessive bleeding around the cannula insertion site, and possible presence of a hematoma. When this situation causes a flap in the arterial vessel with resultant retrograde dissection, it may be possible to recannulate the aorta proximally (i.e., true lumen) and restore antegrade flow patterns to rectify the problem. Use of the TEE may be helpful in diagnosing retrograde aortic dissections.

Because femoral artery cannulae often occlude the entire vessel lumen, distal limb ischemia, and resultant complications (acidosis, compartment syndrome, neuropathy, and necrosis) should be considered. Short periods, usually less than 3–6 h, are tolerated *(59,61)*, but for longer ischemic times, it may be prudent to consider lower limb perfusion techniques. This may be accomplished by using a y connector or luer port in the arterial perfusion line with a small (pediatric) arterial cannula inserted distally to maintain perfusion of the lower leg. In addition to previously discussed complications, femoral artery cannulation may increase the risk for coronary and cerebral atheroembolism. Because flow from conventional femoral artery cannulae is retrograde (i.e., up the descending aorta and arch), patients with extensive atherosclerotic disease are at greater risk for embolization if the plaque is lifted by altered flow patterns *(49,50,62)*. Today, innovative cannula designs are emerging to address some of the issues, risks, and challenges associated with femoral cannulation and minimally invasive operative procedures. These include several variations of long, thin-walled arterial cannulae that are inserted into the femoral artery and are advanced to the aortic arch or ascending aorta. These cannulae offer antegrade flow patterns as well as additional features such as endoaortic balloon cross-clamp and integrated cardioplegia delivery lumen for myocardial preservation during periods of induced arrest. Manufacturers continue to work closely with clinicians to develop innovative cannula options for noncentral arterial cannulation.

Axillary Cannulation

Axillary artery cannulation is being used more frequently as a site for arterial access. The axillary or subclavian artery may be cannulated directly using a host of available cannulae (several specifically designed for this application) or cannulation through a graft (usually 8 mm) sewn end-to-side for extracorporeal arterial perfusion. The axillary artery may have several advantages over other arterial access sites. It is less likely to have atherosclerotic plaques, should not be prone to causing

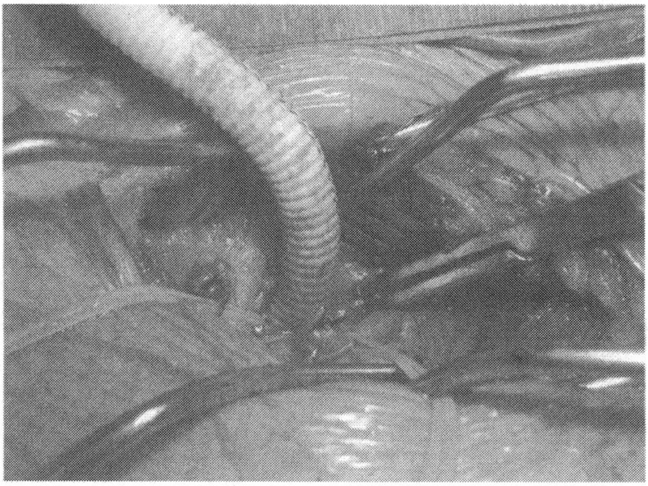

Fig. 2. Axillary cannulation with 8-mm graft.

areas of ischemia or hypoperfusion from vessel occlusion, provides antegrade flow, thus reducing the risk of cerebral embolization, and allows use of hypothermic, selective antegrade cerebral perfusion techniques during repairs of the ascending aorta and aortic arch (Figs. 2 and 3). Often, surgical repair of the aortic arch requires interruption of blood flow to the brain. Extracorporeal options for cerebral protection

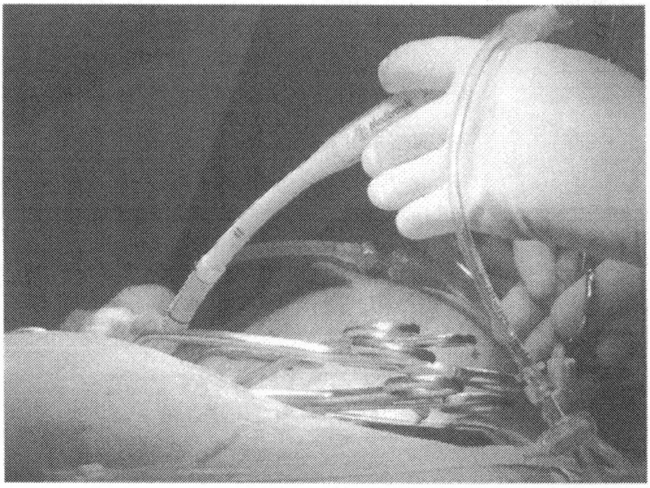

Fig. 3. Axillary graft to CPB circuit connection using an elongated one-piece arterial cannula with luer port and pig tail for deairing.

include deep hypothermia and circulatory arrest (DHCA), retrograde cerebral perfusion (RCP), and antegrade cerebral (or selective) perfusion (ACP). The latter allows operations of the arch to be carried out at moderate hypothermia with adequate cerebral protection *(63)*. Use of axillary artery cannulation facilitates ACP by allowing the surgeon to clamp the brachiocephalic artery during arch repair, while reduced flow rates are used for ACP via the right carotid artery and collateral pathways. During these procedures, arterial pressure should be monitored in the left radial artery and/or groin while on full CPB support, and in the right radial artery during selective cerebral perfusion. Occasionally, right radial artery pressure may be elevated due to the proximity of the cannulation site, and therefore right radial pressure should only be monitored during periods of ACP. Flow rates of 10–20 ml/kg/min are recommended with pressure in the 40–80 mm Hg range. Following surgical repair, full extracorporeal flow may be restored via the axillary artery cannulation technique, thereby avoiding additional cannulation of the repaired vessel or graft. In addition to the previously described cannulae, surgical sites, and operative techniques, use of remote cannulation sites such as the abdominal aorta or left ventricular apex have been reported *(64)*.

Reducing cannulation-related morbidity challenges the surgical community to improve current cannulation techniques and technology. This may include cannulae with improved flow dynamics, automatic insertion devices, bioactive coatings, emboli-catching filters, and a host of innovative ideas to improve care of the cardiac patient.

REFERENCES

1. Peirce ECII. Extracorporeal circulation for open heart surgery. Charles C Thomas, Springfield, IL, 1969.
2. Kirk JW, Barratt-Boyes BE. Cardiac Surgery. Second edition. Churchill-Livingstone, New York, 1993.
3. Riley JB, Hardin SB, Winn BA, et al. In vitro comparison of cavoatrial (dual stage) cannulae for use during cardiopulmonary bypass. Perfusion 1986;1:197–204.
4. Gravlee, Davis, Kurusz, Utley. Cardiopulmonary Bypass: Principles and Practice. Second edition. Lippincott Williams and Wilkins, Philadelphia, 2000.
5. Bennett EV Jr, Fewel JG, Ybarra J, et al. Comparison of flow differences among venous cannulas. Ann Thorac Surg 1983;36:59–65.
6. Reed CC, Stafford TB. Cardiopulmonary Bypass. Second edition. Texas Medical Press, Inc., Houston, 1985.
7. Lake CL. Controversies in the management of cardiopulmonary bypass. In: Cardiothoracic and Vascular Anesthesia Update. Kaplan JA, editor. WB Saunders Co., Philadelphia. 1990:1–21.

8. Casthely PA, Bregman D. Cardiopulmonary Bypass: Physiology, Related Complications, and Pharmacology. Futura Publishing Co., Mount Kisco, NY, 1991.
9. Taylor PC, Effler DB. Management of cannulation for cardiopulmonary bypass in patients with acquired heart disease. Surg Clin North Am 1975;55:1205–1215.
10. Merin O, Silberman S, Bravner R, et al. Femoral- femoral bypass for repeat open heart surgery. Perfusion 1998;13:455–459.
11. Lawrence DR, Desai JB. Forty five degree, two stage cannula: advantages over standard two-stage venous cannula. Ann Thorac Surg 1997;63:253–254.
12. Westaly S. Extrathoracic cannulation for urgent cardiopulmonary bypass in cardiac tamponade: use of internal jugular vein. J Cardiovasc Surg 1998;29:103–105.
13. Flege JB, Jr., Wolf RK. Venous drainage to the heart lung machine via the internal jugular vein. Ann Thorac Surg 1997;63:861.
14. Peters WS, Stevens JH, Smith JA, et al. Minimally invasive right heart operations: techniques for bicaval occlusion and cardioplegia. Ann Thorac Surg 1997;64: 1843–1845.
15. Mongero L, Sistino JJ, Beck J, Smith CR. Current perfusion techniques for repair of giant cerebral aneurysms using deep hypothermia and circulatory arrest. J Extra Corpor Technol 1994;26:13–17.
16. Beck JR, Mongero LB, Goldstein DJ, Oz MC. Perfusion techniques for treatment of right heart failure. Perfusion 1995;10:323–326.
17. Oz MC, Slater JP, Edwards N, et al. Desaturated venous to arterial shunting reduces right heart failure following CPB. J of Heart and Lung Transplantation, Jan 1995;14:172–176.
18. Mongero LB, Beck JR, Kroslowitz RM, Argenziano M, Chabot JA. Treatment of primary peritoneal mesothelioma by hypothermic intraperitoneal chemotherapy. Perfusion March 1999;14:2:141–145.
19. Babka RM. A comparison of the use of venous pumping to gravity return of blood to the oxygenator during cardioplegic arrest. Pro Am Acad Cardiovasc Perfusion 1988;9:47–50.
20. Toomasian JM, Mc Carthy JP. Total extrathoracic cardiopulmonary support with kinetic assisted venous drainage: experience in 50 patients. Perfusion 1998;13: 137–143.
21. Taketani S, Sawa Y, Massai T, et al. A novel technique for cardiopulmonary bypass using a vacuum system for venous drainage with pressure relief valve: an experimental study. Artif Organs 1998;22:337–341.
22. Tamari, Salagub, Beck, Mongero. A new venous bag provides vacuum assisted venous return. Perfusion 2002;17;5:383–390.
23. Sadeghi AM, Rose EA, Michler RE, et al. A simplified method for the occlusion of the vena cavae during CPB. Ann Thorac Surg 1986;41:678.
24. Coselli JS. The use of left heart bypass in the repair of thoracoabdominal aortic aneurysms: current techniques and results. Sem Thorac Cardiovasc Surg 2003;15 (4):326–332.
25. Fusco DS, Shaw RK, Tranquilli M, et al. Femoral cannulation is safe for type A dissection repair. Ann Thorac Surg 2004;78:1285–1289.
26. Svensson LG. Antegrade perfusion during suspended animation? J Thorac Cardiovasc Surg 2002;124(6);1068–1070.
27. Schachner T, Nagiller J, Zimmer A, et al. Technical problems and complications of axillary artery cannulation. Eur J Cardiothorac Surg 2005;27:634–637.
28. Davila RM, Rawles T, Mack MJ. Venoarterial air embolus: a complication of vacuum-assisted venous drainage. Ann Thorac Surg 2000;1369–1371.

29. Beck JR, Mongero LB, Charette KC, et al. Will innovation and change increase gaseous embolization on CPB. Am Acad Cardiovasc Perfusion Proceedings Jan. 2005.
30. Budd J, Isaac J, Bennett J, Freeman J. Morbidity and mortality associated with large bore percutaneous venovenous bypass cannulation for 312 orthotopic liver transplantations. Liver Transpl Surg 2001;7:359–362.
31. Arow KV, Ellestad C, Grover FL, et al. Objective Evaluation of the Efficacy of Various Venous Cannulas. J Thorac Cardiovasc Surg 1981;81:464–469.
32. Beck J. Cannulation and Perfusion Perspective for MICS. July 2004. http://www.ctsnet.org/doc/9270. Accessed July 2004.
33. Souza MH, Decio EO. Weaning from cardiopulmonary bypass. Indian J Extracorpor Tech 1998;6:2.
34. Faulkner SC, Johnson CE, Tucker JL, Schmitz ML, Fasules JW, Drummond-Webb JJ. Hemodynamic troubleshooting for mechanical malfunction of the extracorporeal membrane oxygenation systems using the PPP triad of variables. Perfusion 2003;18:295–298.
35. Herrema IH, Winsser LJA. Flow directed pulmonary artery catheter obstructs venous drainage cannula of cardiopulmonary bypass machine [letter]. Anesthesia 1988;43:799.
36. Bernstein EF, Gleason LR. Factors influencing hemolysis with roller pumps. Surgery 1967;61:432–442.
37. Banbury MK, White JA, Blackstone EH, Cosgrove DM 3rd. Vacuum assisted venous return reduces blood usage. J Thorac Cardiovasc Surg 2003;126(3): 680–687.
38. Jones TJ, Deal DD, Vernon JC, et al. Does vacuum assisted venous drainage increase gaseous mircroemboli during CPB? Ann Thorac Surg 2002;74(6): 2132–2137.
39. Hankei S, Mitsuharu M, Toru M, Suzuki R, Yohu R. Resection of giant right atrial lymphoma using vacuum assisted CPB without snaring the inferior vena cava. Ann Thorac Cardiovasc Surg 2004;10(4):249–251.
40. Jahangiri M, Rayner A, Keogh B, Lincoln C. Cerebral vascular accident after vacuum assisted venous drainage in a fontan patient: a cautionary tale. Ann Thorac Surg 2001;72:1727–1728.
41. Wilcox TW. Vacuum assisted venous drainage: to air or not to air, that is the question. Has the bubble burst? J Extra Corpor Technol 2002;34(1):24–28.
42. Wilcox TW, Simon JM, Gorman DF. Venous air in the bypass circuit: a source of arterial line emboli exacerbated by vacuum assisted drainage. Ann Thorac Surg 1999;68:1285–1289.
43. Almany DK, Sistino JJ. Lab evaluation of the limitations of positive pressure safety valves on hard shell venous reservoirs. J Extra Corpor Technol 2002;34(2): 115–117.
44. Brodman R, Siegel H, Lesser M, et al. A comparison of flow gradients across disposable arterial perfusion cannulas. Ann Thorac Surg 1985;39:225–233.
45. Muehrcke DD, Cornhill JF, Thomas JD, et al. Flow characteristics of aortic cannulae. J Card Surg 1995;10:514–519.
46. Mills NL, Everson CT. Atherosclerosis of the ascending aorta and coronary artery bypass: clinical correlates, and operative management. J Thorac Cardiovasc Surg 1991;102:546–553
47. Blauth CI, Cosgrove DM, Webb BW, et al. Atheroembolism from the ascending aorta. J Thorac Cardiovasc Surg 1992;103:1104.

48. Beique FA, Joffe D, Tousignant G, Konstadt S. Echocardiographic-based assessment and management of atherosclerotic disease of the thoracic aorta. J Cardiothorac Vasc Anesth 1998;12:206.
49. Galletti PM, Brecher GA. Heart-Lung Bypass. Principles and Techniques of Extracorporeal Circulation. Grune & Stratton, New York, 1962, pp. 184–188.
50. Barbut D, Grassineau D, Lis E, et al. Posterior distribution of infarcts in strokes related to cardiac operation. Ann Thorac Surg 1998;65:1656.
51. Drew JA, Cleveland RJ, Nelson RJ. An approach to aortic cannulation with a caution on hemolysis associated with angled cannulas. Rev Surg 1974;31:57–59.
52. Davila-Roman V, Phillips K, Davila R, et al. Intraoperative transesophageal echocardiography and epiaortic ultrasound for assessment of atherosclerosis of the thoracic aorta. J Am Coll Cardiol 1996;28:942–947.
53. Grossi EA, Kanchuger MS, Schwartz DS, et al. Effect of cannula length on aortic arch flow: protection of the atheromatous aortic arch. Ann Thorac Surg 1995; 59:710–712.
54. Stern A, Tunick PA, Culliford AT, et al. Aortic arch endarterectomy increases the risk of stroke during heart surgery in patients with protruding aortic arch atheromas. Circulation 1997;96:1024.
55. King RC, Kanithanou RC, Shockley KS, et al. Replacing the atherosclerotic ascending aorta is a high risk procedure. Ann Thorac Surg 1998;66:396–401.
56. Duda AM, Letwin LB, Sutter FP, et al. Does routine use of aortic ultrasonography decrease the stoke rate in coronary artery bypass surgery? J Vasc Surg 1995;21: 98–107.
57. Biegutay AM, Garamella JJ, Danyluk M, Remucal HC. Retrograde aortic dissection occurring during cardiopulmonary bypass. JAMA 1976;236:465.
58. Carey JS, Skow JR, Scott C. Retrograde aortic dissection during cardiopulmonary bypass: "nonoperative" management. Ann Thorac Surg 1977;24:44.
59. Gates JD, Bichell DP, Rizzu RJ, et al. Thigh ischemia complicating femoral vessel cannulation for cardiopulmonary bypass. Ann Thorac Surg 1996;61:730.
60. Kay JH, Dykstra DC, Tsuji HK. Retrograde ilio-aortic dissection. A complication of common femoral artery perfusion during open heart Surgery. Am J Surg 1966;111:464–468.
61. Van der Salm TJ. Prevention of lower extremity ischemia during cardiopulmonary bypass via femoral cannulation. Ann Thorac Surg 1997;63:251.
62. Svensonn LG. Editorial comment: autopsies in acute type A aortic dissection, surgical implications. Circulation 1998;98:302–304.
63. Panos A, Murith N, Bednarkiewicz M, Khatchatourou G. Axillary cerebral perfusion for arch surgery in acute type A dissection under moderate hypothermia. Eur J Cardiothorac Surg 2006;29:1036–1039.
64. Robicsek F. Apical aortic cannulation: application of an old method with new paraphernalia. Ann Thorac Surg 1991;51:320–322.

9 Ultrafiltration in Cardiac Surgery

Bruce Searles, BS, CCP, *and*
Edward Darling, MS, CCP

Contents

Key Words: Pre-BUF; CUF; Z-BUF; DUF; MUF; dialysis.

INTRODUCTION

Ultrafiltration is the removal of plasma water and its soluble components across a microporous membrane. Various ultrafiltration techniques have been developed for use in cardiopulmonary bypass (CPB). These techniques can be categorized into two rationales: blood concentration and blood filtration. This chapter introduces the reader to the spectrum of ultrafiltration techniques that can be applied to CPB. Special emphasis is placed on the technical considerations for integrating these techniques into clinical practice and a literature review of the reported outcome measures for each technique.

The use of the ultrafilter, which is a porous extracorporeal membrane, for the removal of plasma water and its soluble components is widely used in clinical and laboratory applications. The application of these technologies by the cardiovascular perfusionist can be traced back to the dawn of the profession, when the perfusionist was also the renal dialysis technician and was more generally referred to as an extracorporeal technologist. With applications in renal dialysis, intensive care,

From: *Current Cardiac Surgery: On Bypass: Advanced Perfusion Techniques*
Edited by: L. B. Mongero and J. R. Beck

and cardiovascular medicine, several terms have been used to describe different applications of these devices. Terms such as hemofiltration, hemoconcentration, ultrafiltration, and hemodiafiltration have been used in the literature. Unfortunately, these terms are generally poorly defined and are often used inappropriately as synonyms. Table 1 presents definitions of these terms, as they will be used throughout this chapter.

Because the emphasis of this text is on perfusion techniques, a full presentation of the anatomy and function of an ultrafilter is beyond the

Table 1
Terms used in this chapter

Term	*Definition*
Hemoconcentration	Use of a membrane to concentrate blood components by removing plasma water. This technique is based on convection, which is driven by a transmembrane pressure gradient between the blood and the ultrafiltrate side of the membrane.
Hemofiltration	Use of a membrane in conjunction with fluid replacement to reduce the concentration of water-soluble components of plasma. This technique is based on convection, which is driven by a transmembrane pressure gradient between the blood and the ultrafiltrate side of the membrane.
Hemodialysis	Use of a membrane in conjunction with a fluid dialysate to remove water-soluble components from plasma. This technique is driven by a diffusion gradient across the membrane between the blood and the dialysate solution.
Hemodiafiltration	A technique that combines the diffusion-driven removal of small solutes via a dialysate and the convection-driven removal of larger solutes via a transmembrane pressure gradient. This combined technique has been suggested to provide greater solute moving potential than either technique individually. This technique requires that a replacement fluid is administered to the patient.
Ultrafiltration	A generic term for the removal of plasma water and its soluble components from the blood via convection. The fluid that is removed is called "ultrafiltrate." All of the above techniques can produce an ultrafiltrate, and are therefore specific techniques of ultrafiltration.

scope of this chapter. Several comprehensive and valuable reviews have been prepared on this topic however, and the interested reader is directed to Wheeldon and Bethune *(1)* for a complete, though somewhat dated, discussion of the design characteristics, physical properties, and functional limitations of ultrafilters, as well as Clar and Larson for the most comprehensive discussion of sieving coefficients of these devices for various solutes and drugs *(2)*. Briefly, the ultrafilters standardly applied to CPB consists of a cylinder enclosing a bundle of microporous hollow fiber straws. The pore size is typically between 50 and 65 kD. Blood is directed through the inside of the fibers. Ultrafiltrate is produced by convection that is driven by the pressure gradient between the inside of the fiber and the outside of the fiber. This pressure gradient is described in the literature as the transmembrane pressure (TMP). The outside of the fiber is standardly connected to a controlled vacuum source, and the ultrafiltrate is collected to waste. Fig. 1 illustrates a typical ultrafiltrate fiber.

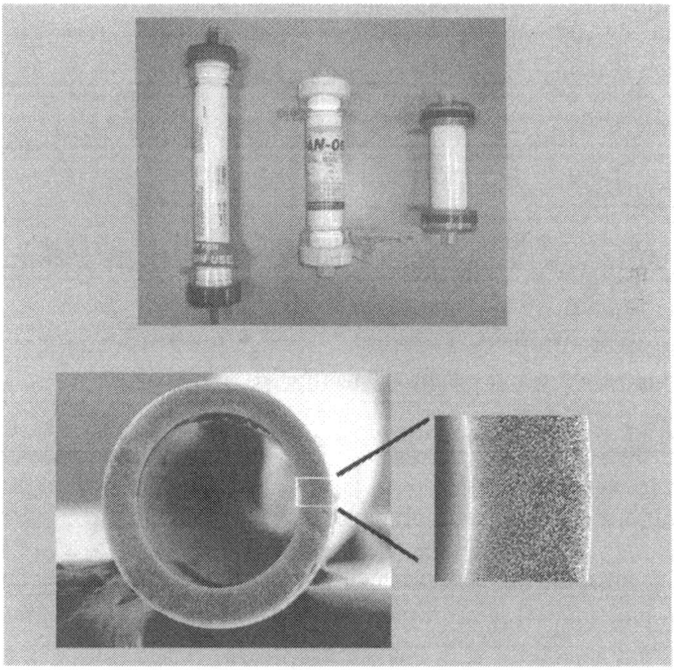

Fig. 1. (Top) Photograph of commercially available ultrafilters. Ultrafilters come in a variety of sizes and are made from various thermoplastics. (Bottom) Close-up of a cross section of an individual ultrafilter hollow fiber (Minntech Corporation; Minneapolis, MN). The inner diameter is approx 200 µm, with a wall thickness of 75–150 µm.

Today, the application of ultrafiltration CPB is commonplace. The myriad of ultrafiltration techniques can be characterized into two primary rationales: volume management and mediator removal. These rationales have emerged successively during the development of ultrafiltration, and they influence the technical integration and use of the ultrafilter with the CPB circuit.

HISTORY

The Volume Management/Concentration Rationale (1976–Present)

The initial use of ultrafiltration in conjunction with CPB was reported in 1976 as a way to concentrate the dilute extracorporeal circuit contents after bypass *(3)*. Soon after, Darup et al. described the first use of ultrafiltration during CPB *(4)*. The bypass circuit was found to be ideally suited for ultrafiltration, as it offers easy access to the blood path and provides either a pump or a positive pressure site to drive blood through the hemoconcentrator. The application of ultrafiltration during CPB was initially reserved for the management of volume overload in patients with renal insufficiency and/or failure. However, as the 1980s progressed, this conventional ultrafiltration (CUF) technique, (i.e., hemoconcentration) became more widely adopted *(5–9)*.

A unique fluid management/blood salvage ultrafiltration technique was first described by the Hospital for Sick Children in London *(1)*. They reported on a modified ultrafiltration (MUF) technique, which was used in the immediate post-CPB period to concentrate the blood volume of their pediatric patients. By 1990, ultrafiltration was well accepted as an important adjunct to CPB that could fulfill a role in fluid balance control and blood conservation.

The Mediator Removal/Filtration Rationale (1990–Present)

While hemoconcentration techniques were experiencing an ever-increasing clinical acceptance in the early 1990s, some clinicians theorized that there was an additional benefit to ultrafiltration. Coraim et al. reported improved hemodynamics in patients following cardiac surgery when continuous arteriovenous hemofiltration (CAVH) was applied. They attributed this observation to the convective removal of myocardial depressant substances *(10)*. Further work by researchers in a septic animal model suggests that left ventricular function improves with ultrafiltration and volume replacement *(11)*. In a 1992 study by Grootendorst et al., when endotoxemic pigs underwent high-volume ultrafiltration (6 L/h in an approximately 80 lb pig), cardiac performance improved *(12)*. This improvement did not occur when the blood passed through the hemoconcentrator with the ultrafiltrate line clamped. In a follow-up study, the same researchers collected and infused the ultrafiltrate from endotoxemic pigs into control animals and found that myocardial performance became depressed in the healthy pigs *(13)*. The work of these researchers fueled the emergence of the conceptual framework that ultrafiltration was doing more than simply removing free water and electrolytes, but rather, it also removes potential deleterious substances from the blood, thereby improving the patient's status.

Unfortunately there have been very few prospective randomized studies comparing the clinical outcomes of patients treated with large-volume ultrafiltration *(14,15)*. Given the shortage of impressive clinical outcome data and the varying results of mediator removal studies, the application of ultrafiltration as a therapeutic technique is still a controversial topic. When considering the varied results on the topic of mediator removal, it is important to consider that different membrane materials may demonstrate different efficacy at removing inflammatory mediators from circulation. Researchers have also suggested that different membrane materials may have significantly different mediator removal potential *(16–19)*.

The purpose of this chapter is to review the technical incorporation of ultrafiltration into the care of the CPB patient before, during, and after CPB.

ULTRAFILTRATION APPLICATIONS

Cardiopulmonary bypass ultrafiltration techniques have been described in context to the operative phase: pre-CPB, peri-CPB, and post-CPB. Overviews of these techniques are described below.

Pre-CPB Ultrafiltration of Pump Prime Pre-BUF

The addition of banked blood to pump prime may elevate prime potassium, glucose, bradykinin, citrate, and lactate levels *(20)*. This may be deleterious, especially to the neonate, whose blood volume is often less than the prime volume. Ridley first described his pre-bypass ultrafiltration (pre-BUF) technique for filtering the CPB prime in 1990 *(21)*. The technique was subsequently reported by Sakurai and Nagatsu in 1998 and 1995, respectively *(22,23)*.

Essentially, Pre-BUF requires the integration of an ultrafilter into the CPB circuit so that primed circuit blood is delivered under pressure into the ultrafilter. The blood may be driven by a dedicated pump, but, more typically, it is driven by the pressure of the arterial side of the circuit. The effluent blood is returned to a low-pressure port in the CPB circuit, such as the venous reservoir or cardiotomy.

Following the addition of blood to the CPB circuit, ultrafiltrate removal is initiated, and volume replacement with a balanced electrolyte solution is titrated to maintain a minimum reservoir level. Typically, for pediatric CPB circuits, whose prime volumes may range from 250–1,000 ml, the circuit prime blood is "washed" with approximately 1 L of a balanced electrolyte solution in this fashion.

This technique has been shown to reduce the levels of bradykinin, Factor XIII, prekallikrein, and high molecular weight kininogen. These same authors suggest that this technique eliminated the initial drop in blood pressure commonly seen with initiation of CPB, reduced the incidence of postoperative edema, attenuated cardiac impairment, and reduced pulmonary dysfunction *(23,24)*.

Technical Considerations of Pre-BUF

- The perfusionist must remain vigilant, as the circuit could be deprimed if the fluid replacement rate is inadequate.
- To avoid removal, addition of certain priming drugs (e.g., mannitol, aprotinin, steroids, buffer, etc.) should not be added to the circuit until after pre-BUF has been completed *(2)*.
- Final prime electrolyte levels should be measured after pre-bypass ultrafiltration and corrected if necessary.

Peribypass Ultrafiltration

Three primary ultrafiltration techniques can be applied during CPB, and each are discussed below.

CUF

Conventional ultrafiltration is the most widely applied ultrafilter technique in the perfusionist's armory. First described by Darup et al. in 1979 as a means of managing circuit volume and increasing hematocrit without bank blood, the technique was not identified as "conventional" until many years later, after multiple other ultrafiltration techniques had been developed *(4)*. The methods of incorporating the ultrafilter into the CPB circuit are as varied and unique as the CPB circuits found at different institutions; however, the ultrafilter is usually positioned in the circuit to receive blood from the high-pressure arterial side of the circuit and to return blood to the low-pressure venous side of the circuit (Fig. 2).

It has been well established that CUF is effective at increasing the hematocrit and concentrating plasma proteins of patients during CPB *(6,25)*. Although the techniques are simple, CUF depends on a volume margin in the venous reservoir to effectively concentrate, and it may not be possible in every case. The extent to which the hematocrit can be raised by CUF is directly related to the ratio of the excess volume of blood in the reservoir (the reservoir volume above the minimum safe operating level) versus the total circulating blood volume (including the patient blood volume and the circuit volume). Consequently, small

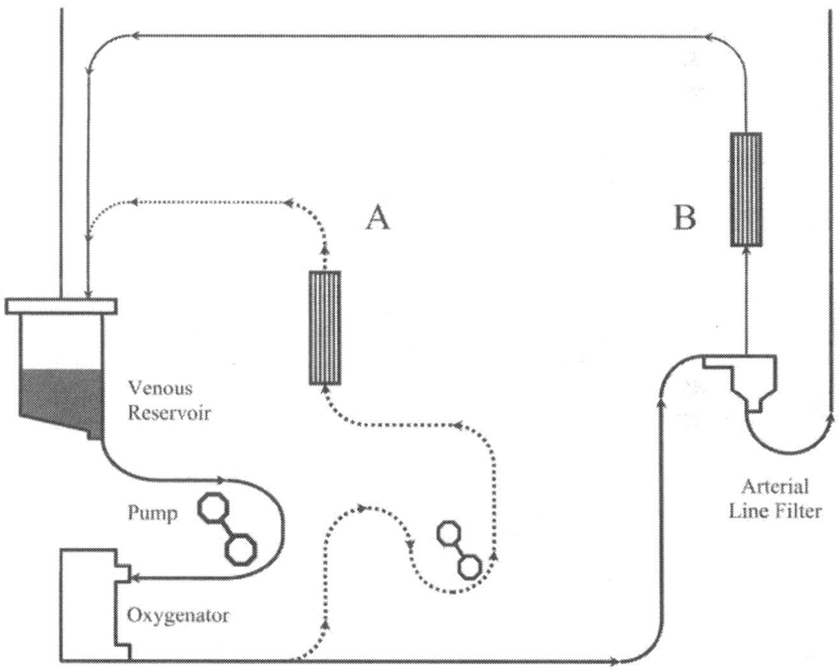

Fig. 2. Pre-BUF, CUF, and DUF circuit diagrams. Conventional ultrafiltration can be done via a dedicated roller pump to shunt blood through the hemoconcentrator (A), or through the pressure in the arterial line (oxygenators recirculation line or filter purge) to drive blood through the hemoconcentrator (B). This setup can also be used before bypass to perform prebypass ultrafiltration (pre-BUF) when blood primes are used. Performance of DUF can be accomplished by removing ultrafiltrate volume and maintaining venous reservoir level by the manual addition of replacement volume.

patients with large reservoir volumes stand to benefit the most from CUF, whereas large patients with low reservoir levels will benefit minimally.

Technical Considerations for Conventional Ultrafiltration

- Must have adequate volume in venous reservoir to safely remove ultrafiltrate.
- The shunt created by diverting arterial blood flow through the ultrafilter must be managed appropriately. Arterial line shunts may reduce the actual blood flow to the patient, and thus increase the risk of accidental exsanguination after CPB termination.
- A level detector with automatic pump shutoff should be used to prevent dangerously low reservoir volumes.
- Overly aggressive CUF could result in an inadequate volume in the venous reservoir to terminate CPB without the addition of significant crystalloid.

Continuous Ultrafiltration Replacement Therapy (CURT) (i.e., Continuous, Zero-Balanced (Z-BUF), Balanced (BUF), High Volume (HVUF) and Dilutional (DUF) Ultrafiltration)

After reports that long-term ultrafiltration in the intensive care setting ameliorated the clinical course of the septic patient, several ultrafiltration techniques were developed for use during CPB. The common element between all these techniques is the removal of a large volume of ultrafiltrate and the subsequent replacement of volume with a balanced electrolyte solution. These techniques are based on the premise that water-soluble inflammatory mediators are removed from circulation during ultrafiltration, so large-volume ultrafiltration may attenuate the inflammatory response to CPB. Although Hakim et al. had reported their ultrafiltration and replacement technique as early as 1985 *(26)*, the application was for the removal of metabolites. Journois et al. was the first to describe this technique applied to the CPB patient *(27)*. In his seminal paper, ultrafiltration was initiated during the rewarming period of CPB at a blood flow rate of 200 ml/min/M^2 and continued through the duration of the CPB run with the goal of removing 3–6 L/M^2 of ultrafiltrate. To maintain the circulating blood volume, fluid replacement was matched to the ultrafiltrate removal through a novel technique, which used a single roller-head pump to remove volume from the ultrafilter and administer replacement solution to the reservoir. Although Journois coined the term Z-BUF, many other authors have applied similar techniques for large-volume ultrafiltration with volume replacement *(28,29)*. The most widely applied technique in the United States seems to be dilutional ultrafiltration (DUF) *(30)*. This technique is similar to Z-BUF in its goals and parameters, except that fluid replacement is managed manually by the perfusionist. Although technically more simple to set up than Z-BUF, DUF requires more user intervention throughout the procedure (*see* Fig. 1, legend). Fig. 3 illustrates the Z-BUF technique.

The use of CURT techniques to correct electrolyte imbalances such as hyperkalemia during CPB has been well documented *(30,31)*. CURT techniques also appear to be effective in the removal and/or attenuation of deleterious mediators. Journois et al. found significant removal of tumor necrosis factor (TNF), interleukin (IL)-10, myeloperoxidase, and

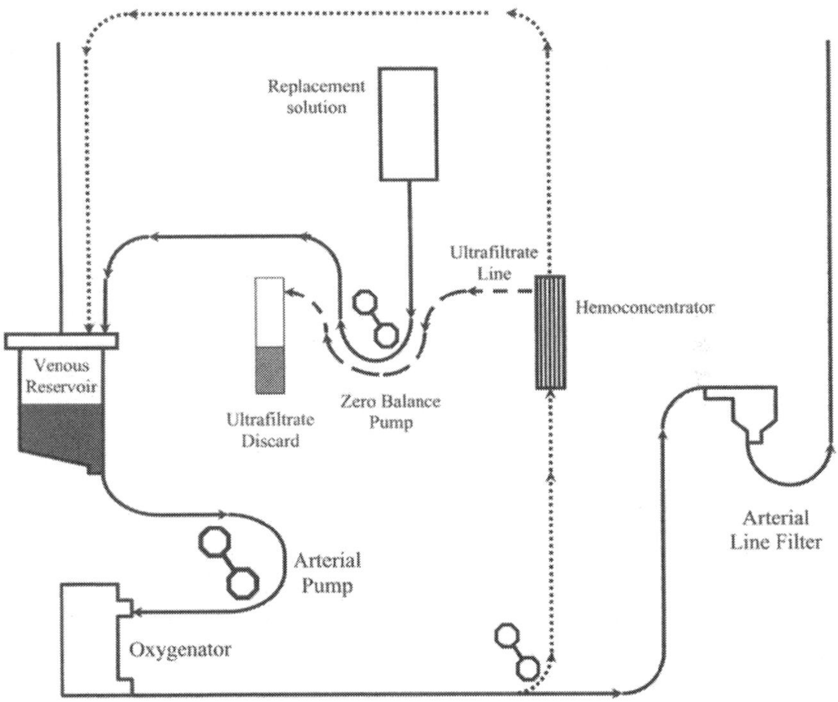

Fig. 3. Z-BUF circuit diagrams. High-volume Z-BUF. Blood is delivered through the hemoconcentrator via pump or high-pressure site. The ultrafiltrate line and volume-replacement line are placed in a double-tubing raceway. As this pump rotates, removal of ultrafiltrate is accompanied by a simultaneous addition of the same volume of replacement fluid to the venous reservoir.

C3a in the Z-BUF group and a significant improvement in postoperative blood loss, time to extubation, and postoperative alveolar–arterial oxygen gradients compared with a control group *(27)*. Subsequent clinical studies have compared a nonultrafiltration control group to a combined DUF/MUF group found significant reductions in plasma endothelin-1 and a decreased pulmonary vascular resistance in the patients who received the DUF/MUF therapy *(28,29)*.

Technical Considerations for CURT

- The shunt created by diverting flow through the ultrafilter must be managed appropriately. Arterial line shunts may reduce the actual blood flow to the patient and increase the risk of accidental exsanguination after CPB termination.
- The type and quantity of the crystalloid replacement solution is important. To avoid unintentional removal, it may be necessary to supplement certain replacement solution (i.e., calcium, glucose, magnesium, or bicarbonate).
- Large volumes may be required to be effective.

Hemodialysis and Hemodiafiltration

In the late 1970s, it was established that dialysis patients could successfully receive cardiac surgery requiring CPB, provided there was judicious preoperative hemodialysis, and aggressive perioperative volume management and postoperative hemodialysis. The dialysis patient suffering from heart failure, however, presented several technical challenges for the cardiac surgeon. They were generally too hemodynamically unstable for the necessary preoperative hemodialysis and, consequently, were poor surgical candidates. Logically, clinicians identified that the extracorporeal circuit of the heart–lung machine could provide both hemodynamic support and unimpeded vascular access at high or low pressures to facilitate CPB-supported perioperative hemodialysis. The interface of a dialysis membrane with the extracorporeal circuit is essentially the same as that used during CUF, with the exception that instead of connecting the ultrafiltrate port to wall suction, it would instead be connected to a supply of dialysate. The dialysate would be recirculated or collected to waste after passing across the membrane. Hemodiafiltration is essentially dialysis with concomitant Z-BUF to broaden the range of solute sizes that can be removed and the efficiency of solute removal. It requires that dialysis be performed with a hemoconcentrator membrane for its larger pore size. In addition to the diffusion-driven removal of solutes inherent with dialysis, the convective removal of larger solutes is performed by removal of ultrafiltrate. A volume of replacement solution equal to the ultrafiltrate is administered to the patient to maintain their fluid balance *(1)*.

The first reports of hemodialysis in conjunction with CPB were authored by Soffer et al. and Beckley et al. in separate articles *(32,33)*. In these papers, the dialysis membrane was interfaced with a standard kidney dialysis machines (Travenol) and dialysis membranes. A shunt line from the extracorporeal circuit was used to supply blood to the dialysis membrane, and the dialyzed blood was returned to the low-pressure side of the extracorporeal circuit. The standard dialysis machine was used to recirculate the dialysate solution between the membrane and the dialysis bath. Early renal dialysis machines offered little functional advantage over a heart–lung machine for circulation of the dialysis solution. Furthermore, the only significant difference between a dialysis membrane and a hemofilter is the size of the membrane pores (10 vs. 50 kD). Consequently, many perfusionists did not use a standard dialysis system, and instead used roller pumps to circulate the blood and/or dialysate *(26,34–36)*. Still others performed dialysis during CPB with a pumpless system that used a high-pressure shunt from the arterial line to drive blood through the hemofilter and gravity to drive the dialysate across the membrane in a single pass *(37)*.

Reports of outcome measures for these studies include decreased blood levels of urea *(26,34,38,39)*, blood urea nitrogen *(34)*, and potassium *(26,34,39)*, as well as increased hematocrit *(35,39)* after CPB.

Technical Considerations for Hemodialysis

- Consultation with a dialysis physician is advised for selection of the appropriate dialysate solution.
- Frequent monitoring of patient's blood concentration of electrolytes and metabolites is required.
- The shunt created by diverting arterial blood flow through the dialysis membrane must be managed appropriately. Arterial line shunts may reduce the actual blood flow to the patient and increase the risk of accidental exsanguination after CPB termination.

Post-CPB Ultrafiltration

MUF

Modified Ultrafiltration was introduced in 1991 by Naik et al. at the Hospital for Sick Children in London as a post-CPB technique in reducing the rise in total body water and tissue edema that often accompanies pediatric CPB *(40)*. In their model, using the CPB circuit, the arterial cannula is left in situ so that blood from the aorta is pumped through the hemoconcentrator and warm hemoconcentrated blood is returned to the right atrium (AV-MUF). As volume is removed, volume remaining in the CPB circuit is titrated into the patient to maintain filling pressures. Since the initial reports, several publications on alternative MUF configurations (VV-MUF, VA-MUF), and on how the technical integration of MUF may be safely accomplished, have been published *(41–48)*.

Fig. 4 illustrates the two basic MUF circuit configurations.

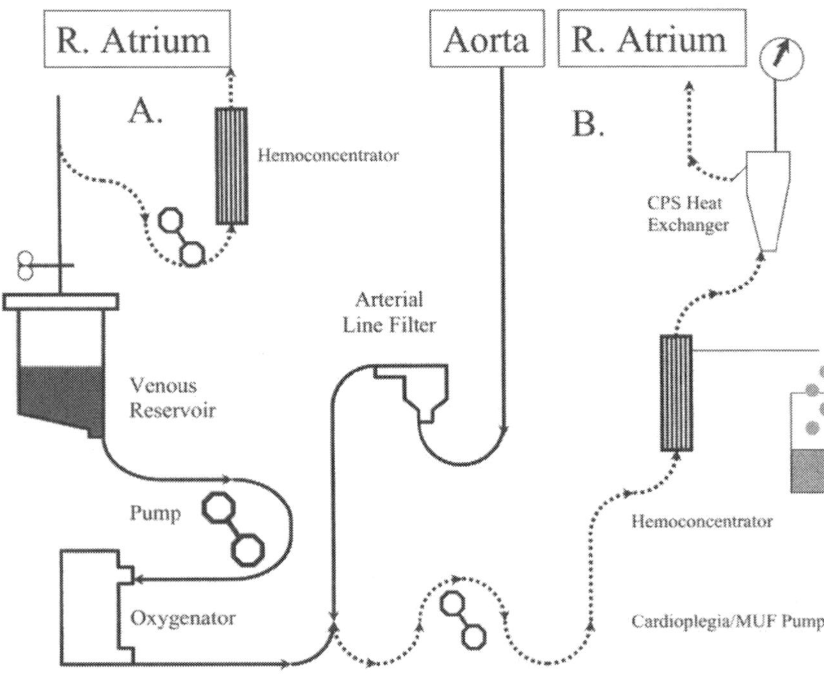

Fig. 4. MUF circuit diagrams. Basic MUF configurations. (A) Venovenous MUF. A dedicated site on the venous line provides access. Blood is pulled from the right atrium, hemoconcentrated, and returned to the right atrium. To maintain patient filling pressures, circuit volume can be titrated into patient via the arterial line. (B) AV-MUF using the blood cardioplegia system. The patient's blood is pulled retrogradely from the aortic cannula by the cardioplegia/MUF pump and pumped through a hemoconcentrator. Concentrated blood passes through, is warmed by the cardioplegia heat exchanger, and then is returned to the right atrium. Patient filling pressures are maintained by titration of circuit contents into the MUF circuit by the arterial pump.

Among the reported benefits of MUF after pediatric CPB are the reduction in total body water, improved hemodynamics, a decrease in blood transfusion requirements, attenuation of dilutional coagulopathy, a decrease in myocardial edema, improvement in cerebral metabolic recovery after circulatory arrest, improved ventricular function, and improved pulmonary compliance and respiratory mechanics *(40, 49–55)*. Some of these benefits, such as pulmonary improvements, may be transient and short-term *(56)*.

The literature suggests that ultrafiltration may reduce circulating mediators *(57,58)*, and thus it may be tempting to attribute these improvements after MUF to this. In other clinical studies, however, the data does not support the idea that improvements reported in MUF patients are the result of a reduction in inflammatory mediators *(59,60)*. In a prospective randomized study of MUF in pediatric patients, Chew and colleagues, although finding evidence of improved clinical outcome, did not see any effect of MUF on TNF, IL-1B, and IL-1ra complement when compared to non-MUF controls *(61)*.

MUF In Adults

Modified ultrafiltration has been applied most commonly to the pediatric CPB patient population. This is primarily due to the disparity in ratio of circuit/patient volume. The effectiveness of MUF is thought to diminish as the patient size increases. Previous experiences with MUF in the adult population report have shown little or no clinical impact *(62,63)*. However, in a well-controlled, prospective randomized study of 573 adult patients undergoing CPB, a significant reduction in morbidity was reported in the MUF group *(64)*.

Technical Considerations for MUF

- Delays protamine administration.
- Air entrapment in AV-MUF mode caused by negative pressure generated in the arterial line *(43)*.
- Patient temperature loss may occur during VV-MUF or when a heat exchanger is not used *(65)*.
- Concentration of heparin into the patient will occur.
- AV-MUF provides oxygenated blood to the pulmonary vasculature.
- Aggressive AV-MUF may result in carotid steal *(66)*.
- Rate of MUF pump should be indexed to patient size (15–30 ml/kg/min).
- Communication with surgeon and anesthesiologist is important regarding filling pressures and MUF end point.

Circuit Salvage by Ultrafiltration

The blood remaining in the CPB circuit at the end of bypass has a significant quantity of red blood cells and plasma proteins. Various methodologies have been used to salvage this blood for patient use, including collection and direct reinfusion, cell saver concentration, and ultrafiltration *(67)*. Romagnoli et al. was the first to describe the use of an ultrafilter to concentrate the residual pump blood after cardiac surgery *(3)*. The blood is generally directed from an arterial shunt line into the ultrafilter and infused directly into the patient *(68)*, collected in the circuit reservoir for recirculation and further concentration, or transferred to a transfer bag for later infusion into the patient. A novel ultrafiltration technique for circuit salvage has been suggested *(69)*. In this technique the entire fluid contents of the circuit are transferred into a large holding bag, and the contents of the bag are then aggressively concentrated. This technique may increase blood product harvest by reducing the amount of blood trapped in the circuit. The use of ultrafiltration of residual circuit volume has advantages over centrifugation and washing methods, as it preserves plasma proteins and coagulation factors *(67–72)*.

Technical Considerations of Circuit Salvage Ultrafiltration

- Heparin will be in the reinfusion product.

CONCLUSION

In summary, there are many clinical applications for the ultrafilter in the CPB patient. Whether the intention is to concentrate the blood proteins, and thereby reduce the need for bank blood, or to filter out potentially dangerous chemical mediators or metabolites, the ultrafilter can be used before, during, and after CPB. Considering that all of these techniques can be performed with the same device, it is logical to conclude that individual patients may benefit from several techniques during their bypass procedure. This is especially true in the pediatric population. It is not uncommon for the pediatric perfusionist to pre-BUF the circuit prime before bypass, apply CUF after CPB initiation and DUF during rewarming, before performing MUF after CPB termination, and, finally, salvage the pump blood through the hemoconcentrator after decannulation *(44)*.

REFERENCES

1. Wheeldon D, Bethune D. Haemofiltration during cardiopulmonary bypass. Perfusion 1990;5(suppl):39–51.

2. Clar A, Larson DF. Hemofiltration: determinants of drug loss and concentration. JECT 1995;27:158–163.
3. Romagnoli A, Hacker J, Keats AS, Milan J. External hemoconcentration after deliberate hemodilution (Abstr). Ann Meet Am Soc Anesthesiol. 1976.
4. Darup J, Bleese N, Kalmer P, et al. Hemofiltration during extracorporeal circulation (ECC). Thorac Cardiovasc Surg. 1979;27:227–230.
5. Moore RA, Laub GW. Hemofiltration, dialysis, and blood salvage techniques during cardiopulmonary bypass. In: Cardiopulmonary Bypass: Principles and Practice. Second edition. Gravlee GP, Davis RF, Kurusz M, Utley JR, editors. Lippincott Williams & Wilkins, Philadelphia, 2000:105–130.
6. Inotoni F, Alquati P, Schiavello R, Alessandrini F. Ultrafiltration during open-heart surgery in chronic renal failure. Scand J Thorac Cardiovasc Surg 1981;15:217–220.
7. Hopeck JM, Lane RS, Schroeder JW. Oxygenator blood volume control by parallel ultrafiltration to remove plasma water. J Extra Corpor Technol 1981;13;267–271.
8. Nelson R, Tamari Y, Tortolani A, et al. Hemoconcentration by ultrafiltration following cardiopulmonary bypass. Surg Forum 1982;32:253–266.
9. Magilligan DJ. Indications for ultrafiltration in the cardiac surgical patient. J Thorac Cardiovasc Surg 1985;89:183–189.
10. Coraim FJ, Coraim HP, Ebermann R, Stellwag FM. Acute respiratory failure after cardiac surgery: clinical experience with the application of continuous arteriovenous hemofiltration. Crit Care Med 1986;14:714–718.
11. Gomez A, Wang R, Unruh H, et al. Hemofiltration reverses left ventricular dysfunction during sepsis in dogs. Anesthesiology 1990;73:671–685.
12. Grootendorst AF, van Bommel EF, van der Hoven B, et al. High volume hemofiltration improves right ventricular function in endotoxin-induced shock in the pig. Intensive Care Med 1992;18:235–240.
13. Grootendorst AF, van Bommel EF, van der Hoven B, et al. Infusion of ultrafiltrate from endotoxemic pigs depresses myocardial performance in normal pigs. J Crit Care 1993;8:161–169.
14. FitzGerald DJ, Cecere G. Hemofiltration and inflammatory mediators. Perfusion 2002;17:23–28.
15. Journois D, Pouard P, Greeley W, Mauriat P, Vouhe P, Sufron D. Hemofiltration during cardiopulmonary bypass in pediatric cardiac surgery. Anesthesiology 1994; 81;1181–1189.
16. Silvester W, Honore P, Sieffert E, et al. Interleukins 6 and 8, tumor necrosis factor alpha and compliment D clearance by polyacrylonitrile and polysulphone membranes during haemofiltration in critically ill patients (Abstract). Blood Purification 1997;15:127.
17. Braun N, Rosenfeld S, Giolai M, et al. Effect of continuous hemodiafiltration on IL-6, TNF alpha, C3a and TCC in patients with SIRS/septic shock using two different membranes. In: Continuous Extracorporeal Treatment in Multiple Organ Dysfunction Syndrome: 3rd International Conference on Continuous Hemofiltration, Vienna, July 8, 1994 (Contributions to Nephrology). Sieberth HG, Strummvoll HK, Kierdorf H, editors. S. Karger AG, Switzerland, 1995: 89–98.
18. Yokohari K, Hirasawa H, Oda S, et al. Comparison of clearances of cytokines with continuous hemodiafiltration using three types of hemofilter/hemodialyser made of different membranes. Blood Purification 1999;17:40.

19. Berdat PA, Eichenberger E, Ebell J, et al. Elimination of proinflammatory cytokines in pediatric cardiac surgery: analysis of ultrafiltration method and filter type. J Thorac Cardiovasc Surg 2004;122(6):1688–1696.
20. Ratcliffe JM, Wyse RKH, Hunter S, Alberti KGMM, Elliott MJ. The role of priming fluid in the metabolic response to cardiopulmonary bypass in children less than 15 kg body weight undergoing open heart surgery. Thorac Cardiovasc Surg 1988;36:65–74.
21. Ridley PD. The metabolic consequences of a "washed" cardiopulmonary bypass pump-priming fluid in children undergoing cardiac operations. J Thorac Cardiovasc Surg 1990;100:528–537.
22. Sakurai H. Hemofiltration removes bradykinin generated in the priming blood in cardiopulmonary bypass during circulation. Ann Thorac Surg Cardiovasc Surg 1998;4:59–63.
23. Nagatsu M. Initial ultrafiltration to the priming solution with preserved blood for cardiopulmonary bypass in infants. Kyobu Geka-Japanese J Thorac Surg 1995;48: 281–285.
24. Nagashima M, Imai Y, Seo K, et al. Effect of hemofiltrated whole blood pump priming on hemodynamics and respiratory function after the arterial switch operation in neonates. Ann Thorac Surg 2000;70:1901–1906.
25. Zhou JL, Gong QC, Guan HP. Effect of ultrafiltration on plasma colloid oncotic pressure and red cell volume during cardiopulmonary bypass. J Cardiovasc Surg 1989;30:40–41.
26. Hakim M, Wheeldon D, Bethune D, et al. Haemodialysis and hemofiltration on cardiopulmonary bypass. Thorax 1985;40:101–106.
27. Journois D, Irael-Biet D, Pouard P, et al. High volume zero balance hemofiltration to reduce delayed inflammatory response to cardiopulmonary bypass in children. Anesthesiology 1996;85:965–976.
28. Sakurai H, Maeda M, Sai N, et al. Extended use of hemofiltration and high perfusion flow rate in cardiopulmonary bypass improves perioperative fluid balance in neonates and infants. Ann Thorac Cardiovasc Surg 1999;5:94–100.
29. Hiramatsu T, Imai Y, Kurosawa H, et al. Effects of dilutional and modified ultrafiltration in plasma endothelin–1 and pulmonary vascular resistance after the fontan procedure. Ann Thorac Surg 2002;73:862–865.
30. Bando K, Vijay P, Turrentine, et al. Dilutional and modified ultrfiltration reduces pulmonary hypertension after operations for congenital heart disease: A prospective randomized study. J Thorac Cardiovasc Surg 1998;115:517–525.
31. Nakamura K, Koga Y, Onitsuka T, Ishii K, Yonezawa T, Shibata K. [Ultrafiltration for hyperkalemia during cardiopulmonary bypass]. [Japanese] Kyobu Geka - Japanese J Thorac Surg 1986;39:771–774.
32. Soffer O, MacDonell RC, Finlayson DC, et al. Intraoperative hemodialysis during cardiopulmonary bypass in chronic renal failure. J Thorac Cardiovasc Surg 1979; 77:789–791.
33. Beckley PD, Erlich LF. The use of concurrent hemodialysis during cardiopulmonary bypass. Dial Transplant 1980;9:768–771.
34. Wiggins DL, Dearing JP. Simultaneous cardiopulmonary bypass and dialysis. JECT 1985;17:117–120.
35. Williams JS, Crawford FA, Kratz JM, Riley JB. Cardiac surgery for patients maintained on chronic hemodialysis. J SC Med Assoc 1991;87:569–573.
36. Niles SD, Sutton RG, Embrey RP. Ultrafiltration/hemodialysis during cardiopulmonary bypass: a case report. JECT 1995;27:104–106.

37. Hamilton CC, Harwood SJ, Deemer KA, et al. Haemodialysis during cardiopulmonary bypass using a haemofilter. Perfusion 1994;9:135–139.
38. Kirby D, Applegate B, Gabrhel W, et al. Renal dialysis during coronary artery revascularization: a case study. JECT 1982;14:424–427.
39. Murkin JM, Murphy DA, Finlayson DC, Waller JL. Hemodialysis during cardiopulmonary bypass: Report of twelve cases. Anesth Analg 1987;66:899–901.
40. Naik SK, Knight A, Elliott ML. A prospective randomized study of modified technique of ultrafiltration during pediatric open-heart surgery. Circulation 1991; 84(suppl 5):422–431.
41. Groom RC, Akl BF, Hill A, et al. Alternate method of ultrafiltration after cardiopulmonary bypass. Ann Thorac Surg 1994;58:573–574.
42. Darling EM, Shearer IR, et al. MUF in pediatric cardio-pulmonary bypass. J Extra Corpor Technol 1994;26:205–209.
43. Darling EM, Nanry K, Shearer IR, et al. Techniques of pediatric MUF: 1996 survey results. Perfusion 1998;13:93–103.
44. Portela FA, Pensado A, et al. A simple technique to perform combined ultrafiltration. Ann Thorac Surg 1999;67:859–861.
45. Aeba R, Matayoshi T, Katogi T, et al. Speed-controlled venovenous MUF for pediatric open heart operations. Ann Thorac Surg 1998;66:1835–1836.
46. Buchholtz BJ, Bert, AA, Price DR, et al. Veno-arterial modified ultrafiltration in children after cardiopulmonary bypass. J Extra Corpor Technol 1999;31: 47–49.
47. Myers GJ, Leadon RB, Mitchell LB, Ross DB. Simple modified ultrafiltration. Perfusion 2000;15:447–452.
48. LaLone BJ, Turrentine MW, Bando K, et al. Modified ultrafiltration after congenital heart surgery: a veno-venous method using a dual lumen hemodialysis catheter. JECT 32:95–102.
49. Naik SK, Balaji S, Elliott MJ. Modified ultrafiltration improves hemodynamics after cardiopulmonary bypass in children. J Am Coll Cardiol 1992;19:37A.
50. Skaryak LA, Kirshbom PM, DiBernardo LR et al. Modified ultrafiltration improved cerebral metabolic recovery after circulatory arrest. J Thorac Cardiovasc Surg 1995;109:744–752.
51. Gaynor JW, Tulloh R, Owen CH, et al. Modified ultrafiltration reduces myocardial edema and reverses hemodilution following cardiopulmonary bypass in children. J Am Coll Cardiol 1995;25:200A.
52. Meliones JM, Gaynor JW, Wilson BG, et al. Modified ultrafiltration reduces airway pressures and improves lung compliance after congenital heart surgery. J Am Coll Cardiol 1995;25:271A.
53. Chaturvedi RR, Shore DF, White PA, et al. Modified ultrafiltration improves global left ventricular systolic function after open-heart surgery in infants and children. Euro J Cardiothorac Surg 1999;15:742–746.
54. Friesen RH, Campbell DN, Clarke DR, Tornabene. Modified ultrafiltration attenuates dilutional coagulopathy in pediatric open heart operations. Ann Thorac Surg 1997;64:1787–1789.
55. Bando K, Turrentine MW, Vijay P, et al. Effect of modified ultrafiltration in high-risk patients undergoing operations for congenital heart disease. Ann Thorac Surg 1998;66:821–828.
56. Keenan HT, Thiagarajan R, Stephens KE, et al. Pulmonary function after modified venovenous ultrafiltration in infants: A prospective randomized trial. J Thorac Cardiovasc Surg 2000;119:501–507.

57. Millar AB, Armstrong L, van der Linden J, et al. Cytokine production and hemofiltration in children undergoing cardiopulmonary bypass. Ann Thorac Surg 1993; 56:1499–1502.
58. Andreasson S, Gothberg S, Berggren H, et al. Hemofiltration modifies complement activation after extracorporeal circulation in infants. Ann Thorac Surg 1993; 56: 1515–1517.
59. Wang MJ, Chui IS, Hsu CM, et al. Efficacy of ultrafiltration in removing inflammatory mediators during pediatric cardiac operations. Ann Thorac Surg 1996;61: 651–656.
60. Pearl JM, Manning PB, McNamara JL, et al. Effect of modified ultrafiltration on plasma thromboxane B2, leukotriene B4, and endothelin-1 in infants undergoing cardiopulmonary bypass. Ann Thorac Surg 1999;68:1369–1375.
61. Chew MS, Brix-Christensen V, Ravn HB, et al. Effect of modified ultrafiltration on the inflammatory response in paediatric open-heart surgery: a prospective randomized study. Perfusion 2002;17:327–333.
62. Grunenfelder J, Zund G, Schoeberlein A, et al. Modified ultrafiltration lowers adhesion molecule and cytokine levels after cardiopulmonary bypass without clinical significance in adults. Euro J Cardiothorac Surg 2000;17:77–83.
63. Tassani P, Richter JA, Eising GP, et al. Influence of combined zero-balanced and modified ultrafiltration on the systemic inflammatory response during coronary artery bypass grafting. J Cardiothorac Vasc Anesth 1999;13:285–291.
64. Luciani GB, Menon T, Vecchi B, Auriemma, Mazzucco A. Modified ultrafiltration reduces morbidity after adult cardiac operations: a prospective randomized clinical study. Circulation 2001;104:I253–I259.
65. Deptula J, Gaynor W, Groneck J, et al. Alleviating heat loss associated with modified ultrafiltration. JECT 2002;34:88–91.
66. Rodriguez RA, Ruel M, Broecker L, Cornel G. High flow rates during modified ultrafiltration decreases cerebral blood flow velocity and venous oxygen saturation in infants. Ann Thorac Surg 2005;80:22–28.
67. Sutton RG, Kratz JM, Spinale FG, Crawford FA. Comparison of three blood-processing techniques during and after cardiopulmonary bypass. Ann Thorac Surg 1993;56:938–943.
68. Smigla GR, Lawson DS, Shearer IR, et al. An ultrafiltration technique for directly reinfusing residual cardiopulmonary bypass blood. JECT 2004;36:231–234
69. Roeder B, Graham S, Searles B, et al. Evaluation of the hemobag: a novel ultrafiltration system for circuit salvage. JECT 2004;36:162–165.
70. Page P. Ultrafiltration versus cell washing for blood concentration. J Extra Corpor Technol 1990;22(3):142–150.
71. Johnson HD, Morgan MS, Utley JR, Leyland SA, Nguyen-Duy T, Crawley DM Comparative analysis of recovery of cardiopulmonary bypass residual blood: Cell saver vs. hemoconcentrator. J Extra Corpor Technol 1994;26(4):194–199.
72. Eichert I, Isgro F, Kiessling AH, Saggau W. Cell saver, ultrafiltration and direct transfusion: comparative study of three blood processing techniques. Thorac Cardiovasc Surg 2001;49(3):149–152.

10 Echocardiography and Cardiopulmonary Bypass

Jack S. Shanewise, MD

Contents

INTRODUCTION

Echocardiography has become indispensable to modern cardiac surgery, particularly since the introduction of transesophageal echocardiography (TEE) approximately 20 years ago. With TEE, an ultrasound transducer attached to a flexible scope (Fig. 1) is positioned in the esophagus or the stomach posterior to the heart. Because it does not interfere with the surgical field, produces high-resolution images of the heart and great vessels, and with Doppler echocardiography demonstrates and measures blood flow, all in real time, TEE has found many uses during heart surgery, as both a diagnostic tool and a monitor of cardiac function. This chapter explores ways in which echocardiography can be of use in patients undergoing cardiopulmonary bypass (CPB). It will begin by considering how echocardiography can be used to prevent complications of CPB by identifying risk factors before cannulation, discuss using TEE to insert and position cannula, and finish up by covering the topic of intracardiac air.

From: *Current Cardiac Surgery: On Bypass: Advanced Perfusion Techniques*
Edited by: L. B. Mongero and J. R. Beck © Humana Press Inc., Totowa, NJ

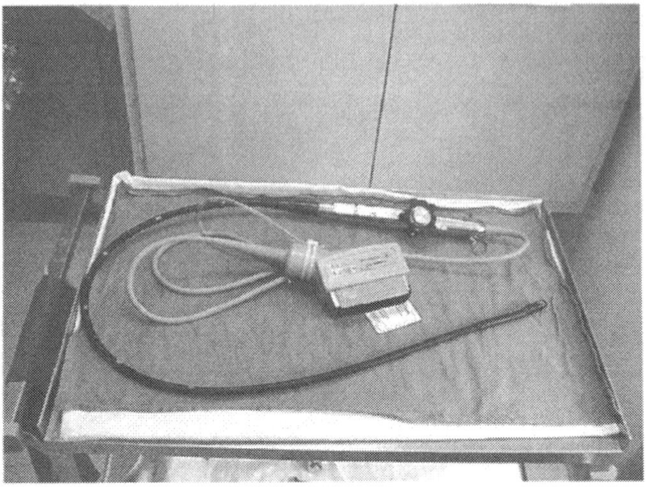

Fig. 1. A transesophageal echocardiography probe. A high-frequency ultrasound transducer is located in the tip, which is placed through the mouth into the esophagus and positioned posterior to the heart. The control wheels on the handle allow manipulation of the probe tip while in the patient.

IDENTIFICATION OF RISK FACTORS BEFORE CARDIOPULMONARY BYPASS

Atherosclerosis of the Ascending Aorta

Perioperative central nervous system (CNS) injury remains one of the biggest risks facing patients undergoing CPB today. A large, multicenter study of coronary artery bypass graft (CABG) patients found that there was a 3.1% incidence of type 1 injuries (focal lesions, stupor, or coma) *(1)*. The risk factors for these injuries were atherosclerosis of the ascending aorta detected by the surgeon, history of a previous neurological injury, and increasing age. Other studies have shown that the risk factors for stroke during heart surgery are risk factors for atherosclerosis: increasing age, hypertension, previous stroke, and carotid bruits *(2,3)*. An autopsy study of 221 patients who died after heart surgery with CPB found that atheroembolism occurred at an increasing incidence with time, reaching over 48% in 1989, which was the last year of the study *(4)*. The incidence of atherosclerosis in the ascending aorta was 55.7%, and was found to increase dramatically with age, with severe disease being present in nearly 75% of the patients over 75 years of age. There was a high correlation between atheroembolism and severe atherosclerosis of the ascending aorta. Transcranial Doppler studies have shown that embolism to the brain occurs when the ascending aorta is manipulated (cannulated, clamped, unclamped, and decannulated) during surgery *(5)*. Thus, it seems reasonable to assume that atheroembolism caused by clamping and/or cannulation of the ascending aorta for CPB is an important cause of CNS injury during heart surgery.

Epiaortic echocardiography (EE) is the best way to diagnose and evaluate patients for ascending aortic atherosclerosis before CPB *(6–10)*. With this technique, a high-frequency ultrasound transducer is placed in a sterile sheath, passed onto the surgical field, and placed directly on the ascending aorta by the surgeon after sternotomy (Fig. 2). TEE has difficulty imaging the distal portion of the ascending aorta and proximal aortic arch because the trachea comes between the esophagus and these regions of the aorta *(11)*. In one study, TEE missed over 70% of palpation and 50% of moderate or severe lesions detected with EE *(7)*.

The equipment needed to perform EE includes an ultrasound machine, a high frequency (5–15 MHz) surface ultrasound transducer, and a sterile sheath. To create an interface through which the ultrasound may pass, sterile water is placed within the sheath and into the pericardial well. To adequately image the anterior wall of the aorta, the

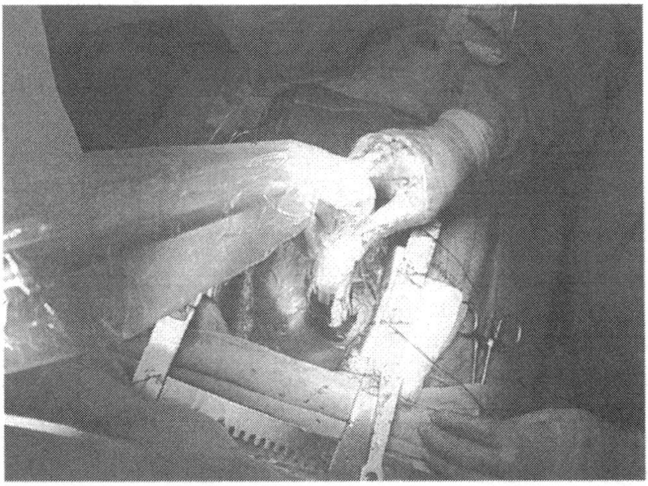

Fig. 2. Epiaortic echocardiography. A high-frequency ultrasound transducer is placed in a sterile sheath, passed onto the surgical field, and placed directly on the ascending aorta. Water has been placed in the sheath and the pericardium to create a fluid interface for the ultrasound.

transducer is held approximately 1 cm above the outer surface of the aorta. This is most easily accomplished by using a stand-off, which is a device that is fitted to the end of the transducer that leaves a gap between it and the anterior wall of the aorta. The depth of the image display is adjusted to center the aorta in the image, usually 6–8 cm. The focus of the instrument is placed at the middle of the aorta. The gain is adjusted so the echoes are just barely visible in the lumen of the aorta. Because the anterior and posterior walls of the aorta are perpendicular to the ultrasound, they will appear to be brighter than the sides, which are more parallel and less reflective. The intima is seen as a thin line less than 2-mm thick around the inner edge of the aorta.

To describe the location of lesions, the ascending aorta is divided into three regions longitudinally and four regions axially, for a total of 12 segments. The proximal third of the ascending aorta is from the aortic valve to the inferior level of the right pulmonary artery. The mid third is that which lies over the right pulmonary artery. The distal third goes from the superior edge of the right pulmonary artery to the aortic arch. Each third is divided into four quadrants: anterior, posterior, left, and right. Right and left are most easily distinguished by identifying the superior vena cava, which is adjacent to the right side of the ascending aorta.

The examination of the ascending aorta should be thorough and systematic. Significant lesions are often highly localized, and may be adjacent to normal appearing aorta. Start by placing the probe over the proximal portion and rotating it until a circular, short-axis image is seen. The transducer is then angled inferiorly until the aortic valve comes into view. Then the probe is slowly moved through the proximal, mid, and distal thirds until the aortic arch is seen. The probe is then rotated 90 degrees until a long-axis image of the aorta is seen, and then the proximal, mid, and distal thirds are imaged once again. The location of lesions in relation to the four axial quadrants is determined with the short axis views and their location proximally or distally with the long axis. The planned locations for manipulation of the aorta (cannulation and clamping sites) are then each carefully examined in short and long axis. The surgeon can determine the location of lesions by noting the position of the probe when the lesion is in the image. Many lesions will also be palpable and can be located in this manner. Calcified lesions of the anterior wall of the aorta may obscure the posterior wall because of acoustic shadowing. Moving the transducer to one side or the other of such a lesion and then angling it to direct the imaging plane under the plaque may allow imaging of the posterior wall in these regions. A

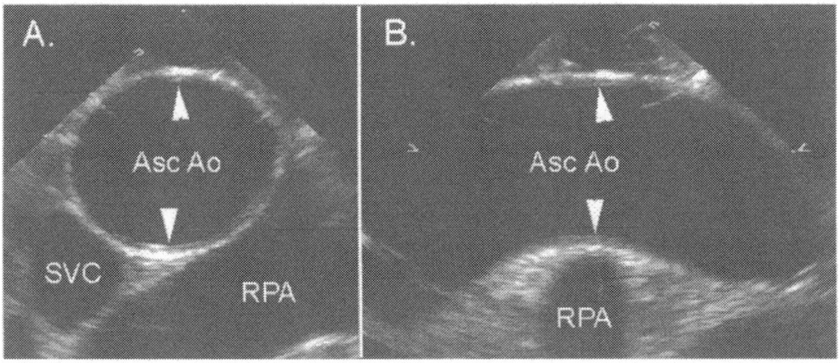

Fig. 3. Short axis (A) and long axis (B) epiaortic views of a normal ascending aorta. The intima (arrowheads) appears as a thin line less than 2 mm thick inside the aorta. Asc Ao, ascending aorta; RPA, right pulmonary artery; SVC, superior vena cava.

five-grade scale is used to indicate the severity of the disease seen: Grade 1 is normal-to-minimal disease, with the intima less than 2 mm in thickness (Fig. 3); Grade 2 is mild disease with intimal thickening of 2–3 mm; Grade 3 is moderate disease with lesions 3–5 mm in thickness (Fig. 4); Grade 4 is severe disease with thickening greater than 5 mm; and Grade 5 indicates that a mobile lesion was seen. In general, Grades 1 and 2 are not considered significant, whereas Grades 3, 4, and 5 may warrant modification of surgical technique.

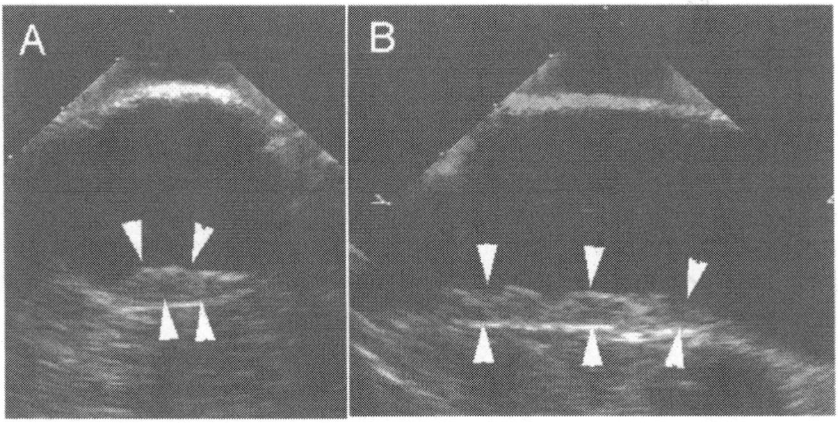

Fig. 4. Short axis (A) and long axis (B) epiaortic views of an ascending aorta with grade 3 atherosclerosis. The posterior aspect of the intima (arrowheads) is thickened and irregular inside the aorta.

Of course, the hope of identifying atherosclerosis within the ascending aorta is that surgical technique can somehow be modified to prevent atheroembolism and stroke. Reported modifications range from simply changing the location of cannulation and clamping sites to replacing the entire ascending aorta when it is severely and diffusely diseased *(12)*. Another approach is to find with EE a suitable location for cannulation, construct the distal anastomoses with cold fibrillatory arrest while cooling the patient, and then construct a proximal anastomosis without clamping the aorta, using a brief period of circulatory arrest. The other vein grafts may be connected to the first as the patient is rewarmed. With the increasing use of off pump techniques to revascularize the myocardium, it is possible to avoid all manipulation of the ascending aorta (no-touch technique) by constructing bypass grafts with arterial conduits, such as the internal thoracic (mammary) arteries, without CPB. Vein grafts and free arterial grafts may be connected to the in situ arterial conduits. There are devices available now that create a proximal anastomosis for a vein graft using staples, without needing to clamp the aorta *(13)*. Some of these modifications may have risks in themselves, and although there are reports of good results using these techniques *(14)*, well-controlled trials proving their efficacy have not been done. It seems unlikely that trials of sufficient size and power to resolve the issue one way or another will be done anytime soon. One would, nonetheless, like to think that we are in a better position to avoid atheroembolism and its consequences knowing when and where such lesions are present.

Intracardiac Thrombus

Another cause of systemic embolization in patients undergoing CPB is dislodgement of thrombus present in the left ventricle or the left atrium *(15,16)*. TEE is an excellent means of identifying such thrombus and, if present, allows the surgeon to avoid dislodging it during manipulation of the heart. Thrombi are much more common in the left heart than the right, and usually have a predisposing cause. Left atrial thrombi are usually associated with chamber enlargement and/or atrial fibrillation and are most often located in the left atrial appendage. Left ventricular thrombi are usually adjacent to a high-grade regional wall motion abnormality caused by myocardial infarction, usually within the apex. Thrombus arising in the right heart is rare, but can occur when devices are present, such as pacemaker electrodes or central venous catheters. Thrombi arising in the veins can be seen in transit through the right heart to the lungs on their way to becoming pulmonary emboli. Such thrombi have, on rare occasion, been seen with TEE passing from the right atrium through a patent foramen ovale (PFO) to the left heart, producing a paradoxical embolus *(17,18)*.

Left heart thrombi that appear on TEE to be fresh or highly mobile may be more prone to dislodgement and embolization than chronic, more organized thrombi. The surgeon may elect to remove the thrombus or not. If left in place, the thrombus should be checked again with TEE before beginning to wean CPB to determine whether it has been dislodged. Dislodged thrombus may obstruct a coronary artery if ejected into the ascending aorta while on CPB, and if large enough, may be visible with TEE.

Aortic Regurgitation

The presence of aortic regurgitation (AR) has important implications for patients undergoing CPB, and TEE is a very sensitive technique for identifying this condition. The best TEE views for seeing AR are the midesophageal aortic valve short- and long-axis views using color flow Doppler *(19)*, which show the regurgitation as high-velocity, turbulent flow at the valve and in the left ventricular outflow tract during diastole (Fig. 5). AR will lead to distention of the left ventricle (LV) on CPB if it stops beating (e.g. with ventricular fibrillation or asystole) or if there is insufficient function of the LV to eject the volume of blood that regurgitates between contractions. Even hemodynamically insignificant, mild AR can cause distention of the LV on CPB if the heart is not beating because the regurgitation will persist until there is equalization of the pressures between the aorta and the LV. This can particularly be a problem immediately after aortic cross-clamp removal in the period before the LV regains adequate function to keep itself emptied out. Knowing that AR is present alerts the surgeon to massage the LV or place a vent in the LV to prevent distention. TEE can be used to monitor the size of the LV to detect distention when it occurs. If severe AR is present, placing a vent in the LV may result in inadequate systemic flow while on CPB if too much of the pump output passes into the LV through the vent back to the pump, bypassing the body. Placing a cross clamp across the ascending aorta is an effective means of preventing ventricular distention from AR. Severe AR may make it difficult to effectively deliver antegrade cardioplegia because much of the cardioplegia solution regurgitates into the LV, preventing an adequate pressure from developing in the proximal aorta to effectively perfuse the coronary arteries.

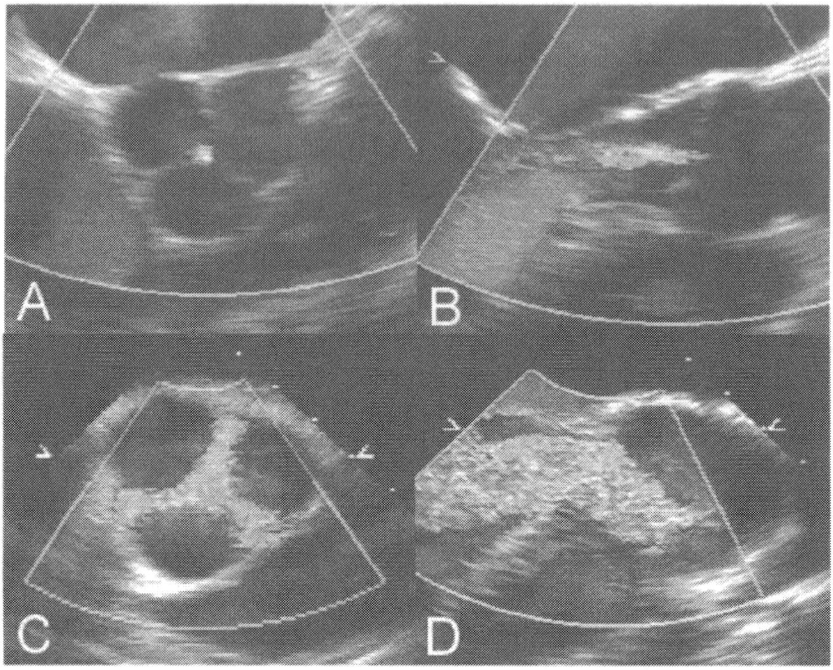

Fig. 5. TEE views of aortic regurgitation (AR). (A) Midesophageal short axis view an aortic valve with mild (1+) AR, showing a small, central regurgitant orifice. (B) Midesophageal long axis view of the same valve as in A, showing a narrow jet of AR confined to the left ventricular outflow tract. (C) Midesophageal short axis view of an aortic valve with severe AR. There is regurgitation visible through the entire surface of cusp coaptation. (D) Midesophageal long axis view of the same aortic valve as in C, showing a wide jet of AR extending into the left ventricle.

Interatrial Shunts

Patients undergoing CPB for open cardiac procedures may develop unexpected problems on CPB if undetected communications between the right and left atria are present. If the left heart is opened, air can enter the right side and cause problems with venous drainage and air lock formation in the venous cannula. Also, blood can pass from the right atrium into the left, making visualization of the left heart structures difficult. If the right heart is opened, air can enter through the communication into the left heart, eventually resulting in systemic air embolization after CPB. To prevent this, TEE can be used to detect interatrial communication before CPB. The most common interatrial communication is a PFO, which is present in 25–30% of the general population *(20)*. PFO can be diagnosed before CPB in some patients by detecting interatrial flow with color flow Doppler, but the most sensitive means of making the diagnosis is with an injection of saline contrast (fluid agitated with a small amount of air) into the venous circulation, using TEE to identify the appearance of contrast in the left atrium, indicating an interatrial communication *(21)*. This may not reveal the presence of a PFO unless the right atrial pressure is somehow elevated above the left, causing the contrast to pass right to left through the PFO. This is usually accomplished with TEE during surgery by applying positive pressure to the lungs for a few seconds and releasing as the contrast is injected. Nonetheless, a saline contrast test is not truly negative for PFO unless the atrial septum is seen to be bowing into the left atrium, indicating that the right atrial pressure was higher than the left, at least transiently. True atrial septal defects can be easily identified with TEE before CPB by examining the atrial septum for visual defects (holes) and interatrial flow with color flow Doppler. Often, the first clue that a patient has an undiagnosed atrial septal defect is enlargement of the right heart caused by the left-to-right interatrial shunt.

Persistent Left Superior Vena Cava

Persistent left superior vena cava (PLSVC) is a relatively common (about 1 in 1,000 in the general population) congenital anomaly that is of no physiologic consequence unless the patient is having heart surgery with CPB *(22)*. It is often undiagnosed before surgery, but is easily detected with intraoperative TEE before CPB. With PLSVC, the venous drainage from the left internal jugular and left subclavian veins enters the right atrium through an abnormally large coronary sinus. This results in two potential problems during CPB if unrecognized. First, if the right atrium is opened, there will be a large amount of uncontrolled venous return entering the surgical field. Second, if retrograde cardioplegia is delivered through a coronary sinus cannula, most of the cardioplegia fluid will regurgitate into the PLSVC, rendering it ineffective *(23)*. PLSVC should be suspected if the coronary sinus appears to be large on TEE. The diagnosis can be confirmed by injecting saline contrast into a vein draining into the left internal jugular or subclavian vein while imaging the coronary sinus. If a PLSVC is present, the contrast will be seen to pass through the coronary sinus into the right atrium, while appearance of the contrast in the right atrium before the coronary sinus rules out the presence of PLSVC.

Systemic to Pulmonary Shunts

Vascular communications between the systemic and pulmonary circulations can create problems in patients on CPB, especially if undetected. Once the heart stops beating effectively, the right side will quickly become distended to systemic pressure, and if the right heart is opened, a torrent of high velocity blood loss may result. The systemic pressures can distend and damage the pulmonary capillary bed and cause distention of the left side of the heart as blood passes through the lungs into the left atrium. The most common congenital systemic–pulmonary connection is a patent ductus arteriosus (PDA), which connects the proximal descending thoracic aorta to the main pulmonary artery and is occasionally undiagnosed in adult patients. Transesophageal echocardiography is an effective means of identifying and measuring the size of a PDA *(24)*, which is usually best seen with color flow Doppler of the proximal descending thoracic aorta. Patients with cyanotic heart disease may have had systemic–pulmonary shunts surgically constructed to increase their pulmonary blood flow. It is important to identify and locate such shunts with TEE so that they can be surgically controlled before initiating CPB. These shunts typically appear on TEE as continuous high velocity flow entering the main, right, or left pulmonary arteries, but the shunting may be balanced, or even right to left, in patients with severe pulmonary hypertension.

INSERTION AND POSITIONING OF CANNULAE USED DURING CARDIOPULMONARY BYPASS

Because TEE provides excellent visualization of the heart and great vessels in most patients, it can facilitate placement and positioning of the various cannulae and catheters that are used during CPB. This has become increasingly important with the use of minimally invasive techniques that limit the ability to directly visualize the heart and great vessels (Fig. 6).

Venous Return Cannulae

Cannulae taking the venous return from the patient to the pump are usually placed in the vena cava or directly into the right atrium. TEE can be used to position cannulae that are inserted at a site remote from the heart, such as the femoral or internal jugular veins. After the vein is accessed, a guide wire is inserted and visualized with TEE to ensure that the cannula is being inserted into the proper blood vessel. After the venous access is enlarged with dilators, the cannula is inserted while

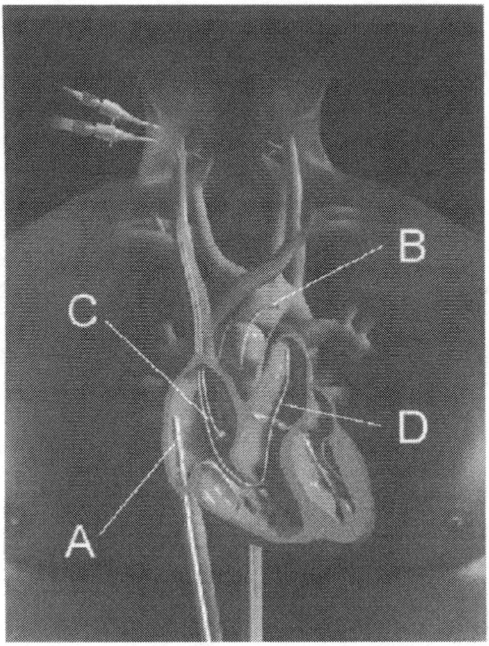

Fig. 6. Cannulae and catheters used for CPB during minimally invasive heart surgery. TEE is used to position these devices. (A) Venous return cannula inserted through the femoral vein and positioned in the inferior vena cava or the right atrium. (B) Aortic balloon occluder catheter inserted through the femoral artery and positioned in the ascending aorta. (C) Coronary sinus retrograde cardioplegia catheter inserted through the right internal jugular vein. (D) Pulmonary artery vent catheter place through the right internal jugular vein.

the position is monitored with TEE. Depending on the surgery and the design of the cannula, venous return cannulae placed through the femoral vein may need to be positioned in the intrahepatic inferior vena cava (IVC) or advanced into the right atrium. The IVC can be visualized with TEE by advancing the probe to the transgastric position and rotating it to the patient's right until the IVC come into view. Increasing the multiplane angle from zero degrees to approximately 50–70 degrees develops a long axis view of the intrahepatic portion of the IVC (Fig. 7). The cannula is easily seen as it is advanced toward the heart (Fig. 8). Once the cannula is in view, the guide wire is pulled back to improve visualization of the tip of the cannula. The midesophageal bicaval view *(19)* is used to position the cannula in the right atrium if needed (Fig. 9). If a PFO is present, the cannula may pass through the right atrium

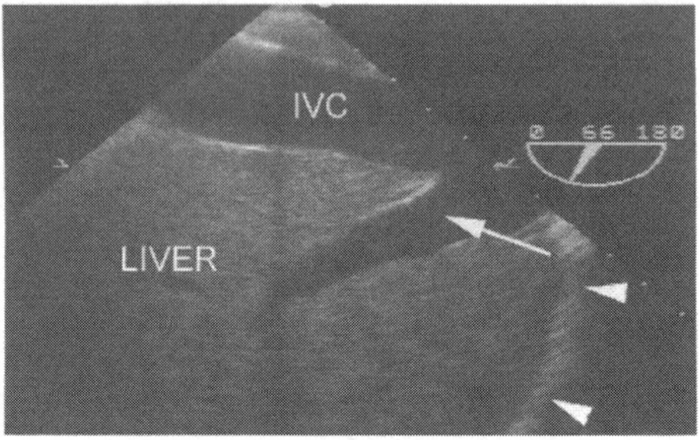

Fig. 7. TEE transgastric long axis view of the intrahepatic portion of the inferior vena cava used to position venous return cannulae inserted through the femoral vein. The arrow indicates the hepatic vein. The arrowheads indicate the diaphragm. IVC, inferior vena cava.

into the left atrium. This is easily detected with TEE and allows withdrawal and repositioning of the cannula into the right atrium (Fig. 10). Cannulae inserted through the internal jugular veins into the superior vena cava (SVC) are best imaged with TEE using a high bicaval view at the level of the right pulmonary artery (Fig. 11).

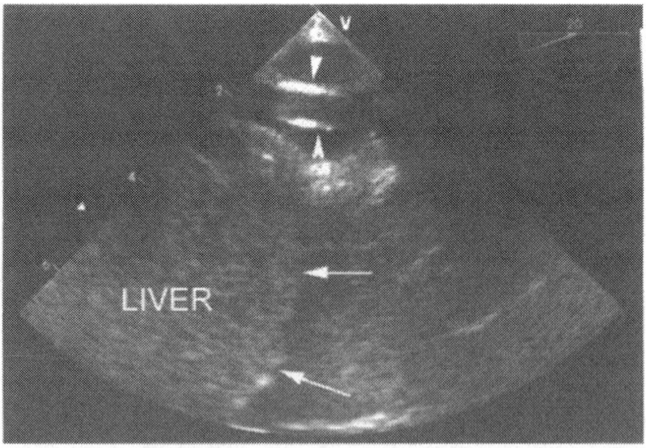

Fig. 8. TEE view of the junction of the inferior vena cava and the right atrium with a venous return cannula (arrowheads) that was inserted through the femoral vein. The arrows indicate the dome of the liver.

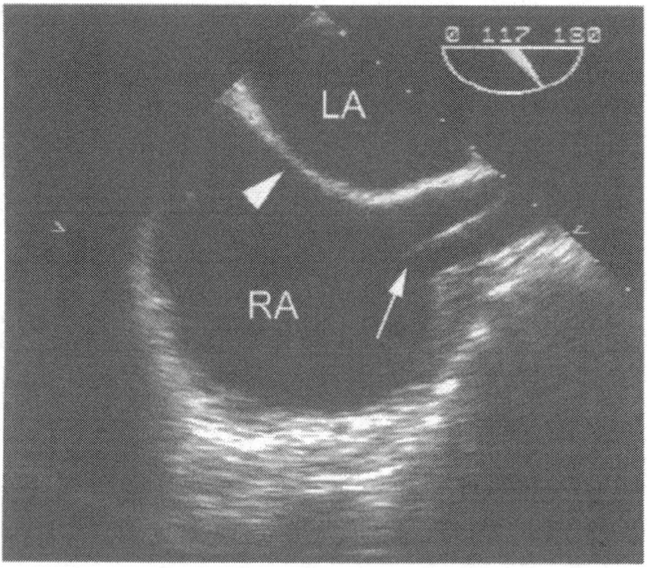

Fig. 9. TEE bicaval view useful for positioning cannulae and catheters in the superior vena cava and the right atrium. The arrow indicates a guide wire entering the right atrium through the superior vena cava. The arrowhead indicates the interatrial septum. RA, right atrium; LA, left atrium.

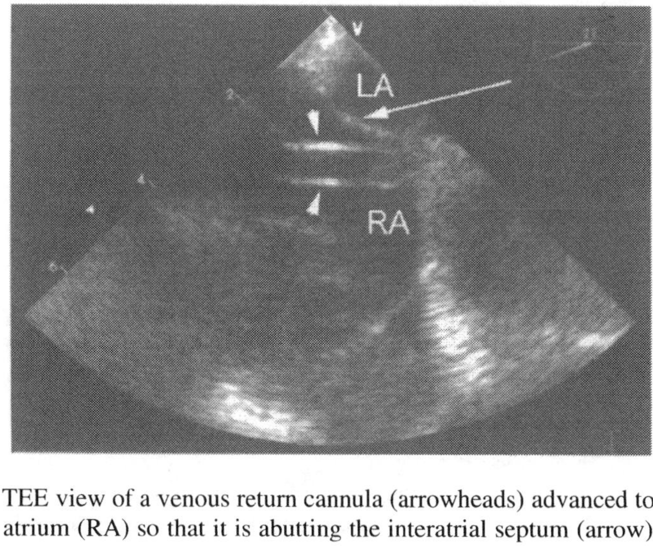

Fig. 10. TEE view of a venous return cannula (arrowheads) advanced too far into the right atrium (RA) so that it is abutting the interatrial septum (arrow). LA, left atrium.

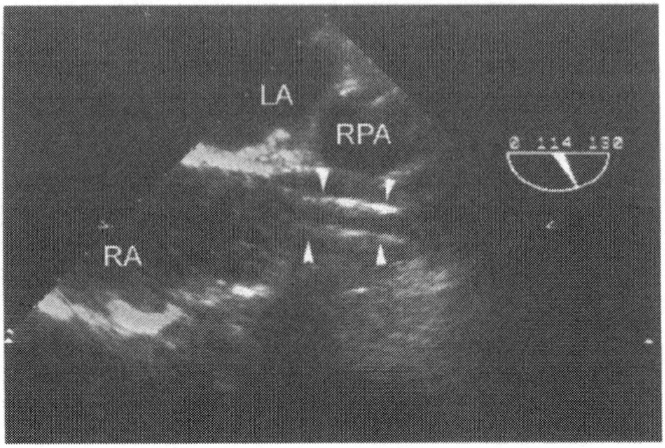

Fig. 11. TEE bicaval view of a venous return cannula (arrowheads) inserted through the right internal jugular vein and positioned in the superior vena cava. RA, right atrium; LA, left atrium; RPA, right pulmonary artery.

Arterial Cannulae and Catheters

Arterial cannulae for CPB are usually inserted directly into the ascending aorta. The location and orientation of the cannula can often be seen with TEE, most often using the midesophageal ascending aorta long axis view *(19)* (Fig. 12). Longer, more flexible arterial cannulae may be inserted through the ascending aorta and positioned in the distal

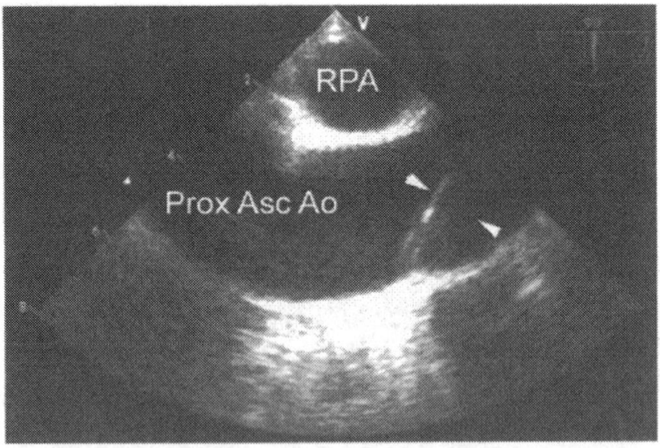

Fig. 12. TEE long axis view of the ascending aorta at the level of the right pulmonary artery (RPA) showing an arterial cannula (arrowheads) properly oriented toward the aortic arch. Prox Asc Ao, proximal ascending aorta.

arch or proximal descending aorta, usually over a guidewire *(14)*. TEE is used to confirm that the wire is not entering a great vessel before inserting the cannula. Alternative sites for arterial cannulation, such as the femoral or axillary arteries, may be used because of limited access through a minimally invasive incision or because of pathology in the ascending aorta, such as atherosclerotic plaquing or dissection *(25)*, which can be detected by intraoperative TEE or EE. If a device is advanced retrograde from the femoral artery into the aorta, TEE examination of the descending aorta is performed to exclude contraindications, such as aneurysm, severe atherosclerosis, and dissection. It can also be used to position cannulae and devices in the descending thoracic aorta *(26)*.

Coronary Sinus Cannulae

Delivery of retrograde cardioplegia through a coronary sinus cannula has become an important part of the myocardial preservation strategy in many patients undergoing heart surgery with CPB *(27,28)*. Although blind insertion of these cannulae through a median sternotomy is usually not difficult, patients with posterior adhesions from previous surgery or minimally invasive incisions may require visualization with TEE to ensure proper positioning of the coronary sinus cannula *(29)*. Some techniques use percutaneous insertion of the cannula through the right internal jugular vein using TEE guidance *(30)*. The coronary sinus is best imaged with TEE in long axis by slightly advancing the probe in the esophagus from the midesophageal four-chamber *(19)* view until the coronary sinus comes into view. Then the multiplane angle is increased until the length of the sinus in the image is maximized (Fig. 13). Echocardiography with myocardial contrast injection has been used to confirm the position of the coronary artery cannula and demonstrate retrograde cardioplegia delivery *(31)*.

INTRACARDIAC AIR

When the heart is opened and blood suctioned from a chamber while on CPB, air inevitably enters the heart. TEE is an excellent means of detecting and locating retained intracardiac air in patients on CPB and is helpful in efforts to remove the air before discontinuing CPB to prevent systemic air embolism *(32,33)*. Air is seen within in the heart in two forms. Most commonly, microscopic bubbles are suspended in the blood, which appear on TEE as tiny white specks moving with blood flow (Fig. 14). The presence of these microscopic bubbles has

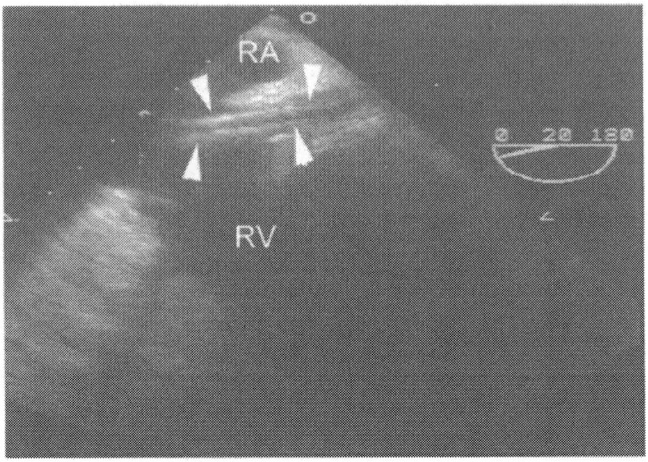

Fig. 13. TEE view of a retrograde cardioplegia cannula (arrowheads) properly positioned in the coronary sinus. RA, right atrium; RV, right ventricle. This image was developed by slightly advancing the probe from the midesophageal four-chamber view until the coronary sinus came into view and increasing the multiplane angle until it opened up in long axis.

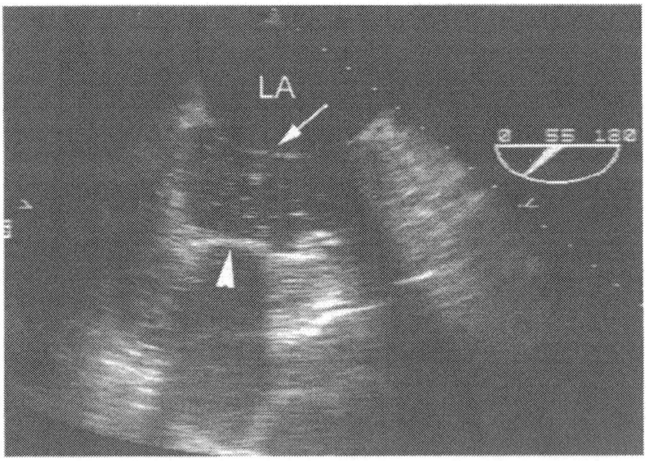

Fig. 14. A TEE view of a patient on CPB with retained intracardiac air in the left ventricle. The mitral valve is indicated by the arrow. The arrowhead indicates the air fluid level of a large pocket of air filling the apex of the ventricle, which is located toward the bottom of the image. The bright, echo-dense spots between the valve and the air–fluid level are caused by microscopic bubbles suspended in the blood. The air–fluid level was seen to wobble as the heart was moving. The echolucent area to the arrowhead side of the air-fluid level is a mirror artifact, and wobbled in synchrony with the air-fluid level.

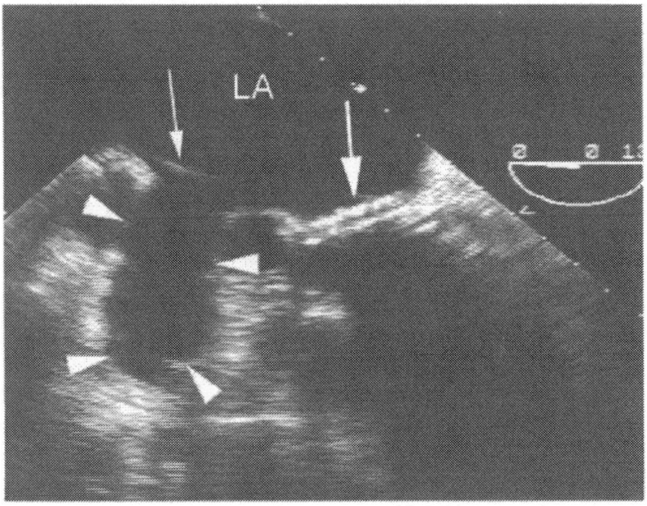

Fig. 15. A TEE view of a patient on CPB with retained intracardiac air in the left atrium (LA). A prosthetic mitral valve is indicated by the large arrow. The small arrow indicates the air fluid level of a pocket of air floating up against the interatrial septum, which was seen to wobble as the heart was moving. The echolucent area indicated by the arrowheads is a mirror artifact, and wobbled in synchrony with the fluid level.

not been associated with adverse events, and should not be a cause for great concern *(34)*. Some patients, however, have macroscopic collections of retained air, which manifest on echocardiography as highly reflective, wobbling lines caused by the air–fluid interface between the blood and the air (Figs. 14 and 15). These lines are typically oriented perpendicular to the direction of gravity (Fig. 16), as one would expect, and echocardiography can be used to estimate the volume of the macroscopic bubble *(35)*. Retained air in the left heart is of primary concern because of its potential to embolize to the systemic circulation, but air in the right heart can cause paradoxical emboli if there is a communication between the right and the lefts sides, such as a PFO.

Precise location with TEE of air pockets facilitates their removal through left heart vent cannulae already in place or direct needle aspiration. Another method of air removal is filling and shaking the beating heart to agitate the bubbles into the blood flow, which carries them to the ascending aorta where they come out a vent site. Turning the right side of the patient down will help passage of the bubbles from the LA into the LV, and then turning the left side down will help passage from

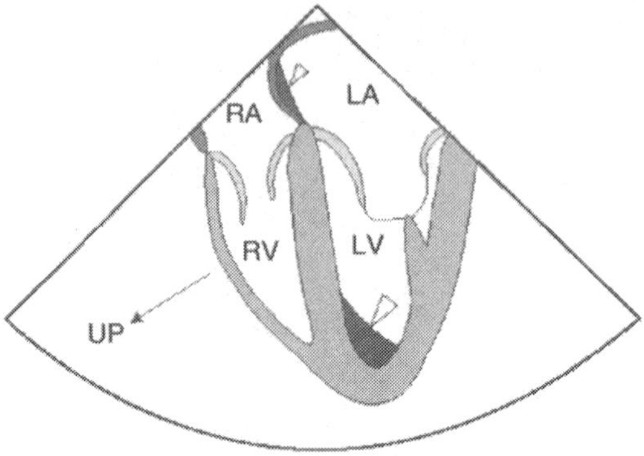

Fig. 16. Diagram of a TEE midesophageal four-chamber view demonstrating typical locations of air collections in the left atrium (LA) and left ventricle (LV). LA air (small arrowhead) layers against the interatrial septum and LV air (large arrowhead) in the LV apex. The arrow indicates the up direction in relation to gravity in a supine patient. RA, right atrium; RV; right ventricle.

the LV to the aorta, progress which can be followed by TEE. Air is often present in the pulmonary veins and does not appear in the heart until flow through the lungs is present as CPB is being weaned, or even sometime after CPB *(36)*. Macroscopic air pockets should be removed from the heart before decannulation to prevent air embolization to the coronary arteries after bypass, which is manifest by acute ST elevation on electrocardiogram ("tombstones"), new regional wall motion abnormalities on TEE, and sudden deterioration in cardiac function. This most often occurs to the right coronary artery because its origin is in the up direction in a supine patient, but left coronary artery embolism can occur, especially through coronary bypass grafts attached to the anterior aspect of the ascending aorta. If the cannulae are still in place, it is a simple matter to go back on CPB until the air passes through the coronaries, which usually takes just a few minutes and is indicated by resolution of the ST elevation and the TEE wall motion abnormalities. If the coronary embolism occurs after decannulation, or even worse, after chest closure or when the patient is moved from the OR table to the bed, the acute right heart failure can quickly lead to cardiac arrest.

CONCLUSION

TEE can provide real-time, high-resolution images of the heart and great vessels of patients undergoing heart surgery without interfering with the progress of the operation. Doppler echocardiography also permits visualization and measurement of blood flow and velocity. EE can be used to identify patients at risk for atheroembolism from cannulating and clamping the ascending aorta, allowing modification of surgical technique to avoid CNS injury. TEE can also be used to help prevent complications of CPB, facilitate insertion and positioning of cannulae used for CPB, and locate and assist with the removal of intracardiac air collections after the heart is opened on CPB.

REFERENCES

1. Roach GW, Kanchuger M, Mangano CM, et al. Adverse cerebral outcomes after coronary bypass surgery. Multicenter Study of Perioperative Ischemia Research Group and the Ischemia Research and Education Foundation Investigators. N Eng J Med 1996;335(25):1857–1863.
2. McKhann GM, Goldsborough MA, Borowicz LM, Jr., et al. Predictors of stroke risk in coronary artery bypass patients. Ann Thorac Surg 1997;63(2):516–521.
3. Gardner TJ, Horneffer PJ, Manolio TA, et al. Stroke following coronary artery bypass grafting: a ten-year study. Ann Thorac Surg 40(6):574–581.
4. Blauth CI, Cosgrove DM, Webb BW, et al. Atheroembolism from the ascending aorta. An emerging problem in cardiac surgery. J Thorac Cardiovasc Surg 1992;103(6):1104–1111; discussion 1111–1112.
5. Barbut D, Hinton RB, Szatrowski TP, et al. Cerebral emboli detected during bypass surgery are associated with clamp removal. Stroke 1994;25(12):2398–2402.
6. Wilson MJ, Boyd SY, Lisagor PG, Rubal BJ, Cohen DJ. Ascending aortic atheroma assessed intraoperatively by epiaortic and transesophageal echocardiography. Ann Thorac Surg 2000;70(1):25–30.
7. Royse C, Royse A, Blake D, Grigg L. Screening the thoracic aorta for atheroma: a comparison of manual palpation, transesophageal and epiaortic ultrasonography. Ann Thorac Cardiovasc Surg 1998;4(6):347–350.
8. Sylivris S, Calafiore P, Matalanis G, et al. The intraoperative assessment of ascending aortic atheroma: epiaortic imaging is superior to both transesophageal echocardiography and direct palpation. J Cardiothorac Vasc Anesth 1997;11(6): 704–707.
9. Davila-Roman VG, Phillips KJ, Daily BB, Davila RM, Kouchoukos NT, Barzilai B. Intraoperative transesophageal echocardiography and epiaortic ultrasound for assessment of atherosclerosis of the thoracic aorta. J Am Coll Cardiol 1996; 28(4):942–947.
10. Nicolosi AC, Aggarwal A, Almassi GH, Olinger GN. Intraoperative epiaortic ultrasound during cardiac surgery. J Card Surg 1996;11(1):49–55.
11. Konstadt SN, Reich DL, Quintana C, Levy M. The ascending aorta: how much does transesophageal echocardiography see? Anesth Analg 1994;78(2):240–244.
12. Wareing TH, Davila-Roman VG, Daily BB, et al. Strategy for the reduction of stroke incidence in cardiac surgical patients. Ann Thorac Surg 1993;55(6):1400–1407; discussion 1407–1408.
13. Calafiore AM, Bar-El Y, Vitolla G, Di Giammarco G, Teodori G. Iaco AL, D'Alessandro S, Di Mauro M. Early clinical experience with a new sutureless anastomotic device for proximal anastomosis of the saphenous vein to the aorta. J Thorac Cardiovasc Surg 2001;121(5):854–858.

14. Gold JP, Torres KE, Maldarelli W, Zhuravlev I, Condit D, Wasnick J. Improving outcomes in coronary surgery: the impact of echo-directed aortic cannulation and perioperative hemodynamic management in 500 patients. Ann Thorac Surg 2004; 78(5):1579–1585.
15. Sharma S, Ehsan A, Couper GS, Shernan SK, Wholey RM, Aranki SF. Unrecognized left ventricular thrombus during reoperative coronary artery bypass grafting. Ann Thorac Surg 2004;78(5):e79–e80.
16. Anderson D, Wibbenmeyer L, Morgan L, Kerber R, Kealey GP. Left atrial thrombus after emergency left atrial cannulation for cardiopulmonary bypass. J Trauma-Injury Infection Critical Care 2000;49(2):345–347.
17. Rinaldi CA, Stewart AJ, Blauth CI. Intracardiac thrombus traversing a patent foramen ovale: impending paradoxical embolism demonstrated by transoesophageal echocardiography. Int J Clin Pract 2002;56(3):230–231.
18. Kessel-Schaefer A, Lefkovits M, Zellweger MJ, et al. Migrating thrombus trapped in a patent foramen ovale. Circulation 2001;103(14):1928.
19. Shanewise JS, Cheung AT, Aronson S, et al. ASE/SCA guidelines for performing a comprehensive intraoperative multiplane transesophageal echocardiography examination: recommendations of the American Society of Echocardiography Council for Intraoperative Echocardiography and the Society of Cardiovascular Anesthesiologists Task Force for Certification in Perioperative Transesophageal Echocardiography. Anesth Analg 1999;89(4):870–884.
20. Schneider B, Zienkiewicz T, Jansen V, Hofmann T, Noltenius H, Meinertz T. Diagnosis of patent foramen ovale by transesophageal echocardiography and correlation with autopsy findings. Am J Cardiol 1996;77(14):1202–1209.
21. Augoustides JG, Weiss SJ, Weiner J, Mancini J, Savino JS, Cheung AT. Diagnosis of patent foramen ovale with multiplane transesophageal echocardiography in adult cardiac surgical patients. J Cardiothorac Vasc Anesth 2004;18(6):725–730.
22. Garduno C, Chew S, Forbess J, Smith PK, Grocott HP. Persistent left superior vena cava and partial anomalous pulmonary venous connection: incidental diagnosis by transesophageal echocardiography during coronary artery bypass surgery. J Am Soc Echocardiogr 1999;12(8):682–685.
23. Roberts WA, Risher WH, Schwarz KQ. Transesophageal echocardiographic identification of persistent left superior vena cava: retrograde administration of cardioplegia during cardiac surgery. Anesthesiology 1994;81(3):760–762.
24. Chang ST, Hung KC, Hsieh IC, et al. Evaluation of shunt flow by multiplane transesophageal echocardiography in adult patients with isolated patent ductus arteriosus. J Am Soc Echocardiogr 2002;15(11):1367–1373.
25. Strauch JT, Spielvogel D, Lauten A, et al. Axillary artery cannulation: routine use in ascending aorta and aortic arch replacement. Ann Thorac Surg 78(1):103–108.
26. Shanewise JS, Sadel SM. Intraoperative transesophageal echocardiography to assist the insertion and positioning of the intraaortic balloon pump. Anesth Analg 79(3):577–580.
27. Gates RN, Laks H. Retrograde cardioplegia. Adv Card Surg 1998;10:115–139.
28. Ruengsakulrach P, Buxton BF. Anatomic and hemodynamic considerations influencing the efficiency of retrograde cardioplegia. Ann Thorac Surg 2001;71(4): 1389–1395.
29. Akhtar S. Off-axis view using a multiplane transesophageal echocardiography probe facilitates cannulation of the coronary sinus. J Cardiothorac Vasc Anesth 1998;12(3):374–375.

30. Plotkin IM, Collard CD, Aranki SF, Rizzo RJ, Shernan SK. Percutaneous coronary sinus cannulation guided by transesophageal echocardiography. Ann Thorac Surg 1998;66(6):2085–2087.
31. Hirata N, Sakai K, Ohtani M, Ohnishi K, Matsuda H. Determination of positioning of coronary sinus cannula for retrograde cardioplegia with intraoperative myocardial contrast echocardiography. J Thorac Cardiovasc Surg 1994;108(6):1157–1158.
32. Wellford AL, Lawrie G, Zoghbi WA. Transesophageal echocardiographic features and management of retained intracardiac air in two patients after surgery. J Am Soc Echocardiogr 1996;9(2):182–186.
33. Dalmas JP, Eker A, Girard C, et al. Intracardiac air clearing in valvular surgery guided by transesophageal echocardiography. J Heart Valve Dis 1996;5(5):553–557.
34. Topol EJ, Humphrey LS, Borkon AM, et al. Value of intraoperative left ventricular microbubbles detected by transesophageal two-dimensional echocardiography in predicting neurologic outcome after cardiac operations. Ame J Cardiol 1985; 56(12):773–775.
35. Orihashi K, Matsuura Y. Quantitative echocardiographic analysis of retained intracardiac air in pooled form: an experimental study. J Am Soc Echocardiogr 1996; 9(4):567–572.
36. Tingleff J, Joyce FS, Pettersson G. Intraoperative echocardiographic study of air embolism during cardiac operations. Ann Thorac Surg 1995;60(3):673–677.

11 Surgical Approach to Aortic Surgery and Perfusion Techniques

Sanjeev Aggarwal, MD,
and Allan Stewart, MD

CONTENTS

INTRODUCTION

The surgical treatment of aortic disease remains a formidable challenge. Only since the advent cardiopulmonary bypass in the early 1950s has the complex repair of aortic aneurysms and dissections become feasible. Today, advances in perfusion methods and surgical techniques have allowed for the treatment of complex aortic disease with ever-improving morbidity and mortality.

DeBakey and Cooley described the first repair of an ascending aortic aneurysm using an aortic allograft in 1956 *(1,2)*. Soon thereafter, the pioneering work of Borst, Barnard, and Shrire led to methods of cerebral protection utilizing hypothermic circulatory arrest (HCA),

From: *Current Cardiac Surgery: On Bypass: Advanced Perfusion Techniques*
Edited by: L. B. Mongero and J. R. Beck © Humana Press Inc., Totowa, NJ

allowing for the treatment of complex aortic arch disease *(3,4)*. In 1975, Griepp and coworkers described a series of patients who underwent repair of aortic arch aneurysms utilizing HCA, leading to widespread interest in modes of cerebral protection during complex aortic surgery *(5)*.

Fundamental to the surgical treatment of aortic disease is the maintenance of end organ perfusion while continuity of the arterial tree is disrupted during the period of repair. Neuroprotective strategies are of particular importance when addressing pathology of the aortic arch. This chapter will discuss different cannulation and perfusion approaches for the treatment of aortic aneurysmal disease in the context of anatomic location. Aortic dissection will be considered in a separate section.

GENERAL CONSIDERATIONS

Cannulation strategies for aortic surgery can broadly be divided as central or peripheral, depending upon the specific anatomy. With central cannulation, the ascending transverse arch, or descending aorta can be cannulated directly. The most common sites for peripheral arterial cannulation include the right axillary and common femoral arteries. Venous drainage is commonly achieved by right atrial cannulation or femoral venous cannulation utilizing a long multiport catheter advanced into the right atrium.

Aortic plaque and mobile atheroma can be a source of systemic embolization during direct cannulation of the aorta. Assessment of the aorta is critical in identifying safe areas for cannulation and for the prevention of embolic stroke and systemic embolization. Traditionally, the modalities most commonly employed include direct inspection and manual palpation, intraoperative transesophageal echocardiography, and epiaortic ultrasonography. Several studies have identified epiaortic ultrasonography as the test of choice *(6,7)*. Direct inspection and palpation has been shown to have a sensitivity of as low as 55% atherosclerotic disease *(8)*. Although TEE has improved sensitivity, it is limited by its difficulty in visualization of the distal portion of the ascending aorta.

ANEURYSMAL DISEASE OF THE AORTIC ROOT AND ASCENDING AORTA

A variety of pathologic entities can lead to aneurysms of the ascending aorta including cystic medial degeneration, connective tissue disorders such as Marfans syndrome and Ehlers-Danlos syndrome, infectious etiologies, poststenotic dilatation, and aneurysm formation associated with bicuspid aortic valves. Surgical considerations include whether or not there is involvement of the aortic root and the distal extent of the disease.

Isolated aneurysms of the ascending aorta with or without involvement of the aortic root are dealt with in a straightforward manner. A standard median sternotomy incision offers optimal exposure. Venous drainage is usually achieved by cannulation of the right atrium using a dual-stage venous cannula. Alternatively, a long venous cannula can be introduced via the femoral vein into the right atrium (Biomedicus cannula 19–21 Fr; Medtronic). Central cannulation of the transverse aortic arch allows for cross clamping at the level of the innominate artery. Moderate hypothermia is usually employed. Extension of the aneurysm into the transverse arch will be discussed in the following section.

ANEURYSMAL DISEASE OF THE AORTIC ARCH

Cerebral Protection

The central concern when operating on the aortic arch is cerebral protection to prevent devastating neurologic injury. Three main techniques exist for cerebral protection: deep HCA, hypothermia with retrograde cerebral perfusion (RCP), and moderate hypothermia supplemented with some form of antegrade cerebral perfusion (ACP).

The value of HCA as a means of cerebral protection was first demonstrated in a canine model by Michenfelder and Theye in 1968 *(9)*. The correlation of increasing cerebral metabolic suppression with decreasing temperature is believed to be the primary protective effect of hypothermia. The first successful clinical application of HCA for the repair of aortic pathology was demonstrated by the early pioneering works of Borst, Shrire, and Barnard *(3,4)*. In 1975, Griepp and colleagues reported a series of four patients undergoing aortic arch replacement utilizing total body hypothermia and HCA *(5)*. Since that time, several large series have validated the use of HCA in aortic repair. As experience with deep HCA has grown, however, so have concerns regarding the safe period of circulatory arrest, optimal cooling temperature, adequacy of neural protection, and long-term neurologic outcomes. Svensson et al. reported on a series of 656 patients undergoing aortic repair with HCA with an overall 30-day incidence of stroke (transient or permanent) of 7% and a 30-day survival of 90% *(10)*. In this series, an increased incidence of stroke was seen when circulatory arrest times exceeded 40 minutes, with a significant increase in mortality after 65 minutes. Ergin and coworkers have defined two distinct categories of neurologic injury *(11)*. First is focal stroke, which is usually caused by embolic injury. Second is a clinical syndrome of "temporary neurologic dysfunction" (TND), which is characterized by delirium, agitation, obtundation, or Parkinson's type symptoms, without localization or abnormalities on imaging studies. In their review of 200 patients undergoing deep HCA for operations on the aorta, TND occurred in 19.3% of patients. The incidence of TND correlated directly with both patient age and duration of circulatory arrest, rising significantly after 40 min *(11)*. To determine the clinical relevance of TND, the Mount Sinai group retrospectively correlated the incidence of TND with abnormalities in neuropsychological testing at 1 and 6 weeks postoperatively *(12)*. Reich et al. also described the association of memory and fine motor deficits, as well as prolonged hospital stay, with circulatory arrest times of greater than 25 minutes *(13)*. As the limitations of HCA have become better characterized, interest has emerged in providing some form of nutritive blood flow to the brain in the hopes of extending the safe period of repair.

The technique of RCP has been described as a means of treating massive air embolism during cardiopulmonary bypass *(14)*. The application of RCP for neural protection became popular after 1990, when Ueda et al. reported the results of a series of eight patients undergoing aortic arch repair under HCA with RCP *(15)*. Since that time, both clinical and experimental data have yielded conflicting results regarding the efficacy of RCP as a means of cerebral protection *(16)*. In a retrospective view of 75 patients undergoing surgery on the proximal aorta, Bavaria and colleagues reported markedly decreased stroke and mortality rates in patients receiving RCP when compared to patients undergoing deep HCA alone *(17)*. Coselli et al., in a series of 290 patients, also demonstrated a decreased incidence of stroke and mortality with RCP versus HCA alone *(18,19)*. Deeb and colleagues reported on the results of 35 patients undergoing complex aortic reconstruction under HCA with a mean RCP time of 63 minutes, with a maximal time of 128 minutes. One patient suffered from a stroke. The authors cited RCP as a useful adjunct to extending the "safe" period of HCA *(20)*. Other series have not demonstrated a clear effect of RCP on neurologic outcomes or mortality *(21)*. Wong and Bonser showed in a series of 130 patients that RCP was associated with long HCA times, and by multivariate logistic regression found it to be a predictor of increased mortality *(22)*. The results of various animal studies have also added to the debate surrounding RCP. Boeckxstaens and Flameng, in a baboon model, were unable to demonstrate significant blood flow to the brain during RCP secondary to venovenous shunting *(23)*. Similar findings were reported by Ehrlich et al. in a porcine model, both with and without clamping of the inferior vena cava. This has led to the postulation that the protective effect of RCP may be due to maintenance of adequate cerebral cooling rather than providing physiologic blood flow for metabolism *(24)*. A worrisome finding was reported by Juvonen and colleagues, where RCP, although effective in flushing particulate embolic debris from the cerebral circulation in a porcine model, also contributed to increased fluid sequestration *(25)*. Anatomic variances in cerebral circulation between these animal models and humans have been a source of criticism of these studies. Nevertheless, they have raised concerns as to potential harmful effects of RCP. Presently, RCP is employed either continuously during the period of HCA, or for a brief period before the termination of HCA to flush the cerebral circulation.

Selective ACP has the appeal of providing physiologic forward flow to the brain during the period of HCA. Early results with antegrade perfusion, however, were poor, being complicated by a significant incidence of embolic stroke *(26–28)*. With improvements in perfusion and surgical techniques, as well as increased awareness of the potential shortcomings of HCA and RCP, there has been renewed interest in providing some form of antegrade cerebral flow to improve outcomes. A recent retrospective multicenter study by Di Eusanio et al. evaluated 588 patients undergoing aortic surgery with selective ACP. The authors reported a permanent neurologic injury rate of 3.8% and a transient neurologic injury rate of 5.6%. The duration of antegrade perfusion had no impact on mortality, or risk of transient or permanent neurologic injury *(29)*. These findings were in accordance with a previous series reported by DiEusanio of 413 patients undergoing selective antegrade perfusion *(30)*. The metabolic effect of ACP compared to HCA alone was evaluated in a prospective randomized controlled trial. Patients receiving antegrade perfusion demonstrated no decrease in jugular venous oxygen saturation and no increase in oxygen extraction upon reperfusion compared to those undergoing circulatory arrest alone. The authors concluded that antegrade perfusion may attenuate the metabolic deficit seen after HCA *(31)*. Several studies have attempted to compare the effects of antegrade perfusion with retrograde perfusion on clinical outcomes. Svensson and coworkers reported the results of a prospective randomized trial comparing the effects of deep HCA alone and with ACP and RCP on neurocognitive testing and serum S-100 levels. This series failed to demonstrate a significant benefit of either ACP or RCP on postoperative neurocognitive testing as compared to circulatory arrest alone *(32)*. Another prospective series reported by Okita et. al compared results of RCP with ACP in patients undergoing total arch replacement. Although outcomes were similar in respect to mortality, patients receiving RCP had a significantly higher rate of TND *(33)*. Similar results were reported by Hagl and colleagues *(34)*. In 453 patients undergoing ascending and aortic arch operations, ACP led to a significant decrease in the incidence of postoperative neurologic dysfunction compared to patients receiving RCP or DHCA alone. There was no difference among groups in respect to the incidence of stroke. More prospective trials will be necessary to better delineate which technique of cerebral protection is optimal for variable clinical scenarios.

Operative Techniques

Exposure of the aortic arch is achieved through a standard median sternotomy incision. The cannulation strategy can be tailored according to the specific type of cerebral protection being used. For deep HCA, the aneurysm can be cannulated directly. Care should be taken to evaluate the aorta for potential atheromatous disease using the previously described techniques. The cannulation site is excised during the repair, and upon completion, reperfusion is initiated either directly through the graft or through a side branch of the graft.

The common femoral artery has long been used as an alternative cannulation site. Particularly in emergent situations, the femoral vessels can be exposed and cannulated quickly. Several cannulas are available for cannulation of the femoral vessels. The authors' preference is the use of 19–21-Fr Biomedicus cannula (Medtronic) for the femoral vein, and a 16–18-Fr EOPA end-hole cannula (Medtronic) for the femoral artery. One potential risk, however, is the embolization of atheromatous debris from the descending thoracic and abdominal aorta retrograde into the cerebral circulation. The femoral artery itself can also be involved in the atherosclerotic process, and may therefore be unsuitable as a cannulation site.

The axillary artery has become a more frequently utilized site for arterial cannulation in recent years, with some considering it the preferred site for aortic arch surgery *(35–38)*. The axillary artery usually is not involved in the atherosclerotic process. It offers the advantage of providing antegrade flow, thereby avoiding the potential risks of retrograde cerebral embolization from a diseased descending aorta.

Complications of axillary cannulation include arterial dissection and brachial plexus injury *(39)*. The axillary artery can either be cannulated directly or through a side graft sewn end-to-side to the artery (8-mm Hemashield). An end-hole cannula (21-Fr EOPA; Medtronic) is then placed and secured into the side graft. Although both techniques have advocates, recent reports seem to suggest a decreased incidence of technically related complications with the use of a side graft (Fig. 1) *(40)*.

Retrograde cerebral perfusion is accomplished by cannulation and snaring of the superior vena cava. Perfusion can be administered either as a continuous cold infusion or for a brief period as a means of flushing the cerebral circulation. The perfusion circuit can be set up with a Y-bridge from the arterial line to the venous return line, as described by Reich and associates *(41)*. Perfusion pressures of approximately 20–25 mmHg are commonly used. Higher perfusion pressures carry the risk of cerebral edema, as previously shown in an animal model *(25)*.

Several technical approaches have been described for the administration of selective ACP during circulatory arrest. Once the aortic arch is exposed, retrograde coronary sinus catheters can be placed directly into the orifices of the innominate and left carotid arteries for antegrade perfusion. Alternatively, selective antegrade perfusion can be accomplished by cannulation and perfusion of the right axillary artery with occlusion of the innominate artery. Spielvogel and colleagues have

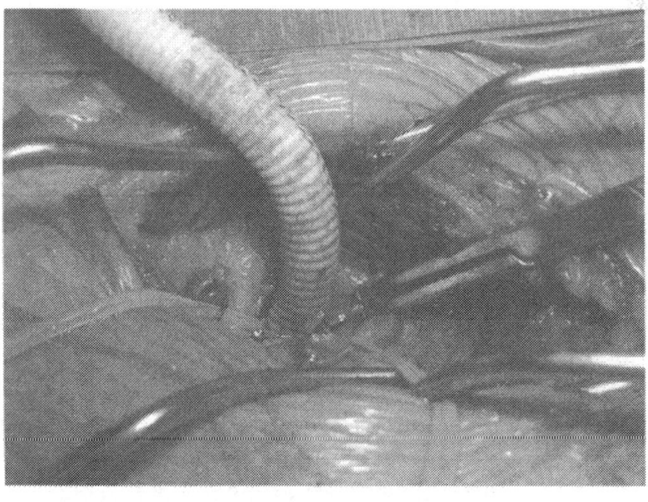

Fig. 1. Axillary artery cannulation utilizing a side graft.

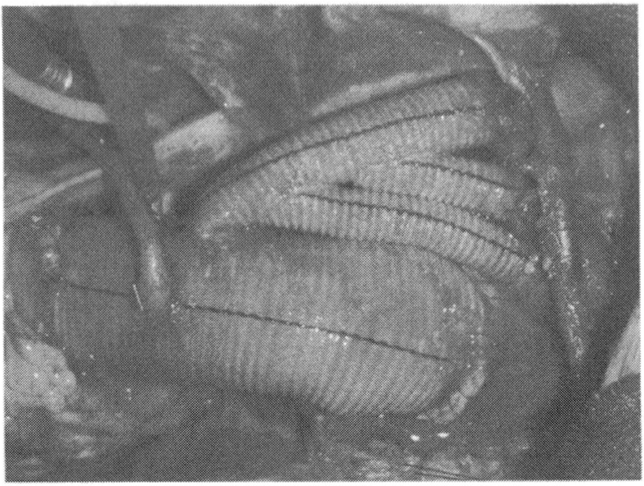

Fig. 2. Complete repair of aortic arch using a trifurcated graft.

described a technique for total arch replacement utilizing right axillary artery cannulation and a trifurcated graft *(42,43)*. Under HCA, the origins of the innominate, left carotid, and left subclavian vessels are transected, and then individually anastomosed to the limbs of the trifurcated graft. The graft is then de-aired and clamped proximally. Flow is restored through the axillary artery, reestablishing perfusion to the head and upper body. After completion of the aortic arch reconstruction, the trifurcated graft is anastomosed in end-to-side fashion to the ascending aortic graft (Fig. 2).

ANEURYSMAL DISEASE OF THE DESCENDING AND THORACOABDOMINAL AORTA

Neurologic and Visceral Protection

Aneurysms of the descending and thoracoabdominal aorta can result from a variety of pathologic entities, including degenerative change, atherosclerosis, infection, inflammatory diseases, and inherited connective tissue disorders. The challenge of repairing thoracoabdominal aortic aneurysms (TAAAs) centers on the avoidance of visceral ischemia and the dreaded complications of paraplegia and paraparesis.

The classification system proposed by Crawford and colleagues provides a standardized method of describing thoracoabdominal aneurysms *(44)*. Crawford type I aneurysms involve the descending thoracic aorta and abdominal aorta without extension to the renal arteries. Type II aneurysms have extension below the renal arteries. Type III aneurysms involve only a portion of the descending thoracic aorta, usually below the level of the sixth rib, and the abdominal aorta. Type IV describes predominantly abdominal aorta aneurysms (Fig. 3).

Svensson and coworkers reported Crawford's 30-year experience of TAAA repair in 1,509 patients *(45)*. This series, published in 1993, reported a 30-day survival of 92%. The incidence of paraplegia and paraparesis overall was 16%. Renal failure occurred in 18% of patients. Over the past several years, advances in surgical and perfusion techniques have led to decreases in mortality, the incidence of renal failure, and neurologic complications of the lower extremities, compared with historical controls. More contemporary series have reported 30-day mortality rates of 5–6%, with paraplegia rates of less than 5% *(46,47)*. The improvement in outcomes is the result of several different advances in surgical, perfusion, and anesthetic management. These include the technique of sequential aortic clamping, reimplantation of intercostal arteries below T7, the use of left heart bypass (LHB) and distal aortic perfusion with moderate hypothermia, cerebrospinal fluid (CSF) drainage, and deep hypothermia and circulatory arrest to achieve neurologic protection of the spinal cord.

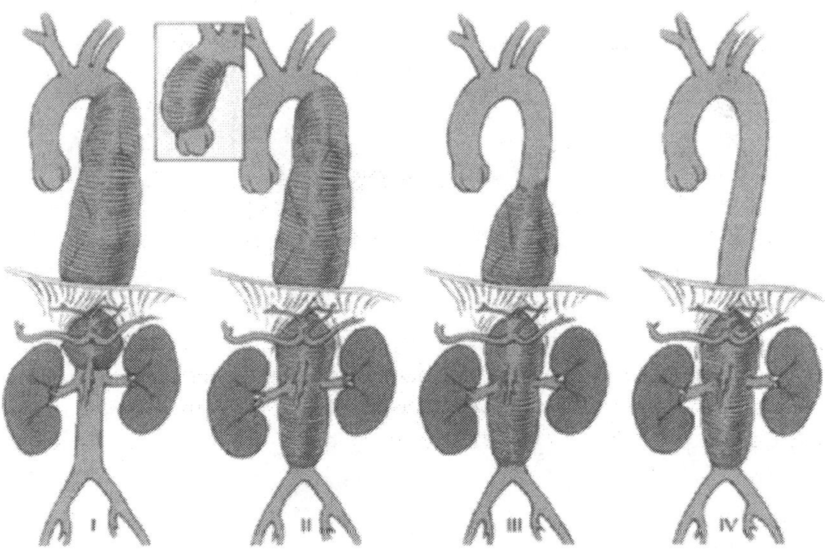

Fig. 3. Crawford classification of thoracoabdominal aortic aneurysms.Reproduced from ref. 44.

The effects of aortic cross clamping and the resultant drop in perfusion pressure distal to the clamp place the viscera and spinal cord at risk for ischemic injury. Partial LHB, or atriofemoral bypass, utilizes a centrifugal pump to provide blood flow to the distal aorta during the period of cross clamping to maintain distal aortic perfusion pressure, potentially avoiding these complications. Safi and colleagues reported early work on the effects of distal aortic perfusion in combination with CSF drainage in 94 patients undergoing repair of Crawford type I and II thoracoabdominal aneurysms *(48)*. When compared to a control group undergoing repair with the "clamp and sew" technique, patients receiving distal aortic perfusion and CSF drainage had a markedly decreased incidence of neurologic complications (9% versus 19%). There was also a beneficial effect on neurologic outcome in patients having prolonged cross clamp times of greater than 45 minutes (13% versus 39%). The beneficial effects of LHB on mortality, incidence of postoperative renal failure, and neurologic outcomes was shown by Schepens et al. in a retrospective analysis of 258 patients undergoing TAAA repair *(49)*. One of the largest series to date has been reported by Coselli and coworkers, in which LHB was used alone without the adjunct of CSF drainage *(50)*. In 1,250 consecutive patients, of whom 666 had LHB, a statistically significant decrease was seen in postoperative paraplegia and paraparesis in patients with Crawford type II aneurysms. Although the incidence of neurologic complications was similar in Crawford type I aneurysms (4.2% without LHB versus 3.1% with LHB), the latter group had significantly longer aortic clamp times, implying that LHB was protective in these patients *(51)*.

Extensive aneurysms of the descending and thoracoabdominal aorta can also be managed by utilizing cardiopulmonary bypass with profound hypothermia and circulatory arrest. This is a useful technique when there is aneurysmal extension into the transverse arch, or when the size of the aneurysm precludes safe placement of a proximal clamp. This approach has been described by Crawford and colleagues *(52)*. More contemporary series by Kouchoukos et al. have provided further validation to this approach. In a series of 211 patients, there was a low incidence of paraplegia, renal failure, and end organ dysfunction, without the need for adjunctive measures such as distal aortic perfusion, selective visceral perfusion, and CSF drainage *(53)*. Concerns regarding increased coagulopathic bleeding and blood transfusion requirement were not seen in this study.

Another important adjunct in spinal cord protection that has previously been mentioned is the use of CSF drainage. The overall perfusion pressure of the spinal cord is the difference between the mean arterial pressure and the CSF pressure. It has been previously shown that aortic cross clamping not only decreases distal arterial perfusion pressure, but also causes a rise in CSF pressure *(54,55)*. Lowering CSF pressure by drainage should augment spinal perfusion pressure and mitigate against ischemic injury. The results of a prospective randomized trial of CSF drainage in patients undergoing repair of Crawford type I and II aneurysms was reported in 1991 *(44)*. This study failed to show a neurologic benefit of CSF drainage. This study has been criticized, however, because only a limited amount of CSF was drained (50 cc). More recent series have titrated CSF drainage to maintain a CSF pressure of 10 mmHg or less. Coselli and colleagues conducted a prospective randomized trial of CSF drainage in 145 patients *(56)*. In patients randomized to CSF drainage, CSF pressures were not allowed to exceed 10 mmHg. The result was a dramatic reduction in the incidence of neurologic deficits (13% control group versus 2.6% in CSF drainage group). CSF drainage is regarded as a useful adjunct in decreasing the incidence of postoperative paraplegia and paraparesis after extensive Crawford type I and II TAAA repairs.

Operative Techniques

After placement of appropriate monitoring lines and a double-lumen endotracheal tube, the patient is placed in a modified right lateral decubitus position *(57)*. A posterolateral thoracotomy incision is performed. Exposure of the thoracic aorta can be through either the sixth intercostal space or through the bed of the resected sixth rib. Alternatively, the aorta can be approached through combined fourth and eighth intercostal space incisions. The skin incision can be extended in a gentle curved fashion over the costal margin towards the umbilicus for exposure of the abdominal aorta.

Left heart bypass utilizes a centrifugal pump to provide flow to the distal aorta. The technique has been previously described by Coselli et al *(50,58)*. Flow rates of up to 3 L/min have been used, while maintaining proximal perfusion pressures in the normal range. Moderate hypothermia is employed. Cannulation for outflow can be achieved either directly into the left atrium via the left atrial appendage, or through the left inferior pulmonary vein. The inferior pulmonary vein has become the preferred approach used by many surgeons because it avoids the potential hazards associated with the often friable and thin tissue of the left atrial appendage. Cannulation of either the femoral artery or distal descending aorta provides inflow from the pump. In addition, a Y-split connected to an octopus tubing arm on the inflow tubing allows for selective renal and visceral arterial perfusion with 9-Fr balloon catheters. The successful conduct of LBP is dependent on coordinated communication between the surgeon, perfusionist, and anesthesiologist. In this way, hemodynamic fluctuations in the upper and lower extremities can be managed appropriately.

The technique of cardiopulmonary bypass with deep HCA has been advocated by Kouchoukos and others for the repair of Crawford type I and II aneurysms *(59)*. Venous outflow is obtained by cannulation of the femoral vein with a long venous catheter advanced into the right atrium under transesophageal echocardiographic guidance. The femoral artery is cannulated for arterial inflow. Alternatively, the descending thoracic aorta can be cannulated directly. Other sites for arterial inflow that have been described include the transverse aortic arch, left axillary artery, and left ventricular apex. After initiation of cardiopulmonary bypass and core cooling, circulatory arrest is employed and the repair performed. In the series reported by Kouchoukos et al., adjunctive measures of CSF drainage and selective visceral and renal perfusion were not used. Deep hypothermia with circulatory arrest has proven to be a safe method for visceral and spinal cord preservation.

AORTIC DISSECTION

Aortic dissection remains the most common surgical emergency affecting the aorta. Dissections are most commonly described using the Stanford classification, with type A dissections involving the ascending aorta, and type B designating dissections of the descending aorta distal to the origin of the left subclavian artery. Pathologically, the intimal disruption and separation of the layers of the aortic wall creates a true and false lumen. This warrants special consideration in respect to perfusion strategies because flow into the false lumen will result in end-organ malperfusion.

Several different approaches to cannulation have been employed with acceptable results. Venous drainage is usually through a dual-stage venous cannula in the right atrium or bicaval cannulation. Alternatively, a long venous cannula can be placed into the right atrium via the femoral vein. For type A dissections, cannulation of the aorta directly at the level of the transverse arch can be done using the Seldinger technique with transesophageal echocardiographic guidance. Care must be taken to ensure cannulation of the true lumen. Another central approach is the cannulation of the ascending aorta through the left ventricular apex. Historically, the femoral vessels have been commonly used for venous return and arterial inflow. The presence or absence of pulses in the femoral vessels can be misleading because, many times, a palpable pulse is the result of perfusion of the false lumen. Frequently, the dissection plane leads to the left femoral vessel being supplied by the false lumen and the right femoral vessel from the true lumen. Although the popularity of axillary arterial cannulation has grown in recent years, a recent series by Fusco et al. demonstrates femoral cannulation to still be a safe approach for perfusion *(60)*. The feasibility of axillary arterial cannulation for aortic dissection has been previously reported *(61)*. It has become increasingly utilized for repair of type A dissections in recent years. An important consideration reported by Svensson, however, is that if the dissection process extends into the subclavian vessels, then there is a high incidence of stroke, and alternative sites for arterial inflow should be considered *(62)*. Moizumi and coworkers recently described their experience with axillary arterial cannulation for type A dissections; they found a decrease in mortality after adopting this as the preferred cannulation strategy *(63)*. Regardless of the strategy used, vigilance must be maintained in detecting evidence of malperfusion intraoperatively, and adjustments in cannulation sites made accordingly to ensure adequate end-organ perfusion.

CONCLUSIONS

The treatment of the wide spectrum of aortic disease remains a significant challenge for caregivers. Advances in surgical, perfusion, and anesthetic techniques have led to a marked improvement in clinical outcomes over the past several decades. Central neurologic injury and visceral ischemic injury with resultant end organ failure remain as significant causes of morbidity and mortality. With the continued aging of the population, the prevalence of aortic disease will likely continue to grow. Endovascular management of aortic disease is becoming an increasingly important mode of therapy and will likely continue to expand in the coming years. Continued basic science research and technological advances will be important in the effort to improve clinical outcomes in the future.

REFERENCES

1. Cooley DA, DeBakey ME. Resection of entire ascending aorta in fusiform aneurysm using cardiac bypass. J Am Med Assoc 1956;162(12):1158–1159.

2. DeBakey ME, Crawford ES, Cooley DA, Morris GC Jr. Successful resection of fusiform aneurysm of aortic arch with replacement by homograft. Surg Gynecol Obstet 1957;105(6):657–664.
3. Borst HG, Schaudig A, Rudolph W. Arteriovenous fistula of the aortic arch: Repair during deep hypothermia and circulatory arrest. J Thorac Cardiovasc Surg 1964;48:443–447.
4. Barnard CN, Schrire V. The surgical treatment of acquired aneurysms of the thoracic aorta. Thorax 1963;18:101–105.
5. Griepp RB, Stinson EB, Hollingsworth JF, et al. Prosthetic replacement of the aortic arch. J Thorac Cardiovasc Surg 1975;70(6):1051–1063.
6. Sylivris S, Calafiore P, Matalanis G, et al. The intraoperative assessment of ascending aortic atheroma: epiaortic imaging is superior to both transesophageal echocardiography and direct palpation. J Cardiothorac Vasc Anesth 1997;11(6): 704–707.
7. Royse C, Rosye A, Blake D, et al. Screening the thoracic aorta for atheroma: a comparison of manual palpation, transesophageal and epiaortic ultrasonography. Ann Thorac Cardiovasc Surg 1998;4(6):347–350.
8. Bolotin G, Domany Y, de Perini L, et al. Use of intraoperative epiaortic ultrasonography to delineate aortic atheroma. Chest 2005;127:60–65.
9. Michenfelder JD, Theye RA. Hypothermia: effect on canine brain and whole-body metabolism. Anesthesiology 1968;29:1107–1112.
10. Svensson LG, Crawford ES, Hess KR, et al. Deep hypothermia with circulatory arrest. Determinants of stroke and early mortality in 656 patients. J Thorac Cardiovasc Surg 1993;106(1):19–28.
11. Ergin MA, Galla JD, Lansman SL, et al. Hypothermic circulatory arrest in operations on the thoracic aorta. Determinants of operative mortality and neurologic outcome. J Thorac Cardiovasc Surg 1994;107(3):788–797.
12. Ergin MA, Uysal S, Reich DL, et al. TND after deep hypothermic circulatory arrest: a clinical marker of long-term functional deficit. Ann Thorac Surg 1999; 67:1887–1890.
13. Reich DL, Uysal S, Sliwinski M, et al. Neuropsychologic outcome after deep hypothermic circulatory arrest in adults. J Thorac Cardiovasc Surg 1999;117(1): 156–163.
14. Mills NL, Ochsner JL. Massive air embolism during cardiopulmonary bypass: causes, prevention, and management. J Thorac Cardiovasc Surg 1980;80:708–717.
15. Ueda Y, Miki S, Kusuhara K, et al. Surgical treatment of aneurysm or dissection involving the ascending aorta and aortic arch, utilizing circulatory arrest and retrograde cerebral perfusion. J Cardiovasc Surg (Torino) 1990;31(5):553–558.
16. Hagl C, Khaladj N, Karck M, et al. Hypothermic circulatory arrest during ascending and aortic arch surgery: the theoretical impact of different cerebral perfusion techniques and other methods of cerebral protection. Eur J Cardiothorac Surg 2003;24(3):371–378.
17. Bavaria JE, Woo YJ, Hall RA, et al. Retrograde cerebral and distal aortic perfusion during ascending and thoracoabdominal aortic operations. Ann Thorac Surg 1995; 60(2):345–352.
18. Coselli JS, LeMaire SA. Experience with retrograde cerebral perfusion during proximal aortic surgery in 290 patients. J Card Surg 1997;12(2 Suppl):322–325.
19. Coselli JS. Retrograde cerebral perfusion is an effective means of neural support duing deep hypothermic circulatory arrest. Ann Thorac Surg 1997;64(3):908–912.

20. Deeb GM, Jenkins E, Bolling SF, et al. Retrograde cerebral perfusion during hypothermic circulatory arrest reduces neurologic morbidity. J Thorac Cardiovasc Surg 1995;109(2):259–268.
21. Okita Y, Takamoto S, Ando M, et al. Mortality and cerebral outcome in patients who underwent aortic arch operations using deep hypothermic circulatory arrest with retrograde perfusion: no relation of early death, stroke, and delerium to the duration of circulatory arrest. J Thorac Cardiovasc Surg 1998;115(1):129–138.
22. Wong CH, Bonser RS. Does retrograde cerebral perfusion affect risk factors for stroke and mortality after hypothermic circulatory arrest? Ann Thorac Surg 1999; 67:1900–1903.
23. Boeckxstaens CJ, Flameng WJ. Retrograde cerebral perfusion does not perfuse the brain in nonhuman primates. Ann Thorac Surg 1995;60:319–328.
24. Ehrlich MP, Hagl C, McCullough JN, et al. Retrograde cerebral perfusion provides negligible flow through brain capillaries in the pig. J Thorac Cardiovasc Surg 2001;122(2):331–338.
25. Juvonen T, Weisz DJ, Wolfe D, et al. Can retrograde perfusion mitigate cerebral injury after particulate embolization? A study in a chronic porcine model. J Thorac Cardiovasc Surg 1998;115(5):1142–1159.
26. Cooley DA, Ott DA, Frazier OH, et al. Surgical treatment of aneurysms of the transverse aortic arch: experience with 25 patients using hypothermic techniques. Ann Thorac Surg 1981;32:260.
27. Frist WH, Baldwin JC, Starnes VA, et al. A reconsideration of cerebral perfusion in aortic arch replacement. Ann Thorac Surg 1986;42:273.
28. Crawford ES, Saleh SA. Transverse aortic arch aneurysm: improved results of treatment employing new modifications of aortic reconstruction and hypothermic cerebral circulatory arrest. Ann Surg 1981;194(2):180–188.
29. Di Eusanio M, Schepens MA, Morshuis WJ, et al. Brain protection using antegrade selective cerebral perfusion: a multicenter study. Ann Thorac Surg 2003;76(4): 1181–1188.
30. DiEusanio M, Schepens MA, Morshuis WJ, et al. Antegrade selective cerebral perfusion during operations on the thoracic aorta: factors influencing survival and neurologic outcome in 413 patients. J Thorac Cardiovasc Surg 2002;124(6):1080–1086.
31. Harrington DK, Walker AS, Kaukuntla H, et al. Selective antegrade cerebral perfusion attenuates brain metabolic deficit in aortic arch surgery. A prospective randomized trial. Circulation 2004;110(Suppl II):231–236.
32. Svensson LG, Nadolny EM, Penney DL, et al. Prospective randomized neurocognitive and S-100 study of hypothermic circulatory arrest, retrograde brain perfusion, and antegrade brain perfusion for aortic arch operations. Ann Thorac Surg 2001;71:1905–1912.
33. Okita Y, Minatoya K, Tagusari O, et al. Prospective comparative study of brain protection in total arch replacement: deep hypothermic circulatory arrest with retrograde cerebral perfusion or selective antegrade cerebral perfusion. Ann Thorac Surg 2001;72(1):72–79.
34. Hagl C, Ergin MA, Galla JD, et al. Neurologic outcome after ascending aorta-aortic arch operations: effect of brain protection technique in high-risk patients. J Thorac Cardiovasc Surg 2001;121(6):1107–1121.
35. Sabik JF, Lytle BW, McCarthy PM, et al. Axillary artery: an alternative site of arterial cannulation for patients with extensive aortic and peripheral vascular disease. J Thorac Cardiovasc Surg 1995;109(5):885–891.

36. Strauch JT, Spielvogel D, Lauten A, et al. Axillary artery cannulation: routine use in ascending aorta and aortic aarch replacement. Ann Thorac Surg 2004;78: 1103–1108.
37. Baribeau YR, Westbrook BM, Charlesworth DC. Axillary cannulation: first choice for extra-aortic cannulation and brain protection. J Thorac Cardiovasc Surg 2000; 119(6):1298.
38. Svensson LG, Blackstone EH, Rajeswaran J, et al. Does the arterial cannulation site for circulatory arrest influence stroke risk? Ann Thorac Surg 2004;78: 1274–1284.
39. Schachner T, Nagiller J, Zimmer A, et al. Technical problems and complications of axillary artery cannulation. Eur J Cardiothorac Surg 2005;27:634–637.
40. Sabik JF, Nemeh H, Lytle BW, et al. Cannulation of the axillary artery with a side graft reduces morbidity. Ann Thorac Surg 2004;77:1315–1320.
41. Reich DL, Uysal S, Ergin MA, et al. Retrograde cerebral perfusion as a method of neuroprotection during thoracic aortic surgery. Ann Thorac Surg 2001;72: 1774–1782.
42. Spielvogel D, Strauch JT, Minanov OP, et al. Aortic arch replacment using a trifurcated graft and selective cerebral antegrade perfusion. Ann Thorac Surg 20002;74:S1810–S18104.
43. Strauch JT, Spielvogel D, Lauten A, et al. Technical advances in total arch replacement. Ann Thorac Surg 2004;77:581–590.
44. Crawford ES, Svensson LG, Hess KR, et al. A prospective randomized study of cerebrospinal fluid drainage to prevent paraplegia after high-risk surgery on the thoracoabdominal aorta. J Vasc Surg 1991;13(1):36–46.
45. Svensson LG, Crawford ES, Hess KR, et al. Experience with 1509 patients undergoing thoracoabdominal aortic operations. J Vasc Surg 1993;17(2):357–370.
46. Coselli JS, LeMaire SA, Miller CC II, et al. Mortality and paraplegia after thoracoabdominal aortic aneurysm repair: a risk factor analysis. Ann Thorac Surg 2000;69:409–414.
47. Coselli JS, Conklin LD, LeMaire SA. Thoracoabdominal aortic aneurysm repair: review and update of current strategies. Ann Thorac Surg 2002;74:S1881–S1884.
48. Safi HJ, Hess KR, Randel M, et al. Cerebrospinal fluid drainage and distal aortic perfusion: reducing neurologic complications in repair of thoracoabdominal aortic aneurysm type I and II. J Vasc Surg 1996;23(2):223–229.
49. Schepens MA, Vermeulen FE, Morshuis WJ, et al. Impact of left heart bypass on the results of thoracoabdominal aortic aneurysm repair. Ann Thorac Surg 1999;67:1963–1967.
50. Coselli JS. The use of left heart bypass in the repair of thoracoabdominal aortic aneurysms: current techniques and results. Sem Thorac Cardiovasc Surg 2003;15 (4):326–332.
51. Coselli JS, LeMaire SA. Left heart bypass reduces paraplegia rates after thoracoabdominal aortic aneurysm repair. Ann Thorac Surg 1999;67:1931–1934.
52. Crawford ES, Coselli JS, Safi HJ. Partial cardiopulmonary bypass, hypothermic circulatory arrest, and posterolateral exposure for thoracic aortic aneurysm operation. J Thorac Cardiovasc Surg 1987;94(6):824–827.
53. Kouchoukos NT, Masetti P, Murphy SF. Hypothermic cardiopulmonary bypass and circulatory arrest in the management of extensive thoracic and thoracoabdominal aortic aneurysms. Sem Thorac Cardiovasc Surg 2003;15(4):333–339.

54. Svensson LG, Stewart RW, Cosgrove DM, et al. Intrathecal papaverine for the prevention of paraplegia after operation on the thoracic or thoracoabdominal aorta. J Thorac Cardiovasc Surg 1988;96:823–829.
55. Blaisdell FW, Cooley DA. The mechanism of paraplegia after temporary thoracic aortic occlusion and its relationship to spinal fluid pressure. Surgery 1962;51: 351–355.
56. Coselli JS, LeMaire SA, Koksoy C, et al. Cerebrospinal fluid drainage reduces paraplegia after thoracoabdominal aneurysm repair: results of a randomized clinical trial. J Vasc Surg 2002;35(4):631–639.
57. Coselli JS, Moreno PL. Descending and thoracoabdominal aneurysm. In: Cardiac Surgery in the Adult. Cohn LH, Edmunds LH Jr., editors. McGraw Hill, 1169–1189, 2003.
58. Coselli JS, LeMaire SA, Ledesma DF, et al. Initial experience with the Nikkiso centrifugal pump during thoracoabdominal aortic aneurysm repair. J Vasc Surg 1998;27:378–383.
59. Kouchoukos NT, Masetti P, Rokkas CK, et al. Safety and efficacy of hypothermic cardiopulmonary bypass and circulatory arrest for operations on the descending thoracic and thoracoabdominal aorta. Ann Thorac Surg 2001;72:699–708.
60. Fusco DS, Shaw RK, Tranquilli M, et al. Femoral cannulation is safe for type A dissection repair. Ann Thorac Surg 2004;78:1285–1289.
61. Yavuz S, Goncu MT, Turk T. Axillary artery cannulation for arterial inflow in patients with acute dissection of the ascending aorta. Eur J Cardiothorac Surg 2002;22:313–315.
62. Svensson LG. Antegrade perfusion during suspended animation? J Thorac Cardiovasc Surg 2002;124(6):1068–1070.
63. Moizumi Y, Motoyoshi N, Sakuma K, et al. Axillary artery cannulation improves operative results for acute type A aortic dissection. Ann Thorac Surg 2005;80: 77–83.

12 ECMO to Artificial Lungs: Advances in Long-Term Pulmonary Support

Brittany A. Zwischenberger, MD,
Lindsey A. Clemson, MD,
James E. Lynch, BS, RRT, *and*
Joseph B. Zwischenberger, MD

CONTENTS

SUMMARY

Lung disease is the fourth leading cause of death (one in seven deaths) in the United States. Acute respiratory distress syndrome (ARDS) affects approx 150,000 patients a year in the US; an estimated 16 million Americans are afflicted with chronic lung disease, accounting for 100,000 deaths per year. Medical management is the standard of care for initial therapy, but is limited by progression of the disease. Chronic mechanical ventilation is readily available, but it is cumbersome, expensive, and often requires tracheotomy with loss of upper airway defense mechanisms and normal speech. Lung transplantation is an option for fewer than 1,000 patients per year because demand has steadily outgrown supply.

From: *Current Cardiac Surgery: On Bypass: Advanced Perfusion Techniques*
Edited by: L. B. Mongero and J. R. Beck © Humana Press Inc., Totowa, NJ

For the last 15 years, our group has studied ARDS and tried to develop viable alternative treatments. Both extracorporeal gas-exchange techniques, including extracorporeal membrane oxygenation (ECMO), extracorporeal carbon dioxide removal ($ECCO_2R$), arteriovenous CO_2 removal ($AVCO_2R$), and intravenous oxygenation (IVOX), aim to allow for a less injurious ventilatory strategy during lung recovery, while maintaining near-normal arterial blood gases but precluding ambulation. The paracorporeal artificial lung (PAL), however, redefines the treatment of both acute and chronic respiratory failure with the goal of ambulatory total respiratory support. PAL prototypes tested on both normal sheep and the LD_{100} smoke/burn-induced ARDS sheep models have shown initial success in achieving total gas exchange. Still, clinical trials cannot begin until bio- and hemodynamic compatibility challenges are reconciled. The PAL initial design goals are for a short-term (weeks) bridge to recovery or transplant, but eventually hope to be used for long-term support (months).

Key Words: Artificial lung; extracorporeal membrane oxygenation (ECMO); intravenous oxygenation (IVOX); Arteriovenous CO_2 removal ($AVCO_2R$); lung transplantation; respiratory failure; acute respiratory distress syndrome (ARDS).

INTRODUCTION

Lung disease is the fourth leading cause of death (one in seven deaths) in the United States. Acute respiratory distress syndrome affects approximately 150,000 patients a year in the US, and is still associated with 30–40% mortality despite recent advances in critical care. An estimated 16 million Americans are afflicted with chronic lung disease, including chronic obstructive pulmonary disease (COPD), accounting for 100,000 deaths per year. Approximately 30,000 children and adults suffer from cystic fibrosis, and 3–5 out of 100,000 Americans have idiopathic pulmonary fibrosis. For emphysema, lung volume reduction surgery (LVRS) has limited application. Medical management is the standard of care for the initial therapy of lung disease, but is limited by the progression of the disease. Chronic mechanical ventilation is readily available, but it is cumbersome, expensive, and often requires tracheotomy with loss of upper airway defense mechanisms and normal speech. Lung transplantation is available to fewer than 1,000 patients per year because demand has steadily outgrown supply. Currently, the average wait for a donor lung is 2 years, with 30% waiting list mortality.

For the last 15 years, our group has studied ARDS to develop viable alternative treatments. We have exploited mechanical ventilation to its limits, including pressure-limited ventilation (permissive hypercapnia), inverse ratio ventilation, high-frequency jet ventilation, high-frequency oscillatory ventilation, intratracheal pulmonary ventilation, and prone position ventilation. In addition, we participated in clinical trials on partial liquid ventilation, inhaled nitric oxide, and surfactant therapy (Fig. 1). All of these therapies have shown promise toward improving arterial blood gases and limiting lung injury in the short term, but none have demonstrated evidence-based survival benefits.

As an alternative to mechanical ventilation, we have explored both extracorporeal gas exchange techniques, including ECMO, $ECCO_2R$, $AVCO_2R$, total artificial lung, and IVOX. All share a common goal: to allow for a less injurious ventilatory strategy during lung recovery while maintaining near-normal arterial blood gases (Table 1). Only the application of ECMO in neonates with severe respiratory failure has shown evidence-based improvement in survival in prospective randomized trials. Until a survival benefit or cost-effective application

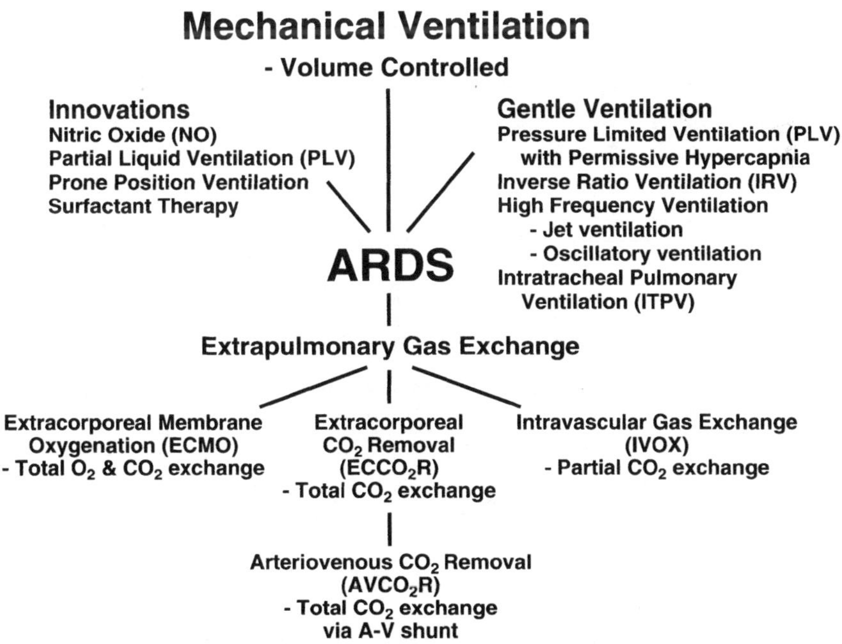

Fig. 1. The spectrum of treatment strategies for the management of ARDS.

Table 1

Comparison of Extracorporeal Membrane Oxygenation (ECMO), CPB Low-Flow Pressure Ventilation With Extracorporeal Carbon Dioxide Removal (LFPPV-ECCO$_2$R), Arteriovenous Carbon Dioxide Removal (AVCO$_2$R), and Artificial Lung

	ECMO	*CPB*	*ECCO$_2$R*	*AVCO$_2$R*	*Artificial Lung*
Setting	Respiratory and/or cardiac failure	Cardiac surgery	Respiratory failure	Respiratory failure (investigational)	Respiratory failure (investigational)
Location	Extrathoracic	Intrathoracic	Extrathoracic	Extrathoracic	Extrathoracic
Type of support	VA (cardiac) VV (respiratory)	VA (total bypass)	VV (respiratory) (CO_2)	AV (respiratory) (CO_2)	PA-PA or PA-LA
Cannulation	VA: neck VV: neck and groin 2 cannulas (surgical or percutaneous) 1 cannula (VVDL)	Direct cardiac 2 cannulas (surgical)	Neck and groin 2 cannulas (surgical or percutaneous)	Groin 2 cannulas (percutaneous)	Transthoracic to major vessels
Blood flow	High (70–80% CO)	Total (100% CO)	Med (30% CO)	Low (10–15% CO)	Total 100%
Ventilatory support	Pressure-controlled ± High PEEP 10–12 breaths/min	None (anesthesia)	High BEEP 2–4 breaths/min High FiO_2	Volume controlled (algorithm driven)	None necessary
Blood reservoir	Small (50 ml)	Yes (>11)	Small (50 ml)	No	No
Arterial filter	No	Yes	No	No	No
Blood pump	Roller or centrifugal	Roller or centrifugal	Roller or centrifugal	None	None
Heparinization	ACT 200–260	ACT >400	ACT 200–260	ACT 200–260	ACT 200–260
Average length of extracorporeal support	Days to weeks	Hours	Days to weeks	Days to weeks	Days
Complications	Bleeding Organ failure	Intraoperative	Bleeding	Bleeding	Bleeding
Cause of death	Support terminated: PAP >75% systemic Irreversible lung disease Cardiac dysrhythmias	Intraoperative Air embolism	Multiorgan failure Septic shock Hemorrhagic	Respiratory failure	Right heart failure

Source: Zwischenberger JB, Alpard SK. Artificial lungs: a new inspiration. Perfusion 2002;17:253–268.

can be demonstrated from these additional extracorporeal techniques, they will remain investigational or niche therapies at a few specialized centers. The focus of this chapter is to chronicle the development of the artificial lung.

ECMO

Today, extracorporeal membrane oxygenation (ECMO) is most commonly associated with neonatal respiratory failure as popularized by Bartlett et al. *(1–3)*. ECMO application in neonates has resulted in a collective experience of over 23,080 patients with an 82% survival rate *(4)*. Three prospective randomized studies have confirmed the efficacy of ECMO for severe respiratory failure in neonates *(5–7)*. As the application of ECMO in children has gained in popularity, ECMO for adult ARDS today still represents a complex, technically demanding treatment, with only 1,909 (5% of total ECMO cases) performed to date *(4)*. Most adult use is on a per case, rescue basis, with spectacular individual successes but little evidence-based outcomes data.

Venoarterial (VA) ECMO, which is similar to classic cardiopulmonary bypass (CPB) for cardiac surgery, allows for both pulmonary and cardiac support. Blood is drained from either the internal jugular vein or the femoral vein, pumped through a gas exchanger where oxygen is added and carbon dioxide is removed, and then pumped back into either the carotid or femoral artery, "bypassing" the native heart and lungs. In venovenous (VV) ECMO, the blood is returned to a large central vein rather than to an artery. Venovenous ECMO is primarily indicated for isolated pulmonary failure because the native heart supplies both pulmonary and systemic blood flow. Both VV and VA ECMO require the patient to be fully anticoagulated with systemic heparin.

Adult ECMO is often viewed as a "last resort" therapy, with center-specific entry and exclusion criteria. Recently, Hemmila et al. *(8)* reported their experience with 255 adult patients with ARDS on ECMO, with 52% of the patients surviving to discharge. This retrospective study only included the most severely ill ARDS patients ($PaO_2/FiO_2 \leq 100$; $A\text{-}aDO_2 > 600$) who failed maximum medical management. This report, as well as others *(9–11)*, has demonstrated the ability of specialized centers to produce better than expected results for patients with ARDS when utilizing ECMO. A randomized controlled adult trial is underway in the United Kingdom and has accrued 86% (154 of 180) of the study population to date. Completion of study accrual and outcomes determinations is expected this year (2007).

The use of ECMO is likely to continue in specialized centers, but is unlikely to become a widespread treatment option for patients with ARDS until the technique is simplified. The ECMO equipment is expensive and requires one-on-one nursing care, as well as either a second nurse, perfusionist, or respiratory therapist specially trained to manage the complex equipment. Many of the ECMO centers were established for neonatal ECMO patients and consist of nurses and respiratory therapists who are not experienced with adults. Also, many programs are located in dedicated children's hospitals that are unable to care for adult patients.

In the late 1970s, Kolobow and Gattinoni developed $ECCO_2R$ using a modified form of ECMO with VV perfusion *(12–14)*. Their focus was CO_2 removal, allowing for a reduction in mechanical ventilatory support. Oxygenation was maintained by simple diffusion across the patient's alveoli, called "apneic oxygenation," using low-frequency, positive-pressure ventilation. Unfortunately, the $ECCO_2R$ system required all of the equipment and expertise of a standard ECMO circuit. Studies in animals *(12–14)* and in humans *(15–17)* demonstrated $ECCO_2R$"s effectiveness in reducing mean airway pressure and minute ventilation. Despite the early success shown by $ECCO_2R$, in a small, prospective, randomized study conducted at a single center comparing $ECCO_2R$ with mechanical ventilation, no difference in mortality was seen *(18)*. Although the results of this study were disappointing for some, other investigators began to look for simpler CO_2 removal devices that would offer the benefits of gentle ventilation without all of the morbidity of ECMO or $ECCO_2R$.

$AVCO_2R$

Gentle ventilation techniques shown to reduce mortality in ARDS patients *(5)* occasionally result in severe respiratory acidosis. Our group developed a technique of simplified $AVCO_2R$ with a new generation of a low-resistance, commercially available, hollow-fiber gas exchanger to remove total CO_2 production and provide lung rest in the setting of severe respiratory failure *(19)* (Fig. 2). The extremely low resistance of the $AVCO_2R$ gas exchange device (<10 mmHg pressure difference) allows blood flows of as much as 25% of cardiac output (>1,300 mL/min) through a simple A-V shunt. The arterial cannula bore size and resistance becomes the determinant of flow. The cannulae are small (12-Fr arterial and 15-Fr venous) in comparison to what would be required for a typical adult venoarterial ECMO patient (22-Fr arterial

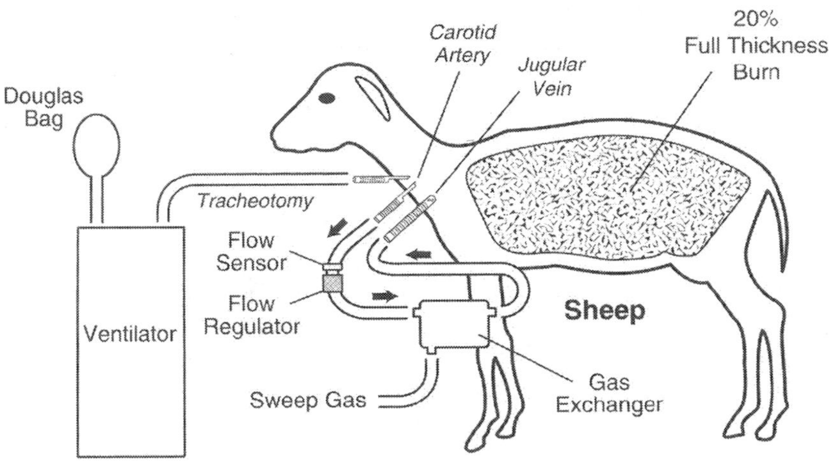

Fig. 2. Schematic of simple arteriovenous circuit with low-resistance membrane gas exchanger in mechanically ventilated sheep. (With permission from Zwischenberger JB, Alpard SK. Artificial lungs: a new inspiration. Perfusion 2002;17:253–268.)

and 30-Fr venous). Percutaneous groin access to the common femoral artery and vein are the preferred routes of vascular access. Commercially available kits allow for rapid percutaneous insertion of these small cannulae. The prime volume of the $AVCO_2R$ circuit is only 200 mL and allows for crystalloid priming, avoiding the need for blood priming (typically necessary in ECMO).

The system removes almost all metabolically produced CO_2 with only a 10–20% shunt, yet allows a significant reduction in mean airway pressures and minute ventilation *(19,20)*. $AVCO_2R$ still requires anticoagulation with heparin, but does not require a pump, a dedicated specialist, or complex equipment. Early phase I human testing confirmed $AVCO_2R$ provides complete removal of CO_2 produced during acute respiratory failure *(21)*. As Phase II clinical trials continue in the US, the European experience with pumpless CO_2 removal (also called pumpless extracorporeal lung assist [pECLA]) has continued to grow. Early reports of the first 70 patients were favorable *(22,23)*. $AVCO_2R$ (pECLA) has also been used for emergency transport of ARDS patients. Although no formal trial has been performed in Europe, a growing patient experience (over 600) with pECLA (70% survival) is starting to make an impact (ASAIO Artificial Lung Club 2005 presentation). The gas exchanger currently used in the pECLA system has not been approved in the United States by the Food and Drug Administration.

This ultra–low resistance (<10 mmHg at 2 l/min blood flow) hollow-fiber gas exchanger with polymethylpentane (PMP) fibers allows days to weeks of support at low levels of anticoagulation before failure. Prospective, randomized-outcome studies will be necessary to establish the risk/benefit of this new technique.

IVOX

The concept of an intravenacaval (intravascular) oxygenation and CO_2 removal device (IVOX) was originally conceived by Mortensen and Berry *(24,25)* for patients with ARDS. The IVOX consisted of multiple hollow fibers placed within the vena cava to provide blood oxygenation and CO_2 removal without the need for extracorporeal circulation or blood transfusion. The fibers were joined together in a potted manifold that communicated with the dual-lumen gas conduit at both its proximal and distal ends. The fibers were silicone (Siloxane®) coated and heparin bonded to create a thin "true" membrane on the previously porous hollow fibers. In the initial design, IVOX was capable of removing up to 30% of CO_2 production in an ovine model of severe smoke inhalation injury *(26–29)*. The average CO_2 removal ranged from 30 mL/min to 55 mL/min. This amount of CO_2 removal represented approximately 30% of the CO_2 production of an adult sheep (150–180 mL/min).

An international multicenter phase I–II clinical trial of IVOX was conducted in major critical care centers in the United States and Europe. From February 1990 to May 1993, 164 IVOX devices were utilized in 160 patients as a means of temporary augmentation of gas exchange. Unfortunately, there was no control arm and no improvement of survival was seen compared to historical controls. Complications or adverse events associated with use of IVOX included: mechanical and/or performance problems (29%), patient complications (bleeding, thrombosis, infection, venous occlusion, and arrhythmia), and user errors. Seven clinically recognized adverse events occurred in four patients, which could have contributed to their death. These complications reflected the learning curve typical of new invasive devices, but also emphasized the difficulties encountered during insertion. Several individual experiences of IVOX were reported from within the collective experience *(30–35)*.

Building on the lessons learned from the *in vitro* testing of the IVOX, the Hattler® Catheter incorporates a small pulsating balloon into the middle of a hollow-fiber bundle. The use of this balloon allows for convective mixing of the blood, which increases the gas exchange capabilities of the device. In a recent report, Hattler et al. (36) characterized *in vivo* and *in vitro* devices. By testing a variety of balloon sizes and pulsation rates, it was determined that larger balloon volumes and high pulsation rates increased both oxygen loading and carbon dioxide removal in a linear fashion in an *in vitro* model. The *in vivo* models, utilizing healthy calves, demonstrated much less consistent results between balloon sizes. Clinical trials are underway in Mexico and China; however, no data has been presented yet.

ARTIFICIAL LUNG

Lung transplantation has proven successful (75% 1-year, 55% 3-year, and 42% 5-year overall survival) in treating chronic irreversible lung disease in select patient populations *(37)*. Unlike dialysis, which often functions as a bridge to renal transplantation, or ventricular assist devices (VADs) that serve as a bridge to cardiac transplantation, no suitable bridge to lung transplantation exists. Since the widespread success of single- and double-lung transplantation in the early 1990s, demand for donor lungs has steadily outgrown supply *(37)*. Median waiting times for a lung transplant have increased during the last decade from less than 200 to over 600 days! The number of lung transplants performed in the United States, meanwhile, has leveled to around 1,100/year. Barring any unexpected change in donor laws, such as implied consent, no increase in donors is foreseen. Death on the waiting list for a lung transplant occurs at the rate of 15%/year; currently, 30% of patients die on the waiting list! Lung transplantation is not currently used to treat irreversible acute lung disease because lung donors are too scarce to be used in acute or emergent situations.

An artificial lung will likely make its first clinical impact either as a short-term bridge to recovery from a fatal but potentially recoverable injury (such as trauma-induced ARDS), or as a short-term (weeks-to-months) bridge to transplant. In the bridge to recovery scenario, the device would lessen ventilator-induced lung injury, converting a lethal lung injury into a recoverable one. In the bridge to transplant scenario, the ideal patient will have already spent several months on the waiting list but be deteriorating and not expected to live to transplant. They should need a single lung transplant, which allows both flexibility in organ acceptance, and a shorter waiting time. At the time of transplant, all artificial lung prosthetic material will be removed (probably during CPB), promoting infection-free recovery. Of course, short-term bridge to transplant will not be the final iteration of the artificial lung. As the artificial lung evolves, it will enter a phase of longer-term bridge to transplant, and the focus will change to patient rehabilitation (much like the evolution of the VAD in the late 1980s, when VADs began to be used for months, restoring patients to ambulatory status, reversing end-organ dysfunction, and allowing rebuilding of muscle mass). Once long-term bridge to transplant becomes a reality, then the artificial lung will enter a final phase in its evolution: alternative to transplant. Ventricular assist devices are currently entering this phase *(38)*. The goal is the stepwise, progressive development of an artificial lung for bridge to recovery, bridge to transplant, and, eventually, as effective palliation for end-stage lung disease.

Basic Design

The basic design of the artificial lung reflects the native lung's function as a gas exchanger. Gas exchange is accomplished by directing deoxygenated blood over a series of hollow fibers that are permeable to oxygen and carbon dioxide. The oxygen diffuses out of the fibers and adheres to hemoglobin for systemic delivery, and carbon dioxide diffuses out of the blood and into the fibers to exhaust or sweep back into the atmosphere. Gas exchange is maximized by increasing the interface between the blood and gas, which is achieved by manipulating several factors in the AL design: internal fiber orientation, surface area, and blood flow rate. First, maximum convective mixing occurs when blood flow is oriented perpendicular to the bundle of hollow fibers that hold a continual supply of oxygen (counter-current flow is an alternative). Secondly, minimizing the diameter and elongating the fibers maximizes the fiber bundle surface area. On the other hand, as surface area is maximized, flow resistance is also elevated. Third, the gas and blood flow rate must be matched for an efficient gas–blood flow relationship (V/Q match) similar to the native lung. Artificial lung engineers use computer modeling to manipulate the operating conditions, such as hemoglobin concentration, viscosity, saturation, CO_2 content, and pressure drop to design prototypes that will achieve the most favorable compromise.

In addition to gas exchange, the artificial lung design must achieve hemodynamic compatibility. Hemodynamic compatibility requires that the AL design have a low blood and gas flow resistance to prevent sheer stress on the blood and pressure on the heart. Resistance can be minimized by two major variables: the material of the device (microporous polypropylene fibers) and the configuration of the device. A notable problem that arises when blood is exposed to an artificial surface, in this case the fiber bundle, is that blood proteins bind to the surface. The proteins subsequently activate both the extrinsic and the intrinsic branches of the clotting cascade and quickly lead to clot formation. Therefore, nonthrombogenic fiber technology is integrated to attenuate the frequency of clot formation. Both the fibers and the encasing housing are made from nonthrombogenic material. Finally, the design must aim to serve as a bridge to transplant, so the AL device must be durable (weeks–months). The material must resist cracking and protect the gas exchange unit from damage as a patient carries the device throughout day-to-day activity.

Development

The concept of an artificial lung is not new. Preliminary efforts to design, fabricate and test prototype implantable artificial lungs have been reported intermittently since 1965 *(39–43)*. Early attempts were focused on the geometry of implantable designs and surgical implantation *(44)* instead of the hemodynamic and gas exchange performance of the device itself *(41–43)*. However, as biomaterials began to improve, so did the gas exchange capacity of the device *(45–47)*. In parallel to the development of the ventricular assist device, the artificial lung was positioned paracorporeally because it allows ambulation and easy access for servicing or exchange.

Artificial lung design and testing requires a large financial commitment by participating centers. Testing facilities must include the ability to test prototypes in large animals, both healthy and diseased, for increasingly longer term studies and employ the manpower to do so. We have completed several series of survival studies of the PAL in sheep, each building on the results of the previous studies. Our group has been working in collaboration with MC3 Corporation® to develop a PAL prototype. We will recall our 15-year effort to illustrate the challenging research and development issues, including future needs.

The PAL was initially attached in-series with pulmonary circulation, pulmonary artery–pulmonary artery (PA–PA) configuration (Fig. 3) because device change-out can proceed without risk of systemic embolization, full metabolic function of the pulmonary bed is preserved, and, most importantly, during periods of intolerance to anticoagulation (e.g., gastrointestinal bleeding), the PAL can be replaced with a C-loop, and the patient can survive temporarily on native lung function. The

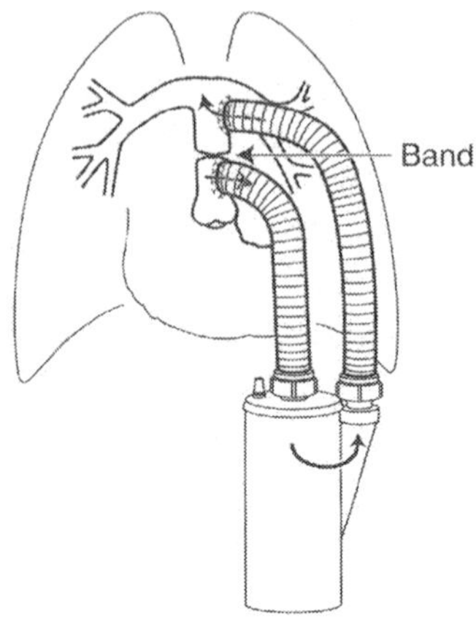

Fig. 3. In-series implantation shunts blood from the proximal PA, through the artificial lung, and back to the distal PA. A band is placed between the two anastomoses to divert 100% of the cardiac output through the artificial lung. Of the various attachment modes, this configuration creates the greatest stress on the right heart.

main disadvantage of the PA–PA configuration is that it relies on the right heart as the driving force of blood through the AL, thereby increasing right heart strain *(48,49)*.

The PAL gas exchange device as initially designed by our collaborator, MC3 Corp *(50)*, was fabricated to have minimal resistance and impedance to right heart flow (Fig. 4, A and B). Conventional CPB oxygenators have blood enter the outside of a rigid housing, flow through the fiber bundle and then exit. The PAL has blood enter through a center channel into the middle of a cylindrical fiber bundle, flow radially around evenly spaced, parallel-wound fibers, and then flow out a tangentially placed outlet. All blood flow must cross gas exchange fibers to reach the PAL outlet. While the mean pressure drop with a conventional CPB oxygenator is around 25 mmHg, bench testing of the initial PAL design showed only 8 mmHg drop at 5 L/min flow.

In the first eight sheep tested, arterial cannulae were anastomosed end-to-side to the proximal and distal main pulmonary artery, and attached to a rigidly housed PAL *(51)*. A pulmonary artery snare between anastomoses diverted total right heart output through the PAL (all survived the operative insertion). Mean pressure gradient across the PAL was 8 mmHg (3 Wood units; 8 mmHg/2.8 L/min) as 4/8 tolerated immediate full diversion of blood flow and then died at 24 and 40 hours (exsanguination) or survived to elective sacrifice at 168 hours. Half of the sheep had serious complications, two died of right heart failure at <8 hours with full flow through the device (full snare), and two survived with partial device flow (partial snare), but the device clotted. The latter two then underwent successful closed-chest cannula thrombectomy and device changeout at 53 and 75 hours, and subsequently tolerated full flow (Fig. 5). We concluded that long-term (up to 7 days) survival with complete diversion of pulmonary blood flow through a noncompliant, low-resistance PAL is possible; however, initial right heart failure in this model was 50% (4/8).

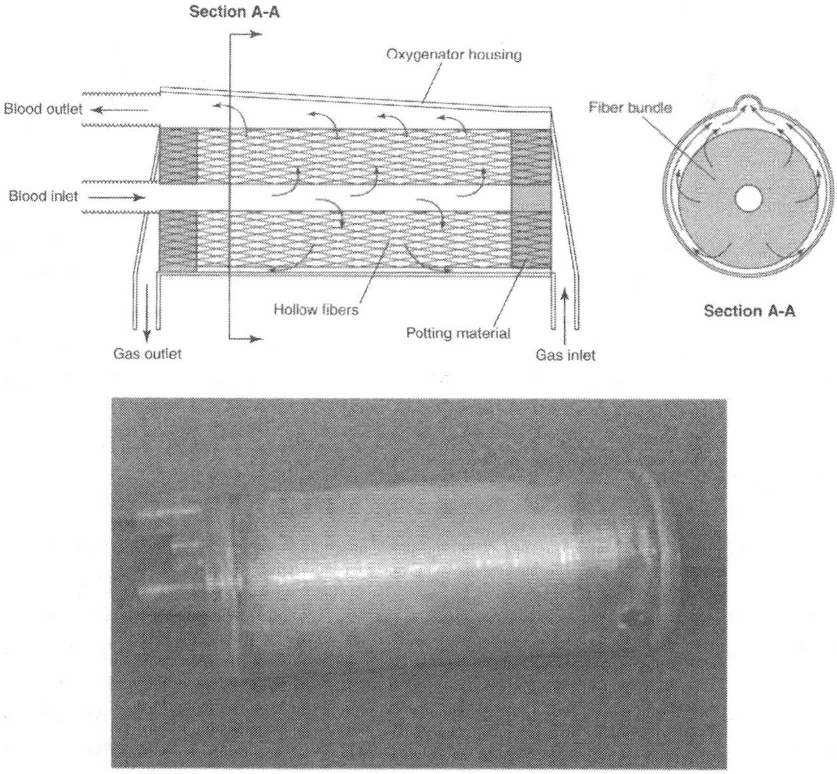

Fig. 4. The MC3 prototype (Ann Arbor, MI) uses radial blood perfusion through a concentrically wound hollow fiber fabric. As the blood flows over the fabric, it generates transverse mixing that is essential for efficient gas exchange. (With permission from Zwischenberger JB, Anderson CM, Cook KE, et al. Development of an implantable artificial lung: challenges and progress. ASAIO J 2001; 47:316–320.)

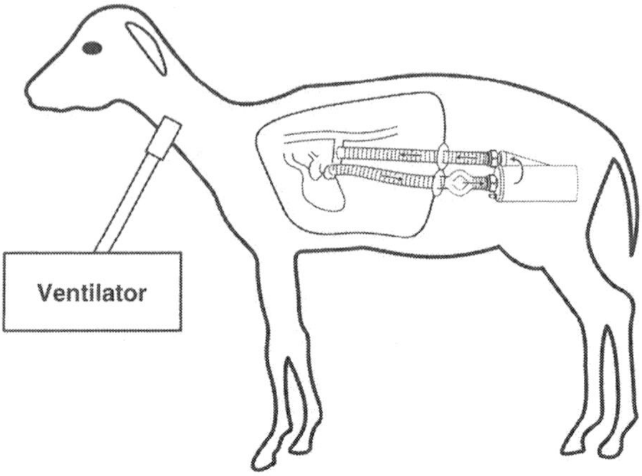

Fig. 5. Illustration of sheep with paracorporeal artificial lung. (With permission from Zwischenberger JB, Wang D, Lick SD, et al. The paracorporeal artificial lung improves 5-day outcomes from lethal smoke/burn-induced acute respiratory distress syndrome in sheep. Ann Thorac Surg 2002;74:1011–1018.)

Hemodynamic modeling shows that right heart work is dependent on PAL impedance, which is minimized by a combination of low resistance and high compliance. The right heart can only tolerate the afterload if compliance is added to the system by way of an elastic chamber or the AL itself *(52,53)*. Mathematical modeling shows that compliance is most effective in lowering impedance if placed on the inflow cannula *(54)* closer to the right heart outflow tract. Based on these sheep studies, three modifications were incorporated into our PAL design: a) the polyurethane compliance chamber was designed to accept the total stroke volume of the right ventricle by filling the chamber without significant elastic expansion; b) an inflow separator was inserted into the center of the fiber bundle to distribute the flow in a progressive pattern; and c) the geometry of the outlet was also altered, thus enlarging its effective diameter along the fiber bundle axis (Fig. 6). These design changes dropped the bench-tested transdevice pressure gradient from 8 to 6 mmHg at 5 L/min of flow. To address our initial problems with disconnections, device ports were modified or altogether removed, and cannula connections were modified to a more secure collet nut configuration.

Input impedance of the MC3 artificial lung (PAL) was compared with that of one with a compliant chamber placed at the inflow to the artificial lung *(55)*. The impedance was measured in an in vitro,

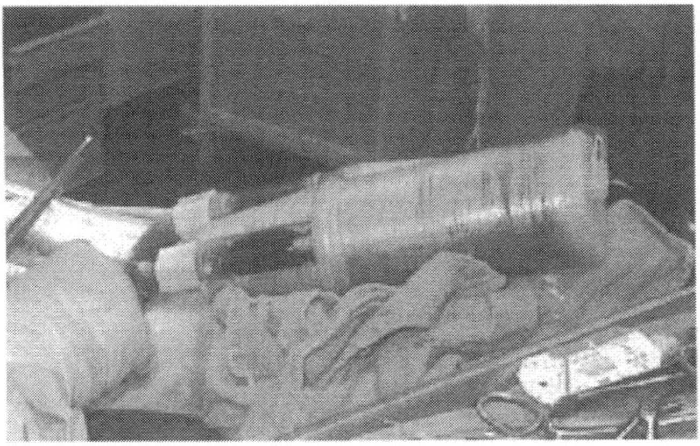

Fig. 6. PAL design was modified to lower right heart impedance. The changes included 1) addition of an in-series compliance chamber, 2) addition of an in-flow separator, and 3) increased diameter of fiber-bundle axis with streamlining.

pulsatile circuit that yielded a flow and pressure profile similar to the pulmonary artery (Fig. 7). The results are for an average flow rate of 5 L/min and a pressure pulse of 22/9 mmHg. We conclude that the modified PAL prototype with an inflow compliance chamber, blood flow separator, and modified outlet geometry greatly improved cardiac function and initial survival in our healthy ovine model.

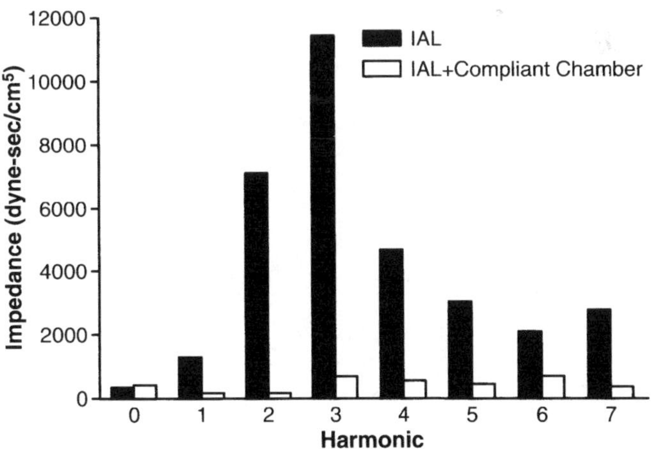

Fig. 7. The MC3 prototype was compared with and without a compliance chamber. Measurements of the flow and pressure profile reflected the right heart impedance generated by the device. The implantable artificial lung (IAL) and compliant chamber lowered impedance at all harmonic levels.

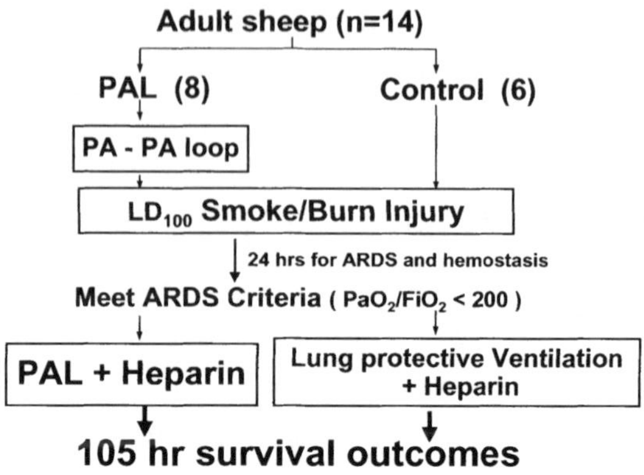

Fig. 8. 105 h-survival outcomes. (With permission from Zwischenberger JB, Wang D, Lick SD, et al. The paracorporeal artificial lung improves 5-day outcomes from lethal smoke/burn-induced acute respiratory distress syndrome in sheep. Ann Thorac Surg 2002;74:1011–1018.)

The modified PAL applied to normal sheep *(50)* showed an increased cardiac output from 2.8 to 4.2 L/min, with mean central venous pressure (CVP) 6.8, and a drop in resistance from 2.5 to 0.79 Wood units *(4)*. Six out of seven normal sheep exhibited good cardiac function throughout the PAL test period: mean CVP 6.8 mmHg, mean CO 4.2 ± 0.1 l/min; before and after device: mean PAP 21.8 and 18.5 mmHg; LAP 10.8 mmHg. Two sheep had technical complications, but 4 survived 48, 48, 72, and 72 hours, respectively, to elective sacrifice. Gas exchange during the first 24 hours averaged 220 mL/min VO_2 and 166 mL/min VCO_2.

Using our LD_{100} smoke/burn-induced ARDS sheep model, we also compared PAL to volume-controlled mechanical ventilation (VCMC) in a prospective, randomized, controlled, unblinded, outcome study *(56)*. To allow for development of a lethal lung injury, the implant technique was changed to a two-stage procedure. Fourteen sheep randomized to PAL ($n = 8$) versus VCMV ($n = 6$) to assess outcomes (Fig. 8). For PAL, arterial cannulae were anastomosed to the proximal and distal main PA with an interposing snare diverting full flow through a paracorporeal loop. An LD_{100} lung injury to produce ARDS was induced in both groups (48 breaths smoke insufflation, third-degree burn 40% total body surface area). When ARDS criteria were met PaO_2/FiO_2 <200, (24–30 h after injury), the PAL was interposed in the paracorporeal loop (Fig. 5). Both groups were managed with a VCMV algorithm minimizing tidal volume, ventilator rate, and FiO_2 *(56)*.

In this study, 6/8 PAL versus 1/6 VCMV sheep survived the 5-day study (Fig. 9). In PAL, CO, MAP, PAP, LAP, and CVP remained stable. Average PAL gas transfer was 218.6 ± 17.7 ml/min O_2 and 183.0 ± 27.8 ml/min CO_2. Ventilator settings 48 h after lung injury in PAL were significantly lower ($p < 0.05$) than VCMV (Table 2). Likewise, PaO_2/FiO_2 was normalized in PAL and still met ARDS criteria in VCMV (Fig. 10). PAL wet/dry ratio was significantly lower than VCMV (6.86 ± 0.63 vs. 11.85 ± 1.54; $p = 0.008$).

In this prospective, randomized, controlled, unblinded outcomes study, PAL decreased ventilator-induced lung injury in a LD_{100} ARDS model to improve 5-day survival. In part, this could be a result of the pulmonary vasodilating effect of oxygenated pulmonary artery blood *(57)*. This sheep ARDS model has only a moderately increased pulmonary vascular resistance (2.4 Wood units vs. 1.5 Wood units before lung injury); however, the human pulmonary vascular bed resistance can be considerably higher in many disease states, and right heart

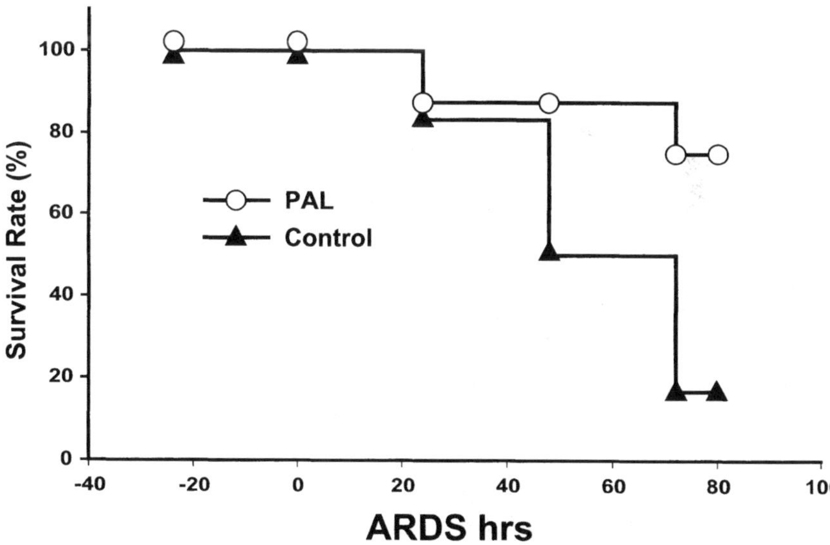

Fig. 9. 75% PAL (6/8) survived 105 hours vs. 17% control (1/6). (With permission from Zwischenberger JB, Wang D, Lick SD, et al. The paracorporeal artificial lung improves 5-day outcomes from lethal smoke/burn-induced acute respiratory distress syndrome in sheep. Ann Thorac Surg 2002;74:1011–1018.)

Table 2
Ventilator Parameters at 48 h After Onset of ARDS

	PAL	*CONTROL*
TV	210 ml	425 ml
RR	5	29
MV	1.2 L/min	10.8 L/min
FiO_2	21%	100%
PaO_2	156 mm Hg	63 mm Hg
$PaCO_2$	34 mm Hg	61 mm Hg

(*Source*: Zwischenberger JB, Wang D, Lick SD, et al. The paracorporeal artificial lung improves 5-day outcomes from lethal smoke/burn-induced acute respiratory distress syndrome in sheep. Ann Thorac Surg 2002;74:1011–1018.)

failure is common. Moreover, near-normal pulmonary vascular resistance can fluctuate into periods of high resistance (pulmonary hypertensive crisis). Although the addition of an inflow compliance chamber, modified outlet geometry and inlet blood flow separator all lowered impedance, we anticipate that, in many patients, right ventricular failure caused by primary or secondary pulmonary hypertension, will still be a potential problem. Indeed, patients with end-stage lung disease

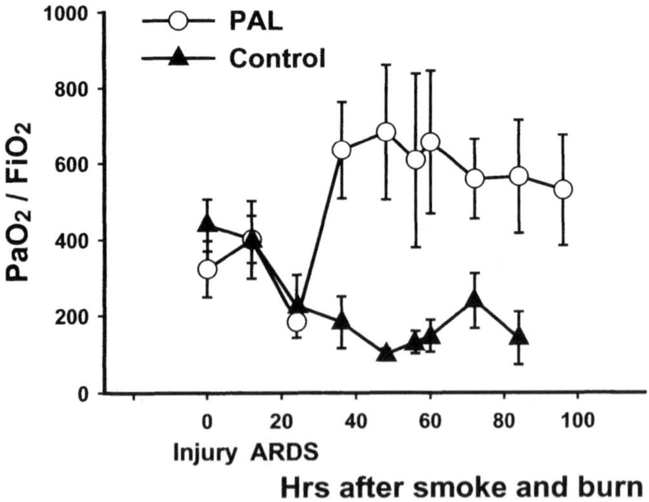

Fig. 10. PaO_2/FiO_2 ratios over 105 h PAL study. (With permission from Zwischenberger JB, Wang D, Lick SD, et al. The paracorporeal artificial lung improves 5-day outcomes from lethal smoke/burn-induced acute respiratory distress syndrome in sheep. Ann. Thorac Surg 2002;74:1011–1018.)

requiring transplantation (pulmonary fibrosis and COPD) often have at least moderately elevated pulmonary artery pressures and resistance at baseline. In some, the oxygenation of pulmonary blood itself will act as a pulmonary vasodilator *(57)*. However, we do not expect that oxygenated blood alone will provide enough vasodilation for many patients *(58)*. Patients with elevated pulmonary resistance would require mechanical assistance to pulmonary blood flow in the PA–PA configuration *(59)*.

Although we have demonstrated the feasibility of the PA–PA configuration in sheep, it is anatomically impractical to implant the PAL into the human in this configuration because the human pulmonary artery (2.5–3 cm) is substantially shorter than that of a sheep (6 cm), leaving inadequate space to successfully attach the PAL with two anastomoses and a snare. Alternative attachment options on the pulmonary artery require CPB during implant and removal, including transecting the common PA, with the proximal segment attaching to the AL inlet and post-AL segment being attached to the distal transected PA, and anatomizing a side graft to the main PA proximally and ligating the main PA distally, to divert all blood flow through the AL to then return to the right PA. Both CPB and the space limitations of the mediastinum are undesirable for long-term implantation, which further lowers the applicability of the PA–PA configuration. The disadvantages of the PA–PA configuration led most groups to focus on the pulmonary artery–left atrium (PA–LA) and right atrium–pulmonary artery (RA–PA) configurations, which are discussed below (Fig. 11).

Biocompatibility Challenges

In addition to improved gas exchange capability, PAL designs must address long-term biocompatibility and hemodynamic requirements. Despite efforts to simulate the design of the native lung, discrepancies between the device and the organ remain. First, the gas must diffuse across a relatively thick material barrier in the AL. The boundaries of fibers in the AL are inherently larger than pulmonary capillaries, therefore creating mass gas transfer resistance.

Second, the artificial material in the AL initiates cell activation and thrombus formation when it interfaces with blood. Prevention of clot formation within any extracorporeal circuit relies on either reducing the activity of circulating platelets or inhibiting the proteins involved in coagulation. Anticoagulation is available in two forms: traditional systemic anticoagulants and recently developed nonthrombogenic fibers. Although nonthrombogenic fiber technology has witnessed

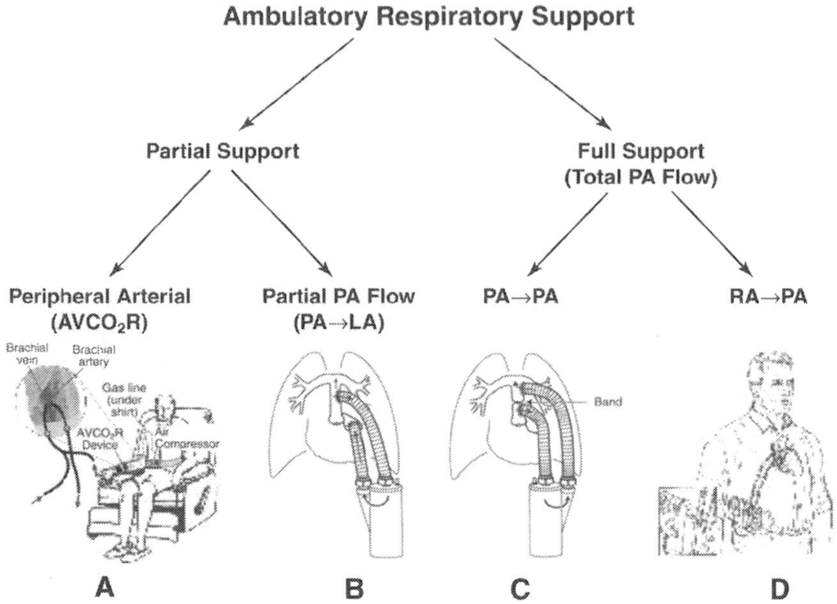

Fig. 11. Long-term ambulatory artificial respiration strategies. (A) Peripheral partial support: arterial venous CO_2 removal. (B) Central partial support: pulmonary artery to left atrium artificial lung. (C) Full support: Pulmonary artery to pulmonary artificial lung. (D) Right atrium to pulmonary artery artificial lung. (With permission from Zwischenberger JB, Lick SD. Artificial lung: bench toward bedside. ASAIO J 2002;50:2–5.)

important advances in the last few years, it cannot completely prevent blood clots. The patient must receive at least some systemic anticoagulants. Unfortunately, anticoagulants are associated with bleeding complications and morbidity.

The final disadvantage of the PAL design is the lack of metabolic or immunologic functions. The native lungs filter small emboli from the venous system and prevent entry into the arterial system. Several vasoactive substances, such as prostaglandins, angiotensin I, and bradykinins, are metabolized in the lungs *(51)*. Acute studies have reported complete pulmonary blood diversion. However, long-term survival completely excluding the pulmonary circulation may not be feasible. The metabolic function of the lungs (clearance of vasoconstrictors, vasodilators, catecholamines, and antidiuretic hormone) decreases with pulmonary flow, reaching a critical level at 10% normal flow *(60)*. Moreover, an excluded pulmonary circulation could potentially lead to diffuse pulmonary bed thrombosis. Partial or full circulation through the native lung is favored.

Configuration Challenges

The currently favored options for implanting the PAL are a) in-series RA–PA or b) parallel PA–LA (Figs. 12 and 13). Although all of the configurations create right heart strain, mathematical modeling by Boschetti and coworkers *(54)* shows that the PA–PA configuration requires the highest increase in right heart power.

Partial support, in the PA–LA configuration, creates a parallel circuit between the AL and the native lung; part of the blood is diverted to the AL, and the rest perfuses the native lung. The pressure gradient between the pulmonary artery and the left atrium passively drives blood flow *(52)*. Flow is resistance-regulated, so as pulmonary vascular resistance increases, more blood is shunted through the low-resistance AL, and right heart impedance is decreased. The PA–LA configuration is particularly suited for patients with fixed hypertension because the amount of blood flow through the device is directly dependent on the resistance of the artificial lung and the lung vascular bed. Initial studies at the University of Michigan utilizing the MC3 prototype AL demonstrated that in healthy (up to 3 d) sheep, an average of 47% of blood flow was diverted through the AL; however, flow varied from 10–90%. This

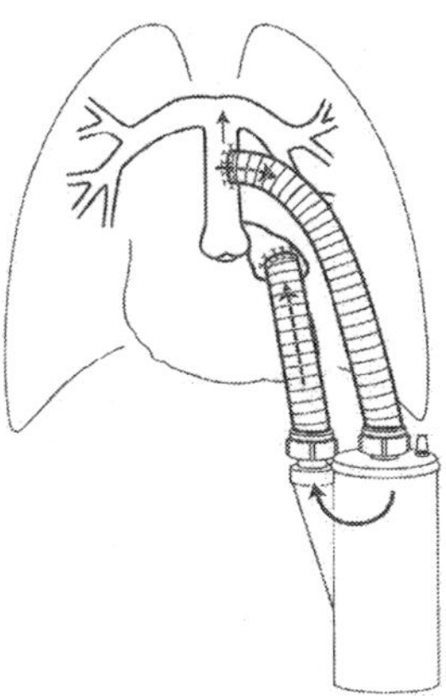

Fig. 12. In-parallel attachment shunts blood from the pulmonary artery (PA),through the artificial lung, to the left atrium (LA). In this arrangement, blood from the right heart is divided between the device and native lungs. This attachment mode creates the least amount of stress on the right heart; thus, it may be best suited for patients who are suffering from pulmonary hypertension.

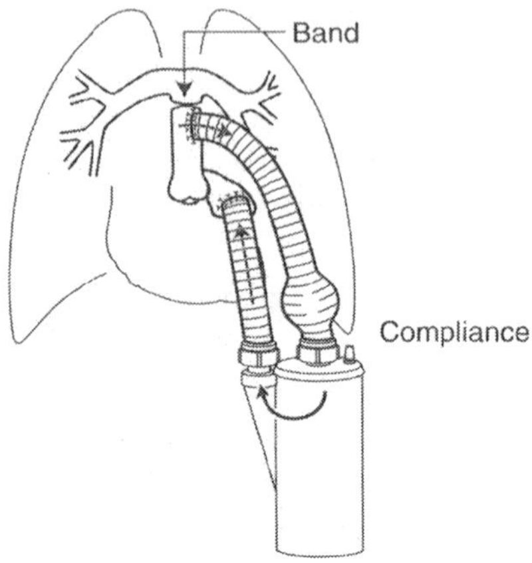

Fig. 13. In parallel attachment following PA-LA configuration. A compliance chamber has been added to reduce right heart impedance. The compliance chamber can be incorporated into any of the attachment configurations in series with the artificial lung.

variable flow, resulting from fluctuating resistance, means that the PA–LA configuration provides an unpredictable level of care. The blood flow may not meet the baseline blood volume requirement for the AL to exchange gas, and blood clots can easily form in the device. Because large animal models of chronic pulmonary hypertension are not currently available, the true benefit (or limitations) of the PA–LA configuration might not be fully realized until human trials of patients with pulmonary hypertension are performed (59). A hybrid PA–LA configuration was also considered, splitting the blood return from the AL to both the distal pulmonary artery and the left atrium (Fig. 14), but experiments demonstrated both variable blood flow and high right heart impedance *(48)*.

The RA–PA configuration bypasses the right ventricle and provides full support, but requires a pump. Designs include using an integrated system that combines the AL and pump into a single unit or using a separate pump and AL (bulkier). Regardless, the AL behaves like a right VAD (RVAD) capable of gas exchange, as the blood first passes through the pump and then through the AL. The single-unit design enhances the goal of ambulation and easy changeout. On the other hand, separating the pump allows easy troubleshooting and changeout of each component separately *(52)*.

Our group has successfully mated a small axial flow pump to a commercially available gas exchange device in a RA–PA configuration for

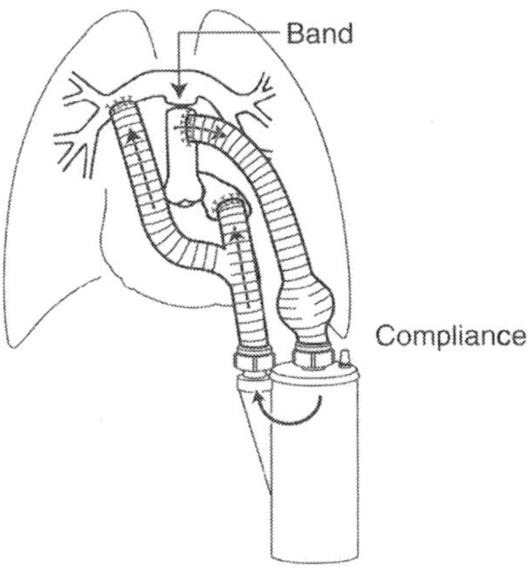

Fig. 14. Hybrid attachment shunts blood from the proximal PA to the artificial lung, with a split return to the distal PA and the LA. A band would be placed on the PA that could shunt as much as 100% of the cardiac output through the artificial lung. This attachment mode is the best compromise between hemodynamic performance and preservation of some portion of the nonrespiratory functions of the natural lungs. The figure also includes an inlet compliance chamber. (With permission from Zwischenberger JB, Anderson CM, Cook KE, et al. Development of an implantable artificial lung: challenges and progress. ASAIO J 2001;47:316–320.)

up to 2 weeks in normal sheep *(61)*. The integrated heart–lung assist device from Japan combines a centrifugal blood pump with a hollow-fiber oxygenator wrapped cylindrically around the pump. The resulting device is ultracompact, with a vaned diffuser between the impeller of the centrifugal pump and the fiber bundle to enhance gas exchange *(62)*. The undulation pump total artificial heart (UPTAH), on the other hand, represents the dual-system model, in which the UPTAH is implantable and connected in series with the ex vivo artificial lung. Two separate undulation pumps (right and left) provide total artificial lung support, but a major disadvantage is the high incidence of atrial suction *(63)*.

Unlike the PA–PA configuration, RA–PA does not require CPB support for insertion. The benefits of RA–PA are improved right heart function and the ability to overcome high pulmonary pressures; however, the risk of mechanical failure increases because the two devices can fail independently or as a unit. The configuration is currently in the early stages of animal testing.

Computer aided engineering technology is proving to be a valuable tool for AL progress. Many of the requirements to develop a successful

AL (low-pressure drop, sufficient gas exchange, and nonthrombogenic surfaces) are dependent on design, specifically housing geometry, and fluid dynamics *(64)*. By examining blood flow patterns, the AL device design can be optimized based on predictions of stagnation areas, which are considered related to many AL complications. Griffith's group at University of Maryland is developing a centrifugal pump/gas exchanger with moving filters that create a vortex pump *(65)*.

Finally, many perceive endothelial seeding or tissue engineering as capable of creating a nonthrombogenic surface or growing functional lung tissue. Use of nonreactive scaffolding to allow lung regeneration or endothelial seeding of gas exchanger macropores also has enthusiasts, despite years of frustration.

In the 30 years since the development of ECMO, much progress has been made. We are on the forefront of an era in which artificial lungs might serve as a "replacement" organ or bridge to transplant or recovery for those crippled by respiratory disease.

REFERENCES

1. Bartlett RH. Extracorporeal life support for cardiopulmonary failure. Curr Probl Surg 1990;27:621–705.
2. Bartlett RH, Gazzaniga AB, Jefferies MR, Huxtable RF, Haiduc NJ, Fong SW. Extracorporeal membrane oxygenation (ECMO) cardiopulmonary support in infancy. Trans Am Soc Artif Intern Organs 1976;22:80–93.
3. ECMO Registry of the Extracorporeal Life Support Organization (ELSO) Ann Arbor Michigan (December, 2005).
4. Bartlett RH, Roloff DW, Cornell RG, Andrews AF, Dillon PW, Zwischenberger JB. Extracorporeal circulation in neonatal respiratory failure: a prospective randomized study. Pediatrics 1985;76:479–487.
5. O'Rourke PP, Crone RK, Vacanti JP, et al. Extracorporeal membrane oxygenation and conventional medical therapy in neonates with persistent pulmonary hypertension of the newborn: a prospective randomized study. Pediatrics 1989;84:957–963.
6. UK collaborative randomised trial of neonatal extracorporeal membrane oxygenation. UK Collaborative ECMO Trail Group. Lancet 1996;348:75–82.
7. Zapol WM, Snider MT, Hill JD, et al. Extracorporeal membrane oxygenation in severe acute respiratory failure. A randomized prospective study. JAMA 1979; 242:2193–2196.
8. Hemmila MR, Rowe SA, Boules TN, et al. Extracorporeal life support for severe acute respiratory distress syndrome in adults. Ann Surg 2004;240:595–607.
9. Kolla S, Awad SS, Rich PB, Schreiner RJ, Hirschl RB, Bartlett RH. Extracorporeal life support for 100 adult patients with severe respiratory failure. Ann Surg 1997; 226:544–566.
10. Lewandowski K, Rossaint R, Pappert D, et al. High survival rate in 122 ARDS patients managed according to a clinical algorithm including extracorporeal membrane oxygenation. Intensive Care Med 1997;23:819–835.

11. Peek GJ, Moore HM, Moore N, Sosnowski AW, Firmin RK. Extracorporeal membrane oxygenation for adult respiratory failure. Chest 1997;112:759–764.
12. Gattinoni L, Kolobow T, Tomlinson T, et al. Low-frequency positive pressure ventilation with extracorporeal carbon dioxide removal (LFPPV-ECCO2R): an experimental study. Anesth Analg 1978;57:470–477.
13. Gattinoni L, Kolobow T, Tomlinson T, White D, Pierce J. Control of intermittent positive pressure breathing (IPPB) by extracorporeal removal of carbon dioxide. Br J Anaesth 1978;50:753–758.
14. Kolobow T, Gattinoni L, Tomlinson T, Pierce JE. An alternative to breathing. J Thorac Cardiovasc Surg 1978;75:261–266.
15. Brunet F, Belghith M, Mira JP, et al. Extracorporeal carbon dioxide removal and low-frequency positive-pressure ventilation. Improvement in arterial oxygenation with reduction of risk of pulmonary barotrauma in patients with adult respiratory distress syndrome. Chest 1993;104:889–898.
16. Gattinoni L, Agostoni A, Pesenti A, et al. Treatment of acute respiratory failure with low-frequency positive-pressure ventilation and extracorporeal removal of CO2. Lancet 1980;2:292–294.
17. Gattinoni L, Kolobow T, Agostoni A, et al. Clinical application of low frequency positive pressure ventilation with extracorporeal CO2 removal (LFPPV-ECCO2R) in treatment of adult respiratory distress syndrome (ARDS). Int J Artif Organs 1979;2:282–283.
18. Morris AH, Wallace CJ, Menlove RL, et al. Randomized clinical trial of pressure-controlled inverse ratio ventilation and extracorporeal CO2 removal for adult respiratory distress syndrome. Am J Respir Crit Care Med 1994;149:295–305.
19. Brunston RL, Jr., Zwischenberger JB, Tao W, Cardenas VJ, Jr., Traber DL, Bidani A. Total arteriovenous CO2 removal: simplifying extracorporeal support for respiratory failure. Ann Thorac Surg 1997;64:1599–1605.
20. Brunston RL, Jr., Tao W, Bidani A, Traber DL, Zwischenberger JB. Organ blood flow during arteriovenous carbon dioxide removal. ASAIO J 1997;43:M821–M824.
21. Conrad SA, Zwischenberger JB, Grier LR, Alpard SK, Bidani A. Total extracorporeal arteriovenous carbon dioxide removal in acute respiratory failure: a phase I clinical study. Intensive Care Med 2001;27:1340–1351.
22. Zwischenberger JB, Conrad SA, Alpard SK, Grier LR, Bidani A. Percutaneous extracorporeal arteriovenous CO2 removal for severe respiratory failure. Ann Thorac Surg 1999;68:181–187.
23. Liebold A, Philipp A, Kaiser M, Merk J, Schmid FX, Birnbaum DE. Pumpless extracorporeal lung assist using an arterio-venous shunt. Applications and limitations. Minerva Anestesiol 2002;68:387–391.
24. Mortensen JD. An intravenacaval blood gas exchange (IVCBGE) device. A preliminary report. ASAIO Trans 1987;33:570–573.
25. Mortensen JD, Berry G. Conceptual and design features of a practical, clinically effective intravenous mechanical blood oxygen/carbon dioxide exchange device (IVOX). Int J Artif Organs 1989;12:384–389.
26. Cox CS, Jr., Zwischenberger JB, Graves DF, Niranjan SC, Bidani A. Intracorporeal CO2 removal and permissive hypercapnia to reduce airway pressure in acute respiratory failure. The theoretical basis for permissive hypercapnia with IVOX. ASAIO J 1993;39:97–102.
27. Cox CS, Jr., Zwischenberger JB, Traber LD, Traber DL, Herndon DN. Use of an intravascular oxygenator/carbon dioxide removal device in an ovine smoke inhalation injury model. ASAIO Trans 1991;37:M411–413.

28. Zwischenberger JB, Cox CS, Jr. A new intravascular membrane oxygenator to augment blood gas transfer in patients with acute respiratory failure. Tex Med 1991;87:60–63.
29. Zwischenberger JB, Cox CS, Graves D, Bidani A. Intravascular membrane oxygenation and carbon dioxide removal—a new application for permissive hypercapnia? Thorac Cardiovasc Surg 1992;40:115–120.
30. Conrad SA, Eggerstedt JM, Morris VF, Romero MD. Prolonged intracorporeal support of gas exchange with an intravenacaval oxygenator. Chest 1993;103: 158–161.
31. Gentilello LM, Jurkovich GJ, Gubler KD, Anardi DM, Heiskell R. The intravascular oxygenator (IVOX): preliminary results of a new means of performing extrapulmonary gas exchange. J Trauma 1993;35:399–404.
32. High KM, Snider MT, Richard R, et al. Clinical trials of an intravenous oxygenator in patients with adult respiratory distress syndrome. Anesthesiology 1992;77: 856–863.
33. Jurmann MJ, Demertzis S, Schaefers HJ, Wahlers T, Haverich A. Intravascular oxygenation for advanced respiratory failure. ASAIO J 1992;38:120–124.
34. Kallis P, al-Saady NM, Bennett ED, Treasure T. Early results of intravascular oxygenation. Eur J Cardiothorac Surg 1993;7:206–210.
35. von Segesser LK, Schaffner A, Stocker R, et al. Extended (29 days) use of intravascular gas exchanger. Lancet 1992;339:1536.
36. Hattler BG, Lund LW, Golob J, et al. A respiratory gas exchange catheter: in vitro and in vivo tests in large animals. J Thorac Cardiovasc Surg 2002;124:520–530.
37. Health and Human Services 1999 Annual Report: UNOS/OPTN Data. 1999.
38. Rose EA, Gelijns AC, Moskowitz AJ, et al. Long-term mechanical left ventricular assistance for end-stage heart failure. N Engl J Med 2001;345:1435–1443.
39. Bodell BR, Head JM, Head LR, Formolo AJ. An implantable artificial lung. Initial experiments in animals. JAMA 1965;191:301–303.
40. Mortensen JD. Afterword: bottom-line status report: Can current trends in membrane gas transfer technology lead to an implantable intrathoracic artificial lung? Artif Organs 1994;18:864–869.
41. Shah-Mirany J, Head LR, Ghetzler R, Formolo AJ, Palmer AS, Bodell BR. An implantable artificial lung. Ann Thorac Surg 1972;13:381–387.
42. Palmer AS, Collins J, Head LR. Development of an implantable artificial lung. J Thorac Cardiovasc Surg 1973;66:521–525.
43. Morin PJ, Gosselin C, Picard R, Vincent M, Guidoin R, Nicholl CI. Implantable artificial lung. Preliminary report. J Thorac Cardiovasc Surg 1977;74:130–136.
44. Trudell LA, Peirce EC II, Teplitz C, Richardson PD, Galletti PM. A surgical approach to the implantation of an artificial lung. Trans Am Soc Artif Intern Organs 1979;25:462–465.
45. Cook KE, Makarewicz AJ, Backer CL, et al. Testing of an intrathoracic artificial lung in a pig model. ASAIO J 1996;42:M604–M609.
46. Galletti PM, Richardson PD, Trudell LA, Panol G, Tanishita K, Accinelli D. Development of an implantable booster lung. Trans Am Soc Artif Intern Organs 1980;26:573–577.
47. Mockros LF, Leonard R. Compact cross-flow tubular oxygenators. Trans Am Soc Artif Intern Organs 1985;31:628–633.
48. Lynch WR, Montoya JP, Brant DO, Schreiner RJ, Iannettoni MD, Bartlett RH. Hemodynamic effect of a low-resistance artificial lung in series with the native lungs of sheep. Ann Thorac Surg 2000;69:351–356.

49. Piene H, Sund T. Flow and power output of right ventricle facing load with variable input impedance. Am J Physiol 1979;237:H125–130.
50. Lick SD, Zwischenberger JB, Wang D, Deyo DJ, Alpard SK, Chambers SD. Improved right heart function with a compliant inflow artificial lung in series with the pulmonary circulation. Ann Thorac Surg 2001;72:899–904.
51. Lick SD, Zwischenberger JB, Alpard SK, Witt SA, Deyo DM, Merz SI. Development of an ambulatory artificial lung in an ovine survival model. ASAIO J 2001; 47:486–491.
52. Lick SD, Zwischenberger JB. Artificial lung: bench toward bedside. ASAIO J 2004;50:2–5.
53. McGillicuddy JW, Chambers SD, Galligan DT, Hirschl RB, Bartlett RH, Cook KE. In vitro fluid mechanical effects of thoracic artificial lung compliance. ASAIO J 2005;51:789–794.
54. Boschetti F, Perlman CE, Cook KE, Mockros LF. Hemodynamic effects of attachment modes and device design of a thoracic artificial lung. ASAIO J 2000;46: 42–48.
55. Haft JW, Bull JL, Rose R, Katsra J, Grotberg JB, Bartlett RH, Hirschl RB. Design of an artificial lung compliance chamber for pulmonary replacement. ASAIO J 2003;49:35–40.
56. Zwischenberger JB, Wang D, Lick SD, Deyo DJ, Alpard SK, Chambers SD. The paracorporeal artificial lung improves 5-day outcomes from lethal smoke/burn-induced acute respiratory distress syndrome in sheep. Ann Thorac Surg 2002;74: 1011–1018.
57. Lazar EI, Weinstein S, Stark CJ. Lung injury does not increase vascular resistance if pulmonary blood is fully saturated. Surg Forum 1993;44:651–652.
58. Haft JW, Alnajjar O, Bull JL, Bartlett RH, Hirschl RB. Effect of artificial lung compliance on right ventricular load. ASAIO J 2005;51:769–772.
59. Haft JW, Montoya P, Alnajjar O, et al. An artificial lung reduces pulmonary impedance and improves right ventricular efficiency in pulmonary hypertension. J Thorac Cardiovasc Surg 2001;122:1094–1100.
60. Takewa Y, Tatsumi E, Taenaka Y, et al. Hemodynamic and humoral conditions in stepwise reduction of pulmonary blood flow during venoarterial bypass in awake goats. ASAIO J 1997;43:M494–M499.
61. Wang D, Zhou X, Lick SD, Zwischenberger JB. Compact oxyRVAD for respiratory and right heart assistance. ASAIO J 2006 (in press);52.
62. Tsukiya T, Tatsumi E, Nishinaka T, et al. Design progress of the ultracompact integrated heart lung assist device-Part 1: effect of vaned diffusers on gas-transfer performances. Artif Organs 2003;27:911.
63. Abe Y, Chinzei T, Isoyama T, et al. Third model of the undulation pump total artificial heart. ASAIO J 2003;49:123–127.
64. Taga I, Funakubo A, Fukui Y. Design and development of an artificial implantable lung using multiobjective genetic algorithm: evaluation of gas exchange performance. ASAIO J 2005;51:92–102.
65. Wu ZJ, Gartner M, Litwak KN, Griffith BP. Progress toward an ambulatory pump-lung. J Thorac Cardiovasc Surg 2005;130:973–978.

13 Policy and Procedure Guidelines*

THE PERFUSION TEAM AT NYPH COLUMBIA CAMPUS

Linda Mongero, CCP, Director Perfusion Services
James Beck, CCP, Chief Perfusionist
Kevin Charette, CCP, Assistant Chief, Pediatrics
Jerry Allen, CCP, Staff Perfusionist
Dana Apsel, Staff Perfusionist
Justin Ashley, CCP, Staff Perfusionist
Trace Baker, CCP, Staff Perfusionist
Alan Becker, CCP, Staff Perfusionist
Thomas Beaulieu, CCP, Staff Perfusionist
Michael Brewer, Staff Perfusionist
Allison Cohen, CCP, Staff Perfusionist
Kelly Derr, CCP, Staff Perfusionist
Neil Edson, CCP, Staff Perfusionist
Christine Farrell, CCP, Staff Perfusionist
Julia Mumm, CCP, Staff Perfusionist
Tom Orr, CCP, Staff Perfusionist
David Park, CCP, Staff Perfusionist
Jeeni Patel, CCP, Staff Perfusionist
Edwin Silver, CCP, Staff Perfusionist
Jeremy Tamari, CCP, Staff Perfusionist
Lori Tomlinson, CCP, Staff Perfusionist
Roger Branch, Materials Manager

*These guidelines are provided for informational purpose only and NYPH and the authors and editors are not liable for its content. Clinicians must accept responsibility for the exercise of sound judgment in the delivery of services and must be responsible for the quality of service provided. Clinicans should not engage in practices beyond their competence of training.

From: *Current Cardiac Surgery: On Bypass: Advanced Perfusion Techniques*
Edited by: L. B. Mongero and J. R. Beck © Humana Press Inc., Totowa, NJ

Policy and Procedure Guidelines

CLINICAL PERFUSION POLICY AND PROCEDURES

Section 1: Special Procedures

CP01 Axillary arterial cannulation
CP02 Buckberg solution—aspartate-glutamate cardioplegia
CP03 Cerebral aneurysm repair
CP04 ECMO—adult
CP05 ECMO—hemoconcentration
CP06 ECMO—neonatal/infant
CP07 ECMO—pediatric
CP08 ECMO—transport
CP09 Laser—CO_2 heart
CP10 Left heart bypass
CP11 Limb perfusion
CP12 Liver procedures
CP12r Liver transplants
CP13 Lung transplant—leukodepletion
CP14 Peritoneal perfusion—hyperthermic
CP15 Retrograde cerebral perfusion
CP16 Right to left shunt
CP17 Robotic procedures/mini MVR, AVR
CP18 Vacuum-assisted venous return

Section 2: Daily Procedures

CP19 Aprotinin
CP20 Autotransfusion
CP21 Intraaortic balloon pumps
CP22 Battery backup
CP23 Blood administration
CP24 CPB adults
CP25 Cardioplegia warm delivery
CP26 Clear prime replacement
CP27 Formulae
CP28 Hemochron response
CP29 I-STAT
CP30 Nitric oxide

CP31 Oxygenator changeout
CP32 Protamine administration and reaction
CP33 Standby and backup procedures
CP34 HCU 30 maintainence

Section 3: Pathologies

CP35 Antithrombin III deficiency
CP36 Cold agglutinins
CP37 Disseminated intravascular coagulation
CP38 Gas embolism
CP39 Hyperkalemia
CP40 Malignant hyperthermia
CP41 Pregnant patient perfusion
CP42 Sickle cell anemia

*Section 4: Ventricular Assist Devices (VADs)** Note: These guidelines change frequently and clinicians must refer to current manufacterers guidelines before performing ventricular assist implant procedures.

CP43 Abiomed
CP44 Bio Medicus
CP45 Heartmate TCI, I, II
CP46 Novacor
CP47 Thoratec
CP48 DeBakey
CP49 Impella VAD

Section 5: Children's Hospital

CP75 Babies circuits
CP76 Pediatric primes
CP77 Pediatric cardioplegia
CP78 Pediatric cannula
CP79 Pediatric blood
CP80 Pediatric aprotinin
CP81 Pediatric MUF
CP82 ABO incompatibility
CP83 Apheresis policy and procedure
CP84 CPB procedures for pediatrics
CP85 NOi setup & transport
CP86 Sickle cell & isoantibody for pediatrics
CP87 Pediatric pump calibration
CP88 Washing PRBCs with the Cell Saver

Policy and Procedure Guidelines

CP01

AXILLARY ARTERIAL CANNULATION, ANTEGRADE CEREBRAL PERFUSION (ACP), AND ELEPHANT TRUNK

Antegrade cerebral perfusion through the axillary artery, in combination with hypothermic circulatory arrest, provides protection to the brain during operations that involve the aortic arch. Axillary artery cannulation may be used as an alternative aortic cannulation site in the presence of a highly calcified aorta or in procedures that the surgeon deems necessary for repair of the aorta and its branches. For example, the total aortic arch replacement with elephant trunk procedure requires the following equipment:

Standard adult perfusion circuit
Standard two-stage venous cannula
Dacron graft (8 mm) for end-to-side anastomosis to axillary artery
Two appropriately sized arterial cannulae, softflow or EOPA (22 or 24 F); confirm choice with surgeon
At times, an additional 3/8″ arterial line is inserted into the arterial limb of the circuit for arterial flow into the distal graft

PROCEDURE

1. Dacron graft is attached to the axillary artery.
2. Appropriate size arterial cannula is inserted into the graft and tied so tip of cannula is within wound to prevent kinking.
3. Dual-stage cannula is used for venous drainage.
4. Arterial pressure should be monitored in the left radial artery and/or groin while on cardiopulmonary bypass (CPB), and in the right radial artery during selective cerebral perfusion.
5. Cool per surgeon's request (18–28°C).
6. Aortic cross clamp and deliver cardioplegia solution.
7. Hypothermic circulatory arrest. Clamp arterial line, drain venous line, and leave open.
8. Initiation of ACP. Surgeon should tell you to flow 10–20 cc/kg/min. Right radial pressure should be monitored at this time. Values should be in the 40–80 mm Hg range.

9. Open the venous line to allow continuous drainage of the cerebral vasculature and monitor CVP.
10. Set appropriate FIO_2 and sweep gas and forane if used.
11. Arch replacement with graft and increase in flow to all head vessels (20 cc/kg).
12. Surgeon replaces distal graft and elephant trunk into descending thoracic aorta, and then cannulates the distal graft for perfusion with second arterial line and cannula.
13. Proximal graft is sewn to aortic root.
14. The proximal and distal grafts are sewn together.
15. Surgeon will tell you to come off ACP.
16. Head vessels are clamped, and the graft is deaired by surgeon.
17. Full flow will begin, and rewarming through both aortic lines commences.
18. The preferred pressure to monitor during full CPB is left radial or groin pressure. Right radial pressure will often be elevated because of proximity of the cannulation site.

Policy and Procedure Guidelines
CP02

PROCEDURE FOR "ASPARTATE-GLUTAMATE ENRICHED" CARDIOPLEGIA

Purpose

The use of the amino acid "enriched" cardioplegia solutions formulated by Dr. Gerald Buckberg is now available from CAPS Pharmacy for delivery to NYP. These solutions are used to replace Kreb's cycle intermediates and reduce reperfusion injury.

One group of patients that can benefit from this solution is acute infarction patients, where the solution is delivered with a high KCl level for warm cardioplegic induction. The other group of patients includes those with long aortic x-clamp times. In this group, the warm cardioplegia delivered just before the release of the aortic x-clamp contains a low KCl "glutamate-aspartate enriched" cardioplegia solution.

Method

"Buckberg Solution"

THAM (0.3 M)	225 ml
CPD	225 ml
Dextrose 50% in water	40 ml
Glutamate/Aspartate	250 ml (prepared as a 0.458 M solution)
Potassium Chloride (30 mEq)	15 ml

Dextrose 5% in water qs to 1,000 ml total volume

1. **Acute Infarction Protocol**—"Warm Cardioplegic Induction"
    1. To 500 ml of *Buckberg Solution* add 12.5 ml (25 mEq) of KCl to increase the concentration to 80 mEq/L for warm induction. Add 200 mg of $CaCl_2$ to pump prime.
    2. With a 4:1 blood/cardioplegia delivery system, warm to 37°C and deliver with a flow rate of 250–350 ml/min until the heart is arrested.

3. Reduce the flow rate to 150 ml/min and continue for 2 min of warm induction.
4. Switch to retrograde for 3 min of warm cardioplegia.
5. Change the cardioplegia bag to the non–amino acid standard low K^+ solution (60 mEq/L).
6. Lower the temperature of the cardioplegia to 4°C.
7. Increase the flow rate to 250–350 ml/min and deliver approximately 500 ml of cold blood cardioplegia antegrade.
8. Switch to retrograde and deliver an additional 500 ml at 150 ml/min, limiting coronary sinus pressure to below 50 mm Hg.

2. **Reperfusion Protocol**

1. Use the standard Buckberg Solution with the 4 : 1 blood/cardioplegia delivery system.
2. Warm cardioplegia solution to 37°C and deliver at 150 ml/min for 3–5 min retrograde.
3. Discontinue the infusion and remove the aortic x-clamp.

Policy and Procedure Guidelines

CP03

PERFUSION TECHNIQUE FOR REPAIR OF GIANT INTRACEREBRAL ANEURYSMS DURING TOTAL CIRCULATORY ARREST UNDER DEEP HYPOTHERMIA

Intracerebral aneurysms unapproachable with conventional techniques can be clipped during total circulatory arrest under deep hypothermia. The perfusion circuit was modified to apply centrifugal pump suction to the venous line without sacrificing the ability to rapidly add and subtract volume, incorporating protection against air embolism by suction entrainment. Protection of the fibrillating heart during hypothermia was facilitated by transesophageal echo monitoring of the ventricular volume to detect distention.

MATERIALS

2 Bio-Medicus consoles
1 Roller pump
2 disposable Bio-Medicus centrifugal heads
1 Medtronic cerebral aneurysm custom tubing pack
1 Cardiotomy reservoir
1 Heater–cooler unit
1 Waterloo cart

EQUIPMENT

Preparation of the perfusion circuit by the perfusionist is as follows:

Connect venous return line (3/8″ × 3/32″ wall tubing) to the biohead inlet with the biohead outlet in the upright position (venous suction pump). The pump outlet should be directed into the BMR 1,900 soft reservoir bag. A hard-shell cardiotomy should be attached to the reservoir bag at the usual port.

The outlet of the BMR 1,900 should be connected via 3/8″ × 3/32″ wall tubing to the arterial Biopump inlet. The Biopump outlet should be directed to the inlet of the oxygenator. The oxygenator outlet will connect to the arterial filter. The arterial filter outlet will be attached to the arterial side of the AV loop.

A roller suction line with a one-way vacuum relief valve will return purge dair from the top of the BMR to the cardiotomy reservoir.

PROCEDURE

Double Biopump System: The femoral vein is cannulated under direct vision using a modified Seldinger technique. The venous cannula (19–21 F) have 1 end hole, 12 side holes, and are constructed of polyurethane with wire reinforcement that resists collapse under high negative pressures. The 3/8″ I.D. venous tubing (3/16″ wall) is attached to the venous centrifugal pump (Bio-Medicus) that is operated with the outlet in the upward position to facilitate the removal of air from the venous line. Output from the venous pump enters a 1,900-ml collapsible venous reservoir bag (Cobe Cardiovascular), which then empties into the inlet of the arterial centrifugal pump. The arterial limb of the circuit also consists of 3/8″ tubing and is connected to the outlet of the arterial centrifugal pump. The arterial pump is operated in the normal downward position to protect against air embolism. Output from this pump is directed to a low-prime (220 ml) adult membrane oxygenator, and then to an arterial filter before being returned to the patient. Connected to the top of the reservoir bag is a 1/4″ tubing passed through a roller pump, through which air can be easily aspirated from the system. The venous reservoir is protected against excessive suction with a pressure-relief valve. Volume is returned to the circuit by gravity through the cardiotomy drain line. The double Biopump circuit is primed with a 1,500-ml nonblood prime consisting of 1,000 ml 6% hetastarch (Hespan) and 500 ml of balanced electrolyte solution (Plasmalyte). The venous line pressure is monitored with a pressure display box (DLP) attached to the inlet of the venous Biopump. Flow is regulated by adjusting the revolutions per minute (RPM) of the venous pump to maximize venous flow and increasing the flow of the arterial pump to match the venous return. The venous pump is operated at the lowest RPM necessary to achieve the desired blood flow rate and limit negative venous line pressure (usually <100 mmHg).

A transesophageal echocardiogram is continuously displayed to ensure adequate monitoring of cardiac function and filling. Absence of distention of the ventricles is confirmed by viewing the left ventricular cross sectional area and comparing it to the prebypass end-diastolic volume. Myocardial protection is ensured with a bolus potassium infusion (20–40 mEq) into the central venous pressure catheter during periods of fibrillation.

Temperatures are measured and recorded continuously throughout the procedure. A 30-gauge needle probe is inserted into the temporal lobe. In addition to brain temperature, the following temperatures are monitored to ensure adequacy of cooling and rewarming: tympanic membrane, esophageal, axillary, rectal, arterial blood, and venous blood. The patient is cooled to a brain temperature of 16–18°C before circulatory arrest.

During circulatory arrest, blood is drained into the venous and cardiotomy reservoirs to shrink the cerebral vessels and aneurysm for direct, bloodless surgical repair under the neurosurgical microscope. Intermittent transfusion from the circuit, under the direction of the neurosurgeon, tests the clipped aneurysm for bleeding. Rewarming of the patient begins at full flow once the neurosurgeon determines that bleeding is absent at the aneurysm site.

Caution: During periods of circulatory arrest, the inlet and the outlet of the oxygenator may need to be clamped to prevent negative pressure on the oxygenator fibers with resultant air entrainment. This may happen if the oxygenator is positioned higher than the patient.

Blood conservation is maximized with the use of an autotransfusion device. The autologous blood recovery device is used to wash the cells from the perfusion circuit after discontinuation of cardiopulmonary bypass (CPB).

Alternative Method for Conduct of CPB Utilizing Vacuum-Assisted Venous Return

Vacuum-assisted venous return (VAVR) offers some alternatives to conventional CPB techniques. It uses negative pressure to assist or augment venous return over traditional siphon drainage technique. This technique utilizes a wall suction source to generate a vacuum and enhance venous drainage during open heart surgery. Using VAVR allows smaller venous cannulae, smaller venous line size, and reduced prime.

VAVR with a Hard-Shell Venous Reservoir

Initial Setup before Going on Bypass

- Assemble CPB circuit as per standard procedure. Test and install the positive pressure relief valve onto a vacuum-assist capable hard-shell venous reservoir. Place occluding plugs on all unused ports.
- Properly occlude all roller pump heads. If using a centrifugal arterial head, make sure a one-way valve is placed between the centrifugal head and the oxygenator to prevent air from being pulled across the oxygenator fiber in the event of centrifugal pump stoppage.
- Attach the "To Vacuum" connector of Bentley Vacuum Controller to a reliable hospital-grade (NFPA-U.S.) vacuum source.
- Attach a calibrated means of monitoring negative pressures to the venous line and/or cardiotomy reservoir. Set and use alarms whenever possible.
- Verify that the "Conversion Module" vacuum line is connected to the moisture trap.
- Attach the Conversion Module vacuum line to the To Reservoir connector of the Bentley Vacuum Controller, and the moisture trap to the vent port of the appropriate venous reservoir.
- Clamp the venous reservoir drain line between the arterial pump head and the venous reservoir.
- Clamp the venous line just distal to its connection to the venous reservoir pressure-monitoring site.
- Verify that all other ports and lines to the venous reservoir are closed to the atmosphere.
- Verify that all roller pumps are off.
- Clamp the "To Reservoir" vacuum line just below the Bentley Vacuum Controller.
- Increase vacuum level to beyond –90 mmHg to test the Safety Vacuum Interrupter.
- Remove the clamp from just below the To Reservoir line and place it on the vacuum vent line of the Conversion Module.
- Observe the venous drain line pressure and verify that it is at least –60 to confirm system vacuum integrity.
- Remove all unnecessary line clamps.
- Clamp the To Reservoir vacuum line just below the Bentley Vacuum Controller.
- Reduce vacuum level to –45 mmHg.
- Unclamp the To Reservoir vacuum line.

Initiating Bypass

- Clamp arterial and venous lines.
- Connect the extracorporeal circuit to the patient's cannulae (follow current protocol).

- To initiate bypass, verify that the arterial line is air free and unobstructed. Unclamp line and slowly initiate arterial flow.
- Place clamp on the vacuum vent line of the Conversion Module, and unclamp the venous return line.
- Adjust vacuum to achieve an appropriate and consistent rate of venous return and arterial flow.
- Open arterial filter purge port when appropriate.
- Verify that no air is trapped in the venous return line. (If air remains in the venous line, transiently increase the vacuum applied to the reservoir. Once the air is removed, readjust the vacuum to an appropriate level.)
- The roller pumps driving the vent and suckers may be started when required.
- To achieve the desired venous return flow rate, adjust the vacuum using the Bentley Vacuum Controller suction regulator knob.

Warnings

1. Obstruction of the vent/vacuum port could result in pressurization of the reservoir and, potentially, gaseous bubbles passing to the patient, and/or damage to the device.
2. Do not allow the venous reservoir to become overpressurized, as this could obstruct the venous drainage, force air retrograde into the patient, or cause air to enter the blood path of the oxygenator.
3. Do not allow the vapor trap to become completely filled during use. This may allow fluid to enter the vacuum controller or may prevent the reservoir from being vented to atmosphere when no vacuum is applied.
4. The cap must be removed from the vent/vacuum port to prevent inadvertent pressurization of the reservoir. The vent/vacuum port must remain open at all times during the operation of the reservoir or be attached to a regulated vacuum source not to exceed –90 mmHg in procedures that utilize VAVR.
5. Ensure that the cap on any unused port is airtight before initiating VAVR.
6. Do not let anesthetic agents, such as isoflurane, come into direct contact with this device. These agents may jeopardize its structural integrity.
7. Utilization of VAVR can lead to negative pressures in the oxygenator and the potential for air to be pulled across the oxygenator membrane into the blood pathway. The sample system, the arterial purge line, a hemoconcentrator, a nonocclusive roller pump, a centrifugal pump, or any other connection between the patient arterial line and the reservoir may provide a conduit for the vacuum to be applied to the arterial side of the oxygenator.

8. Do not infuse fluids or drugs to the arterial side of the sample system.

Concluding Bypass At the conclusion of bypass, reducing vacuum level will reduce the rate of venous return. When arterial flow is reduced to an acceptable level, disengage vacuum by removing the clamp from the vacuum vent line and wean the patient from CPB, as per standard procedure.

Policy and Procedure Guidelines
CP04

CENTRIMAG ECMO WITH QUADROX D

The recently FDA-approved Quadrox D oxygenator may be utilized for extracorporeal membrane oxygenation (ECMO) support of the patient in the setting of biventricular support with a centrifugal pump.

The use of this oxygenator will be cut into the outlet of the centrimag pump and on right-sided support only. It may not be used in left-sided support because of the risk of air embolism.

Equipment Needed

1. Quadrox D
2. Pressure monitoring for inlet/outlet pressure
3. Temperature monitoring
4. Oxygen blender
5. Clamps
6. Heater–cooler
7. Gas line
8. Pump record
9. ECMO checklist

HOLLOW AND DIFFUSION FIBER OXYGENATORS

A membrane oxygenator is an oxygenator that has a gas-permeable membrane interposed between the oxygenating gas and the blood (Fig. 1). Fiber oxygenators (artificial lungs) transfer gas by diffusion across a membrane or through small micropores in the membrane. Sweep gas is the gas that is used to oxygenate the blood and remove CO_2. Sweep gas is adjusted to obtain the desired gas parameters, similar to ventilator function. Faster sweep gas flow rate is like a higher rate of ventilation, which removes more CO_2. Higher FiO_2 will yield higher pO_2 in the blood exiting the oxygenator. The sweep gas is delivered to the oxygenator through a blender (Fig. 2) and 1/4″ tubing.

All oxygenators exhibit some resistance to blood flow. Pressure drop is the resistance to blood flow produced by any membrane oxygenator.

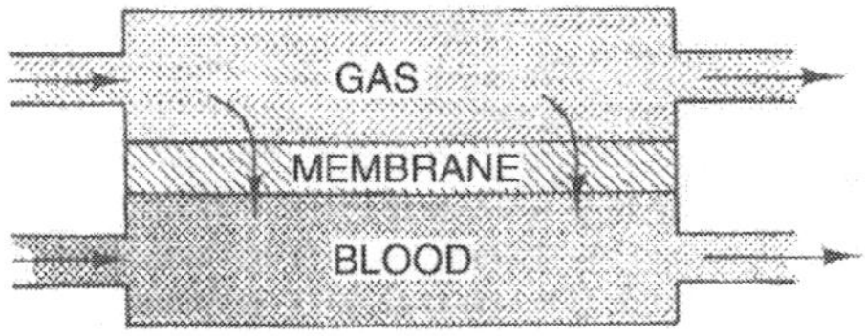

Fig. 1.

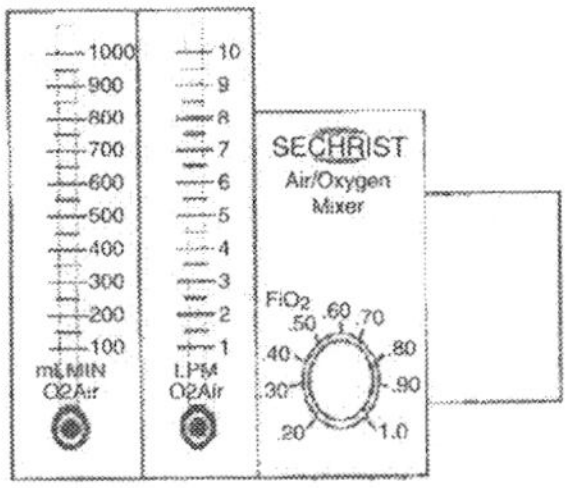

Fig. 2.

The difference between the inlet and outlet pressure is how we calculate pressure drop.

The pressure of the blood on the inlet side of the oxygenator will always be higher than the blood path on the outlet side of the oxygenator. Many factors may affect pressure drop such as tubing length and size, cannula size, gas pressure, flow rate, blood viscosity, hematocrit, and temperature. Do not be too alarmed by the absolute number, but rather changes in pressure drop over time.

Most membrane oxygenators also incorporate a heat exchanger that allows for thermal regulation of the blood as it passes through the oxygenator. This is usually accomplished by passing warm or cool water through a series of small, stainless steel tubes that contact the blood, thus facilitating the exchange of heat.

Monitor patient/device parameters; temperature, blood gases, flow rates, oxygenator inlet and outlet pressures, sweep rate, and FiO_2 (Figs. 3 and 4).

Trouble Shooting

Trouble	*Possible cause*	*Action*
Blood leak	displaced tubing	Clamp, reconnect tubing (air free). Resume flow
Oxygenator blood leak	Broken fiber (slow leak)	Contact perfusionist for Changeout
Blood not oxygenated	Check gas lines from wall & blender	Reconnect, call perfusionist
Pressure drop change	possible oxy failure	Contact perfusionist
Pressure/temp. alarm	Pressure/temp out of range	Check heater/cooler, call perf.

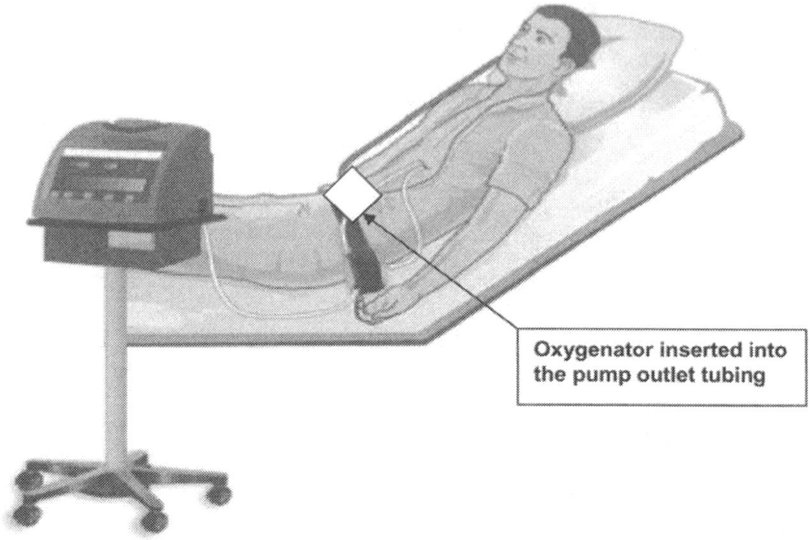

Fig. 3. Oxygenator inserted into the pump outflow tubing for pulmonary support.

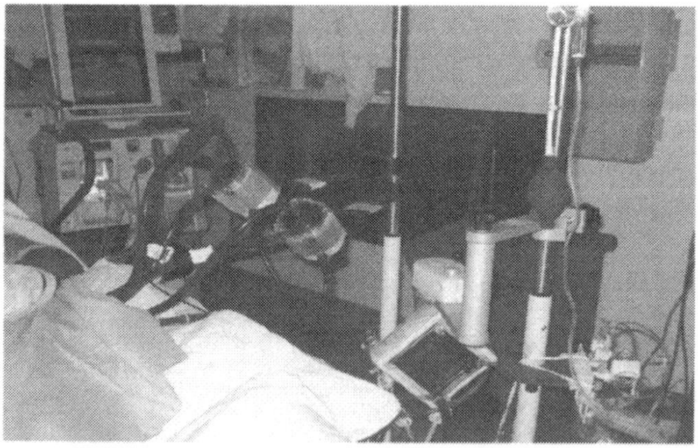

Fig. 4.

Policy and Procedure Guidelines
CP05

ECMO HEMOCONCENTRATION PROTOCOL

Equipment

Hemocor HPH Mini Hemoconcentrator with 2 accessory connector packs
(4) Tubing clamps
(4) Scalpel blades and alcohol swabs
(2) DLP perfusion adapters (1/4″-male)
(2) DLP perfusion adapters (1/4″-female)
(1) 1/4″ × 1/16″ × 8′ Tubing
(1) 1 liter Plasmalyte
(2) DLP Rapid Prime Set #10021
(2) Large-bore stopcocks
(1) Pediatric urimeter bag
(1) Baxter solution set
(1) Ureteral drainage bag (Ref 7,000)

Assembly

1. Attach female perfusion adapters (found in accessory pack) with 1/4″ ends to hemoconcentrator.
2. Attach 1 piece of 6″ × 1/4″ tubing to connectors previously placed on hemoconcentrator.
3. Place 2 male perfusion adapters with 1/4″ connectors to 1/4″ lines with large-bore stopcocks on each end.
4. Attach 1/4″ female connector to other end of stopcock.
5. On inflow of hemoconcentrator, attach 6′ × 1/4″ tubing and place in rollerhead. Attach 1/4″ female perfusion adapter to 1/4″ line, and then to quick-prime line. Clamp and spike plasmalyte bag.
6. On outflow of hemoconcentrator, attach 12″ × 1/4″ line from stopcock to DLP perfusion adapter (1/4″ female) to quick-prime line, to plasmalyte bag.
7. Prime and debubble blood path.
8. Attach Baxter solutions set to effluent port with leur lock connection.

9. Place ureteral drainage bag on spike port of Baxter solution set and clamp.
10. Deair effluent side of the hemoconcentrator, Baxter solution set, and ureteral drainage bag.
11. Once properly deaired, place hemoconcentrator in ECMO circuit, utilizing large-bore stopcocks.
12. Place hemoconcentrator inflow post pump, outflow prepump, and pre-bubble detector.
13. Insert effluent line in I.V. pump to pull *from* hemoconcentrator.
14. Set to desired effluent pull rate (not to exceed 35 ml/h).
15. Increase arterial pump flow to compensate for shunting across hemoconcentrator.

Policy and Procedure Guidelines

CP06

NEONATAL/INFANT ECMO CIRCUIT ASSEMBLY

1. **Turn on the master power switch on the console O.** Turn on the monitor system switch "**M**" on the lower left face of the pump console. Make sure the console is plugged in and confirm that all circuit breakers in the rear of the pump are in the "on" position. The yellow "C" light indicates the battery is charging. The yellow "B" light means the console is being powered by the backup battery (see the Jostra operators manual, battery section). Turn on the power button for the individual pump head being used (P1, P2, etc.). Set the pump mode to Arterial "**art**" and set the tubing size to the appropriate tubing being used in the arterial raceway.

Warning: Do not cover the console when connected to the mains; restricted air flow may overheat batteries.

2. **Set pump stop selectors:** In the rear of the pump, check and set the "pump stop selectors" for the air bubble detection system and the pressure modules so that each will stop the "art" pump. Confirm that all delay adjustments are set to the minimum delay position (completely counterclockwise).

3. **Assembly of circuit.** The tubing pack is preassembled by the manufacturer and includes all items. An appropriately sized membrane oxygenator is also used. Sterile technique must be observed during setup.

a. Remove circuit, place onto the mounting bracket, and secure heat exchanger and bladder. Do not put tubing through the roller head at this time. Place the "Better Bladder" (BB) in the venous limb of the extracorporeal membrane oxygenation (ECMO) circuit between the SAT/Hct cell and the roller pump inlet. Be sure to use a 1/4″ × 1/4″ leur lock connector on the connection closest to the roller pump. (This port will be used for a backup negative-pressure shutoff.)
b. Connect heat exchanger and test for leaks.
c. Tighten all pigtails and replace with PRN adapters when necessary.
d. Connect vacuum source to both vent and O_2 for priming of circuit.
e. Flush circuit with 100% CO_2 for a minimum of 3 min at a rate of 1–2 liters/min, with an unobstructed exhaust for the CO_2.

f. After flushing with CO_2, the system should be totally closed to the atmosphere. Open the vacuum and create suction for 3 min. At this point, the cardiotomy has been primed with 1 liter of plasmalyte solution.
g. Clamp the tubing between the oxygenator and the heat exchanger. Speed prime the system (the vacuum in the system will assist priming of the tubing and oxygenator).
h. Release the clamp from between the oxygenator and the heat exchanger, and the vacuum will prime the rest of the circuit.
i. When the system is primed, insert tubing into the roller head and begin recirculation through the AV loop. Continue to tap bubbles through circuit and deair. Be sure to vent all pigtails.
j. With vacuum still on the system, begin to flow and gradually increase flow to maximum. Do not exceed maximum flow, or a shift in the membrane material may occur, compromising gas exchange.
k. Add 1 g of Ancef.

4. **Occlusion:** Set the roller head occlusion, utilizing a column of clear fluid 30″ high that drops 1–2 cm/min.

5. **Pressure transducers:** Set up four pressure transducers: #1 premembrane, #2 postmembrane, #3 negative-pressure shutoff (must be located between the BB and the roller pump, as close to the BB as possible), and #4 negative-pressure shutoff on the BB (*see* CP05). Place transducers #1–3 in the pole-mounted transducer holder and "zero" these transducers. Fill with fluid, close the stopcocks to the circuit, open the transducer to air, and hold the zero button and the safety key (with the folded green corner) for 3, until the long tone confirms adequate zero.

6. **Setting the BB for negative-pressure shut off (#4):**

a. With the pump primed, stop arterial head, visualize the BB, and confirm that the bladder is full. Connect the pressure transducer stopcock directly to the BB leur fitting (do not use the 48″-long thin tubing). Open the stopcocks to air and zero the transducer (hold the zero button and the safety key with the folded green corner for 3 s until the long tone confirms zero). Place a 5-cc syringe on the distal stopcock and set the proximal stopcock to *close it to atmosphere*. Draw back on the syringe and put –5 mmHg (negative pressure) on the area around the BB lumen and *close the stopcock to both the syringe and atmosphere*. Make sure the BB is completely full during this step. Set the negative-pressure pump-stop alarm limit to −100 mmHg. Use channel #4 for BB monitoring (*means negative pressure, do not change*). The pressure on the BB should never read more positive than –5 mmHg. A reading of "0" may indicate a leak to atmosphere, probably at a BB stopcock fitting connection, or possible line drift. A leak of this nature *must* be corrected or the bladder will collapse with the slightest negative pressure.

b. **Note:** The BB zero and –5 mmHg setting procedure should be performed every 8 h to correct for loss of gas in the BB chamber as a result of PVC tubing permeability. Please be sure to override the pressure shutoff for the BB while performing this procedure on cardiopulmonary bypass (CPB) and rearm the pressure shutoff when complete. While performing this procedure, the direct venous return negative–pressure alarm (usually p3) must remain active to provide excessive negative–pressure protection.

7. **Procedure for going on bypass.** Call for patient blood (**3 units packed cells**).

a. **Heater unit.** Turn the heater on and set temperature to 37.5°C.
b. **Alarm.** Confirm proper function of each alarm before initiation of CPB.
c. **Albumin.** The circuit must be coated with albumin (50 ml/25%), which is added through the cardiotomy reservoir, displacing the clear fluid into a discard container. Recirculate albumin before adding blood through the nonfiltered return to the cardiotomy reservoir.
d. **Blood.** All pump prime blood must be washed (via Cellsaver 5 or Cobe brat) before administration. The prime usually takes 1.5 U of adult packed cells. Each unit requires 200 U (0.2 ml) of **heparin**. **Calcium gluconate** is added to the circuit once primed (300 mg or 94 mg/ml).
e. The priming sequence is completed by displacing the albumin with the heparin-treated packed cells added to the filtered cardiotomy reservoir. Again, displace all clear fluid into a discard container.
f. **Recirculate.** Blood gases should be done on the prime, and appropriate changes should be made to match the pH of the prime to the infant. Sodium bicarbonate should be added at this time.
g. Gas flow should be turned on to arterialize the circuit. Do not exceed gas phase pressure over blood phase. The air/O_2 mixture should be 70% for institution of ECMO.
h. The nurses will prepare a heparin drip for the patient at a concentration of 60 U/kg. The patient will be systemically heparinized for insertion of the cannulae before going on bypass (50–75 U/kg).
i. **Antithrombin III administration.** One vial (approximately 500 IU) of Thrombate III should be added to the pump prime before initiation of ECMO. Confirm use of antithrombin III supplementation with the surgeon before administration. Please order Thrombate III from the pharmacy utilizing the patient's unit number.
j. **Cannulation.** Arterial cannulation is usually done first. The cannulae in the ECMO stock room will be used after discussion with the surgeon

to assess size and flow requirements. #14 F VV or 10 arterial, 12 venous (Elecath), and, in special situations, 8–10 arterial (Bio-Medicus) 10–12 (Bio-Medicus) and Jostra 12 F VV.

k. **On bypass.** The patient is placed on ECMO circulation at 50 cc/min, gradually increasing to calculated flow. Check with surgeon about flow and cannulae placement. Communicate. Stabilize patient and begin chart.

PRIMING THE ECMO PUMP (QUICK REFERENCE)

A. Prime pump with 900 ml of Normosol-R (add 1 g of Keflex [Ancef] if left on standby)

B. If decision is made to go on ECMO, then do the following: (will take approximately 30 min)
   1) Add 50 ml albumin 25%.
   2) Add 2 U PRBC and 200 U heparin/U (should bring pump hematocrit to approximately 40%).
   3) Turn on O_2 to arterialize the system.
   4) Do ACT and blood gas of prime.
   5) Add $NaHCO_3$ to adjust pH to patient's pH pre-ECMO.
   6) Add 300 mg of Ca gluconate after ACT is more than 300.
   7) Go on bypass—Good Luck!!

THE BETTER BLADDER

Description

The BB is made from a single length of PVC perfusion tubing, a portion of which has been processed to form a sausage-shaped balloon with a thin wall. The thin-walled balloon is sealed within a clear, rigid housing. The pressure of blood flowing inside the tubing is transmitted across the thin wall to the chamber formed by the housing, and then via a pressure port to a pressure sensor (Figs. 1 and 2). The BB thereby serves as an inline blood reservoir that provides compliance at the pump inlet, much like the silicone bladders used at the inlet of a roller pump. The pressure measured at the pressure port allows noninvasive pressure measurements, which in turn can be used as input signals to control pump speed.

Intended Use

The BB is used as an inline reservoir to provide compliance between the venous cannula and the pump inlet during routine bypass and long-

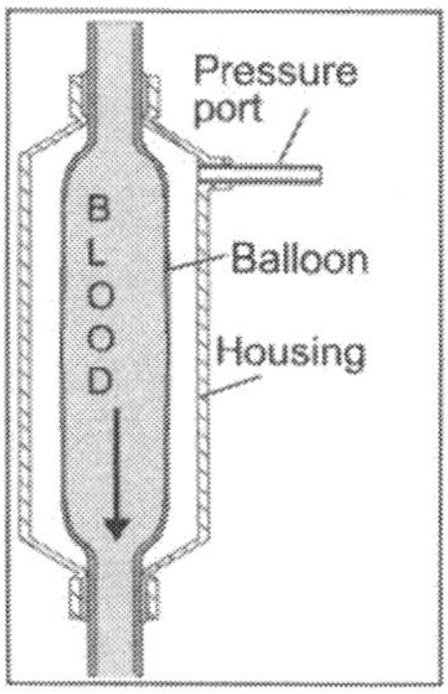

Fig. 1. Better Bladder (BB).

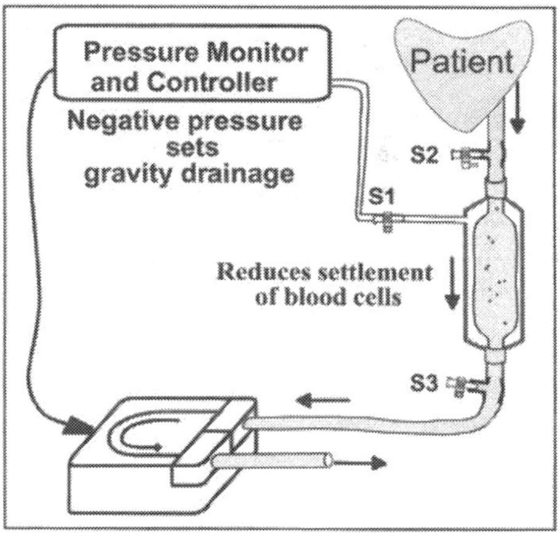

Fig. 2. The Better Bladder (BB) at pump inlet.

term extracorporeal pumping procedures, such as ECMO. It also can be used to measure the blood pressure in the venous line noninvasively. The compliance provided by the BB reduces the pressure pulse at the pump inlet, allowing for smoother control of pump speed as a function of inlet pressure. Pump control can be ON/OFF or continuous (Table 1).

Table 1
Nominal specifications for the BB.

Model	BB14
Tubing ID × OD	1/4″ × 3/8″
Volume	25 ml
Pressure port	Female Luer
High pressure limit	500 mm Hg
Low pressure limit	–250 mm Hg

Instructions for Use[1]

The BB is sterile if its package is not opened or damaged.

CAUTION: It is the responsibility of the surgical team to ascertain the suitability of the BB relative to the pumps and circuit components used.

CAUTION: For pressure measurements, use ONLY pressure transducer. Do not use mechanical gauges.

CAUTION: Do not allow the ballooned section of the BB to collapse to the extent that it may impede pump flow.

CAUTION: Orient the BB vertically in the circuit with its inlet facing up and blood flow directed downward. This minimizes gravitational collection of red cells and reduces stagnation.

Setup

1. Remove BB from its package.

2. Connect the BB with a 1/4″ perfusion connector having a Luer fitting to the inlet side of the pump. Attach stopcocks to each Luer fittings (S2 and S3 in Fig. 2). Orient the BB such that blood flow is downward (i.e., toward the floor). When using the BB14 holder, snap the BB14 into position, making sure that the flow is directed downward (Fig. 2).

3. Connect a three-way stopcock to the pressure port of the BB. Connect a pressure transducer to the stopcock (S1 in Fig. 2) and an empty 10-cc syringe to the side port of S1.

4. Check the seals and connections of the bladder as follows: isolate the BB from the rest of the circuit by clamping off (using tubing clamps) its inlet and outlet tubing, turn stopcock S1 to connect all three ports, pull on the 10-cc syringe until the pressure monitor indicates a negative pressure of at least −100 mmHg. Turn the stopcock off to the syringe, but open between the BB and the transducer. Maintain that negative pressure for at least 1 min. Observe the pressure indicator to assure its reading does not drift upward (from a negative value toward atmosphere) from its initial pressure reading. A change in pressure indicates that air is leaking into the housing (not the blood path) of the BB. A slight initial increase in pressure may occur due to contraction of the components. If the pressure continues to drift upward, you have a leak. Ensure that all gas connections are tight and retest. If a leak persists, close the stopcock to the pressure transducer. If the pressure continues to increase, then replace the stopcocks or trans-

[1]Always check our website at cirtec.com for newer versions of the Instructions for Use.

ducer. If there is no pressure loss, then one of the seals of the BB may be leaking and the BB must be replaced.

5. Turn S1 to connect all its ports and, using the 10-cc syringe, adjust the volume in the housing to assure that the bladder is full and the pressure is slightly negative (e.g., 5 mmHg). Close S1 to atmosphere, but open between the pressure transducer and BB pressure port.

6. Prime the circuit as usual, ensuring that all air is removed from the BB. Remove air as follows: place a 30-cc or 50-cc empty syringe to the open port of the inlet stopcock (S2 in Fig. 2), turn S2 to connect the syringe to the blood path, temporarily stop the flow, and pull on the syringe to draw the air from the top of the BB into the syringe. When the air is cleared, close S2, and resume the flow.

7. The BB should be rezeroed at least once every 8 h. Turn S1 to close the BB, but have the transducer connected to the open port, and zero the transducer. Attach a 10-cc syringe with its plunger at the 5-cc mark to S1, turn S1 to connect the syringe to the pressure transducer and the BB, stop the pump, adjust the volume in the BB until the pressure is between –5 and –10 mmHg. Close S1 off to the syringe, but open between the pressure transducer and the BB, and restart the pump.

Conduct during Use

8. Air entering the venous line tends to accumulate at the top of the BB (blood velocity in the BB is 10% of that in the 1/4″ tubing, allowing bubble buoyancy to overcome drag). Follow step 4 to eliminate that air.

WARNING: When re-zeroing the pressure transducer, be sure that the BB is not exposed to atmospheric pressure. Either plug up the middle open port (e.g., an empty 5-cc syringe) or rotate the stopcock such that its center port is closed to atmosphere.

CAUTION: Monitor the blood pressure between the BB and the pump inlet via stopcock S3 at the outlet of the BB. A very negative readout would indicate that the bladder may be collapsed and obstructing flow. It is recommended that an alarm be set to the maximum negative pressure acceptable. This pressure can also be used to control pump speed using the newer pumps (e.g., Stockert's SIII or Jostra's HL20). Here, the BB provides the compliance required for smooth pump control.

CAUTION: The integrity of the connection between the BB and the pressure transducer must be secured. Any leak or accidental opening in that line may allow additional air to enter the housing, thereby losing the suction and causing the bladder to collapse. This will happen if the housing is exposed to atmosphere and the pump inlet pressure is negative. Should that happen, stop the pump and repeat step 6 given in Setup.

CAUTION: The user should be aware that whenever negative pressure is applied to a blood line, any opening in that line would introduce air into the blood line. Use caution and extreme care to assure that during use, no port in the pump inlet line is open to atmosphere.

CAUTION: The BB must be placed in clear view of the user. The user must periodically examine the collapsed state of the bladder to assure that it does not obstruct flow. Should this happen, repeat step 6.

Policy and Procedure Guidelines
CP07

PEDIATRIC ECMO CIRCUIT ASSEMBLY

1. **Turn on the master power switch on the console O.** Turn on the monitor system switch **M** on the lower left face of the pump console. Make sure the console is plugged in and confirm that all circuit breakers in the rear of the pump are in the on position. The yellow "C" light indicates the battery is charging. The yellow "B" light means the console is being powered by the backup battery (see the Jostra operator's manual, battery section). Turn on the power button for the individual pump head being used (P1, P2, etc.). Set the pump mode to Arterial "**art**" and set the tubing size to the appropriate tubing being used in the arterial raceway.

Warning: Do not cover the console when connected to the mains, restricted air flow may overheat batteries.

2. **Set pump stop selectors.** In the rear of the pump check and set the "pump stop selectors" for the air bubble detection system and the pressure modules so that each will stop the "art" pump. Confirm that all delay adjustments are set to the minimum delay position (completely counterclockwise).

3. **Assembly of circuit.** The tubing pack is preassembled by the manufacturer and includes all items. A membrane oxygenator is also used. Sterile technique must be observed during setup.

a. Remove circuit and place onto the mounting bracket and secure heat exchanger and bladder. Do not put tubing through roller head at this time. Place the Better Bladder (BB) in the venous limb of the extracorporeal membrane oxygenation (ECMO) circuit between the CDI cell and the roller pump inlet. When using a 3/8″ × 3/8″ venous return line you must insert a 1/4″ bridge with a better bladder to allow adequate negative pressure control. The 3/8″ side and the 1/4″ side with the BB should both be left open to prevent areas of stagnation in the circuit. Be sure to use a leur lock connector on the connection closest to the roller pump. (This port will be used for a backup, negative pressure shutoff).
b. Connect heat exchanger and test for leaks.
c. Tighten all pigtails and replace those necessary with PRN adapters.
d. Connect vacuum source to both vent and O_2 for priming of circuit.

e. Flush circuit with 100% CO_2 for a minimum of 3 min at a rate of 1–2 liters/minute with an unobstructed exhaust for the CO_2.
f. After flushing with CO_2 the system should be totally closed to the atmosphere. Open the vacuum and create suction for 3 min. At this point the cardiotomy has been primed with 1 liter of plasmalyte solution.
g. Clamp the tubing between the oxygenator and the bridge. Speed prime the system (the vacuum in the system will assist priming of the tubing and oxygenator).
h. Release the clamp from between the oxygenator and the bridge and the vacuum will prime the rest of the circuit.
i. When the system is primed, insert tubing into roller head and begin recirculation through AV loop. Continue to tap bubbles through circuit and deair. Be sure to vent all pigtails.
j. With vacuum still on the system, begin to flow and gradually increase flow to rated maximum. Do not exceed maximum flow or a shift in the membrane material may occur, compromising gas exchange.
k. Add 1 g of Ancef.

4. **Occlusion:** Set the roller head occlusion utilizing a column of clear fluid 30″ high that drops 1–2 cm/min.

5. **Pressure transducers:** Set up four pressure transducers: #1 premembrane, #2 postmembrane, #3 negative pressure shutoff (must be located between the BB and the roller pump as close to the BB as possible), and #4 negative pressure shutoff on the Better Bladder (*see* CP05). Place transducers #1–3 in the pole-mounted transducer holder and "zero" these transducers. (Fill with fluid, close the stopcocks to the circuit, open the transducer to air, and hold the zero button and the safety key (with the folded green corner) for 3 s, until the long tone confirms adequate "zero."

6. **Setting the BB for negative pressure shutoff (#4) (Fig. 1):**

a. With pump primed, stop arterial head and visualize BB, and confirm that the bladder is full. Connect the pressure transducer stopcock directly to the BB luer fitting (do not use the 48″-long thin tubing). Open the stopcocks to air and zero the transducer (hold the zero button and the safety key with the folded green corner for 3 s, until the long tone confirms "0"). Place a 5-cc syringe on the distal stopcock and set the proximal stopcock to *close it to atmosphere*. Draw back on the syringe and put −5 mmHg (negative pressure) on the area around the BB lumen; *close the stopcock to both the syringe and atmosphere*. Make sure the BB is completely full during this step. Set the negative-pressure pump-stop alarm limit to −100 mmHg. Use channel #4 for BB monitoring. The pressure on the BB should never read more positive than −5 mmHg. A reading of "0" would indicate a possible leak to

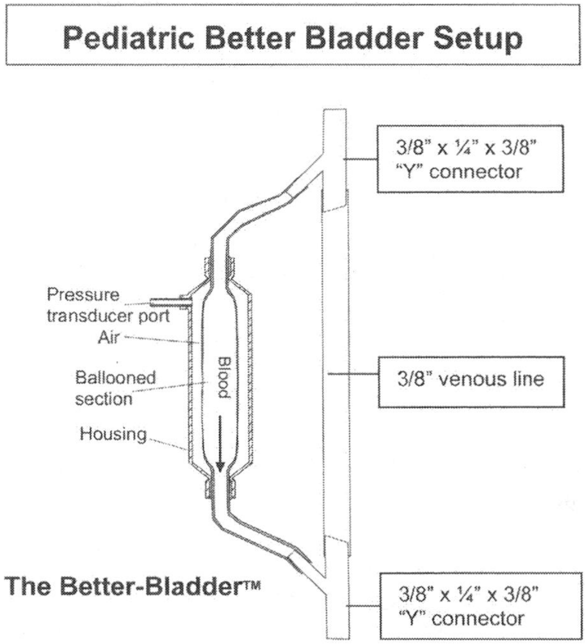

Fig. 1. Typical pediatric Better Bladder setup with tubing bypass.

atmosphere, probably at a BB stopcock fitting connection, or possible line drift. A leak of this nature *must* be corrected or the bladder will collapse with the slightest negative pressure.

b. **Note:** The BB "0" and –5 mmHg setting procedure should be performed every 8 h to correct for loss of gas in the BB chamber as a result of PVC tubing permeability. Please be sure to override the pressure shutoff for the BB while performing this procedure on CPB, and to rearm the pressure shutoff when complete. While performing this procedure, the direct venous return negative pressure alarm (usually p3) must remain active to provide excessive negative pressure protection.

7. **Procedure for going on bypass.** Call for patient blood (**3 U packed cells**).

a. **Heater unit.** Turn the heater on and set temperature to 39°C.
b. **Alarm.** Confirm proper function of each alarm before initiation of CPB.
c. **Albumin.** The circuit must be coated with albumin (50 ml/25%) and is added through the cardiotomy reservoir, displacing the clear fluid into

a discard container. Recirculate albumin before adding blood through the nonfiltered return to the cardiotomy reservoir.

d. **Blood.** All pump prime blood must be washed (via Cellsaver 5 or Cobe Brat) before administration. The prime usually takes 1.5 U of packed cells. Each unit requires 200 U (0.2 ml) of **heparin**. **Calcium gluconate** is added to the circuit once primed (300 mg or 94 mg/ml).
e. Completion of the priming sequence is by displacing the albumin with the heparin-treated packed cells added to the filtered cardiotomy reservoir. Again, displace all clear fluid into a discard container.
f. **Recirculate.** Blood gases should be done on the prime, and appropriate changes should be made to match the pH of prime to the infant. Sodium bicarbonate should be added at this time.
g. Gas flow should be turned on to arterialize the circuit. Do not exceed gas phase pressure over blood phase. The air/O_2 mixture should be 70% for institution of ECMO.
h. The nurses will prepare a heparin drip for the patient at a concentration of 60 U/kg. The patient will be systemically heparinized for insertion of the cannulae before going on bypass (50–75 U/kg). Check ACT before initiation of CPB (400 s).
i. **Antithrombin III administration.** One vial (approximately 500 IU) of Thrombate III should be added to the pump prime before initiation of ECMO. Confirm use of antithrombin III supplementation with the surgeon before administration. Please order Thrombate III from the pharmacy utilizing the patient's unit number.
j. **Cannulation.** Arterial cannulation is usually done first. The cannulae in the ECMO stock room will be used after discussion with the surgeon to assess size and flow reqiirements.
k. **On bypass.** The patient is placed on ECMO circulation at 50 cc/min, gradually increasing to calculated flow. Check with surgeon about flow and cannulae placement. Communicate. Stabilize patient and begin chart.

PRIMING THE ECMO PUMP (QUICK CHECKLIST)

A. Prime pump with 900 ml of Normosol-R (add 1 g of Keflex [Ancef] if left on standby).

B. If decision is made to go on ECMO, then do the following: (will take approximately 30 min).

   1) Add 50 ml albumin 25%.
   2) Add 2 U PRBC and 200 U heparin/Unit (should bring pump hematocrit to approximately 40%).
   3) Turn on O_2 to arterialize the system.
   4) Do ACT and blood gas of prime.

5) Add $NaHCO_3$ to adjust pH to patients pH pre-ECMO.
6) Add 300 mg of Ca gluconate after ACT is >300.
7) Go on bypass—Good Luck!!

THE BETTER BLADDER

Description

The Better-Bladder™ (BB) is made from a single length of PVC perfusion tubing, a portion of which has been processed to form a sausage shaped balloon with a thin wall. The thin walled balloon is sealed within a clear, rigid housing. The pressure of blood flowing inside the tubing is transmitted across the thin wall to the chamber formed by the housing and then via a pressure port to a pressure sensor (Figs. 2 and 3). The BB thereby serves as an inline blood reservoir that provides compliance at the pump inlet, much like the silicone bladders used at the inlet of a roller pump. The pressure measured at the pressure port allows noninvasive pressure measurements, which in turn can be used as input signals to control pump speed.

Intended Use

The Better-Bladder™ (BB) is used as an inline reservoir to provide compliance between the venous cannula and the pump inlet during routine bypass and long-term extracorporeal pumping procedures such as ECMO. It also can be used to measure the blood pressure in the venous line non-invasively. The compliance provided by the BB reduces the pressure pulse at the pump inlet, allowing for smoother control of pump speed as a function of inlet pressure. Pump control can be ON/ OFF or continuous.

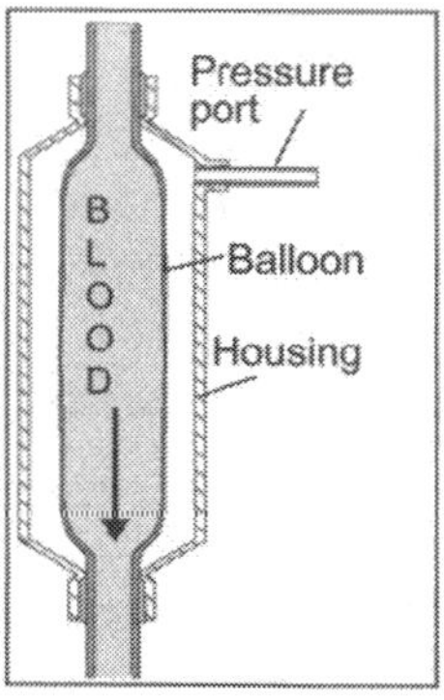

Fig. 2. Better-Bladder™.

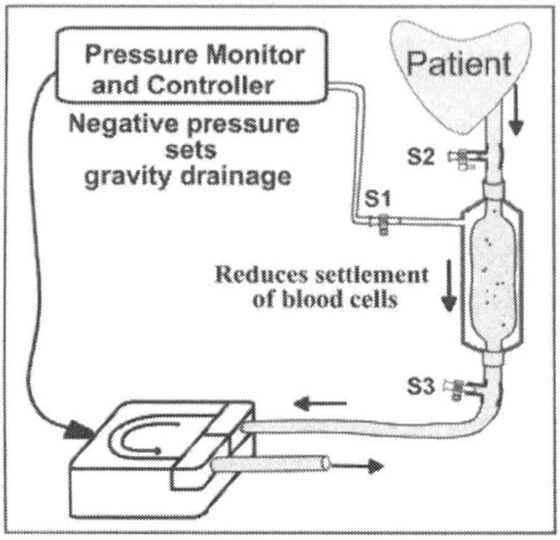

Fig. 3. The **BB** at the pump inlet.

Instruction for Use[1]

The BB is sterile if its package is not opened or damaged.

CAUTION: It is the responsibility of the surgical team to ascertain the suitability of the BB relative to the pumps and circuit components used.

CAUTION: For pressure measurements, use ONLY pressure transducer. Do not use mechanical gauges.

CAUTION: Do not allow the ballooned section of the BB to collapse to the extent that it may impede pump flow.

CAUTION: Orient the BB vertically in the circuit with its inlet facing up and blood flow directed downward. This minimizes gravitational collection of red cells and reduces stagnation.

Setup

1. Remove BB from its package.
2. Connect the BB with a 1/4″ perfusion connector having a Luer fitting to the inlet side of the pump. Attach stopcocks to each Luer fittings (S2 and S3 in Fig. 3). Orient the BB such that blood flow is downward (i.e. towards the floor). When using the BB14-Holder, snap the BB14 into position making sure that the flow is directed downward (Fig. 3).
3. Connect a 3-way stopcock to the pressure port of the BB. Connect a pressure transducer to the stopcock (S1 in Fig. 3) and an empty 10cc syringe to the side port of S1.

[1]Always check our website at cirtec.com for newer versions of the Instructions for Use.

4. Check the seals and connections of the bladder as follows: isolate the BB from the rest of the circuit by clamping off (using tubing clamps) its inlet and outlet tubing, turn stopcock S1 to connect all three ports, pull on the 10cc syringe until the pressure monitor indicates a negative pressure of at least −100 mmHg. Turn the stopcock off to the syringe but open between the BB and the transducer. Maintain that negative pressure for at least 1 minute. Observe the pressure indicator to assure its reading does not drift upward (from a negative value towards atmosphere) from its initial pressure reading. A change in pressure indicates that air is leaking into the housing (not the blood path) of the BB. A slight initial increase in pressure may occur due to contraction of the components. If the pressure continues to drift upward, you have a leak. Ensure that all gas connections are tight and retest. If a leak persists, close the stopcock to the pressure transducer. If the pressure continues to increase, then replace the stopcocks or transducer. If there is no pressure loss, then one of the seals of the BB may be leaking and the BB must be replaced.

5. Turn S1 to connect all its ports and, using the 10cc syringe, adjust the volume in the housing to assure that the bladder is full and the pressure is slightly negative (e.g., −5 mmHg). Close S1 to atmosphere but open between the pressure transducer and BB pressure port.

6. Prime the circuit as usual, ensuring that all air is removed from the BB. Remove air as follows: place a 30cc or 50cc empty syringe to the open port of the inlet stopcock (S2 in Fig. 3), turn S2 to connect the syringe to the blood path, temporarily stop the flow, and pull on the syringe to draw the air from the top of the BB into the syringe. When the air is cleared, close S2, and resume the flow.

7. The BB should be re-zeroed at least once every 8 hrs. Turn S1 to close the BB but have the transducer connected to the open port, and zero the transducer. Attach a 10cc syringe with its plunger at the 5cc mark to S1, turn S1 to connect the syringe to the pressure transducer and the BB, stop the pump, adjust the volume in the BB until the pressure is between −5 and −10 mmHg. Close S1 off to the syringe but open between the pressure transducer and the BB, and restart the pump.

Conduct during Use

8. Air entering the venous line tends to accumulate at the top of the BB (blood velocity in the BB is 10% of that in the 1/4″, tubing allowing bubble buoyancy to overcome drag). Follow step 4 to eliminate that air.

WARNING: When re-zeroing the pressure transducer, be sure that the BB is not exposed to atmospheric pressure. Either plug up the middle open port (e.g., an empty 5 cc syringe) or rotate the stopcock such that its center port is closed to atmosphere.

CAUTION: Monitor the blood pressure between the BB and the pump inlet via stopcock S3 at the outlet of the BB. A very negative readout would indicate that the bladder may be collapsed and obstructing flow. It is recommended that an alarm be set to the maximum negative pressure acceptable. This pressure can also be used to control pump speed using the newer pumps (e.g., Stockert's SIII or Jostra's HL20). Here the BB provides the compliance required for smooth pump control.

CAUTION: The integrity of the connection between the BB and the pressure transducer must be secured. Any leak or accidental opening in that line may allow additional air to enter the housing, thereby losing the suction and causing the bladder to collapse. This will happen if the housing is exposed to atmosphere and the pump inlet pressure is negative. Should that happen, stop the pump and repeat Step 6 given in Setup.

CAUTION: The user should be aware that whenever negative pressure is applied to a blood line, any opening in that line would introduce air into the blood line. Use caution and extreme care to assure that during use, no port in the pump inlet line is open to atmosphere.

CAUTION: The BB must be placed in clear view of the user. The user must periodically examine the collapsed state of the bladder to assure that it does not obstruct flow. Should this happen, repeat step 6 above.

Policy and Procedure Guidelines

CP08

EMERGENCY ECMO TRANSPORT PROTOCOL FOR THE EAST CAMPUS

Overview

The Cardiac Perfusion program at the East campus will initiate therapy for infant/pediatric patients requiring either postcardiotomy or pulmonary support. Within 12 h, these patients will be transferred to the West campus.

Request for Support

The perfusion team, as requested by the attending surgeon, will initiate ECMO support. At this time, the circulating nurse will contact the ECMO coordinator at the West campus (telephone: 52565). It is expected that the patient will be transported to the West campus within 12 h.

Personnel

The perfusion team from the East campus will assemble the ECMO circuitry and initiate ECMO. Their perfusionists will maintain patients on the original ECMO system as per the physician's request, and transport of the patient to the West campus where they will be met by the receiving perfusion personnel at the receiving unit.

Equipment

A circuit consisting of a centrifugal console/pump, heparin-coated tubing, and a hollow-fiber oxygenator with integral heat exchanger will be used. Arterial inlet pressure will be measured via a fluid separator pressure-monitoring system. Pump flow will be provided via a Bio-Medicus console. Temperature will be maintained via an external heater–cooler.

Contingencies

If transfer is not possible, extended maintenance of ECMO at the East campus will be necessary. In this event, rooms for the next day's cardiac schedule may need to be closed. Based on current staffing, three perfusion staff members would be required per day of ECMO. This would allow only three rooms to be run for cardiac surgery.

Necessary Equipment

Disposables
Miami Circuit with oxygenator and pump (CB1P01R1)
Hardware
Bio Console 550 (#95208)
Flow Probe TX50P (#95185)
Bio Cal Heater 95161-000

Policy and Procedure Guidelines

CP09

ECLIPSE TRANSMYOCARDIAL REVASCULARIZATION (TMR) HOLMIUM LASER SYSTEM, LASER OPERATORS ROLE

1. Place laser signs on entrances and cover all windows.
2. Test fire the laser into a basin of N/S before the patient is brought into the room, using the test fiber.
3. Fifteen to twenty minutes before the surgeon is ready to do TMR, turn the laser key to the on position. The pulse counter will count down to 0000 as the system cools to the appropriate temperature.
4. Ensure all lights on the interlock panel go off, except the fiber light.
5. Move the laser to the side opposite the surgeon and place the foot pedal at the surgeon's right foot.
6. Open the SoloGrip° II package and hand to Scrub nurse.
7. Cut out the SoloGrip° II label and place on top of laser console, noting the calibration factor 8. After the Laser Pulse counter window shows 0000, remove the black protective cap from the end of the lager fiber, and connect the fiber to the connection port behind the sliding door on the laser front. Screw in the fiber until it is finger tight. The "fiber" light on the interlock panel will go out.
9. Enter the "calibration factor" from the packaging for the fiber that is being connected.
10. Ask the surgeon for the correct power setting of 6, 7, or 8 W and select in the power setting window.
11. Check to be sure at this time that every one in the room is wearing the correct safety glasses or goggles, specific to the wavelength 2,100 pm and with optical density of 3, 4, 5, or 6.
12. Check that the patient's eyes are protected with moistened gauze, towel, safety goggles, or glasses.
13. Keep the laser in standby, unless enabled is requested by the surgeon.
14. Enable the laser for testing when instructed by the surgeon.
15. After testing, reset the pulse counter to 0000.

16. Repeat aloud each time the laser is enabled or placed on standby.

17. At the end of the TMR procedure, disconnect the fiber from the laser, placing the protective cap on the fiber, and allow the connector "to hang" off of the sterile field.

18. Record all necessary information, i.e., pulses, channels with their location, watts, etc., and if the case is performed as part of a protocol, record the information on the CRF.

19. Turn off the key switch and move laser away from the table.

20. If more channels are needed, the laser can be turned on again, rolled into place, and the fiber reconnected.

Policy and Procedure Guidelines

CP10

LEFT HEART BYPASS

Left heart bypass is utilized to remove oxygenated blood from the left atrium and return it to the distal descending aorta or femoral artery. This procedure allows repair or replacement of the descending thoracic aorta while regulating blood flow, minimizing surface area contact activation, and reducing heparin requirements.

Equipment

E-pack (carmeda coated)
Cardiotomy reservoir
#26 Bard right-angled, wire-reinforced aortic cannula or an appropriate-sized cannula for left aorta drainage
#20 Bard right-angled, wire-reinforced aortic cannula or an appropriate-sized cannula for pump return into the distal aorta or femoral artery.
2 3/8″ × 3/8″ leur lock connectors (if not already in the line of the E-pack)
Large-bore stopcocks
Cellsaver Citrate drip may be required instead of heparin
Rapid infusion capability
Heparin (100 U/kg)
Perfusion of the renal vessels
  1-multiple perfusion cannula (14,000 DLP)
  cardioplegia line
  perfusion adaptor
  large-bore stopcock on 3/8″ × 3/8″ leur tubing connector
Medtronic heat exchanger and 3/8″ bypass bridge may be included

Procedure

Set up and prime the bypass circuit. A Medtronic heat exchanger and 3/8″ bypass may be included in the system should heat loss become a problem necessitating active rewarming. Place the large-bore stopcock on one of the 3/8″ × 3/8″ leur connectors for perfusion of the visceral or renal vessels if necessary. Recirculate prime until circuit is needed. Before initiating bypass, remove the outflow from the cardiotomy reservoir and connect to the 3/8″ connector to complete the loop with the patient. Pass loop to the table for separation and cannulation by the surgeon. Heparin (100 U/kg) is given before initiation of bypass. ACTs should be maintained between 180–200 s.

Notes

- Flows are generally maintained between 1.5–3.0 liters/min.
- Monitoring of upper and lower extremity pressures is ideal to assess flow requirements.
- 2 mEq/kg/h of sodium bicarbonate drip may be given by anesthesia.
- Visceral and renal perfusion may be facilitated by using 9-F Pruitt irrigation occlusion catheters, a 3/8″ × 3/8″ × 1/4″ Y connector, a 1/4″ male leur hemoconcentration line, and a DLP multiple perfusion adaptor. The 3/8″ arterial line can be cut at the table and the 3/8″ × 3/8″ × 1/4″ Y connector is added with the 1/4″ hemoconcentration line connected to the 1/4″ arm of the connector, and the male leur end of the hemocon-

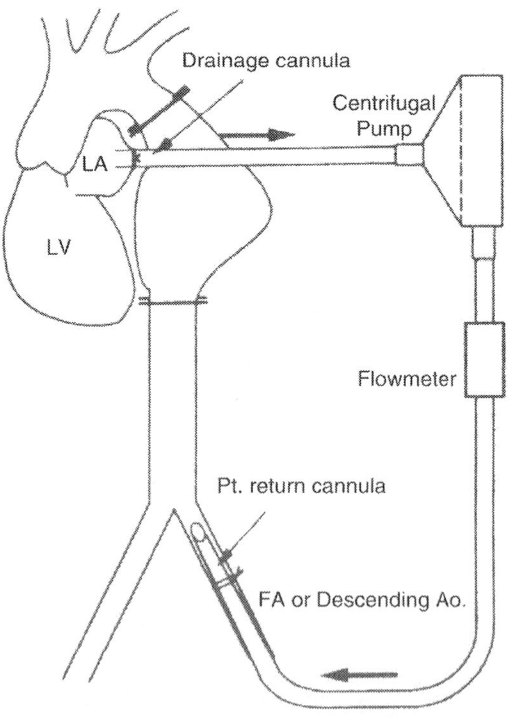

Fig. 1. Typical left heart bypass configuration.

centration line is secured to the multiple perfusion adaptor. Individual arms of the multiple perfusion set are connected to the Pruitt catheters for individual vessel perfusion.

- Rapid infusion may be necessary following bypass after the distal aortic clamp is removed. This can be accomplished by adding a cardioplegia line to the luered port of the 3/8″ connector on the arterial line along with a perfusion adaptor and large-bore stopcock for anesthesia to allow us to infuse volume to the patient via an anesthesia access. When bypass is terminated, pump volume should be chased or carefully recirculated to prevent stagnation and thrombus formation. Please double clamp all lines and use extreme caution when using an open cardiotomy for volume infusion. An Ozomiser (custom rapid infusion system) may also be used for rapid infusion (Fig. 1).

Policy and Procedure Guidelines
CP11

ISOLATED LIMB PERFUSION

Definition

The purpose of Isolated Limb Perfusion (ILP) is to deliver chemotherapeutic agents using 6–10 times the usual systemic dose, with minimal systemic toxicity. The use of an oxygenator in the circuit provides a means of delivering the chemotherapeutic drug, oxygenating the limb, and hyperthermia.

Malignant melanomas are the most commonly treated tumors, with sarcomas being the second most common. Melanomas account for 20% of all skin cancers; are more common in older age groups; occur more frequently in the Caucasian race; and are found more frequently on the head and neck of males and the lower extremities of females.

Isolated limb perfusion is indicated for:

1. Invasion beyond the papillary level.
2. Any degree of vascular involvement.
3. Tumor diameter greater than 1 cm.
4. Ulceration of the tumor.

Chemotherapeutic Agents Used

Alkylating Agents or Nitrogen Mustard Agents

Primarily target the DNA molecule; however, the normal cell's DNA repair system makes it resistant to alkylating agents with selectivity of action against cancer cells.

Nitrogen mustards were used as a nerve gas during WWII, and have the ability to interfere with normal mitosis and cell division in all rapidly proliferating tissues.

Natural Products

Actinomycin-D or Dactinomycin is one of the most powerful antitumor agents. This drug inhibits rapidly proliferating cells of normal and neoplastic origin by binding to DNA and inhibiting DNA-dependent RNA synthesis.

Cardiopulmonary Bypass

The use of a 1/4″ × 1/4″ infant circuit for the arm, and 3/8″ × 3/8″ pediatric circuit is used for the legs. This will limit the amount of hemodilution. A pediatric oxygenator is incorporated into the circuit.

- Flow is determined by using the *"rule of the nines"*; the leg is approximately 18% of the BSA and the arm is approximately 9% of the BSA.
- Cannulation is achieved by using a 10–20-F arterial cannula, and the largest single-stage venous cannula possible to ensure good drainage.
- Upper limb cannulation is via the brachial artery and axillary vein. Lower limb cannulation is via the femoral artery/vein or popliteal artery/vein.
- Full-body heparinization with 300 U/kg. is achieved.
- Maintain PaO_2 of greater than 400 mmHg for tumoricidal effect.
- Water bath is set to 42°C to increase the limb temperature to 40°C for increased metabolic rate.
- Keep the patient's diastolic pressure greater than the limb pressure to avoid systemic leak. Leakage can occur from the systemic circulation to the limb circulation or vice versa, with complete isolation insured only for the axillary and popliteal vessels. An *Esmarch tourniquet* is used in ILP.
- To correct leakage during ILP, it may be necessary to try all the following:
  1. Reposition the cannulae or tourniquet.
  2. Change or lower the pump flow rate.
  3. Alter the resistance of the circulation, e.g., lower the patient's diastolic pressure.
- It will be necessary to have a Y connecter in the venous line to remove the chemotherapeutic agent during limb washout. Washout is achieved by using a hyperosmotic agent, such as Hespan or Dextran 40. Approximately 6 liters will be needed to ensure the return is clear.
- Replace volume with 2 U PRBCs and isotonic solution. Oxygenate and recirculate through the limb until limb pressure is equal to systemic pressure.

The most accurate method for determining leakage from the isolated circulation to the systemic circulation during ILP is by the use of a radioactive tracer such as iodinated serum albumin or technetium-labeled albumin. A collimator is placed over the ventricles. The use of fluorescin dye and UV lamps is another method to determine proper cannulae placement.

Policy and Procedure Guidelines
CP12

VENO-VENOUS BYPASS FOR LIVER TRANSPLANTATION

Definition

Veno-venous (VV) bypass allows for venous circulation that normally drains through the portal vein and inferior vena cava (IVC), to return to the right side of the heart. During liver resection and transplantation, these vessels are clamped and, without venous bypass, venous congestion occurs, resulting in increased venous pressures and decreased venous return. This protocol is for partial VV bypass with cannulation of the femoral vein and return to the internal jugular vein.

Equipment Needed

—Bio-Medicus BP-80 Blood Pump, and 3/8″ × 38″ Flow Probe, *Carmeda coated E pack,* Bio-Medicus Pump Console and handcrank
—1–2 L Lactated Ringers
—4 clamps
—Cannulae: femoral vein #15, 17, 19, 21 Bio Medicus arterial; internal jugular vein or axillary #15, 17 Bio Medicus arterial; Medtronic EOPA 18, 20, 22 F
—Venous saturation monitor and inline sensor (in pack)
—Consider rapid infuser, if necessary
—Autotransfusion device
—3/8″ Biotherm Heat exchanger

Procedure

—Unpack the liver bypass circuit. If the Bio head and flow probe are not already in the circuit, make the necessary connections. Under strict aseptic conditions, set up the E pack.
—Prime circuit.
—Place the Biohead into the console with the outlet facing up, and the flowprobe into the flow sensor. Recirculate through the system while judiciously removing all air bubbles. Turn the Biopump outlet to the downward position.

—Calibrate the CDI 100, and check the Biomedicus console for properly set alarms, flow ranges, flow probe, pressures, etc.
—Aseptically hand the "double-wrapped" loop up to the operative field. When asked to do so, clamp and stop recirculation for loop division.
—Obtain patient's height, weight, and prebypass labs and pressures.
—Calculate your flow (30% of the cardiac output). Flows should be expected in the 2.5–3.5 LPM range.

Operative Procedure

—Once the femoral vein is cannulated, connect to the inlet side of the Bio Medicus. The internal jugular vein or axillary vein is connected to the outlet side of the Bio Medicus.
—Flow will be ~1–2.5 L/min. This is partial bypass.
—The donor organ is implanted and anastomosed in the following sequence: 1 suprahepatic IVC; 2 infrahepatic IVC; 3 portal vein; 4 hepatic artery; 5 bile duct.
—The donor organ is then flushed with cold plasmalyte to remove the high-potassium Wisconsin solution. This usually avoids a high K+ in the patient.
—The first two anastomoses are performed on full bypass.
—Before the portal vein anastomosis, the portal vein cannula is clamped and removed. Venous return to the pump may be reduced, so pump flow must also be reduced accordingly, to avoid overfilling of the right heart.
—Monitor right heart filling pressures. Continue low flow bypass until the portal vein anastomosis is complete.
—Some bleeding may occur after removal of the portal vein clamp. When this is under control, bypass is terminated. The remaining cannulae will be removed.
—The hepatic artery and bile duct anastomoses are completed off bypass.
—Blood loss during the procedure is scavenged and processed in the CellSaver or Brat autotransfusion system and returned to the patient via an "Ozomiser" or other Rapid Infusion Device.

Use of a heparin-bonded circuit may allow for heparinless bypass and eliminates the inability to adequately reverse the effect of heparin. Assess activated clotting time to remain at or above 200 seconds.

Policy and Procedure Guidelines

CP12r

LIVER TRANSPLANTS

We have been notified of a change to our liver preservation solution and technique for living-related liver transplants. We will continue to assist with intraoperative cell saving and organ preservation and flush. The Viaspan solution for live donor transplantation is replaced with Custodial HTK solution, as described below.

PROTOCOL FOR PRESERVATION SOLUTIONS FOR LIVER TRANSPLANTATION

Live Donor Liver Transplantation

1. Donor liver back table flush: custodial HTK solution 2 L bags
2. Preparation: add 20,000 U heparin to the 2-L bag
3. No hespan is required for preimplantation flush during recipient transplantation

Cadaver Donor Liver Transplantation

1. Viaspan (UW) solution 1 L bags available if necessary for cadaver procurements
2. Hespan 500 cc bags for preimplantation flush during recipient transplantation

Before connection to the organ, the solution container should be suspended from a sufficient height to allow for a steady stream of solution and to produce flow rates of at least 30 ml/min, while flushing the liver. Flushing should be continued until the organ is uniformly pale and the effluent is relatively clear.

Suggested Minimum

Adults, 1,200 ml
Infants, 50 ml/kg

Policy and Procedure Guidelines
CP13

LEUKODEPLETION/LUNG TRANSPLANT

Recent documentation suggests clinical benefit from leukocyte filtration on cardiopulmonary bypass (CPB). Neutrophils are proposed to be activated by two major immunogenic mechanisms: (a) contact of circulating leukocytes with artificial surfaces and (b) ischemia and reperfusion after release of the cross-clamp. A growing body of evidence exists for a beneficial role of leukocyte filters placed in the arterial and reperfusion lines of the extracorporeal circuit.

Arterial and pulmonary (plegia) reperfusion leukocyte filtration should be set up on all lung transplants. Leukofiltration will be facilitated with the Pall LG6B leukoguard arterial blood filter placed distal to the one-way duckbill valve and proximal to the oxygenator/arterial filter combination and one or two Pall BC2B cardioplegia leukocyte reduction filters used in conjunction with the Sorin Vanguard BCD cardioplegia delivery set (cardio plegia system [cps]) for individual lung reperfusion.

CIRCUIT MODIFICATIONS

When assembling the CPB circuit for lung transplant cases, circuit modifications are necessary. The Pall LG6B leukoguard arterial filters (2) with filter bypass should be inserted into the extracorporeal circuit between the one-way duckbill valve (3/8″) and the oxygenator/arterial filter combination (Cobe Synthesis) currently being used for standard CPB cases. Tie bands should be placed on all connections of the LG6B filter and Medtronic quick-connect Hansen fittings. Pressure monitoring of this filter is also necessary. This configuration allows the systemic blood to be leukofiltered, as well as the lung reperfusate blood being delivered via the cardioplegia administration set.

PROCEDURE

The extracorporeal circuit should be primed in the standard fashion, ensuring all circuit components, including leukodepletion filters, are air free. The LG6B leukoguard arterial filter bypass should be clamped out, allowing systemic flow through one leukoguard filter. The standard arterial filter should be used in the usual fashion during the procedure. Careful monitoring of the LG6B pressure should be followed, to allow identification of a clogged or obstructed filter should this situation arise. If the leukoguard arterial filter becomes obstructed, the attending surgeon must be notified immediately, and the first leukoguard filter bypass should be clamped out and the second leukoguard filter should be opened and used. In the unlikely event that the second filter becomes clogged, that leukoguard filter should be clamped out and the leukoguard filter bypass bridge opened. **Note:** The LG6B leukoguard arterial filter is a self-venting arterial filter, and appropriate precautions must be observed when using this feature. Any negative pressure on this filter can allow air to be pulled into the filter and embolized systemically. This filter must be run below the fluid level in your reservoir, or the vent port must remain securely closed to avoid air entrainment and embolization.

Pulmonary plegia or pulmonary reperfusion may be used to reperfuse the transplanted lung before cross-clamp removal. This will be facilitated by delivering warm blood via the cardioplegia set, utilizing the following technique.

The bypass circuit may be modified to allow delivery of controlled reperfusion to the transplanted lung(s). The Sorin BCD Vangard CPS delivery set is modified by adding two short sections of 1/4″ tubing with plastic screw type Cobe/Sorin cardioplegia connectors (Fig. 1) into the CPS delivery line (Fig. 2). One or two (cut second filter into bypass bridge if necessary) BC2B cardioplegia leukofilters with 1/4″ tubing and 1/4″ bypass bridge are used. These filters are placed in the cardioplegia delivery line, utilizing Cobe screw-type connectors and 1/4″ tubing (Fig. 3). The Pall Leukoguard BC2B filter(s) should be placed in the outlet line of the standard blood cardioplegia set and CO_2 flushed. Carefully deair the Pall leukoguard BC2B blood cardioplegia filter(s) with crystalloid prime (NOT CARDIOPLEGIA) and recirculate into the cardiotomy reservoir. Once deaired, cps recirculation must be discontinued to prevent air entrainment. The cardioplegia pump must not be flowing without ensuring positive pressure and forward flow from the CPB circuit. Pressure monitoring of this filter is also necessary (cardioplegia line pressure can be utilized).

The cps blood draw line (i.e., yellow clamp) from the oxygenator allows arterial blood reperfusate from the bypass circuit to be drawn into the Sorin Vanguard CP system, additional luekocyte reduction

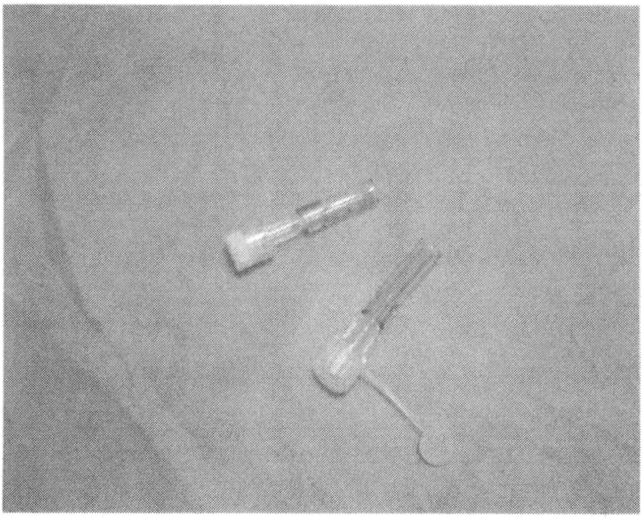

Fig. 1. Cobe cardioplegia connection tubing.

with the Pall BC2B filter, and delivery of pulmonary reperfusate to reduce reperfusion injury. The plastic clamps on the CPS are positioned to allow delivery of whole blood reperfusate in the standard fashion, with an appropriate-sized cannula. Currently the 9-F Pruitt cannula

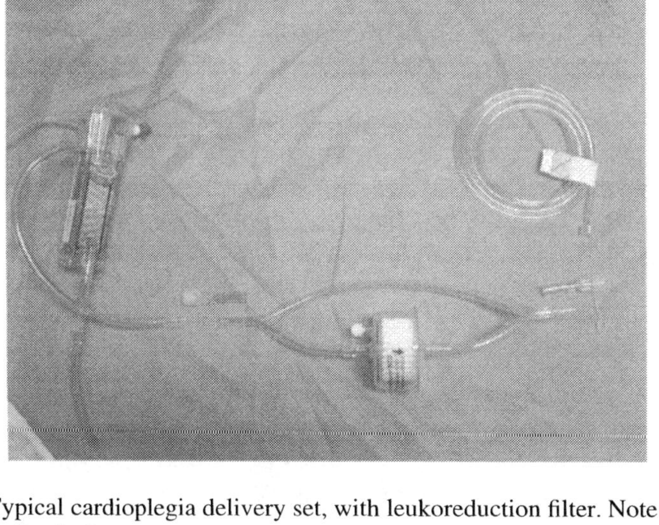

Fig. 2. Typical cardioplegia delivery set, with leukoreduction filter. Note connectors to cardioplegia set.

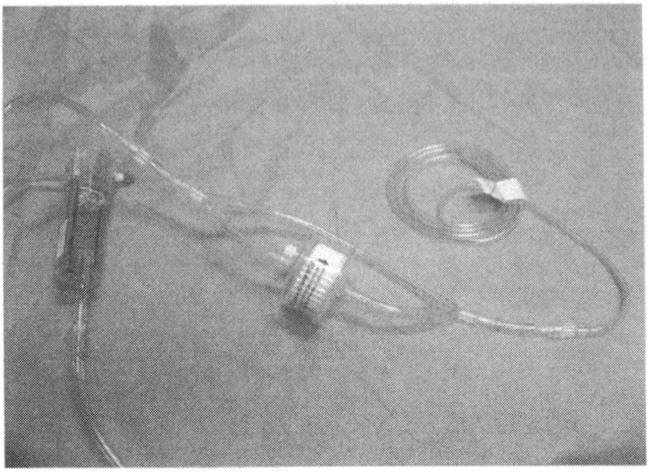

Fig. 3. Complete setup, with tubing, filter, and delivery line.

appears to be adequate for this procedure. Upon the surgeon's command, a cps delivery line can be handed off the sterile field, connected to the Pall BC2B filter outlet, primed, and debubbled, and warm blood can be delivered at the desired flow and pressure as prescribed by the attending surgeon (commonly a flow of 100 cc/min for 10 minutes is utilized). Pressure and flow should be carefully monitored at all times.

LEUKODEPLETION/LUNG TRANSPLANT (REPERFUSION PROTOCOL FOR NON-CPB CASES)

Recent documentation suggests clinical benefit from leukocyte filtration on CPB. Neutrophils are proposed to be activated by two major immunogenic mechanisms: (a) contact of circulating leukocytes with artificial surfaces, and (b) ischemia and reperfusion after release of the cross clamp. A growing body of evidence exists for a beneficial role of leukocyte filters placed in the arterial and reperfusion lines of the extracorporeal circuit.

Controlled reperfusion of the transplanted lung (on non-CPB cases) using white cell filtered and/or nutrient-enriched blood has been shown recently to significantly ameliorate reperfusion damage in a porcine model. Approximately 1,000–1,500 ml of arterial blood is slowly collected into a cardiotomy reservoir or IV infusion bag. This blood is passed through a leukofilter and returned into the transplanted pulmonary artery. This technique has been adopted by some transplant centers and applied to human lung transplantation with impressive results. A conventional blood cardioplegia administration set and Pall leuko-reducing filter will be utilized.

TECHNIQUE

When requested by the surgeon, on non-CPB lung transplants, the bypass circuit may be modified to allow delivery of controlled reperfusion to the transplanted lung. The Sorin BCD Vangard CPS delivery set is modified by adding two short sections of 1/4″ tubing with plastic screw type Cobe/Sorin cardioplegia connectors (Fig. 1) into the cps delivery line (Fig. 2). One or two (cut second filter into bypass bridge if necessary) BC2B cardioplegia leukofilters with 1/4″ tubing and 1/4″ bypass bridge are used. These filters are placed in the cardioplegia delivery line utilizing Cobe screw-type connectors and 1/4″ tubing (Fig. 3). Each filter should be primed and debubbled using clear prime (NOT CARDIOPLEGIA). The cps blood draw line from the oxygenator is double clamped, and the arterial blood reperfusate is spiked on the cps IV spike line of the Sorin Vanguard PC system. The plastic clamps on the cps are positioned to allow delivery of whole blood re-perfusate at 37°C from the IV bag, as described below.

Technique for controlled reperfusion of the transplanted lung in humans as described by Lick, MD, Brown, MD, and Kurusz, CCP, The University of Texas Medical Branch, Galveston, Texas. Patients are given 10,000 U of heparin intravenously just before native lung pneumonectomy. Bronchial anastomosis is completed in the usual fashion. Before beginning the pulmonary vascular anastomoses, an arterial drainage catheter is passed to the perfusionist. This may be facilitated through an 8-F cardioplegia cannula placed in a convenient spot in the aorta, a femoral arterial access, or via anesthesia arterial access. Blood should be collected into a 1,000-ml IV bag containing 1,500 U heparin. While the pulmonary venous and arterial anastomoses are constructed, approximately 1,000 ml of blood is slowly allowed to fill the bag or reservoir by intermittently clamping and unclamping the drainage line; during this time, the anesthesiologist must maintain an appropriate patient blood volume with colloid or blood volume replacement.

Once the vascular anastomoses are completed (but left untied), the leukofiltered whole blood is delivered to the operative field at 37°C into an appropriate cannula, (Pruitt or retrograde coronary sinus catheter), which is inserted through the untied pulmonary artery anastomosis, and the anastomotic suture is snared. The warm blood reperfusion solution is delivered at approximately 100–150 ml/min and is adjusted to keep the pulmonary artery pressure below 20 mmHg. Currently the 9 F Pruitt cannula appears to be adequate for this procedure. Warm blood can be delivered at the desired flow and pressure as prescribed by the attending surgeon (commonly a flow of 100 cc/min for 10 min is utilized). Pressure and flow should be carefully monitored at all times.

The atrial cuff anastomosis is propped open, allowing unimpeded egress of wash out into the thorax, which is aspirated into the cell salvage system. The salvaged blood is then washed, and the packed red blood cells are returned to anesthesia for reinfusion.

Policy and Procedure Guidelines

CP14

Continuous hyperthermic peritoneal perfusion (CHPP) is administered via infusion catheters placed in the cephalad portion of the abdominal cavity and effusion catheters placed deep within the pelvis that are attached to a roller pump circuit and heat exchanger. The catheters are positioned after resection of the primary tumor, when peritoneal metastases have been detected, and/or after appearance of primary tumor. All peritoneal adhesions are lysed to ensure uniform distribution of fluid over all the peritoneal surfaces. The abdomen is temporarily closed and the peritoneal cavity is filled with approximately 2 L of perfusate (chemotherapy: e.g., Cisplatin) until it is slightly distended. The occluding clamp on the outflow catheter is then removed, and a recirculating perfusion through the closed peritoneal cavity is begun (Fig. 1).

Sodium thiosulfate is administered to the patient intravenously at the start of the perfusion, 7.5 g/m^2 diluted in 150 ml of saline given over 20 min, and CHPP is followed by a total dose of 25.6 g/m^2 diluted in 1,000 ml of saline and infused over the next 12 h. (optional).

Supplies

1/4″ × 3/8″ AV bridge
Cardiotomy reservoir
Ozomiser custom pack from Sarns
VAD cannulae #34 DLP right-angle spiral tipped (Medtronic) 3/8″ Y connector
CellSaver waste bag for chemotherapy disposal at end of case
Heater/Cooler (Sarns silver hyperthermia unit)
Roller pump, tubing clamps
Drugs and chemotherapy ordered by surgeon
Paperwork: NYPH Cardiopulmonary
Bypass Orders Sheet, Signed by physician in charge. Write the surgical procedure and drugs used, and add to the Cell Saver database as chemoperfusion. Keep a perfusion chart recording every 15 min.
Bill in the pyxis for a CellSaver

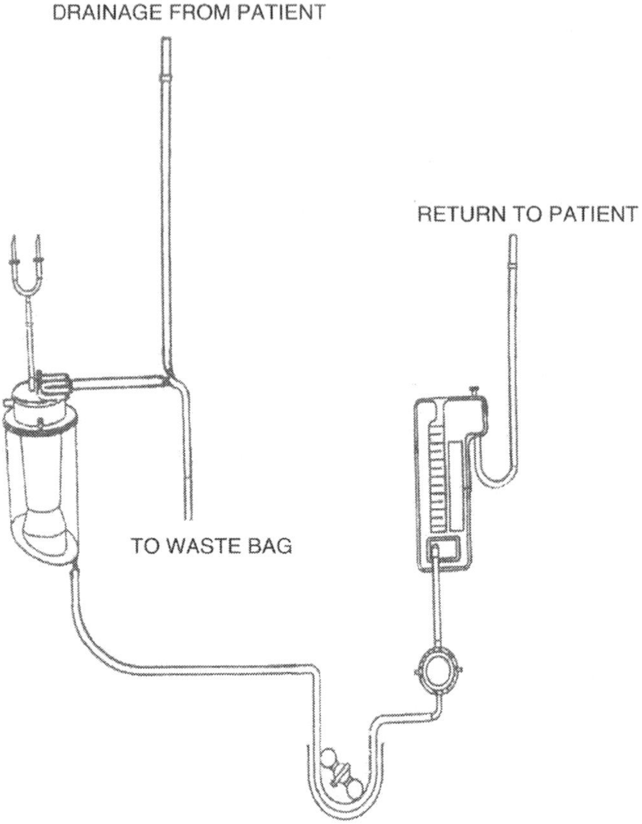

Fig. 1. Typical peritoneal perfusion circuit utilizing a cardiotomy reservoir and cardioplegia set for heating of the chemotherapy fluid.

Set up and prime the circuit (Fig. 1) according to the manufacturer's recommendations for each product. Use saline or plasmalyte and warm to 40°C. Continuously recirculate solution until chemotherapy agent is provided by pharmacy. Add to the circuit and warm to 40°C.

The circuit is run below the level of the peritoneal cavity to ensure adequate siphon from the 3/8 line to the cardiotomy. Hand AV loop to surgeon and separate.

After cannulation of the peritoneal cavity, begin to fill the cavity until air is completely removed by surgeon. Connect the second cannula and begin recirculation for 1 h at 40°C.

During recirculation of chemotherapy agent, leakage may occur near or along the incision. The addition of a floppy sucker for salvage of chemotherapy agent may be utilized. Just add the suction to the same roller pump you are using for recirculation. Use double inserts in raceway.

Once chemotherapy is completed, use the 3/8″ Y connector and waste bag to dispose of agent. Chase circuit with 2L of normal saline.

Caution: Do not increase perfusion temperature over 42°C.

Policy and Procedure Guidelines
CP15

PROCEDURE FOR RETROGRADE CEREBRAL PERFUSION

Retrograde cerebral perfusion through the superior vena cava (SVC), in combination with hypothermic circulatory arrest, provides protection to the brain during operations that involve the aortic arch.

EQUIPMENT

Standard adult perfusion circuit

24-F DLP venous cannula or suitable sized cannula for the SVC

PROCEDURE

1. Establish circulatory arrest at 18°C or 20°C, with the arterial line clamped before the oxygenator and the venous line clamped just below the venous reservoir.
2. Double clamp arterial line distal to the bridge.
3. Leave venous line clamped just below venous reservoir.
4. Remove clamps from the arterial–venous (AV) bridge.
5. Inferior vena cava cannula is clamped by the surgeon.
6. Central venous pressure should be monitored using the cordis (side port of the Swan-Ganz introducer).
7. Check for air in the venous line and SVC cannula.
8. Establish retrograde cerebral perfusion at 500 ml/min. Do not exceed CVP greater than 25 mmHg. Use 1 : 1 or less gas, blood flow ratio and appropriate FiO_2 for temperature.
9. To reestablish total body CPB, clamp the arterial line proximal to the oxygenator, double clamp AV bridge, remove clamps from the arterial line distal to the AV bridge, and go on full bypass.

Policy and Procedure Guidelines
CP16

RIGHT TO LEFT SHUNT PROTOCOL

This circuit can be used as an alternative therapy to treat right-sided circulatory failure. Desaturated venous blood is shunted to the left-sided circulation to increase systemic blood pressure at the expense of saturation. We will use a heparin-bonded circuit with mimimal tubing to create a femoral vein to femoral artery shunt.

EQUIPMENT

1. Bio-Medicus pump console
2. Sterile disposable pediatric pump head
3. Electromagnetic flow probe
4. Sterile custom tubing pack (heparin bonded) (ped. VAD pack)
5. Tubing clamps
6. 1 L double-spiked bag of balanced electrolyte solution

Preparation of the assist device by the perfusionist is begun by inserting the 1/4″ × 3/32″ wall tubing with spike into the bag of solution. Debubble the circuit up to and including the Biohead by gently applying positive pressure to the bag of solution while venting through the other spike. Once the pump head is filled with solution, a clamp is placed on the tubing distal to the outflow of the Biopump. Hang the solution on an IV pole and engage the pump head to the console. The pump is turned on. Spike the solution bag with the other spike, completing the bypass loop. Continue recirculating and debubbling until all air is removed. The system is now ready to be passed into the sterile field, divided, and connected to the appropriate cannula.

CANNULATION

1. Femoral vein (using a 12 or 14 F Bio-Medicus heparin-bonded cannula) for inflow to the pump.
2. Femoral artery (using a 10 or 12 F Bio-Medicus heparin-bonded cannula) for outflow from the Biohead to the patient.

INITIATION OF ASSIST

The perfusionist will begin flow after confirmation of an air-free circuit, including both cannula connection sites. This device should only be used at flows exceeding 500 cc/min. Anticoagulation will be at the discretion of the attending physician.

Policy and Procedure Guidelines
CP17

VACUUM ASSISTED VENOUS RETURN (VAVR) FOR REOPERATIONS: ROBOTIC MVR AND ASD WITH VAVR

General Description

Cardiopulmonary bypass (CPB) is used to support the patient's circulation during the period of surgical intervention. This can be achieved with various pump/oxygenator combinations, and the system used in this hospital will be described in detail. Attempts will be made to evaluate and update the system whenever new and improved equipment is available. In addition, there are times when the venous return is indicated through a venous cannula in the groin and neck, and smaller cannulae may be used that require vacuum-assisted venous return (VAVR).

Indications

Reoperations with femoral cannulation, or minimally invasive and robotic procedures requiring remote access.

Procedure

Blood flow is determined by the patient's body surface area (BSA). A calculated blood flow at an index of 2.4 L/min/m^2 is used to determine the size of the circuit.

Adult pack: available in a sterile component that contains the adult tubing pack, the oxygenator, and an integrated cardiotomy reservoir. The arterial line is 3/8″ and the venous line is 1/2″. An adult arterial line filter with a 3/8″ bridge may be included. The configurations of these disposable products are reviewed, and changes are made to improve as necessary. The arterial limb of the circuit also consists of 3/8″ tubing, and if is connected to the outlet of the arterial centrifugal pump with a one-way duckbill valve to help protect the oxygenator from negative pressure. Output from this pump is directed to an adult membrane oxygenator, and then to an arterial filter, before being returned to the patient. The venous reservoir is protected against excessive suction with a positive and negative pressure relief valve. Volume is returned to the circuit by gravity or VAVR through one or more venous drain lines. Flow is regulated by adjusting the negative pressure regulator for VAVR (maximum is 90 mmHg) to maximize venous flow, and then increasing the flow of the arterial pump to match the venous return. The VAVR is operated at the lowest negative pressure necessary to achieve the desired blood flow rate and limit negative venous line pressure (usually <80 mmHg).

In anticipation of alternate cannulation site usage, modification of the existing CPB circuit is required. This is accomplished by inserting a 1/2″ × 3/8″ × 1/2″ connector into the venous drainage line and connecting this to the neck or superior vena cava (SVC) drainage cannula with 3/8″ tubing. This will allow for the use of a "second" venous line, augmented by VAVR, to facilitate adequate venous drainage from accessory drainage sites using small cannulae. When possible, a Transonic flow probe should be used to assess neck or SVC cannula drainage.

EQUIPMENT

Arterial cannulae: Bio-Medicus, Medtronic EOPA, and Femflex for reoperations and mini mitrals; Estech (with accessory pack) for robotic ASD

Venous cannulae: Bio-Medicus (groin) for reoperations

Bio-Medicus (groin) and arterial Bio-Medicus (neck) for all robotic procedures and mini mitral. Small central cannulae may include DLP metal right-angle 18–30 F, single lighthouse tip straight 14–32 F, and Medtronic maleable, lighthouse tip 20–24 F.

—(1) extra pigtail
—(1) 1/2″ × 3/8″ × 1/2″ connector
—(1) sterile scissors
—(1) 4′ 3/8″ tubing
—(4) alcohol wipes

Neck supplies:

—(1) L lactated Ringer's (LR) with 5,000 U of heparin (i.e., 5 U heparin/ml)
—(1) Vented tubing set from anesthesia for LR heparin drip (10 drops/ml)
—(1) 60 cc syringe with 5 U/cc of heparin in LR drawn from the 1 L bag you made up

—(1) 10 cc syringe with 5,000 units of heparin in 10 cc of solution (i.e., 500 U/ml)
—(1) 3/8″ tubing for neck extension to the venous return tubing
—(1) 15 F arterial Bio-Medicus cannula for the internal jugular
—(1) pigtail for leur lock on cannula

Procedure for Neck Cannulation Under Sterile Technique

After choosing the correct size cannula, give the scrub nurse the percutaneous cannula kit and pigtail for preparation. It is recommended that the perfusionist obtain a baseline activated clotting time (ACT) before neck cannulation. The cannula should be flushed with heparinized saline before it is introduced into the patient. Surgeon/anesthesiologist will introduce cannula into internal jugular vein with transesophageal echo guidance. After advancing the cannula, the obturator is taken out and the cannula is clamped. The 3/8″ tubing is now connected and clamped distal to the pigtail. Through the pigtail, the 5,000 U heparin is given, and then flushed to clear. Move the clamps proximal to the pigtail and attach the heparin drip to the pigtail. Fill the 3/8″ tubing with solution to prime, and move clamps distal to pigtail. Establish a slow drip of heparinized LR through the percutaneous neck cannula into patient to maintain patency. Secure 3/8″ tubing to the table or bed before connection to 1/2″ × 3/8″ × 1/2″ Y connector for venous drainage.

Once the AV loop is handed up to table, place 1/2″ × 3/8″ × 1/2″ connector into venous line, after the AV bridge. Connect 3/8″ line from neck cannula to connector. After systemic heparinization and cannulation, remove clamp from neck tubing at head of table, only after confirming both venous lines are clamped on the pump end of circuit. Upon initiation of CPB, start with only head cannula drainage and observe flow through the Transonic flow probe. Now add VAVR and observe flow. After adequate flow is obtained through the neck cannula under VAVR, open femoral venous line and observe flows. Be sure to adjust centrifugal pump RPMs when turning vacuum on and off, as flow rate will be affected. When putting volume in, reducing forward flow, and/or weaning from CPB, always remove VAVR first to prevent accidental entrainment of air into the extracorporeal circuit.

Notes

1. An extra pigtail is needed for the CO_2 insufflation line from the robot monitor.

2. A third transducer is needed when using the Estech RAP cannula to connect to the aortic occlusion balloon. Set up the transducer as usual, keeping an extension on the transducer that will connect to a pressure line handed from the table. (You may need to give this to the scrub nurse—a 48″ extension from anesthesia). Flush and zero the transducer. This will read the pressure in the occlusion balloon, which should be between 250 and 300 mmHg.

3. Cardioplegia delivery through the Estech RAP cannula may be difficult, with line pressures over 350 mmHg.

Reoperations

1. Femoral vein cannulation: The 1/2″ venous line must be downsized to attach to the 3/8″ connector on the percutaneous cannula. The 1/2″ × 3/8″ connector from the table pack is connected to the venous line and a short piece of 3/8″ tubing (from a portion of the discarded AV loop) is used to connect the percutaneous cannula to the venous drainage line. If possible, an air-free connection is best.

2. Transonic flow meter and probe are used to determine the flow from the SVC catheter via the jugular vein site or central cannulation site when smaller cannulae are used for minimally invasive procedures.

3. Aprotinin is used for all reoperations.

Policy and Procedure Guidelines
CP18

VACUUM-ASSISTED VENOUS RETURN PROCEDURE

Vacuum-assisted venous return (VAVR) offers some alternatives to conventional cardiopulmonary bypass (CPB) techniques. It uses negative pressure to assist or augment venous return over traditional siphon drainage technique. This technique utilizes a wall suction source to generate a vacuum and enhance venous drainage during open heart surgery. Using VAVR allows smaller venous cannulae usage, smaller venous line size, and reduced prime. It can be used on hard-shell venous reservoirs, as well as soft venous bags enclosed in a rigid, sealed, non-disposable housing.

VAVR WITH A HARD-SHELL VENOUS RESERVOIR

Initial setup before going on bypass:

1. Assemble CPB circuit as per standard procedure. Test and install the positive pressure relief valve onto a vacuum-assist–capable hard-shell venous reservoir. Place occluding plugs on all unused ports.
2. Properly occlude all roller pump heads. If using a centrifugal arterial head, make sure a one-way valve is placed between the centrifugal head and the oxygenator to prevent air from being pulled across the oxygenator fiber in the event of centrifugal pump stoppage.
3 Attach the "To Vacuum" connector of Bentley Vacuum Controller to a reliable hospital-grade (NFPA-U.S.) vacuum source.
4. Attach a calibrated means of monitoring negative pressures to the venous line and/or cardiotomy reservoir.
5. Verify that the "Conversion Module" vacuum line is connected to the moisture trap.
6. Attach the Conversion Module vacuum line to the To Reservoir connector of the Bentley Vacuum Controller, and the moisture trap to the vent port of the appropriate venous reservoir.
7. Clamp the venous reservoir drain line between the arterial pump head and the venous reservoir.
8. Clamp the venous line just distal to its connection to the venous reservoir pressure monitoring site.

9. Verify that all other ports and lines to the venous reservoir are closed to the atmosphere.

10. Verify that all roller pumps are off.

11. Clamp the To Reservoir vacuum line just below the Bentley Vacuum Controller.

12. Increase vacuum level to beyond –90 mmHg to test the Safety Vacuum Interrupter.

13. Remove the clamp from just below the To Reservoir line and place it on the vacuum vent line of the Conversion Module.

14. Observe the venous drain line pressure and verify that it is at least –60 mmHg to confirm *(neg. pressure, needs to be here)* system vacuum integrity.

15. Remove all unnecessary line clamps.

16. Clamp the To Reservoir vacuum line just below the Bentley Vacuum Controller.

17. Reduce vacuum level to –45 mmHg.

18. Unclamp the To Reservoir vacuum line.

Initiating Bypass:

1. Clamp arterial and venous lines.
2. Connect the extracorporeal circuit to the patient's cannulae. Note: The venous return line need not be primed (follow current protocol).
3. To initiate bypass, verify that the arterial line is air free and unobstructed. Unclamp line and slowly initiate arterial flow.
4. Place clamp on the vacuum vent line of the Conversion Module, then unclamp the venous return line.
5. Adjust vacuum to achieve an appropriate and consistent rate of venous return and arterial flow.
6. Open arterial filter purge port when appropriate.
7. Verify that no air is trapped in the venous return line. (If air remains in the venous line, transiently increase the vacuum applied to the reservoir. Once the air is removed, readjust the vacuum to an appropriate level.)
8. The roller pumps driving the vent and suckers may be started when required.
9. To achieve the desired venous return flow rate, adjust the vacuum using the Bentley Vacuum Controller suction regulator knob.

Warnings

1. Obstruction of the vent/vacuum port could result in pressurization of the reservoir and, potentially, gaseous bubbles passing to the patient and/or damage to the device.

2. Do not allow the venous reservoir to become overpressurized, as this could obstruct the venous drainage, force air retrograde into the patient, or cause air to enter the blood path of the oxygenator.
3. Do not allow the vapor trap to become completely filled during use. This may allow fluid to enter the vacuum controller or may prevent the reservoir from being vented to atmosphere when no vacuum is applied.
4. The cap must be removed from the vent/vacuum port to prevent inadvertent pressurization of the reservoir. The vent/vacuum port must remain open at all times during the operation of the reservoir or be attached to a regulated vacuum source not to exceed −90 mmHg in procedures that utilize VAVR.
5. Ensure that the cap on any unused port is airtight before initiating VAVR.
6. Do not let anesthetic agents, such as isoflurane, come into direct contact with this device. These agents may jeopardize its structural integrity.
7. Utilization of VAVR can lead to negative pressures in the oxygenator and the potential for air to be pulled across the oxygenator membrane into the blood pathway. The sample system, the arterial purge line, a hemoconcentrator, a nonocclusive roller pump, a centrifugal pump, or any other connection between the patient's arterial line and the reservoir may provide a conduit for the vacuum to be applied to the arterial side of the oxygenator.
8. Do not infuse fluids or drugs to the arterial side of the sample system.

Concluding Bypass:

At the conclusion of bypass, reducing vacuum level will reduce the rate of venous return. When arterial flow is reduced to an acceptable level, disengage vacuum by removing the clamp from the vacuum vent line and wean the patient from CPB as per standard procedure.

VACUUM-ASSISTED VENOUS RETURN WITH A VENOUS BAG

Augmented venous return allows the perfusionist to use a venous line having a smaller inner diameter, thereby reducing prime volume, and allows the surgeon to use a smaller venous cannulae, resulting in easier insertion, better surgical view, and a smaller surgical incision. Currently, augmented venous return is achieved either by applying vacuum directly to a hard-shell venous reservoir (vacuum-augmented venous drainage [VAVD]). The former does not allow use of a closed-bag reservoir, whereas the latter requires an additional pump. Therefore, users who prefer the safety of venous bags (VBs) and would

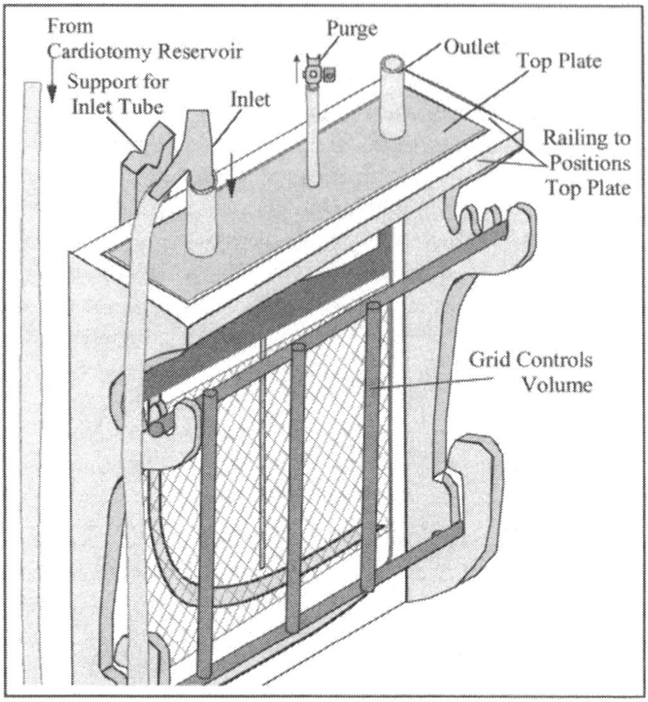

Fig. 1. The V-Bag Holder for non-VAVD applications.

like to augment venous return without using a venous pump are unable to do so or must compromise.

Vacuum can be applied to a soft-shell venous reservoir by enclosing it within a rigid housing (Fig. 1). Once the bag is sealed within the rigid structure, vacuum applied to the space surrounding the bag is transmitted across the flexible wall of the bag to the blood. It is as if the vacuum is applied directly to the blood, but without contacting it. Thus, whatever negative pressure is in the housing (P housing), this is also the blood pressure in the bag (P blood), P housing » P blood. A vacuum regulator controls the degree of vacuum of P housing, similar to a hard-shell reservoir. The system allows the user to make the "atmospheric" pressure around the bag negative, and the negative pressure in the bag provides vacuum-assisted drainage.

WARNINGS/PRECAUTIONS

- Read all instructions for use before setup.
- Only trained, qualified medical professionals familiar with its operation should use the VB.

- CAUTION: Federal (U.S.A.) law restricts this device to sale by or on the order of a physician.
- The VB is intended for single use only. Do not resterilize.
- Use aseptic techniques during setup and connection procedures.
- It is the responsibility of the surgical team to ascertain the suitability of the VB relative to the pumps, circuit components, and pumping conditions used.
- Tubing should be attached in such a manner as to prevent kinks or restrictions that may alter blood flow.
- The use of safety/warning devices for detecting and eliminating gaseous bubbles in the extracorporeal circuit, as well as a level sensor, an arterial filter, and a prebypass filter are recommended.
- Ensure that the bottom of the VB is positioned above the highest point in the membrane compartment of the membrane oxygenator. This helps ensure that the blood side pressure remains greater than the gas side pressure.
- Ensure that the tube connecting the cardiotomy to the VB inlet loops ***below*** the bottom of the VB holder. This minimizes the chance of air siphoned into the venous line via that tube when the cardiotomy is empty.
- Ensure that the support for the inlet tube in the back of the holder lines up with the venous line (see holder's instructions for use.)
- Adequate heparinization must be maintained before and during bypass.

SETUP

1. Remove the VB from its package. The VB is sterile if its package is not opened or damaged.
2. Place the VB in its holder. The VB can be placed with the outlet on the left or right side, as desired. Because the VB is loaded into its holder from the top, the front plate need not be removed between cases. Instead, the front plate can be maintained at the desired position from case to case.
3. Remove the aerator cap from the upward facing port of the Y connector of the VB and connect the venous line to that port.
4. Remove the aerator cap from downward facing port of the Y connector of the VB and connect the cardiotomy outlet line to that port.

WARNING: Avoid siphoning air from an empty cardiotomy to the VB via the venous line by looping the tubing between the cardiotomy and the VB ***below*** the bottom of the VB holder.

5. Remove the aerator cap from outlet connector and connect the inlet tubing of the arterial pump to it.

6. Remove the leur fitting off the top leur of the stopcock and connect it, via a purge line with a one-way valve, to the inlet of a suction pump. Rotate the stopcock handle to form fluid communication between the VB and the suction pump.

PRIMING

Note: For easier debubbling, add noncrystalloid solutions only after priming and debubbling are complete.

1. Ensure that all tubing connections are secure, all leur fittings are tightly closed, and all stopcocks are closed before priming.
2. Prime the venous reservoir before priming the pump and oxygenator system.
3. Clamp the cardiotomy outlet tube.
4. Fill the cardiotomy reservoir with enough priming solution to prime the entire extracorporeal circuit.
5. Clamp the venous blood inlet to the VB.
6. Remove the clamp from the cardiotomy blood outlet tube and allow the priming solution to fill the VB.

CAUTION: Ensure that the suction pump is rotating in the correct direction and the stopcock on the purge line is open.

7. Turn on the suction pump connected to the purge line of the VB and remove all bubbles in the VB.
8. To prime a centrifugal pump, lower the pump head below the VB and propel the prime up the outlet tube of the VB and into and beyond the pump head by compressing the front wall of the VB. Once the head is filled, clamp its outlet, place it back into its drive, turn the pump on, and unclamp outlet tubing.
9. During bypass, thorough mixing of drugs added to the venous blood is ensured when adding them through the leur port on the venous inlet connector.

ADDITIONAL INSTRUCTIONS WHEN USING VACUUM-ASSISTED VENOUS DRAINAGE

Warnings

1. Be sure to read the instructions for use of the Vac-Box.
2. Obstruction of the vacuum port could result in pressurization of the reservoir and, potentially, bubbles passing to the patient.
3. Do not allow the venous reservoir to become pressurized, which may obstruct the venous drainage.

4. The vacuum port of the Vac-Box must remain open at all times or be attached to a regulated vacuum.

5. Do not apply a vacuum greater than –60 to the vacuum port.

6. Do not apply vacuum to the Vac-Box without having a forward flow. Without flow, the negative pressure may reach the blood side of the oxygenator and pull air across the membrane into the blood pathway. Use a one-way valve at the outlet of the arterial pump to minimize that possibility.

7. Prevent anesthetic agents, such as isoflurane, from contacting the VB or Vac-Box. These agents may jeopardize the structural integrity of the VB or Vac-Box.

8. Use only cardiotomy reservoirs that incorporate a pressure relief valve and a vacuum relief valve.

PRECAUTIONS

1. Operating in the VAVD mode can lead to negative pressures in the oxygenator and to the potential for air to be pulled across the oxygenator membrane into the blood pathway. The sample system, the arterial purge line, a hemoconcentrator, a nonocclusive roller pump, a centrifugal pump, or any other connection between the patient arterial line and the reservoir may provide a conduit for the vacuum to be applied to the arterial side of the oxygenator. Be sure that one-way valves are incorporated where necessary to prevent retrograde flow.

2. Do not connect patient vent lines to the filtered ports of the cardiotomy reservoir unless some means of preventing retrograde flow toward the patient is located between the patient and the cardiotomy reservoir (Fig. 2).

3. Ensure that the bottom of the venous reservoir is positioned above the highest point inside the membrane compartment of the oxygenator. This will reduce the possibility of pulling gas from the gas side into the blood side of the membrane oxygenator.

4. Be sure to monitor the pressure at the inlet to the venous bag. Set the alarm to no higher than –60 mmHg.

5. Use only a reliable wall suction and calibrated vacuum regulator specified for VAVD. Be sure to follow the instruction for use associated with that regulator (e.g., use of vapor trap).

CAUTION: Never apply vacuum to only the cardiotomy or only the Vac-Box.

6. Use caution when infusing drugs or any other fluid during VAVD. The vacuum can increase the rate of infusion into the reservoir significantly higher than clinically desirable.

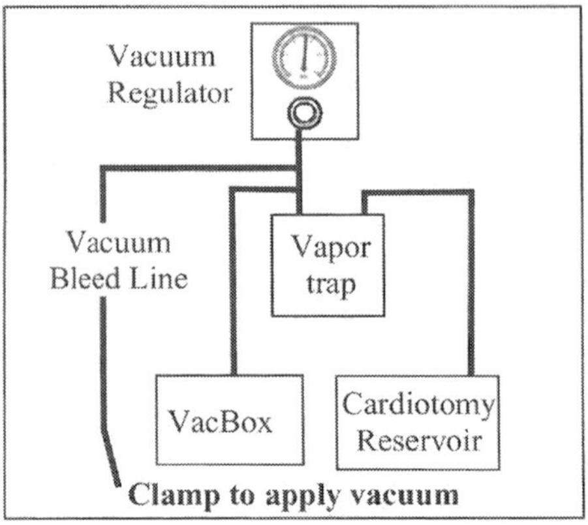

Fig. 2. Vacuum Regulation/Application.

SETUP PROCEDURES

1. Ensure that the mounting bracket of the Vac-Box is securely fastened to the pump console and oriented to provide maximum visibility during use.
2. Rotate the volume adjustment levers (Fig. 3) to retract the back pusher-plate to its open-most position to allow easy insertion of the VB.
3. Lift and rotate the retaining knobs, located along the left and right top of the Vac-Box, to allow insertion of the VB.
4. Insert the VB into the Vac-Box by angling the front portion lower than the back to allow the white plate to of the VB to slip under the lip of the front railing of the Vac-Box (Fig. 3). Align this white plate within the space provided by the railing of the Vac-Box. This will assure a proper seal.
5. Rotate the retaining knobs, located along the left and right top of the Vac-Box, 180° until they push against the sides of the white top-plate of the VB.
6. Connect a 1/4″ Y connector to the outlet of the vacuum regulator and attach a 1/4″ tubing to one of its open ends. This tubing, referred to as the vacuum bleed line, should be easily reached. Clamp this bleed line to apply vacuum and unclamp it to relieve the vacuum.

CAUTION: The same vacuum must be applied to the cardiotomy reservoir as is applied to the Vac-Box. Equalizing the vacuum applied to the VB and the cardiotomy reservoir assures that operation of the cardiotomy relative to the venous bag will be the same as without vacuum. This is achieved by step 7.

7. Connect a second 1/4″ Y connector to the open end of the first Y connector. Connect the one open end of the second Y connector to the Vac-Box and the other end to the cardiotomy reservoir via a vapor trap.

The vapor trap should be replaced for each case. This arrangement provides same vacuum to the cardiotomy reservoir as is applied to the Vac-Box.

CAUTION: Use only a cardiotomy with pressure and vacuum relief valves and follow the instructions for use associated with that unit for VAVD mode (e.g., plugging all unused ports).

8. Be sure that all pumps are off.
9. Clamp the outlet tubing of the venous reservoir.
10. Clamp the inlet tubing to the venous reservoir above the location of the pressure sensor.
11. Verify that all other ports and lines to the cardiotomy reservoir are closed to the atmosphere.
12. Clamp the vacuum bleed line—this directs the vacuum to the Vac-Box and cardiotomy reservoir.
13. Increase the vacuum via the vacuum regulator beyond –80 mmHg and observe that the vacuum reading on the vacuum gauge does not increase beyond –100 mmHg. If –100 mmHg is exceeded, replace the Vac-Box.

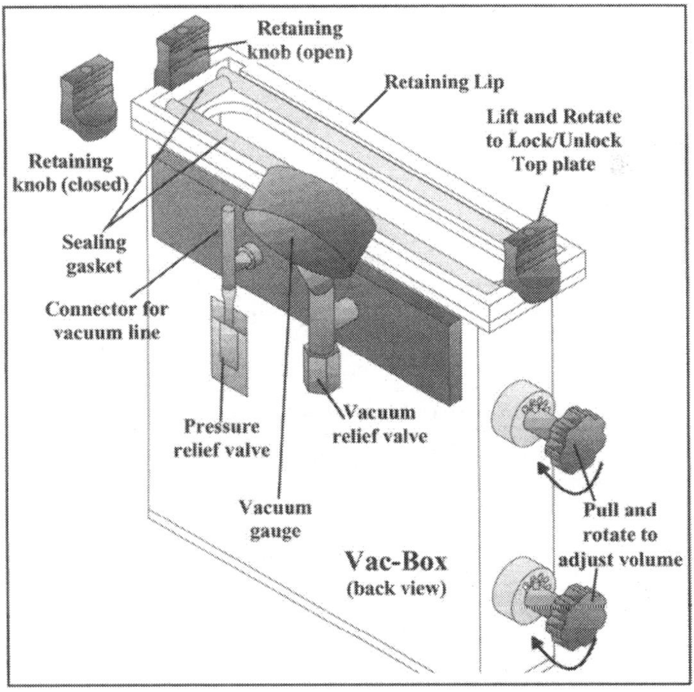

Fig. 3. The Vac-Box (back view).

14. Remove all unnecessary line clamps.

15. Clamp off the vacuum line exiting the vacuum controller. Use the vacuum regulator to reduce vacuum to −45 mmHg.

16. Unclamp the vacuum bleed line—this removes vacuum from the Vac-Box.

Initiating Bypass

17. Initiate bypass per your protocol.
18. Place clamp on the vacuum bleed line.
19. Adjust the vacuum regulator until venous drainage is as desired.

CAUTION: DO NOT exceed a vacuum of −60 mmHg.

20. Rotate the volume adjustment levers (Fig. 3) to adjust the back pusher-plate to adjust the maximum volume the VB accommodates. The filling volume can be adjusted between a minimum of 880 ml and a maximum of 1,750 ml.

Concluding Bypass:

At the conclusion of bypass, reduce vacuum level to reduce venous drainage until arterial flow is reduced to an acceptable level, until vacuum is no longer needed. Disengage the vacuum by removing the clamp from the vacuum bleed line, and wean the patient from CPB as per standard procedure.

CLEANING/DISINFECTING THE VAC-BOX

CAUTION: The Vac-Box is made of Lucite (an acrylic) and therefore contact with solutions containing chlorine, ammonia, or solvents must be avoided (Box 1).

The Vac-Box can be cleaned using mild soap and warm water. It can be disinfected by wiping its surface with 70% isopropyl alcohol.

Routine Maintenance

The Vac-Box should be visually inspected to assure that it is crack free and that the seal along the top opening is intact.

Unit Specifications

Model # Vac-Box15
A rigid housing for use with the VB for VAVD applications.
IFUVB-0102
US Pat. 6,337,049, others pending.

BOX 1. VAC-BOX: NOMINAL SPECIFICATIONS

Material	Acrylic
Inside Height	30 cm
Inside Width	25 cm
Outside Depth	4.5 cm
Weight	4 kg
Vent/Vacuum Port	1/4 in (6.4 mm)
Vacuum relief valve	Opens at −85 ± 5 mmHg
Pressure relief valve	Opens at >–5 mmHg
Vacuum gauge	0 to −110 mmHg
VB18 Max Fill Volume	1,750 ml
VB18 Min. Fill Volume	890 ml

Policy and Procedure Guidelines

CP19

PROCEDURE FOR USE OF TRASYLOL (APROTININ)

Aprotinin is a broad spectrum protease inhibitor that modulates the systemic inflammatory response (SIR) associated with cardiopulmonary bypass (CPB) surgery.

Administration

1. Loading dose/test dose: One vial (200 ml, 2.0 million KIU). After induction of anesthesia, but before the skin incision, 1.0 ml of loading dose is withdrawn and given through a central venous catheter. After 10 min have elapsed without evidence of hypersensitivity, the loading dose is given through a central venous catheter over 20–30 min.
2. Pump prime: One vial (200 ml) is added to the pump prime after discarding an aliquot of the priming solution.
3 Constant infusion dose: After the loading dose is complete, a constant infusion of 50 ml/h (500,000 KIU/h) should be administered IV through a central line until the operation is completed. Aprotinin dosage: 1 cc = 1.4 mg.

Adult: 1/2 Hammersmith protocol may be used upon request of the surgeon. The load would be (100 ml, 1.0 million KIU), a constant infusion of 25 ml/h (250,000 KIU/h), and the pump dose is (100 ml, 1.0 million KIU) added to the pump prime in same manner as above.

Anticoagulation

1. The Hepcon HMS will be used to evaluate the patient's heparin/dose response (red and white striped cartridge). A level of 4 mg/kg will be the minimum target level unless assessed differently by the HDR. This level will be maintained during the CPB procedure. A yellow cartridge will assay this level during heparinization.
2. Sodium heparin (4 mg/kg, unless otherwise specified by HMS protocol) will be given as directed by the cardiac surgeon.

3. Kaolin ACT tubes will be used for measurement of activated clotting times during aprotinin procedures. The activated clotting times (ACTs) will be kept above 480 s.

Heparin-Resistant Patients

We will be performing heparin dose response tests on all patients who are more likely to be heparin resistant. Those patients are defined as anyone on IV heparin within 24 h of surgery. This will allow us to obtain a therapeutic ACT faster, and perhaps use less AT-III.

Pediatric Protocol

Children:	*Full dose*	*Half dose*
Loading	4 mg/kg	2 mg/kg
Pump prime	4 mg/kg	2 mg/kg
Constant infusion	1 mg/kg	0.5

Policy and Procedure Guidelines
CP20

PROCEDURE FOR INTRAOPERATIVE AUTOTRANSFUSION

I. General Description

Intraoperative autotransfusion is used to recover shed blood from the surgical site or post-bypass pump volume. The blood is centrifuged and rinsed with normal saline in a Cell Saver (Haemonetics) or Cobe BRAT (Cobe Cardiovascular), with the plasma and wash solution being discarded. The resulting washed red blood cells with a hematocrit of 50–55% may then be reinfused to the patient. More than 99% of the heparin is removed during the washing procedure when 1,000 ml of wash solution is used. In addition to cardiac surgery, intraoperative autotransfusion may be used for vascular surgery, orthopedic surgery, neurosurgery, and trauma. The use of intraoperative blood autotransfusion must be restricted to use by a clinical perfusionist. It must be operated, assembled, and maintained under strict supervision. Training is required by the hospital through the Technical Services department of the manufacturer.

II. Indications

The procedure is used on the order the of an attending physician for recovery of intraoperative red cells. Because of the expenses involved with both personnel, disposable supplies, and equipment maintenance, the device is usually ordered when a blood loss equivalent to two or more units of red cells is expected. Intraoperative autotransfusion is contraindicated in the presence of Avitene or other clotting adjuncts, Betadine, and antibiotics not licensed for parenteral use, infection or malignancy in the operative field, or contamination of operative field with bowel contents. The risk/benefit ratio of blood salvage must be determined on an individual basis by the surgeons, anesthesiologists, and transfusion medicine specialists involved in the patient's care. The responsibility for the use of this device belongs solely to the physician in charge.

III. Procedure

Supplies needed: adult or pediatric cell recovery kit, 1,000 ml bag of normal saline with 30,000 U heparin, 3,000 ml bag of normal saline for wash, Pall blood transfusion filter, and Fenwal 600 ml transfer bags. ***There are no additives to the processed blood.***

Setup

1. Inject 30,000 U heparin into 1,000 ml normal saline. Label bag, and hang it on IV pole.
2. Place cardiotomy reservoir in holder.
3. Open cell recovery pack, record lot #, and place bowl in centrifuge.
4. Hang waste bag and attach line from bowl outlet (save caps).
5. Place color-coated tubing in corresponding clamps and attach the blue line to collection bag. Close two small clamps on the drainlines from the collection bag. Attach a Pall transfusion filter and transfer bag to the outlet of one of the drain lines.
6. Attach adapter line to the bottom of the cardiotomy reservoir and connect red line from the bowl inlet.
7. Attach the yellow line to the 3 L normal saline irrigation bag.
8. Turn on the device and check operation of all systems, i.e., computer function, bowl spin, and pump operation.
9. Open sterile suction assembly and pass suction tubing to scrub nurse, or give it to circulating nurse to pass to the sterile field. When the suction line is passed off the sterile field, connect to the left 1/4″ inlet of the cardiotomy reservoir. Attach sterile suction tubing to the vacuum port of the cardiotomy reservoir and suction source of −150 mmHg.
10. Prime the suction line and cardiotomy reservoir with 100 ml of the heparin solution, and regulate the heparin drip to 60 drops/min for routine surgery; increase during periods of rapid blood loss.

Processing

Fill bowl in automatic mode, wash with 1,000 ml normal saline in automatic mode, and after washing empty bowl into the collection bag. Drain by gravity through a Pall transfusion filter into a transfer pack. Label with a patient sticker that includes the patient's name and unit number. In addition, note blood volume, date of collection, and expiration time that is 6 h from collection time on the sticker. The time and volume of this collected blood should be recorded on the patient's transfusion record.

IV. Storage

After 4 h, if the blood is not reinfused, it should be discarded in a hazardous waste container.

V. Reinfusion

The processed blood can be retransfused though an intravenous line by an anesthesiologist in the operating room or by a physician or nurse during the postoperative period. Proper identification of the blood unit with the patient's name and unit number is mandatory. Under no circumstances should the collection bag of the Cell Saver be connected directly to a patient's intravenous line during intraoperative autotransfusion. The risk of a massive air embolism exists through a direct connection. The blood must be drained by gravity through a filter into a transfer bag that, after being properly deaired and tied off, is handed to the anesthesiologist. During bypass, the cells can be reinfused directly into the heart–lung machine by the perfusionist if needed. All reinfusion must be recorded on the patient's transfusion record including date, time, volume, and signatures.

VI. Recording Autotransfusion

An autotransfusion form will become part of the patient's medical record to document collection and reinfusion of the patient's own blood. This includes Cell Saver, Plasma Saver, Cobe BRAT, presurgical autologous donation, and postoperative autotransfusion. This can be compared with the use of exogenous blood products to document and evaluate the effectiveness of these procedures.

VII. Centralized Recordkeeping and Reporting

The Clinical Perfusion Department will be responsible for all recordkeeping regarding autotransfusion. This includes the date of service, surgical procedure, number of units collected, lot number and serial number of equipment, and identity of the operator. A quarterly report will be sent to the Blood Bank Director summarizing this data. Reinfusion data will be available on the transfusion record in the patient's chart.

VIII. Preventative Maintenance and Quality Control

Preventive maintenance is performed by a representative of the device manufacturer who will inspect the device on a yearly basis or whenever called by a hospital representative. An unlimited service contract is maintained on all autotransfusion equipment and is renewed on a yearly basis to ensure optimal maximum performance and safe operation of these devices. In addition, Biomedical Engineering will inspect these devices for electrical safety, and will renew these safety stickers before expiration. This will be monitored by Clinical Perfusion Quality Assurance.

Policy and Procedure Guidelines
CP21

DATASCOPE INTRAAORTIC BALLOON PUMP (IABP)

The IABP is an intravascular volume counterpulsation device that augments the circulation by the displacement of aortic blood volume in diastole and reduces the work load of ventricular ejection in systole. Expanded use of the IABP now includes the following:

1. Unstable angina refractory to medical therapy.
2. Preoperative and intraoperative assist in the patient presented with cardiogenic shock.
3. Circulatory stabilization in patients with sudden development of ventricular septal defect and mitral regurgitation.
4. Postoperative interim organ support.

EQUIPMENT

1. Datascope IABP console 97/97E/cs100/300
2. Datascope balloon (with or without central lumen), including percutaneous insertion kit
3. Catheter extension
4. Pressure cable
5. Five-lead patient cable with electrosurgical interference suppresser filter blocks
6. Slave cable for both electrocardragrion (ECG) and pressure monitoring
7. Silver-Silver chloride ECG skin electrodes
8. Fiberoptic sensation balloon if using CS 300

PROCEDURE

CAUTION: Before operating the Equipment the user must be familiar with controls and functions of the datascope IABP console.

1. Establish power. Console will automatically go through self test.
2. Perform safety chamber leak test (refer to operators manual for instructions on performing this test), if applicable.
3. Open helium cylinder (close when system is not in use).

4. Acquire ECG either with skin leads or via slave of existing monitor.

5. Acquire pressure trace either through central lumen of IABP catheter, arterial line, or via slave of existing monitor.

6. Select trigger. ECG usually safest and best trigger. Pressure trigger is useful during operation of electrosurgical (bovie) equipment, but requires periodic adjustments with the timing of the console and changes in the patient's rate of rhythm. Pacer trigger is only operational if the ECG is being monitored directly by the IABP from electrodes placed on the skin. The pacer trigger may not work while slaving from an external source.

7. Initiate assist. Best to start at an assist rate of 1:2 so that proper timing adjustments can be made.

8. Adjust timing. The system automatically establishes correct timing of the IABP in the autotiming mode. The inflation and deflation controls may be adjusted to optimize IABP timing, following the manufacturer's guidelines.

Policy and Procedure Guidelines
CP22

EMERGENCY MANAGEMENT

In the event of a pump failure, two emergency back-up modalities exist. The first choice for emergency backup is operation of the pump by battery power source. These procedures are discussed in detail in the following paragraphs (Table 1). The second choice of backup is manual pump operation utilizing hand crank systems. Emergency backup modalities should be implemented immediately once a pump failure has been recognized by the perfusionist. Backup operation should be continued until the problem has been rectified, pump has been replaced, or patient has been weaned from bypass. Any failed equipment must be removed from service immediately and labeled defective with the time, date, and nature of the problem. A perfusion supervisor should be promptly notified and an incident report should be filled out according to hospital policy and procedures.

BATTERY BACKUP OPERATION

A. Jostra Pump

Turn on the master power switch on the console O. Turn on the monitor system switch M on the lower left face of the pump console. Make sure the console is plugged in and confirm that all circuit breakers in the rear of the pump are in the on position. The yellow "C" light indicates the battery is charging. The yellow "B" light means the console is being powered by the backup battery (see the Jostra operator's manual, battery section). Note, batteries only charge when console base is plugged in and turned on. Turn on the power button for the individual pump head being used (e.g. P1, P2, etc.). Set the pump mode to Arterial (art) and set the tubing size to the appropriate tubing being used in the arterial raceway.

Warning: Do not cover the console when connected to the mains; restricted air flow may overheat batteries

Jostra Rotaflow system automatically switches to battery operation when the external power supply (mains voltage or Jostra Heart–Lung

Table 1
Battery Quickcheck List

	Device	*Operation*	*Fully Charged*	*Low Alarm Message*	*Recharge Time*
A.	Stockert Pumphead	Manual	1.5 h	red LED	24 h
B.	Biomedicus console	Automatic	30–60 min	Bar graph alarm	24 h
C.	Sarns 8000 console	Automatic	25–40 min	red light	24 h
D.	Abiomed BVS 5000	Automatic	1 h	Battery on low	16 h
E.	Heartmate TCI Assist Device	Automatic	15 min	Lo Batt	?
F.	Datascope IABP's	Automatic	90T-2 h 90 50–90 min	Flashing charge light	24 h

machine console) is interrupted. If power returns, the Rotaflow system switches back to the external power supply. New, fully charged batteries at 5 LPM and normal load will provide approximately 1.5 h of operation.

Battery voltage during battery operation, the status display flashes "BAT XX.X" (XX.X: current battery voltage), and the acoustic alarm sounds during battery operation.

1. 27.4 V (fully charged battery) >20.0 V. The acoustic alarm can be switched off with the "audio off" button.
2. 20.0 V greater than 19.0 V. The speed and flow display flashes "LOW BAT" and the acoustic alarm cannot be switched off.
3. 19.0 V. The system switches off.

Warning: When the voltage has sunk to 20.0 V, there is only power left for a very short time.

B. Bio-Medicus Battery Backup

The Bio-Medicus console switches automatically to battery backup when alternating current (AC) power is lost. Check all plugs and outlets in the event of loss of AC power. A LED "AC power off" alarm will illuminate when the console switches to battery mode. An audible alarm will accompany battery operation (do not override this alarm). Several factors affect battery life. A new, fully charged battery at a flow of 3.5–4.5 L/min, a Hct of 42%, and 3,500 RPMs will last 29 min, at 3,000 RPMs 39 min, and at 2,500 RPMs 59 min. Note that the round metal plug at the rear of the console must remain inserted for battery operation.

C. Sarns 8000 Modular system

After the system has completed its startup tests, check the battery indicators while using AC power. A green indicator light signals that the battery charger is functioning. Both DC indicators should be off, as the battery supply is not being used. The three battery supply indicators should be off, as the battery supply is not in use. When the system begins operating in battery backup, both direct current power supply indicators will light, the battery supply indicator will light green, yellow, and red, and every 2 min a short audible tone will sound. The battery supply indicators are a relative indication of the operating time available to use battery power. Green indicates that the battery supply is charged, yellow indicates that the battery power is dropping, and red indicates a discharged battery. A fully charged battery will operate 2 pumps for 25 min or 1 pump for 40 min. If possible, decrease the number of devices dependent on the battery to prolong its life. Turn off the light, place the cardioplegia pump in stop mode, etc. Leave the safety monitors on. The battery backup is automatic when AC power is lost.

D. The Abiomed BVS 5000

Internal battery power is automatically activated whenever AC power is interrupted. The battery will last for 1 h when fully charged. The BATTERY ON message is displayed whenever battery power is engaged. When operating on battery power and less than 10 min of charge remains, BATTERY ON LOW is displayed. If the battery has less than 80% capacity, the BATTERY CHARGING message is displayed.

E. The Heartmate TCI Assist Device Console

The Heartmate console will operate on battery automatically when AC power is interrupted. The message "BATT" appears in the lower right quadrant of the display. Fully charged batteries will operate the console for at least 15 min. This is a conservative rating for battery function. When approximately 10 min of power is left, the LO BATT message will appear in the lower right of the display and the audio alarm will sound. To recharge the battery, plug console in and make sure white circuit breaker switch is in AC on position 1.

F. The Datascope System

The system will operate on battery automatically when removed from AC power. When the charge light is illuminated, the battery is charging. If the charge light is flashing, less than 30 min of portable time is available on the battery. The battery on the 90T has approximately 2 h of portable time when the battery is fully charged. Fully depleted batteries will require approximately 24 h for return to full charge. The flashing charge light will remain steady when the batteries are at full charge. A fully charged battery on the system will last approximately 50–95 min. The CS 300 will last about 3 h on battery.

G. Thoratec Ventricular Assist Device

Low battery alarms when the module batteries have less than 30 min of power remaining. The AC light (yellow) should always be on unless the console is unplugged from an electrical source during patient transportation or ambulation. The battery light flashes when the console is unplugged from the electrical outlet. Uninterruptable Power Supply (UPS) status panel is displayed on the lower front portion of the console and provides approximately 40 min of battery time. When the UPS is operating during transportation, or power outage, it gives a brief audible signal every few seconds. As discharge of the battery continues, four green battery lights disappear one at a time. A red battery alarm light and continuous audible alarm indicates less than 5 min of UPS battery operation. The UPS AC light should be on unless the UPS is in use.

Policy and Procedure Guidelines

CP23

DEPARTMENT OF NURSING CARDIOTHORACIC SURGERY INTENSIVE CARE UNIT

BLOOD AND BLOOD COMPONENT ADMINISTRATION PROCDURE

Purpose

To outline the nurse's responsibility in the safe set-up of blood products.

Levels

Interdependents (* indicated MD order required)

Equipment Needed

250 cc normal saline solution
IV administration set appropriate for blood or blood component being infused
Transfusion slip
Blood or blood products
Three-way stopcock
CAP

PROCEDURE	KEY POINTS
1. Check MD order for blood or components solution to be infused.	
2. Set up saline solutions before, during, and ofter administration at keep vein open/or as ordered.	IV solutions that include 5% dextrose cause hemolysis of the erythrocytes.
3. Place the three-way stopcock between the twin site and IV administration set.	
4. Match patient identification form to unit of blood or blood component supplied by MD.	

5. Two people need to verify: Patient Name ID number ABO and RH type Expiration date	If any discrepancies are noted, blood to be returned to the blood bank.
6. Set up blood or blood component according to chart.	(See chart)
7. Attach unit to primed saline solution, maintaining sterility of system.	
8. Infuse slowly for first 15 min.	Observe for adverse reactions. (See chart for time chart).
9. Adjust infusion based on MD order.	
10. Discontinue after completion. a. Flush with saline solution. b. Resume parenteral infusion as ordered.	
11. Transfusion form to be completed by two RNs and/or RN and MD and placed in chart.	
12. Document patient's response to the transfusion in nurses notes.	

BLOOD COMPONENTS	ADMINISTRATION SET/FILTER	INFUSION RATE	COMMENTS
Store whole blood	—	2–4 h	Invert bag several times to give uniform suspension
Fresh whole blood	Pall blood filter + Hemoset 100 × 10 Cair Clamp	2–4 h	
Packed cells	Pall blood filter + Hemoset 100 × 10 Cair clamp or Bloodset 64	2–4 h	Do not mix, must be used in 24 h.

(Continued)

BLOOD COMPONENTS	ADMINISTRATION SET/FILTER	INFUSION RATE	COMMENTS
Platelet	Components filter or Venoset 78	Rapidly	Must be given with 24–72h of preparation. Infuse 15–30min.
Fresh frozen plorar	Bloodset 64 or 20–40M or component filter + Hemoset 100 × 10 with Cair clamp	rapidly	Must be within 6h of thawing.
Cryoprecipitated antihemophilic factor (Cryo)	Component filter	Rapidly	Administer rapidly approximately 4U in 15min.
Antihemophilic of Factor PHF	Component filter	Rapidly	Use within 60min of preparation. Administration should be complete 3h after mixing.
25% normal serum albumin	Special ADM Set with Vial.		Compatible with IV solutions. common

TRANSFUSION REACTION

Transfusion reaction is any unfavorable response by the patient that occurs as the result of or during transfusion of blood or blood products.

I. TRANSFUSION REACTION CATEGORIES:

Hemolytic
Febrile
Allergic
Anaphylactic
Circulatory overload
Sepsis

II. INVESTIGATION OF TRANSFUSION REACTION:

When floor/doctor notified the Blood Bank of a possible transfusion reaction, ask the following questions:

a. Has transfusion been stopped? If "no" then advise them to stop it.
b. Has a posttransfusion sample been drawn? (necessary for complete workup)
c. Has urine sample been collected?
d. Get patient's name, unit number, location, diagnosis, and reactions symptoms.

Request that posttransfusion sample and donor bag suspected of causing reaction be returned immediately to the blood bank. Urine sample is to be sent to Urinalysis lab for test.

Fill in transfusion reaction form with all information.

III. LAB TEST WORKUP

A. Recheck all clerical data and initial form that this has been performed.
B. In case of hemolytic transfusion reaction, notify supervisor immediately.
C. Spin down patient's posttransfusion specimen and check serum for hemolysis. Compare to serum of pretransfusion sample.
D. Do ABO and RH typing on post transfusion specimen and donor bag. If results are not the same as pretransfusion result, repeat tests on retransfusion results.
E. Do direct and indirect Coombs on posttransfusion sample. If either is positive, repeat tests on pretransfusion sample to determine if it was a preexisting condition.
F. If patient's indirect Coombs was positive in pretransfusion testing, run panel on post specimen to determine if it was preexisting condition.
G. Run major compatibility testing with posttransfusion sample using 1-h incubation. If results are positive, repeat compatibility testing with pretransfusion sample.
H. Record all results on transfusion reaction form and submit to supervisor for review.
I. If febrile reaction is suspected to be caused by bacterial contamination of donor blood, send remaining donor unit to microbiology for sterility check. Advise floor to send blood culture sample from patient to microbiology.

Policy and Procedure Guidelines
CP24

CARDIOPULMONARY BYPASS PROCEDURE FOR ADULTS

General Description

Cardiopulmonary bypass (CPB) is used to support the patient's circulation during the period of surgical intervention. This can be achieved with various pump oxygenator combinations, and the system used in this hospital will be described in detail. Attempts will be made to evaluate and update the system whenever new and improved equipment is available.

Indications

Cardiopulmonary bypass is indicated for patients who undergo heart or major vessel surgery and require that the blood flow to these organs be diverted to the heart–lung machine for artificial oxygenation and circulation and to provide a safe and effective exposure during surgical repair. Hypothermia and hemodilution provide safe periods of low flow and/or circulatory arrest when necessary. This is determined by the attending surgeon, depending on the complexity of the operation.

Procedure

Circuits

Blood flow is determined by the patient's body surface area (BSA). A calculated blood flow at an index of $2.4\,L/min/m^2$ is used to determine the size of the circuit.

Adult Pack

Available in a sterile component that contains the adult tubing pack, the oxygenator, and an integrated cardiotomy reservoir. The arterial line is 3/8″ and the venous line is 1/2″. An adult arterial line filter with a 3/8″ bridge may be included. The configurations of these disposable products are reviewed and changes are made to improve as necessary.

The arterial limb of the circuit also consists of 3/8″ tubing, and it is connected to the outlet of the arterial centrifugal pump with a one-way duckbill valve to help protect the oxygenator, from negative pressure. Output from this pump is directed to an adult membrane oxygenator and then to an arterial filter, before being returned to the patient. The venous reservoir is protected against excessive suction with a positive and negative pressure relief valve.

Circuit Design and Safety Considerations

The perfusion circuit has been designed to maintain adequate blood flow with minimal hemolysis and avoid accidental air embolism. The latter is achieved with the combination of a centrifugal pump, a vented arterial filter, and an inline air bubble detector. Various devices to reduce the risk of accidental air and offer a greater margin of safety are utilized. These include level detection with pump stop, positive and negative pressure monitoring of arterial line pressure, cardiotomy/venous reservoir pressure, and cardioplegia delivery pressure. In addition, one-way vacuum relief valves are used on the suction lines to guard against reverse pump direction and to reduce hemolysis.

All equipment is maintained within operating specifications by the manufacturer, and preventive maintenance is carried out according to their schedule. Preventive maintenance contracts are maintained on all equipment, and periodic monthly inspections by the Bioengineering Department are completed before expiration to insure electrical safety.

Priming the Circuit

After setting up the circuit and flushing with 100% CO_2 through a sterile gas filter, priming of the circuit can begin. 1,000 ml lactated Ringer's and 1,000 ml 6% Hextend is used as the priming solution, and the circuit is debubbled and recirculated before use. The oxygenator is ventilated with 100% O_2 to reduce the CO_2 level before the final priming. A predicted postdilutional pump hematocrit of <20% may require that packed red cells be added to the perfusion circuit. This decision is surgeon directed, and is usually based on the complexity of the surgical procedure and preoperative condition of the patient.

Packed cells should be refrigerated in the blood refrigerator after being checked by the perfusionist and a physician. Proper identification of the blood with the patient's name, birth date, hospital number, blood type, donor number, and expiration date is mandatory before addition to the pump. This must be witnessed by another member of the open heart team, and both signatures must be recorded on the transfusion form. One copy of the blood transfusion form is placed on the patient's chart, and the other is returned to the blood bank. In some instances, blood will be leukodepleted as needed (i.e., transplants).

Additional prime constituents include 4,000 U heparin, 50 mEq sodium bicarbonate, and 12.5 g Mannitol. If blood is added to the prime, then the prebypass filter (if present) must be either removed from the circuit, or recirculation can be only through the AV bridge. Crystalloid priming volume should be reduced by the additional blood volume. Hemoconcentration is available during bypass to increase the hematocrit when excess circulating blood volume is present.

Documentation of the Perfusion Procedure

At the beginning of each procedure, the following forms are necessary:

- Perfusion record (original + 3 copies)
- Perfusion summary record
- NY state form
- Transfusion record
- Charge cards
- Patient labels

After calculating the patient's BSA, flow rate, heparin dose, and postdilutional hematocrit, the rest of the preoperative data and history should be recorded on the appropriate forms. Serial numbers for disposables and equipment should be noted, and the prebypass checklist completed. During bypass, documentation of the blood flow rate, arterial blood temperature, esophageal temperature, axillary or rectal temperature, mean arterial blood pressure, and central venous pressure must be made on the perfusion record at least every 15 min. Additional information is recorded in the "Events" column.

In addition to continuous monitoring of the venous oxygen saturation by the perfusionist, blood gases and electrolytes should be monitored at least once during hypothermia, and once during rewarming. Blood gas and electrolyte values are obtained by use of the iSTAT handheld blood gas analyzer. Blood gases and electrolytes should be adjusted by the perfusionist to maintain normal levels, as determined by the attending physicians. For longer bypass procedures, these studies should be done at least once an hour and recorded on the perfusion record.

Cardioplegia

FLUSHING (PRIMING) THE CARDIOPLEGIA DELIVERY SYSTEM

Once cardioplegia system (cps) components are assembled in the surgical field, proper assembly and clamp orientation should be confirmed by the perfusionist and surgical staff. Anesthesia personnel should connect, fill, and flush the pressure monitoring line before connection of the cps set with the aortic root needle. This procedure may also be reconfirmed at the surgeon's command during the perfusion priming sequence. This line should never be flushed while connected to the patient, unless extreme caution is used and clear direction is given by the surgeon to prevent possible air embolism.

The perfusionist should check the cps set before initial priming to ensure all clamps are properly placed and one cardioplegia bag is open with a clear blood path to the table. The red sucker must be on and connected to the cardioplegia "Y" at the table. The Y connector should not be connected to the aorta until after the cps system is primed and air free. If connected, the aortic limb of the Y must be clamped until priming is complete. Both surgical staff and perfusionists should communicate and confirm proper clamp orientation before "open connection" of the root needle and aortic root.

Flushing between cardioplegia doses should no longer be necessary. The Sorin Vangard cps set has a very low prime volume, allowing more efficient delivery of cold or warm cardioplegia with very little lag time. Should flushing be necessary during the case, the surgical and perfusion staff must clearly communicate to avoid possible air embolization.

Cardioplegia is delivered with a blood cardioplegia delivery system. There are various disposable units that include a temperature indicator, a pressure monitor, and a bubble trap. The cardioplegia solution is provided by the pharmacy and contains 120 mEq/l of potassium chloride, for high-dose administration and 60 mEq/l of potassium for low-dose administration. 20 U of regular insulin are added to the low-dose bag just before CPB. It is manufactured under a prescription by the Chief Cardiac Surgeon. Once potassium arrest is achieved, the concentration is reduced to 60 mEq/L concentration. Because the cardioplegia is mixed with 4 parts blood, the actual concentration delivered to the coronary circulation is approximately 28 mEq/L in the initial solution and 14 mEq/l in the low-concentration solution. Cardioplegia is delivered between 4–8°C, and the flows and pressures are determined by route of administration.

Route of delivery	*Flow*	*Line Pressure*	*Delivery Pressure*
Antegrade:			
Aortic Root	300 ml/min	200–300	100–150
Left Coronary	150–200	200–300	100–150
Rt Coronary	100–200	200–300	100–150
Retrograde:			
Coronary sinus	100–300	150–300	40–50

Because of the danger of rupturing the coronary sinus, delivery pressure of retrograde cardioplegia is measured directly from the coronary sinus (Fig. 1). Low or high pressure at normal flow rates may indicate that the catheter is not properly positioned, and the surgeon must be notified immediately.

Antegrade or retrograde cardioplegia delivery is selected by the surgeon by using a DLP switch. On the antegrade outlet of the switch there is a DLP Y for recirculation of the cardioplegia through the "red" pump sucker. This allows for cooling of the cardioplegia between doses, if necessary. Cardioplegia is usually given approximately every 20 min, and the surgeon should be notified when this period has elapsed.

ANTICOAGULATION

A prebyass activated clotting time (ACT) is obtained before heparinization to determine the baseline coagulation before initiating bypass. Adequate heparinization is achieved when the ACT reaches 480 s. On bypass, the ACT should be maintained >480 s, with additional heparin

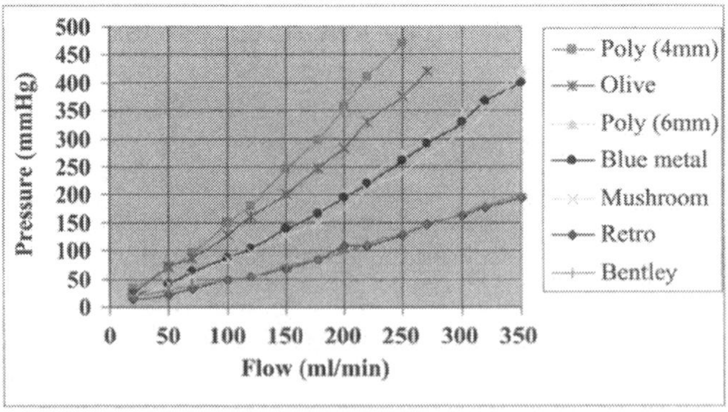

Fig. 1. Typical pressure flow characteristics of various cardioplegia delivery cannulae.

administration when necessary. An ACT should be monitored every 20 min on bypass, and more frequently during rewarming, when the ACT may decrease rapidly. After the end of bypass, a protamine dose is calculated by measuring the heparin level with an automated protamine titration using a Hepcon HMS System. 1.3 mg of protamine is given by the anesthesiologist to neutralize each 100 U of circulating heparin. Ten minutes after protamine, an ACT and heparin level is performed to assure complete neutralization of the heparin and that the ACT has returned to the prebypass baseline.

Recovery of Pump Volume

At the end of bypass, all blood is recovered from the perfusion circuit. This is accomplished by first clamping the arterial line to the patient, attaching a purge line from the sampling manifold to the cell recovery reservoir, and slowly pumping volume into the autotransfusion reservoir. Additional crystalloid solution is added to the pump to replace this volume until the pump is completely diluted and red cell recovery is no longer possible. Once the aorta is decannulated, aggressive flushing of the circuit with a balanced electrolyte solution can be carried out. All blood is processed in the autotransfusion device and transfused to the patient according to the "Protocol for Intraoperative Autotransfusion."

Circuit Breakdown/Disposal

Pump circuit breakdown should not begin until **all** lines have been separated from the patient and surgical field. This includes arterial lines, all venous lines (central, femoral, neck, etc.), and cardioplegia lines (central, aortic, coronary sinus, steerable neck cannula, etc.). Once all lines have been disconnected from the patient and returned to the perfusionist, pump circuit disassembly may begin when directed by the surgeon. The HCU 30 takes approximately 5 min to prime and achieve a normothermic operating temperature should reinitiation of CPB become necessary. The HCU 30 heater–cooler should remain connected and recirculating until instructed to discard the pump circuit, at which time the lines may be deprimed, valves closed, and cps lines removed from the delivery set.

Cardiopulmonary Support System

A closed system for emergent cardiopulmonary support is (CPS) available to facilitate rapid-response CPB outside the operating room area. Use of a single centrifugal pump head provides propulsive force for arterial blood flow, as well as negative pressure to aspirate patient blood volume (provide venous return). This system consists of a venous drainage line (3/8″) into a centrifugal head out to an oxygenator/arterial filter combo, and back to the patient via a 3/8″ arterial line. The system uses a cardiotomy reservoir for priming only. The lack of a venous reservoir for drainage minimizes exposure to nonendothelial foreign surface area, silicone oil/silica particle antifoam, and blood gas interface, and aids in reducing inflammatory response.

Supplies and Equipment Needed

1. CPS cart, which includes the centrifugal pump console (with backup) and hand crank, heater–cooler unit, oxygen blender and O_2 tank, and SAT/Hct monitor.
2. 1 each: a coated tubing pack that includes a coated E-Pack, A Cobe Synthesis oxygenator-filter combination with a cardiotomy reservoir for priming (Fig. 2), and appropriate size arterial and venous cannulae.
3. Backup of all the above.

Procedure

1. The system is assembled by attaching the circuit lines to the oxygenator and recirculating with priming solution after flushing with CO_2.

(No albumin in the prime because it may decrease the activity of the heparin coating).

2. All connections must be tie banded because the coating may make the tubing slippery on the connectors.

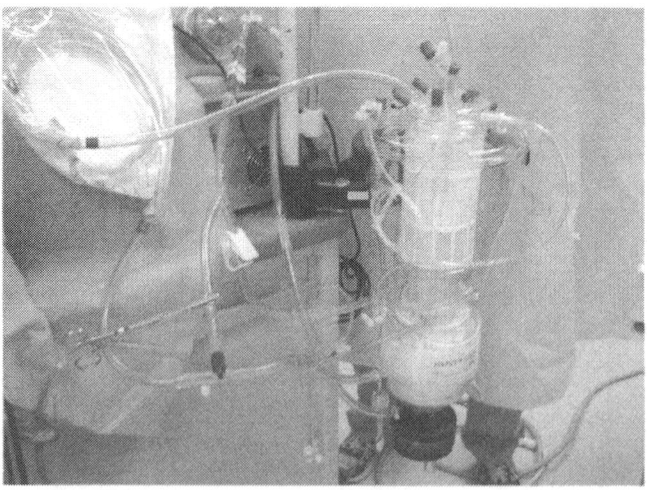

Fig. 2. Adult Synthesis.

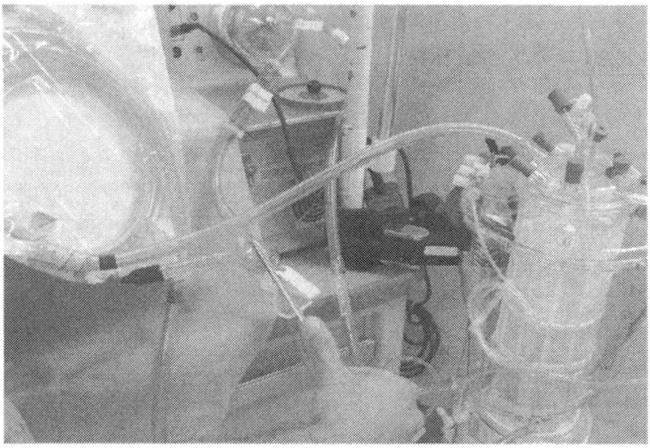

Fig. 3. Patient inflow will be removed and placed into inflow of centrifugal head.

3. For peripheral arterial cannulation, Bio-Medicus cannulae are available coated with heparin. For peripheral venous cannulation, Bio-Medicus cannulae are also available coated with heparin.
4. Heparin must be administered before initiation of CPB in accordance with institutional guidelines.
5. ACT will be monitored hourly.
6. A checklist must be completed before initiation of CPB.

Equipment Selection and Setup

An adult bypass tubing pack (E-Pack) is used with a Bio-Medicus or Rotaflow centrifugal pump and a Cobe Synthesis membrane oxygenator. Please refer to the diagram below for proper setup of the E-Pack circuit. An oxygenator should be selected to provide a minimum of full flow for the patient. Pigtails may be attached to the leur locks on the inflow and outflow lines for pressure monitoring but should not be used for circuit access. The setup is then flushed with CO_2 before priming. The priming volume of 1,200–2,000 ml consists of 6% Hextend and lactated Ringer's (in equal amounts). 4,000 U heparin and 50 ml sodium bicarbonate are added to 2,000 ml prime. Blood prime should be used if the estimated postdilutional hematocrit is below 20%. A blood gas on the prime should then be performed, and the prime should be adjusted as close to normal physiologic values as possible. After deairing the circuit, the venous inflow tubing to the cardiotomy reservoir is removed and connected to the inflow of the centrifugal pump (Fig. 3). Recirculation is continued until just before attachment to the cannulas. The cardiotomy reservoir MUST be double clamped before bypass to ensure a closed system and prevent exsanguination. **Note: The oxygenator to cardiotomy shunt must be closed to prevent exsanguination into the cardiotomy reservoir. However, this shunt may be utilized intermittently to remove air from the arterial filter if necessary. The shunt may also be used to briefly translocate volume (i.e., unload the heart) if necessary** (Fig. 4).

Vascular Access and Cannula Selection

Venoarterial cannulation is used for combined cardiac and respiratory support. Venous drainage may be accomplished via the femoral vein, the internal jugular, or direct right atrial cannulation. Arterial inflow may be accomplished via the femoral artery, internal carotid artery, axillary artery, or ascending aorta. Other cannulation sites may be required as per the surgeon's request. Consult cannula flow chart for appropriate cannula size.

Cardiopulmonary support Initiation and Management During Bypass

Before cannulation, the patient should be systemically heparinized with 100 U kg sodium heparin, with ACT of more than 300 s (minimum). The sterile AV loop is passed up to the surgical field, and recirculation

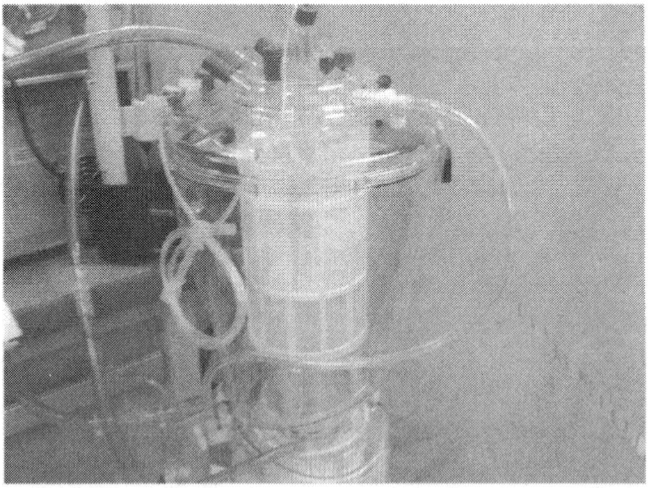

Fig. 4. Typical oxygenator to cardiotomy shunt line.

is discontinued. Tubing clamps are placed distal to the centrifugal head and distal to the oxygenator. The venous inflow tubing to the cardiotomy reservoir is removed and connected to the inflow of the centrifugal pump. Upon adequate anticoagulation, cannulation is performed by the surgeon. CPS is initiated by removing both arterial and venous clamps and increasing blood flow to the desired rate. Gas flow is then immediately instituted to the recommended gas to blood flow ratio of 1:1 for the oxygenator, used as per manufacturer's recommendations. Line pressures should be checked immediately to ensure adequate venous drainage and arterial return and to rule out the possibility of arterial dissection. Volume may be given through the CPS circuit via the cardiotomy reservoir by opening the double clamps on the cardiotomy line. The perfusionist must ensure that there is adequate volume in the reservoir while doing this because this volume is being infused into a closed system with negative pressure on the venous side. Extreme care must be exercised to ensure air-free addition of volume. As soon as hemodynamic stability is achieved, all volume management should be completed via patient lines, the cardiotomy should remain double clamped, and circuit integrity should not be compromised. Blood gases are sampled routinely at the bedside, and the patient is managed using an alpha-stat protocol to maintain values within normal acceptable ranges. ACTs are sampled hourly and maintained at >180 s. All ACT and blood gas samples should be obtained by the nurse via the patient's arterial line. Blood gases should not be drawn from the pump, except for the purposes of checking oxygenator performance or for calibrating the oxygen saturation analyzer. The perfusionist is required to document patient and CPS pump parameters on the pump record on an hourly basis, and all significant events as they occur.

CONVERSION

On occasion, conversion to conventional CPB in the operating room (OR) or extended care extracorporeal membrane oxygenation (ECMO) may be necessary. If conversion to conventional CPB is needed, transport to the OR will be facilitated with the mobile closed system CPS cart with a full oxygen tank, adequately charged centrifugal pump battery, and backup console. CPS tubing will be aseptically prepped in the OR. Once stable in the OR, CPB will be briefly discontinued to allow the sterile surgical team to divide the arterial and venous lines and reconnect (in an air-free fashion) to arterial and venous lines of a conventional CPB circuit, respectively. Note: To ensure a delay-free conversion, make sure you have the proper tubing connectors before terminating CPS support. This allows you to reinitiate CPB in a conventional manner with the ability to provide cardiotomy suction, left vestries venting, aortic root venting, cardioplegia delivery, and rapid hypothermia, as well as level, bubble temperature, and pressure protection. Any remaining volume in the discontinued circuit may be returned to the cell recovery device for processing.

If extended term support (i.e., ECMO) is needed, an adult EMCO circuit is set up and primed on the Adult ECMO Cart, as per our adult ECMO protocol. Conversion to adult ECMO is performed by the cardiothoracic surgeon. However, conversion to the adult ECMO circuit may be delayed until the Hollow Fiber Synthesis Oxygenator begins to show signs of failure (poor gas exchange capability or plasma leakage). Be sure to complete a prebypass and on-bypass checklist each time you convert to a new circuit, as per protocol.

Policy and Procedure Guidelines
CP25

WARM-DOSE CARDIOPLEGIA OR BLOOD-ONLY DELIVERY VIA THE CARDIOPLEGIA SET

Materials

1. Jostra/Maquet heater–cooler unit, HCU-30
2. Cardioplegia delivery set with conducer
3. Cardioplegia water lines with valves

Procedure

A simple system is utilized by the West campus perfusion staff to allow delivery of cardioplegia at normothermia. The same system is easily adapted to allow delivery of warm blood to the heart before unclamping the aorta (i.e., warm reperfusion). Upon the surgeon's request, warm cardioplegia or warm blood reperfusion may be administered via the cardioplegia delivery set. The cardioplegia side of the HCU-30 may be set to deliver warm water to the heat exchanger of the cardioplegia delivery set. We are currently using a Sorin BCD Vangard 4:1 blood cardioplegia set with a 1/8″ delivery line. Because the post–heat exchanger volume is very small (approximately 15 ml), flushing should not be necessary. An alternative method is to close the HCU-30 cardioplegia system (cps) water valves and allow warm blood from the oxygenator to be utilized for reperfusion.

Delivery of either warm cardioplegia or warm blood reperfusion is accomplished by proper placement and orientation of clamps, as outlined in the manufacturer's instructions for use. To deliver only warm blood to the heart, the following procedure should be observed. Clamp both the high- and low-dose cardioplegia spike lines. Open the blood-only bridge clamp on the cardioplegia delivery set to allow blood-only delivery from your oxygenator to your cps system. Extreme care must be used while repositioning clamps and valves for warm or cold cardioplegia delivery.

During all delivery of cardioplegia or warm reperfusion, the perfusionist should monitor delivery pressure and temperature and utilize pressure and temperature alarms whenever possible (Fig. 1).

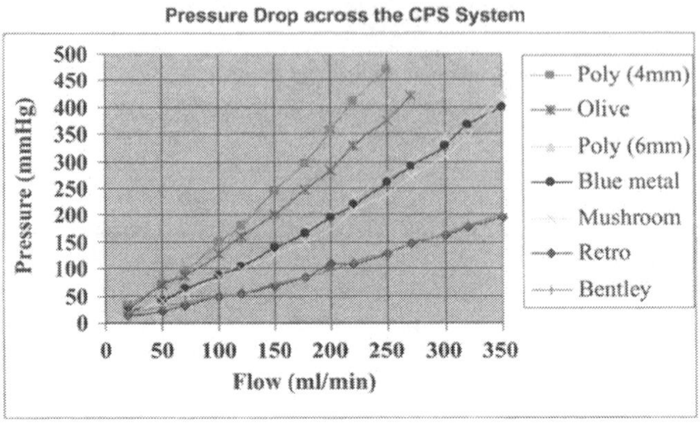

Fig. 1. Typical pressure flow characteristics of various cardioplegia delivery cannulae.

Please return all valves to the cold position after any delivery of warm blood or cardioplegia and reposition all appropriate clamps to allow delivery of cold, high-potassium concentration cardioplegia should an additional arrest period become necessary.

Policy and Procedure Guidelines
CP26

CLEAR PRIME REPLACEMENT

Definition

Replacement of extracorporeal clear prime with patient autologous blood before commencement of cardiopulmonary bypass (CPB). The obligatory hemodilution resulting from crystalloid priming of the CPB circuit represents a major risk factor for blood transfusion in cardiac operations. Autologous priming of the bypass circuit may result in decreased hemodilution and red cell transfusion.

Methods

The CPB circuit should be assembled and primed according to protocol, with the addition of Mannitol withheld. After heparinization (adequate activated chaffing time), arterial and venous cannulation, administration of a test dose, and consultation with the surgeon and anesthesiologist, the autologous replacement of clear prime is started. The anesthesia team may start some background vasoconstriction to promote maintenance of vaso tone. The arterial line distal to the arterial filter is double clamped. The venous line is partially occluded to allow very slow exchange of patient volume, while pumping clear prime to the arterial filter and out of the manifold into a properly labeled collection bag. Patient parameters should be closely monitored to prevent hypotension. This procedure should be continued (patient parameter permitting) until blood reaches the collection bag. Once complete, the venous line should be clamped, the centrifugal pump outlet line clamped, the manifold turned off, and, after careful inspection of the pump circuit (air-free, all clamps properly placed, etc.), the double clamps distal to the arterial filter may be removed in preparation for initiation of CPB. The mannitol dose should be administered at this time. Commencement of CPB will be on command of the surgeon, as per protocol.

Policy and Procedure Guidelines

CP27

USEFUL FORMULAE

A. Body Surface Area (BSA) (m^2)

1. $$\frac{\text{Ht.(cm)} \times \text{Wt.(kg)/square root}}{3600}$$
2. Ht. (cm) .725 × Wt. (kg) .425 × .007184

Conversions: Ht. (inches) × 2.54 = cm
Wt. (lbs)/2.2 = kg

B. Post Dilutional Hct

Blood volume: Adult = 65 cc/kg
Adult = 80 cc/kg with cyanosis
Pediatric = 80 cc/kg
Infant = 85 cc/kg
—kg × cc/kg = blood volume
—Blood volume × Pre Dil Hct = Estimated Red Blood Cell Volume (ERBCV)

$$\frac{\text{ERBCV}}{\text{Total Circulating Volume (Pt. B.V. + Pump Prime)}} = \text{Post Dil. Hct.}$$

If a low Hct is expected, and you plan to add blood to the prime:

If packed red blood cells are used: EST Hct. = 55%
If Whole Blood is used: EST Hct = 35%

1. Est. RBCV of Exogenous Blood Product = Est. Hct. × ml of product given

$$\frac{\text{Pt.RBCV.} + \text{Blood RBCV}}{\text{Total Circulating Volume}} = \text{New Est. Post Dil Hct.}$$

2. Total Circulating Volume (TCV) × Desired Hct. % –Pt. RCBV = ml. of RBC's required.

C. O_2 Transfer/O_2 Consumption:

$$O_2 \text{ Consumption } (VO_2) = \text{C.O.} \times CaO^2 - CvO_2$$

—normal O_2 consumption of an adult = 250 ml O_2/min
—anesthesia reduces O_2 consumption by ≈ 1/3 = 165 ml/min

O_2 Content (CaO_2) or (CvO_2) = The amount of O_2 the blood is actually carrying (Vols%).

—O_2 dissolved in plasma = .003 × PaO_2
—.003 = solubility coefficient at 37°C
—Normal CaO_2 = 20 Vols%
—Normal CvO_2 = 15 Vols%

$$CaO_2 = (\text{Hgb.} \times 1.34 \times SaO_2) + (PaO_2 \times .003)$$

O_2 Capacity = The amount of O_2 the blood is capable of carrying

$$(\text{Vols\%}) = (\text{Hgb.} \times 1.34 \times 100\%) + (PaO_2 \times .003)$$

$$O_2 \text{ Saturation} = \frac{O_2\text{Content}}{O_2\text{Capacity}}$$

$$O_2\text{Transfer} = \frac{(\text{Art. Sat.} - \text{Ven. Sat.}) \times (\text{Hgb.} \times 1.34) \times \text{Flow (lpm)}}{100}$$

$$= \text{ml/kg/min}$$

Basal Metabolic Rate = 4 ml/kg/min

D. Desired Gas Flow:

$$\frac{\text{Present } PcO_2}{\text{Desired } PcO_2} \times \text{Present Gas Flow} = \text{New Gas Flow}$$

E. Correction For Bicarbonate Deficit:

$$\frac{\text{Wt. (kg)} \times \text{Base Deficit} \times 0.3}{2} = \text{mEq of } NaHcO_3 \text{ to give}$$

Policy and Procedure Guidelines
CP28

HEMOCHRON QA

Hemochron Quality Control products are intended to verify proper instrument and test performance, as well as operator technique. Control Plasma is manufactured using nonhuman plasma and provides tests results similiar to those obtained clinically. This institution utilizes Control Plasma Level 2 (CPL-2), which contains both normal and abnormal controls. It is reccomended that both a normal and abnormal control be performed once per shift each day the Hemochron is used clinically. The results are recorded, and the data may be analyzed to establish quality assurance of routine testing. Hemochron Quality Control products verify the accuracy, precision, and reliability of coagulation test values obtained during cardiopulmonary bypass.

EQUIPMENT:

2 vials of distilled, de-ionized water (2.5 cc)
2 vials of 0.025 M calcium chloride (1.5 cc)
1 vial tan-labeled normal nonhuman plasma (2.0 cc dried)
1 vial red-labeled abnormal Level 2 nonhuman plasma (2 cc dried)
Hemochron machine
2 plastic syringes
Hemochron coagulation test tubes

PROCEDURE

1. Withdraw 2 cc from distilled water vial. Transfer to plasma vial by direct puncture of stopper. Depress Hemochron start button.
2. Vigorously agitate plasma vial for 30 s. Restart timer and allow vial to stabalize for 60 s.
3. During stabilization, fill a syringe with 1 cc of $CaCl_2$.
4. After 60 s, dispense 1 cc $CaCl_2$ into stabilized vial. While firmly holding syringe in place, vigorously agitate 5 times. Do not remove syringe and needle from vial.

5. With same syringe, withdraw 2 cc of the mixture and dispense into the test tube, while depressing the Hemochron start button. Agitate vigorously from end to end 10 times.
6. Insert tube into Hemochron and turn clockwise until green light appears. Turn one additional revolution to assure illumination of green light.
7. At buzzer, record result.

This procedure is followed for both the normal and abnormal controls.

Note: If kept refrigerated, allow plasma, water, and calcium vials to reach room temperature for at least 20 min before use.

Now performed by Point of Care Testing.

Policy and Procedure Guidelines
CP29

DETERMINATION OF STAT BLOOD GASES AND CHEMISTRIES BY PERFUSIONISTS USING THE I-STAT PORTABLE CLINICAL ANALYZER

The policies and procedures contained in this manual are to be strictly followed. For additional information or assistance call Point of Care Testing.

Warning! The Policy of Universal Precautions must be followed during all laboratory procedures. This is mandated by OSHA.

PURPOSE OF TEST

The I-STAT Chemistry Analyzer is used in patient care areas:

1. where results are needed urgently (e.g., intensive care unit/emergency room/operating room)
2. where there is requirement to reduce the specimen size (e.g., nurseries)
3. where patient treatment regimes require it (e.g., dialysis or CPB).

Regulatory Considerations/Responsibilities

Note: Only personnel with documented training on this instrument may operate it. Violations of these regulations of the policies and procedures that follow will result in the removal of the system from the patient care area until satisfactory remedial action is taken.

INTRODUCTION

The I-STAT system incorporates comprehensive components needed to perform blood analysis at the point of care. Just 2–3 drops of fresh whole blood is all that is required, and the portable battery-operated analyzer displays quantitative test results in approximately 2 min. The system consists of the following: the cartridge, the analyzer, and a central data station.

PRINCIPLES OF THE TESTS

A single-use disposable cartridge contains a microfabricated sensor array, a calibrant solution, fluidics system, and a waste chamber. Sensors for analysis of sodium, potassium, chloride, ionized calcium, pH, PCO_2, PO_2, urea nitrogen (BUN), glucose, and hematocrit are available in a variety of panels. A whole blood sample of approximately 2–4 drops is dispensed into the cartridge sample well.

A handheld analyzer into which the blood-filled cartridge is placed for analysis automatically controls all functions of the testing cycle, including fluid movement within the cartridge, calibration, and continuous quality monitoring. Analyzers with thermal control capability for testing at 37°C and cartridges requiring thermal control are labeled with a 37°C symbol.

A dedicated desktop computer, called the I-STAT Central Data Station, provides the primary information management capabilities for the I-STAT system. IR Links allow for transmission of patient records from a widely distributed network of analyzers to the central data station. Data can be stored, organized, edited, and transferred to a laboratory information system or other computer.

SUPPLIES AND STORAGE REQUIREMENTS

Cartridges

Store the main supply of the cartridges at 2 and 8°C (35–46°F.) Do not allow cartridges to freeze. Cartridges may be stored at room temperature (18–30°C or 64–86°F) for 14 d. Cartridges should never be returned to the refrigerator once they have been at room temperature, and should not be exposed to temperatures above 30°C (86°F). Mark the calendar on the box to indicate the 2-wk room temperature expiration date. Cartridges should remain in pouches until time of use. Do not use after the labeled expiration date.

Blood Collection and Transfer Equipment

Plastic syringe or blood gas syringe.

Controls

Electronic Simulator. Store at room temperature and protect contact pads from contamination by placing the electronic simulator in its protective case.

Liquid controls will be stored and performed by the Point of Care Testing laboratory.

BLOOD SPECIMENS

Suitable Specimens

Fresh whole blood collected in plastic syringe without anticoagulant (test within 3 min of collection).

Fresh whole blood collected in a syringe with lithium and sodium heparin anticoagulant (fill tubes to capacity; fill syringes for correct blood to heparin ratio). Test within 10 min of collection.

Specimen Labeling

Unless the specimen is analyzed immediately after collection and then discarded, the specimen container must be labeled with the following information:

Patient name, sex, age
Patient ID number
Time and date of collection
Phlebotomist ID
Doctor's name

SPECIMEN COLLECTION

Arterial Specimens

Fill blood gas syringe to the recommended capacity or use the least amount of liquid heparin anticoagulant that will prevent clotting. Underfilling syringes containing liquid heparin will decrease results due to dilution and decrease ionized calcium results due to binding. For ionized calcium, balanced or low-volume heparin blood gas syringes are recommended.

Mix blood and anticoagulant by rolling syringe between palms for at least 5 s, and then inverting the syringe repeatedly for at least 5 s. Avoid or remove immediately any air drawn into the syringe to maintain anaerobic conditions. A blood sample should be tested within 10 min after it has been obtained.

Venous Specimens

If a cartridge cannot be filled immediately, collect sample into an evacuated blood collection tube or a syringe containing heparin (sodium, lithium, or balanced) anticoagulant. For ionized calcium measurements, balanced heparin or 10 IU/ml of sodium or lithium heparin is recommended. Fill tubes to capacity; fill syringes for correct blood to heparin ratio. Incomplete filling causes higher heparin to blood ratio, which will decrease ionized calcium results and may affect other results.

Mix blood and anticoagulant by rolling syringe between palms for at least 5 s, and then inverting the syringe repeatedly for at least 5 s. If possible, test samples immediately after they are drawn; samples should be tested within 10 min (remix before testing).

Criteria for Specimen Testing

Evidence of clotting
Specimens collected in vacuum tubes with anticoagulant other than lithium or sodium heparin.
Syringe for pH, PCO_2, PO_2 with air bubbles in sample
Other sample types, such as urine, Cerebrospinal Fluid, and pleural fluid

Avoid the following circumstances:

Hemolysis (a traumatic draw)
Icing before filling cartridge
Time delays before filling cartridge
Exposing the sample to air when measuring pH, PCO_2, and PO_2

PROCEDURE FOR ANALYSIS

Preparation for Use

Cartridges requiring thermal control (i.e., blood gases) should stand at room temperature for 4 h before use (individually or an entire box). Individual cartridges that do not require thermal control can be used after standing just 5 min at room temperature. An entire box should stand for 1 h at room temperature before use.

Procedure

1. Remove the cartridge from the pouch. Avoid touching the contact pads or exerting pressure over the calibrant pack in the center of the cartridge.
2. Direct the syringe tip containing the blood into the sample well.
3. Dispense the sample until it reaches the fill TO mark on the cartridge. Leave some sample in the well.
4. Close the cover over the sample well until it snaps into place. (Do not press over the sample well.)
5. Insert the cartridge door until it clicks into place.
6. Enter a 6-digit operator ID number. Repeat the number for verification.
7. Enter the 7-digit patient ID number. Repeat the number for verification.

8. Enter the parameters (if required) for cartridges requiring thermal control. Patient temperature can be entered as degrees Centigrade or Fahrenheit. Use the * key for decimal point.

%FIO_2 can be entered as the number of liters or as a percentage of the oxygen a patient is receiving.
Field 1 and 2 are user-defined fields for up to 6 digits, typically used for ventilator settings such as PIP or PEEP.
Choose the number corresponding to the type of sample used when prompted at the sample type field.
Press the SAVE soft key to record the blood gas parameters entered.

9. View results shown on analyzer's display screen.

Alternative Procedure

Should the I-STAT system become inoperable for any reason, specimens should be collected and submitted to the Laboratory in accordance with the Laboratory Procedure Manual.

RESULTS

Calculations

The I-STAT analyzer contains a microprocessor that performs all calculations required for reporting results.

Note that results outside the expected ranges should be repeated on another I-STAT analyzer, or a sample should be sent to the laboratory for confirmation. No clinical decisions should be made on a questionable result until it is confirmed.

Suppressed Results

There are three conditions under which the I-STAT system will not display results:

1. Results outside the system's reportable ranges are flagged with ">" or "<", indicating that the result is below the lower limit or above the upper limit of the reportable range, respectively.
2. Results that are unreportable based on QC rejection criteria are flagged with "*****"
   Action:
   Analyze the specimen again, using another cartridge. The results that are not suppressed should be reported in the usual manner. If the result is suppressed again, send specimen(s) to the laboratory for analysis in accordance with the Laboratory Procedure Manual.

3. Results will not be reported if a test cycle has a problem with a sample, calibrant solution, sensors, mechanical, or electrical functions of the analyzer.
   Action:
   Take the action displayed with the message that identifies the problem. Refer to the I-STAT system manual's troubleshooting section if necessary.

Reporting Results

Transmitting Results to the Central Data Station

1. Place the analyzer in the cradle of the IR Interface of Link. The IR status light must be green.
2. To transmit the displayed test record, press the * key.
3. To transmit all stored test records, access stored results from the menu. Press the 3 key on the analyzer to transmit all test records.
4. Do not move the analyzer while "transmitting" is displayed. During transmission, the IR Status light will blink alternately red and green. If transmission is successful, the IR Link will emit a single high-pitched beep, and the light will return to green. An unsuccessful transmission is indicated by three low tone beeps. In this case, repeat the transmission process. If unsuccessful the second time, notify the I-STAT Program Coordinator.

QUALITY CONTROL

Daily Procedures

Analyzer Verification

Verify the performance of each analyzer in the I-STAT system using an electronic simulator once on each day of use.

If PASS is displayed on the analyzer screen remove the electronic simulator after the LCK message disappears from the display screen. Transmit the result to the central data station. Use the analyzer as required.

If FAIL is displayed on the analyzer screen repeat the procedure with the same electronic simulator. If PASS is displayed, use the analyzer as required. If FAILED is displayed, repeat the procedure with a different electronic simulator.

If PASS is displayed with the second electronic simulator use the analyzer as required and deliver the questionable electronic simulator to the I-STAT system coordinator.

If fail is displayed with the second electronic simulator, DO NOT analyze patient samples with the analyzer. Transmit the result to the central data station and deliver the faulty analyzer to the I-STAT system coordinator.

Verification of Cartridge Storage Conditions

Refrigerated Cartridges

1. Verify that the cartridges stored in the refrigerator are all within the expiration date printed on the boxes. Deliver any expired cartridges to the I-STAT system coordinator.
2. Verify that the refrigerator did not exceed the limits of 2–8°C (35–46°F). Use cartridges as required. If the temperature of the cartridge storage refrigerator is within the range of 2–8°C (35–46°F), use cartridges as required. If the temperature is outside the range of 2–8°C (35–46°F), quarantine the cartridges in the storage refrigerator. Notify the I-STAT system coordinator immediately. Do not use the cartridges from the out of control refrigerator.

Room Temperature Cartridges

Verify that all boxes of cartridges at room temperature have been out of the refrigerator for less than 2 wk. Deliver any expired cartridges to the I-STAT System Coordinator. If the measured temperature of the room has been continuously below 30°C (86°F), use cartridges as required. If the measured temperature of the room has exceeded 30°C (86°F) for any period of time, quarantine the cartridges and notify the I-STAT system coordinator immediately.

INTEGRITY TESTING

To be performed by Point of Care Testing laboratory.

CALIBRATION

Calibration is automatically performed as part of the test cycle on each cartridge. Operator intervention is not necessary.

PRINCIPLES OF MEASUREMENT

Sodium, potassium, chloride, ionized calcium, pH, and PCO_2 are measured by ion-selective electrode potentiometry. Concentrations are calculated from the measured potential through the Nernst equation.

Urea is first hydrolyzed to ammonium ions in a reaction catalyzed by the enzyme urease. The ammonium ions are measured by an ion-selective electrode, and the concentration is calculated from the measured potential through the Nernst equation.

Glucose is measured amperometrically. Oxidation of glucose which is catalyzed by the enzyme glucose oxidase, produces hydrogen peroxide. The liberated hydrogen peroxide is oxidized at an electrode to produce an electric current that is proportional to the glucose concentration.

PO2 is measured amperometrically. The oxygen sensor is similar to a conventional Clark Electrode. Oxygen permeates through a gas-permeable membrane from the blood sample into an internal electrolyte solution, where it is reduced at the cathode. The oxygen reduction current is proportional to the dissolved oxygen concentration.

Hematocrit is determined conductometrically. The measured conductivity, after correction for electrolyte concentration, is inversely related to the hematocrit.

Policy and Procedure Guidelines

CP30

Nitric oxide (NO) protocol is maintained by respiratory therapy. For full protocol guidelines, please refer to the manual for NO use in the Respiratory Therapy Department.

SETUP AND PRE-USE PROCEDURE FOR THE OHMEDA I-NOVENT DELIVERY SYSTEM

Purpose

To ensure the safe delivery of NO, an inhalationl gas, through the I-NOvent delivery system.

Supportive Data

1. When inhaled in concentrations as low as 1–20 parts per million (ppm), NO has been shown to be a selective vasodilator of the pulmonary artery bed in patients suffering from pulmonary hypertension.
2. Nitric oxide has improved arterial oxygenation by selectively vasodilating capillaries in well-ventilated alveoli, thereby reducing shunting.
3. Nitric oxide does not cause systemic vasodilation.
4. When exposed to oxygen, NO can form nitric dioxide (NO_2) and other toxic oxides of nitrogen. These gases can cause lung damage. In addition, when NO and NO_2 are exposed to moisture, nitric acid and nitrous acid can form. Both acids can cause interstitial pneumonitis.
5. Therefore, the I-Novent is the preferred system for NO delivery because it provides accurate dosage and measurement of NO and NO_2.

Equipment Needed

1. Ohmeda I-NOvent Delivery System (includes: injector module, size **D** NO cylinder)
2. Mechanical ventilator
   —7200AE/model 840
   —Siemens 900C/model 300
   —Infant Star 500
3. Oxygen source

Procedure

Confirmation of connections and leak test/purge and performance system

1. Connect one end of black hose to 50 psi oxygen supply source (H tank or wall outlet).
2. Turn I-Novent on and confirm the buzzer and speaker sound.
3. Turn each NO cylinder on and off one at a time to assure they pressurize. Wait 30 s and check for pressure decrease, indicating a leak. If there is a pressure drop, check for leaks around the connections and tighten NO cylinder valves.
4. Press calibration button and then press Control wheel to perform a low calibration of NO, $N0_2$, and 0_2 sensors on room air. Wait for message "Calibration Complete." Now press Control wheel to confirm and "Exit to Normal Display."
5. Connect thin, green oxygen tubing to flowmeter outlet and turn flow to 15 LPM.
6. Press "SET NO" button and turn Control wheel to the right, increasing NO level to 80 ppm. Press Control wheel to confirm it. Observe that each NO cylinder pressure gauge drops to zero one at a time. Wait for message "Low NO/N2 Pressure, Delivery Failure."

Key Point: This procedure washes $N0_2$ out from the system. This step also confirms the function of audible and visual alarm condition.

7. Turn on the one tank you intend to use (turn all the way on).
8. Press "SET NO" button, decrease NO level to 40 ppm by turning Control wheel to the left and confirm it. Wait for acceptable ranges:

02% +/– 3%: 95%
$N0_2$ ppm max: 1.5 ppm
NO ppm min/max: 32/48 ppm

Key Point: This is to confirm accuracy of delivered and measured gases.

9. Turn off oxygen flow from 15 to 0.
10. Press "SET NO" button and turn NO to zero. Press Control wheel to confirm. Do not turn off NO tank until manual system performance test is completed.

Key Point: If the system is not used within 5 min you must purge NO_2 from the system.

Key Point: When using INOvent in the operating room, the fresh gas flow must exceed minute volume (BPM × TV).

A. Ohmeda Manual NO Delivery Purge and Performance:

1. Disconnect oxygen tubing from auxiliary oxygen flow meter and connect it to back nozzle of INOvent (marked NO/02).
2. Connect green high-pressure oxygen hose to auxiliary oxygen flow meter outlet.
3. Take sample line sensor T-adapter and connect to purple adapter with oxygen tubing.
4. Increase oxygen flow to 15 and make sure black float for NO/02 rises midway in column window.
5. Make sure NO reading is 20 (+/– 8 ppm) and the $N0_2$ reading is <1 ppm.
6. Reduce oxygen flow to 1 L/min and make sure black float drops to bottom of NO/02 column window.
7. Reduce oxygen flow to 0.
8. Turn off NO tank.
9. After performing the test, the INOvent will be ready for patient use.

B. "Purge Test" must be performed 5 min *before* the start of NO therapy.

1. Make sure NO tank is turned off.
2. Disconnect the (short) black low-pressure hose quick-connect fitting from the NO/N2 input on the rear of the INOvent Delivery System.
3. Purge or bleed the cylinder by putting the quick-connect fitting into the purge manifold (NO pressure will drop to zero on manometer).
4. Reconnect the low-pressure black (short) hose.
5. Open the NO cylinder and confirm a steady pressure on manometer.
6. Set NO as per physician orders and confirm by pressing the Control wheel. Wait approximately 3 min for stabilization.

C. Alarm Setting for Low and High NO

1. Set Low and High NO alarms as follows:
   Low = 5 below set NO level
   High = 10 above set NO level
2. Select alarm setting by pressing Alarms button and turning the Control wheel to select Low and High levels.
3. Press Control wheel to select low alarm (display reads OFF). Turning Control wheel to the right increases alarm level. Press Control wheel to confirm desired alarm limit.

4. Turn Control wheel to the right to set High alarm level. Press Control wheel to begin adjusting. Turning Control wheel to the left decreases alarm level to desired limit. Finally, press Control wheel to confirm.

Key Point: I-NOvent does not have a memory backup for operator set values, including alarms, once machine is turned off. Only factory-installed default parameters remain. For patient safety, if I-NOvent is turned off (even if briefly) while on a patient, the NO parameters must be reset, including alarms.

Taken from the Ohmeda Operation and Maintenance Manual and Module 4 of the Training Manual.

CHANGING NO THERAPY CYLINDERS AND PURGING THE REGULATOR ASSEMBLY ON THE OHMEDA INOVENT

Supportive Data

You MUST purge the regulator assembly immediately before using a new NO cylinder to make sure the patient continues to receive the correct NO concentration and does not receive high NO_2 concentrations.

A purge manifold is provided to allow purging the regulator assembly. It is located either between the regulators on the transport cart or attached to the wall mount regulator inlet fitting.

Key Point: Refer to the Ohmeda INOvent operation and maintenance manual, section 6–11.

Procedure

Key Point: Replace an NO therapy gas cylinder when its pressure is 500 or less. (Call INOTherapeutics to deliver replacement cylinder)

To purge the regulator assembly before using a new NO therapy gas cylinder:

a. Determine which regulator assembly is not being used and requires purging. The cylinder valve should be closed on the regulator assembly, which is not being used.
b. On the regulator assembly that requires purging, disconnect the low-pressure hose quick-connect fitting from NO/N2 input on the rear of the INOvent Delivery System.

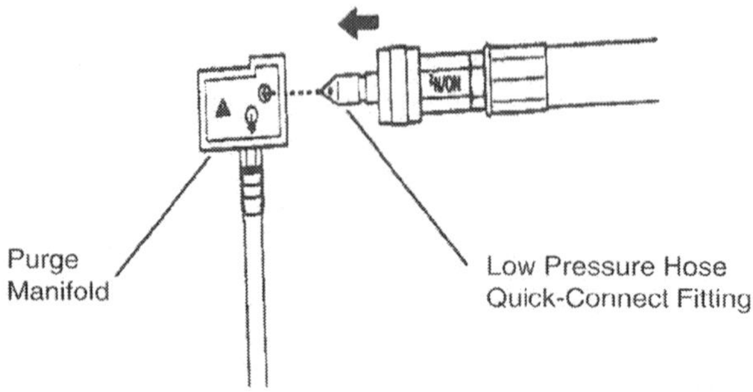

Fig. 1. Connecting to the purge manifold for regulator assembly purging.

c. Open the cylinder valve on the new NO therapy gas cylinder.
d. Close the cylinder valve on the "empty" NO therapy gas cylinder.
e. Check for leaks at the cylinder valve outlet connection of the new therapy cylinder with soapy water.
f. Insert the low-pressure hose quick-connect fitting into the purge manifold (Fig. 1).
g. Firmly push and hold the quick-connect fitting in place while the pressure drops to zero on the regulator gauge.
h. After the pressure drops to zero (approximately 15 s), reconnect the low-pressure hose quick-connect fitting to the NO/N2 input on the rear of the INOvent Delivery System.
i. Open the cylinder valve on the new cylinder.
j. Close the cylinder valve on the empty cylinder and label appropriately.
k. Replace the empty NO therapy gas cylinder. Leave the cylinder valve on the replacement cylinder turned off until needed. The purge procedure will be performed on this cylinder immediately before its use.

Taken from the Ohmeda Operation and Maintenance Manual and Module 4 of the Training Manual.

INOVENT MANUAL DELIVERY SYSTEM SETUP AND USE

Purpose

To ensure the continued delivery of NO in the event of INOvent system failure and to provide continued NO Therapy during manual resuscitation.

Policy

The INOvent Manual NO Delivery System must be set up and available for use at all times.

Supportive Data

1. The manual NO delivery system permits continued NO delivery if the ventilator or the main INOvent Delivery System fails. The manual system is completely pneumatic and is not linked to the primary delivery system.

2. The Manual NO Delivery System is used in conjunction with a Pressure Compensated Oxygen Flowmeter and a manual resuscitator bag to **deliver a concentration of 20 ppm NO 6 ppm to the patient with an oxygen flowrate of 15 L/m.**

3. The oxygen flowmeter provides the ON/OFF function and is used to set the oxygen flow at 15 L/min. A shutoff valve in the delivery system prevents NO flow if there is insufficient oxygen flow.

4. When the manual NO delivery system is operating correctly, the float in the NO Flow Indicator Window will be in the middle.

Procedure

Key Point: When setting a patient up on nitric oxide in the Critical Care Unit, always ensure the Ohmeda Nitric Oxide Manual Delivery System is setup and confirmed ready for use (Fig. 2).

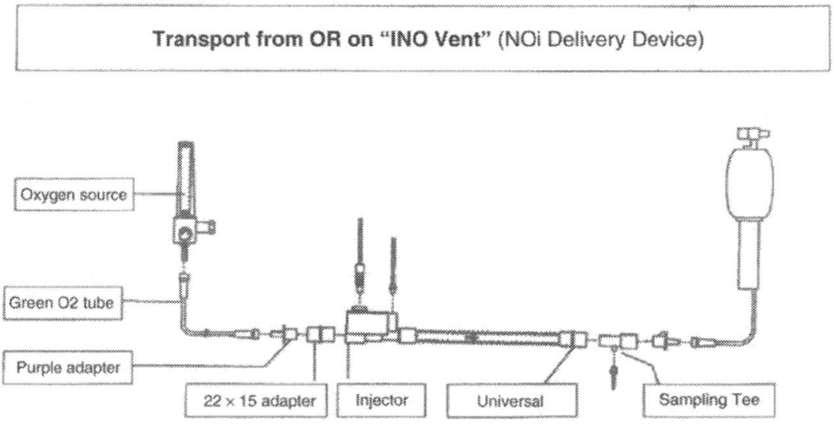

Fig. 2. Typical setup for transport of a patient from the operating room on an INOvent.

Key Point: A "purge test" must be performed 5 min before the start of NO therapy (Refer to policy and procedure topic: Set-up and Preuse Procedure for the Ohmeda INOvent Delivery System). **If you need to use the Ohmeda Manual Delivery System emergently, remember to purge the system by squeezing the resuscitator bag 5–6 times before attaching to the patient.**

INOVENT MANUAL DELIVERY SYSTEM SETUP

A. Connect oxygen tubing attached to the manual resuscitator bag to the NO/O2 output connector on the back of the INOvent Delivery System.

B. Attach the green oxygen high-pressure tubing to the oxygen port on the back of the INOvent and attach the other end to the flow meter on the side of the INOvent. The black high-pressure tubing attached to the flow meter "T" will then be attached to the wall oxygen outlet in the patient's room. (You could also attach to an oxygen cylinder).

C. To use the manual system, turn the oxygen flow meter on to 15 L/min and make sure black float for NO/O2 rises midway in column window.

Remember to purge system by squeezing the manual resuscitator bag at least 5–6 times before attaching to the patient.

Key Point: Remember to turn the oxygen flow meter off when not using the manual system.

PERFUSION INOVENT CHECKLIST

A. Preuse System Setup and Performance Test

1. Connect one end of black hose to 50 psi oxygen supply source (H tank or wall outlet) (Fig. 3).
2. Turn INOvent on and confirm the buzzer and speaker sound.
3. Turn each NO cylinder on and off one at a time to pressurize. Wait 30 s and check for pressure decrease, indicating a leak. If there is a pressure drop, check for leaks around the connections and tighten NO cylinder valves.
4. Press calibration button and then press Control wheel to perform a low calibration of NO, $N0_2$, and 0_2 censors on room air. Wait for message "Calibration Complete." Now press Control wheel to confirm and "Exit To Normal Display."
5. Connect thin, green 0_2 tubing to flowmeter outlet, and turn flow to 15 L/mm.

ANESTHESIA MACHINE CONNECTION FOR NITRIC OXIDE DELIVERY
(OHMEDA INO-VENT)

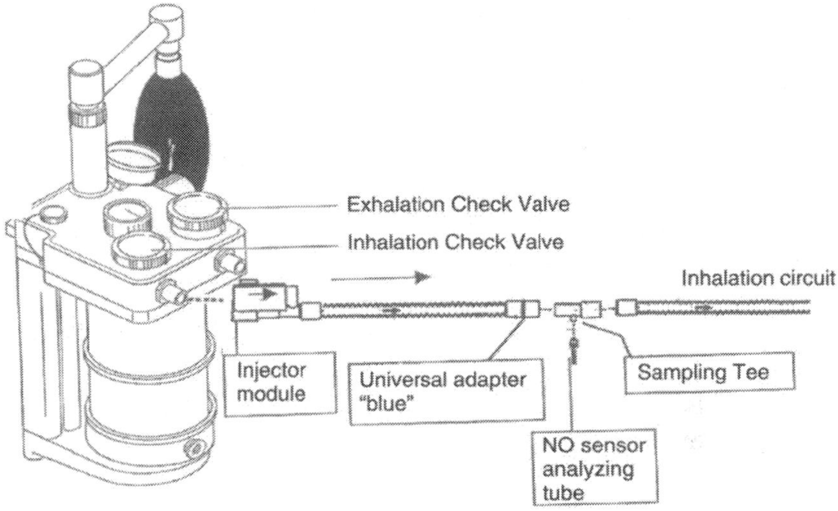

Fig. 3. Typical setup from the INOvent to the anesthesia machine.

6. Press SET NO button and turn Control wheel to the right, increasing NO level to 80 ppm. Press Control wheel to confirm it. Observe that each NO cylinder pressure gauge drops to zero one at a time. Wait for message: Delivery Failure, Low NO/N2 Pressure.

Key Point: This procedure washes $N0_2$ out from the system. This step also confirms the function of audible and visual alarm condition.

7. Turn on the one tank you intend to use.
8. Press SET NO button, decrease NO level to 40 ppm by turning Control wheel to the left, and confirm it. Wait for acceptable ranges:
   02% +/− 3%: 95%
   $N0_2$ ppm max: 1.5 ppm
   NO ppm min/max: 32/48 ppm

Key Point: This is to confirm accuracy of delivered and measured gases.

9. Turn off O_2 flow from 15 to 0.

10. Press SET NO button and turn NO to 0. Press Control wheel to confirm. Do not turn off NO tank until manual system performance test is completed.

*Note: If the system is not used within 5 min you must purge NO_2 from the system (**see** Purge Test)*

B. Alarm Setting For Low and High NO

1. Set Low and High NO alarms as follows: Low = 5 below set NO level and High = 10 above set NO level.
2. Select alarm setting by pressing Alarms button and turning the Control wheel to select Low and High levels.
3. Press Control wheel to select low alarm (display reads OFF). Turning Control wheel to the right increases alarm level. Press Control wheel to confirm desired alarm limit.
4. Turn Control wheel to the right to set High alarm level. Press Control wheel to begin adjusting. Turning Control wheel to the left decreases alarm level to desired limit. Finally, press Control wheel to confirm.

Key Point: **INOvent does not have a memory backup for operator set values, including alarms, once machine is turned off. Only factory-installed default parameters remain. For patient safety, if INOvent is turned off (even if briefly) while on a patient, the NO parameters must be reset, including alarms.**

C. Purge Test (Purge Test must be performed 5 min *before* the start of NO therapy)

1. Make sure NO tank is turned off.
2. Disconnect the black low-pressure hose quick-connect fitting from the NO/N2 input on the rear of the INOvent delivery system.
3. Purge or bleed the cylinder by putting the quick-connect fitting into the purge manifold (NO pressure will drop to 0 on manometer).
4. Reconnect the low-pressure hose.
5. Open the NO cylinder and confirm a steady pressure on manometer.
6. Set NO as per physician orders and confirm by pressing the Control wheel. Wait for approximately 3 min for stabilization.

D. Manual NO Delivery System Purge and Performance Test

1. Disconnect thin, green oxygen tube from auxiliary oxygen flowmeter and connect it to the manual output nozzle on the back of INOvent (marked NO/O2)

2. Connect heavy, reinforced green oxygen hose to auxiliary oxygen flowmeter outlet.
3. Take sample line censor T-adapter and connect to purple adapter with oxygen tubing.
4. Increase oxygen flow to 15 and make sure black float for NO/02 rises midway in column window.
5. Make sure NO reading is 20 (+/– 8 ppm) and the $N0_2$ reading is <l ppm.
6. Reduce oxygen flow to 1 and make sure black float drops to bottom of NO/02 column window.
7. Reduce oxygen flow to 0.
8. Turn off NO tank.
9. After performing the above test the INOvent will be ready for patient use.

Policy and Procedure Guidelines
CP31

PROCEDURE FOR OXYGENATOR CHANGEOUT

Is your oxygenator failing? Mechanical considerations need to be evaluated before oxygenator changeout (Fig. 1).

1) Is oxygen being delivered to the oxygenator?
2) Is the gas path obstructed?
3) Is the gas connected to the correct port?
4) Are FiO_2 and gas flow appropriate?

Patient considerations need to be evaluated

1) Is the hematocrit adequate?
2) What is the temperature?
3) Is blood flow adequate?
4) Are anesthesia and relaxant levels adequate?

Calculate O_2 transfer of your oxygenator.

(arterial O_2 content – venous O_2 content) × (10) × (flow in LPM)

$$\text{Art. Content} = [(\text{art. sat.}\%) \times (1.34\,\text{ml } O_2) \times (\text{Hgb gm }\%)] + [(PaO_2)(.003)]$$

$$\text{Ven.Content} = [(\text{ven. sat.}\%)(1.34\,\text{ml } O_2)(\text{Hgb gm }\%)] + [(PvO_2)(.003)]$$

Maximum Value = 360 ml/min @ blood flow 6 L/min
gas flow 15 L/min
blood temp 37°C
hemoglobin 12 g/dl

ADDITIONAL EQUIPMENT

1) Oxygenator
2) Tubing clamps—4
3) 400 ml of prime solution
4) Sterile scissors

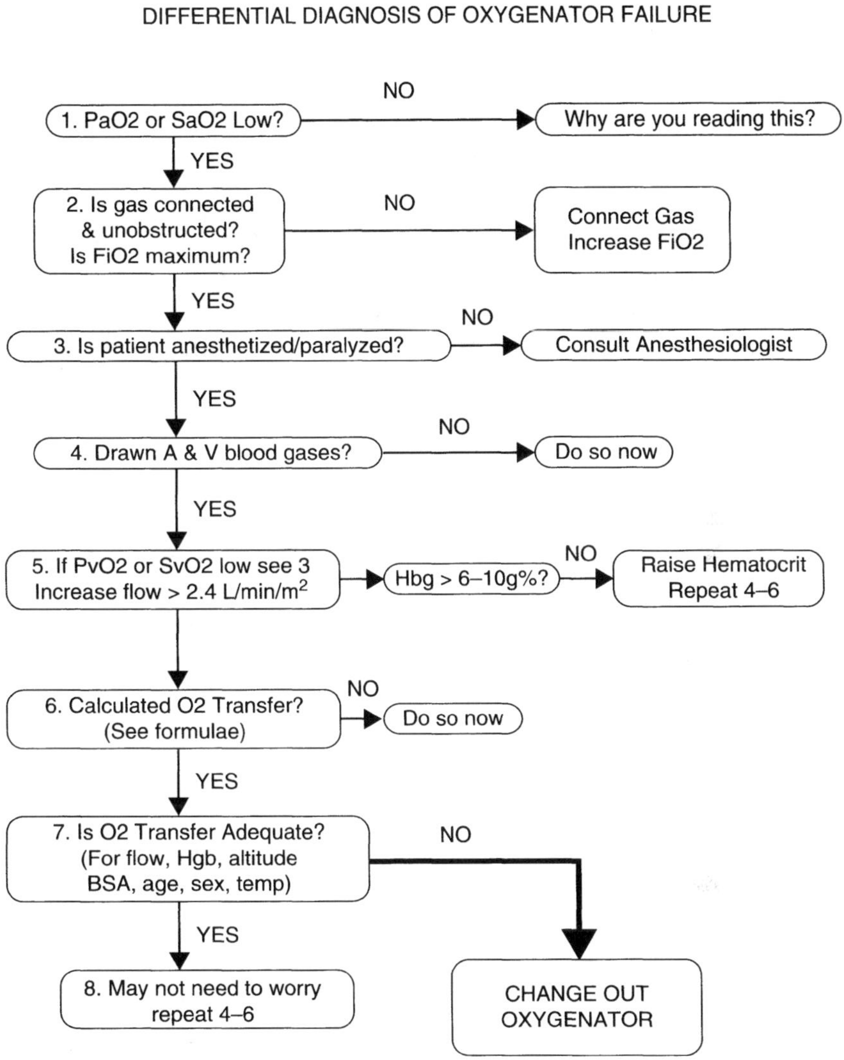

Fig. 1. Differential diagnosis of oxygenator failure.

PROCEDURE

Prepare to change out the oxygenator by getting any necessary extras into the room, including additional perfusionists, oxygenators, clamps, sterile scissors, etc. Notify the surgical team of your intentions and discuss your plans. If possible, terminate cardiopulmonary bypass (CPB) and remind anesthesia to ventilate. If changeout during bypass is unavoidable, then the following protocol should be observed. Turn off water lines and disconnect from oxygenator. Prep lines for sterile severance (alcohol). Remove new oxygenator from package. Come off bypass and clamp the arterial and venous lines to the patient and open the AV bridge. Clamp out the arterial filter and/or open the filter bypass. Double clamp all inlets and outlets of the oxygenator where you have previously prepped. Using sterile scissors, cut inlet and outlet tubings and remove the failed oxygenator. Insert new oxygenator into circuit and deair through the bridge. Replace oxygen delivery line to air/O_2 inlet on new oxygenator. Open the arterial filter and clamp/close the arterial filter bypass while recirculating. Deair filter. Come off recirculation and clamp the AV bridge. Reinitiate CPB as soon as possible. Reconnect water lines and open valves. Reuse checklist to confirm adequate reinitiation of CPB.

Policy and Procedure Guidelines
CP32

PROTAMINE ADMINISTRATION/REACTION—D

Protamine is a basic protein originating from salmon sperm that effectively neutralizes heparin. A number of hemodynamic effects are suggested after protamine neutralization of heparin. Guffin et al. showed a 50% reduction in postoperative bleeding with protamine doses adjusted to unneutralized heparin, suggesting an advantage to avoiding protamine overdosing and its anticoagululant and proinflammatory effects. This is accomplished with use of a heparin–protamine titration assay utilizing a Hepcon analyzer.

After the patient is off cardiopulmonary bypass (CPB) and is hemodynamically stable, heparin is reversed with protamine sulfate. This is accomplished by utilizing a Hepcon analyzer. If protamine titration assay is not available, a dosage of 1.3 mg protamine/mg of heparin is used. Before starting protamine, the perfusionist should be notified by anesthesia and all pump suctions should be turned off. If not notified, ask if protamine has been started.

Protamine is associated with a wide variety of cardiovascular responses that do not appear to be related to speed or total dose of administration. However, it seems prudent to administer protamine slowly in patients with impaired cardiovascular function or previous exposure to protamine. Some commonly seen hemodynamic profiles are:

1) No change.

2) Systemic vasodilatation with decreased arterial blood pressure and decreased ventricular filling pressures (volume, $CaCl_2$, or a peripheral alpha agonist are useful treatments).

3) With pulmonary artery vasoconstriction, there is an elevation in PA pressure, the heart dilates, and CVP increases. If right ventricle failure occurs, systemic BP and left-sided ventricular filling pressures decrease. (The treatment consists of inotropic support until right heart function returns to normal. Rarely, reinstitution of CPB may be necessary).

4) Myocardial depression and left ventricular failure manifested by increases in left ventricle (LV) filling. This may be more common in patients with preexisting LV dysfunction. (Additional inotropic and/or vasodilator support may be required).

Policy and Procedure Guidelines
CP33

POLICY FOR PERFUSION SETUP FOR STANDBY CASES AND EMERGENCY BACKUP

Emergency Procedure

The heart–lung machine and all disposable equipment needed are set up under sterile technique. The disposable setup is dry and not primed until needed by the perfusionist. The setup is moved to an area within the sterile confines of the operating room. The setup should remain ready for use within 72h. The setup is marked with time and date, as the same perfusionist may not be using this equipment.

Standby Procedures: OPCABs, Renal Tumor, Pericardiectomy, Type III Aneurysms, etc.

The heart–lung machine and all disposable equipment needed are setup under sterile technique. The disposable setup is CO_2 flushed and draped until needed by the perfusionist. The setup is moved into an operating room suite and draped to maintain sterility. If the pump is not primed and used, the setup is used for additional standby procedures and remains ready for use within 72h.

The surgeon may want to prime the heart–lung machine for the procedure and will proceed to cardiopulmonary bypass. In the event that the pump is then wet with prime, but not used, it must be used within 36h. The setup is marked with time and date, as the same perfusionist may not be using this equipment.

This policy is a guideline for use by the perfusionist. In the event that the pump setup is not clearly defined for a sterility time line, then the setup is disposed of and a new setup is required.

Off-Pump Coronary Artery Bypass (OPCAB)

The heart–lung machine and all disposable equipment needed are setup using strict aseptic technique. The disposable setup is CO_2 flushed and primed according to the manufacturer's instructions for use and departmental protocol. A CO_2 blower assembly is setup for OPCAB procedures. Heparin is administered at the surgeon's request at an initial dose of 150 U/kg. Activated clotting times (ACTs) are monitored 3 min after heparinization and, subsequently, every 30 min, with a target ACT of 300 s. After notification of the surgeon, additional heparin may be administered as needed to maintain a safe level of anticoagulation. Postprocedure heparin reversal may be accomplished by protamine administration using the Bull Curve heparin level technique or Medtronic Hepcon protamine titration assay. Heparin reversal should be confirmed by postprotamine ACT.

Policy and Procedure Guidelines

CP34

Refer to User's Manual for complete operating instructions

The Jostra Heater–Cooler Unit HCU 30 supplies temperature-controlled water for cardioplegia heat exchangers, for blood heat exchangers in extracorporeal circulation and for blankets with which patients can be warmed or cooled. The water temperature is adjustable from 1°C to 41°C. A 26L tank with ice and approximately 1°C cold water assures quick cooling of the patient. Two independent circuits with separate temperature controls can be attached (one of the circuits has two connections). A safety system monitors the regulation to prevent the temperature from rising above 42°C. The growth of algae, fungus, mold, bacteria, and other microbes are effectively prevented by the routine maintenance of heating the internal water path to 90°C utilizing the system's cleaning protocol.

FRONT VIEW OF THE HCU 30 (FIG. 1)

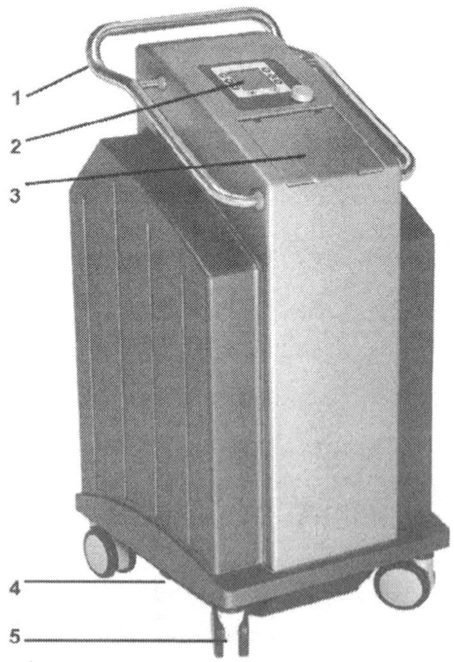

Fig. 1.

1. Handrail
2. Display panel
3. Lid over the funnel for the water tank
4. Opening for tank overflow/emptying
5. Wheels with foot-lever operated brake

REAR VIEW OF THE HCU 30 (FIG. 2)

1. Socket for remote control and service terminal.
2. Stopcock for the 1st patient circulation (open in vertical position).
3. Stopcock for the 2nd patient circulation (open in vertical position).
4. Stopcock for the cardioplegia circulation (open in vertical position).
5. Inlet (suction side) of the 1st patient circulation.
6. Outlet (pressure side) of the 1st patient circulation.
7. Inlet (suction side) of the 2nd patient circulation.
8. Outlet (pressure side) of the 2nd patient circulation.
9. Inlet (suction side) of the cardioplegia circulation.

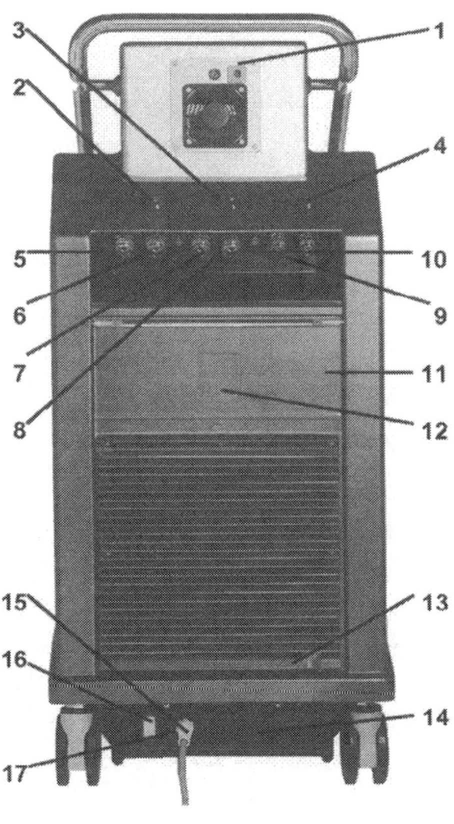

Fig. 2.

10. Outlet (pressure side) of the cardiplegia circulation.
11. Cleaning door.
12. Type label.
13. Drain lever. Remove the filter and lift the lever to empty the water tank.
14. Connection for potential equalization.
15. Mains cable.
16. Mains circuit-breaker.
17. Secondary circuit-breaker.

3/8″ connections are standard for the cardioplegia circulation and 1/2" for the patient circulation.

DISPLAY PANEL (FIG. 3)

1. Menu button, Press to switch between the menus "Main," "Status," "Daily maintenance," and "Maintenance & service."
2. Main menu button, Press to return to the main menu.
3. Set buttons. These buttons have different functions in different menus.
4. Cardioplegia circulation on/off button. The green light is lit when circulating.
5. Patient circulation on/off button. The green light is lit when circulating.
6. Adjustment knob.

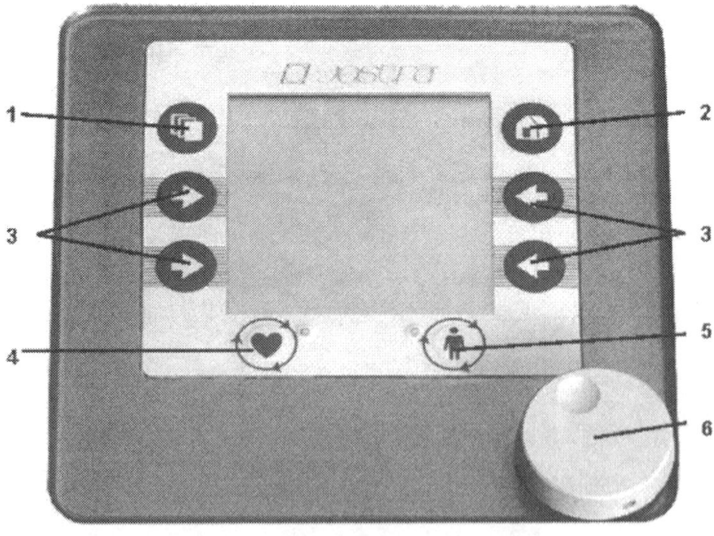

Fig. 3.

Fig. 4.

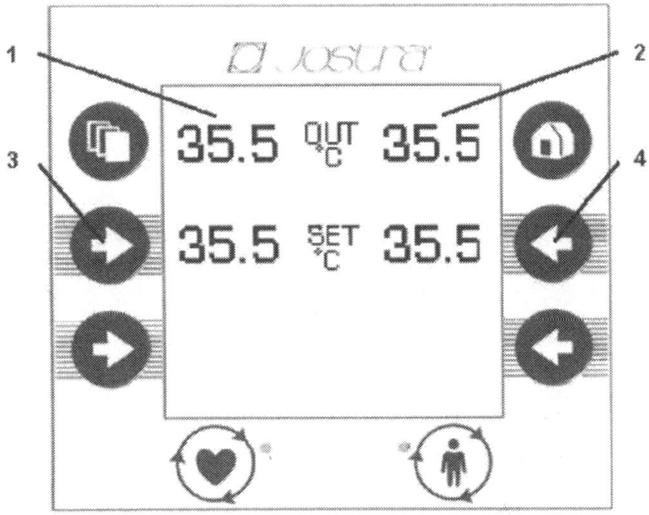

MAIN MENU ON DISPLAY PANEL (FIG. 4)

	Cardioplegia circulation	*Patient circulation*
Outlet water Temperature	1	2
Set button	3	4

Hold down the respective set button and turn the adjustment knob to set a temperature. Check that the outlet water temperature adjusts sufficiently fast and accurate to the set value.

STATUS MENU (FIG. 5)

1. Water level. Shows the water level graphically in four steps Fig. 6.
2. Ice level. Shows the amount of ice graphically in four steps Fig. 6.
3. Temperature of the cold water in the tank.
4. Compressor button. Press to start the compressor (before the autostart). The symbol flashes when the compressor is on. Press again to stop the compressor (before the autostop).

Cold water from the tank is pumped around the circulations during deairing. It stops automatically after 1.5 minutes. Water from the circulations is pumped to the tank during emptying. It stops automatically when dry or after a maximum of 1.5 min.

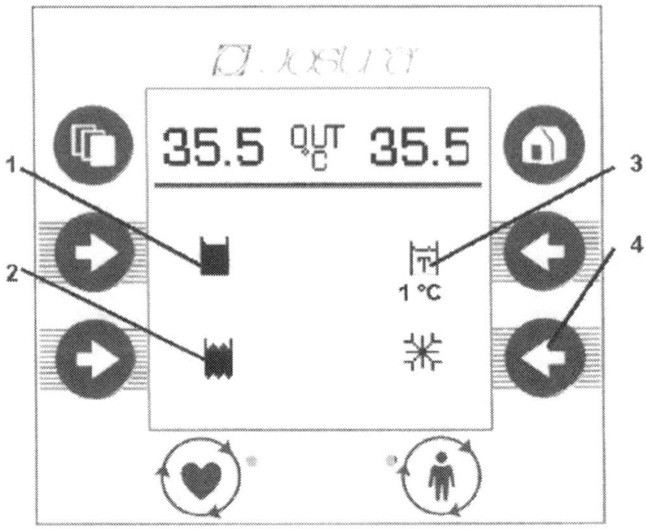

Fig. 5.

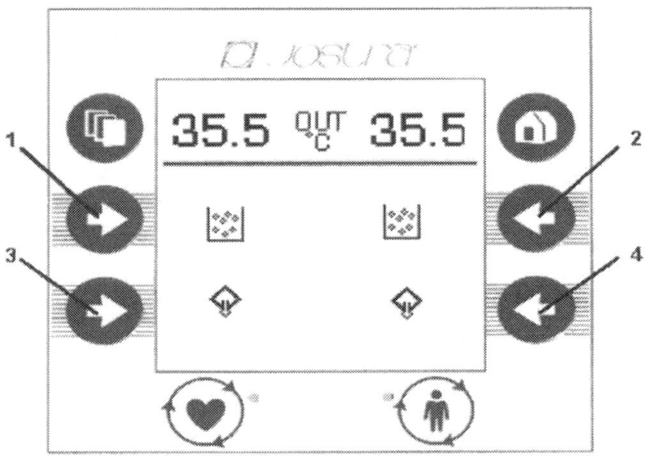

Fig. 6.

Daily maintenance menu
On/off button Cardioplegia circulation Patient circulation
De-airing 1 2 Emptying 3 4

MAINTENANCE AND SERVICE MENU (FIG. 7)

1. Timer page button. Press to enter the timer page (*see* Timer).
2. Cleaning page button. Press to enter the cleaning page (*see* Cleaning).

Fig. 7.

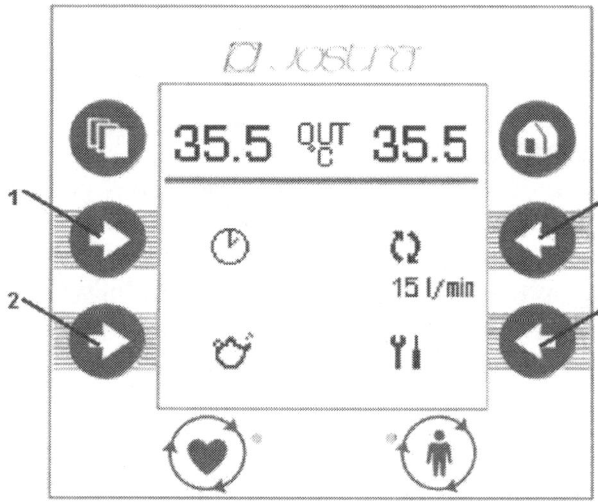

3. Set flow button. Hold down this button and turn the adjustment knob to set the patient circulation flow between 10 and 23 L/min.
4. Service button. Press to enter the service pages (*see* Service)

The patient circulation flow is also limited by the maximum pressure set in the service pages (and will, in practice, never reach 23 L/min). A higher flow gives a higher warming/cooling capacity (also depending on the heat exchanger), but also a higher outlet pressure.

PREPARATION FOR OPERATION

1. The HCU 30 should always be connected to the mains supply and switched on so that there is a sufficient amount of ice in the tank.

2. Switch off and switch on the mains circuit-breaker to let the HCU 30 run a self-test. The display shows a room glass during the test.

3. Connect the circulations to be used from the respective outlet to the respective inlet. (The 1st and 2nd patient circulation is intended for the blanket and the arterial heat exchanger, and the cardioplegia circulation for the cardioplegia heat exchanger.)

4. Open the stopcocks for the connected circulations.

5. Press the deairing button in the Daily maintenance menu for the connected circulations (patient and/or cardioplegia circulation). Run until the circulations are sufficiently free of air.

6. Set the start temperature to be used in the "Main menu" for the connected circulations (patient and/or cardioplegia circulation).

7. Press the circulation button for the connected circulations (patient and/or cardioplegia circulation). Circulate until the actual temperature has reached the set value.

⚠ Check that the outlet water temperature adjusts sufficiently fast and accurate to the set value.

Starting with 20°C, it takes approximately 4 h until there is a normal amount of ice in the tank. In an emergency, ice can be thrown directly into the tank for additional cooling capacity.

If the water tank is overfilled, or if a maximum filled unit is moved, the superfluous water is released through the opening for tank overflow (underneath).

AFTER OPERATION

1. Open the stopcocks for the connected circulations.
2. Press the emptying button in the "Daily maintenance menu" for the connected circulations (patient and/or cardioplegia circulation). Run until the circulations are sufficiently free of water.
3. Disconnect the emptied circulations.
4. Leave the HCU 30 switched on to maintain the ice in the tank.

REMOTE CONTROL UNIT (OPTIONAL) (FIG. 8)

The remote control unit works the same way as the display panel.

1. Attach holder, e.g., to a mast of a heart–lung machine.

Fig. 8.

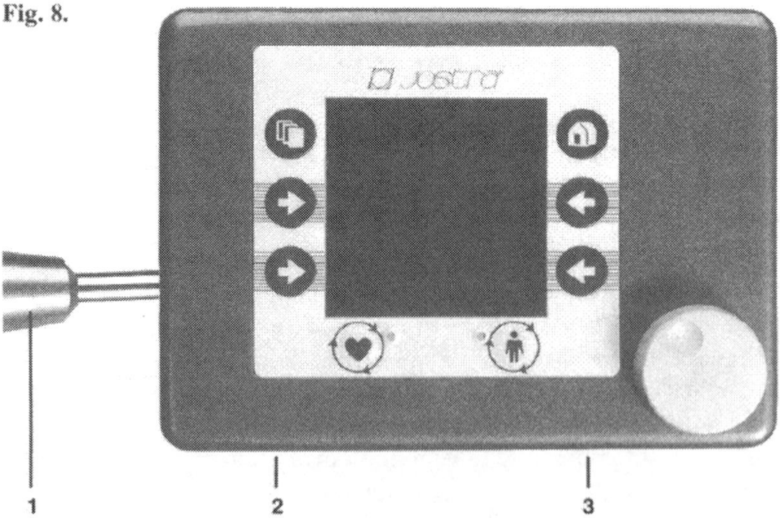

2. Temperature sensor socket for the cardioplegia circulation (underncath).
3. Temperature sensor socket for the patient circulation (underneath).
4. Remote control cable socket (rear side). Connect to the socket for remote control on the rear side of the HCU 30 with the remote control cable.
5. Socket for service terminal and programming (rear side).

GRADIENTS

As soon as a temperature sensor is connected to the remote control unit, the corresponding circulation will work in gradient mode. In gradient mode, the outlet water temperature deviates from the set value according to the relation described the following paragraph. Check that the outlet water temperature holds this relation to the set value, the measured temperature, and the gradient. Use insulated thermistor temperature probes of the YSI 400 series by Yellow Springs, or other compatible probes.

The functions for the patient circulation are pointed out in Fig. 9. The cardioplegia circulation works correspondingly.

1. Gradient (warming or cooling).
2. Set gradient button. Hold down this button and turn the adjustment knob to set the gradient.
3. Measured temperature.

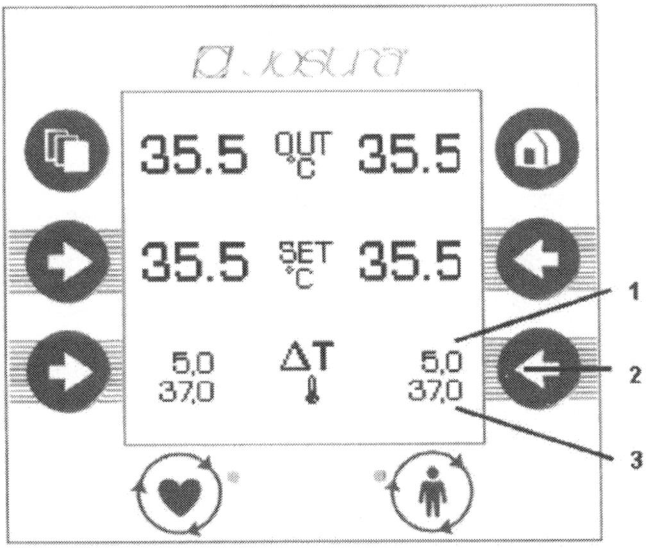

Fig. 9.

The patient will be warmed (or cooled) to the set temperature, but the water temperature, Tw, will not exceed (or fall below) the measured temperature, Tp, by more than the gradient, Tgrad.

$$Tw(max) = Tp + Tgrad \text{ (warming)}$$

or

$$Tw(min) = Tp - Tgrad \text{ (cooling)}$$

Example:

You want to warm a patient who has a current temperature of 27°C to the normal temperature of 37°C. In the "Main menu" the temperature is set to 37°C and the gradient to 8°C.

The water temperature is calculated: 27°C + 8°C = 35°C.

The water temperature now rises, keeping the gradient of +8°C constant, in relation to the patient temperature, until it reaches the preset upper limit of 41°C. The water now remains at this temperature until the patient has reached the set temperature of 37°C.

MAINTENANCE

CAUTION Do not use any fully desalinated or distilled water.

Daily

- Check that the water level is approximately 1 cm above the cooling spirals.
- Check that air can circulate unobstructed to the condenser (rear side) to ensure good cooling capacity. The unit must be at least 30 cm from walls or cupboards.

Weekly

- Clean the internal circulation (*see* Cleaning).
- If the internal circulation is not cleaned, remove the filter and lift the drain lever to empty the water tank. Refill with new softened water (through the funnel on top).

Every Other Week

- Remove the filter and lift the drain lever to empty the water tank. Refill with new softened water (through the funnel on top).

Monthly

(or after every 100 h of operation)

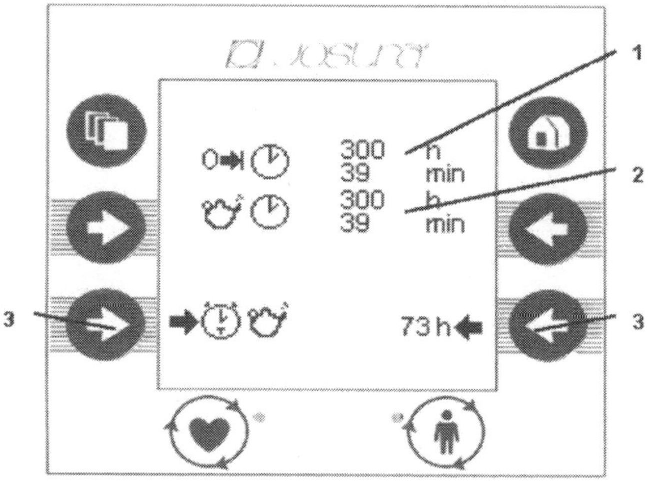

Fig. 10.

- Remove the filter at the back and clean the filter and the compressor with a soft brush.

Every 6 Mo

- A complete service by a service engineer is recommended.
  CAUTION △

Only use a household dishwashing liquid to clean the cover.

Do not flush the system with excessive water, as this could damage the electronics.

Do not use chemical solvents (such as alcohol, ether, and acetone) and do not spill anaesthetics (such as Forane [isoflurane], as this could damage the machine.

1. Operating hours. (Fig. 10)
2. Operating hours since the last cleaning.
3. Cleaning timer buttons. Hold down the right button and turn the adjustment knob to set the remaining time until the cleaning will start. Press both buttons to enter the cleaning page (*see* Cleaning).

Cleaning (Fig. 11)

Press both cleaning timer buttons in the timer page or the cleaning page button in the "Maintenance and service menu" to enter this page.

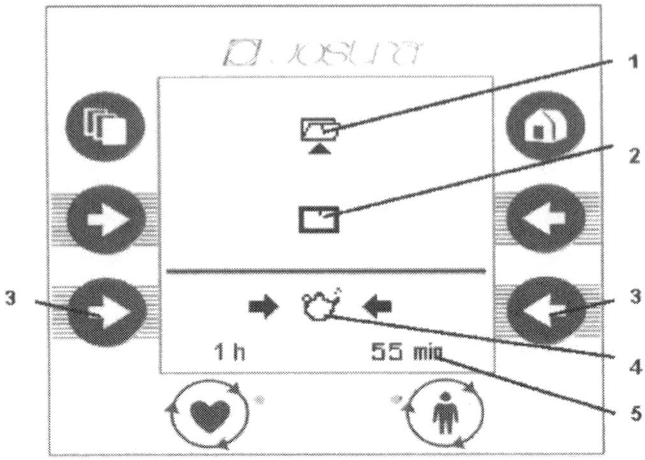

Fig. 11.

1. Cleaning door open symbol. Indicates that before cleaning all tubes must be disconnected from the HCU 30 and the cleaning door closed.
2. Cleaning door closed symbol. If the symbol flashes, open and close the cleaning door again (it must be closed while this page is visible).
3. Cleaning buttons. If the timer has not been set, press both these buttons to start the cleaning directly.
4. Countdown symbol. Alternates between a teapot and a clock to indicate countdown.
5. Remaining time until cleaning.

In the cleaning process, the internal water path will be heated to 90°C, followed by an automatic cooling down and ice building. A complete cleaning program takes approximately 10 h, until there is a normal amount of ice in the tank again.

WARNING ⚠ The circulation cannot be started until the tank temperature has sunk below 41°C after the cleaning. A warning is still appropriate. Heating the patient above 42°C can cause death or severe injury. Do not get into contact with hot water or steam from the tank during cleaning.

After cleaning, large ice crystals might cause the system to indicate an amount of ice that is normal or too much, although there is too little. This will improve during the next compressor cooling cycle.

As a suggestion, start the cleaning in the end of the working day once a week and the HCU 30 will be ready for operation directly the next day.

To interrupt the cleaning press the "Menu" or the "Main menu" button. An automatic cooling down starts.

START CLEANING WITH TIMER

1. Disconnect all tubes from the HCU 30.
2. Set the timer in the timer page.
3. Press both cleaning timer buttons to enter the cleaning page.
4. (Open and) close the cleaning door while the cleaning page is visible. Check that the cleaning door closed symbol is steadily visible.
5. The cleaning will start after the set time.

START CLEANING IMMEDIATELY

1. Disconnect all tubes from the HCU 30.
2. Make sure the timer is set to zero.
3. (Open and) close the cleaning door while the cleaning page is visible.
4. Press both cleaning buttons. Check that the cleaning starts.

- Contrast button. Hold down this button and turn the adjustment knob to set the contrast.
- Background light button. Hold down this button and turn the adjustment knob to set the background light.

Error messages (Fig. 12)

1. Menu button
2. Main menu button
3. Error symbol
4. Error mute buttons

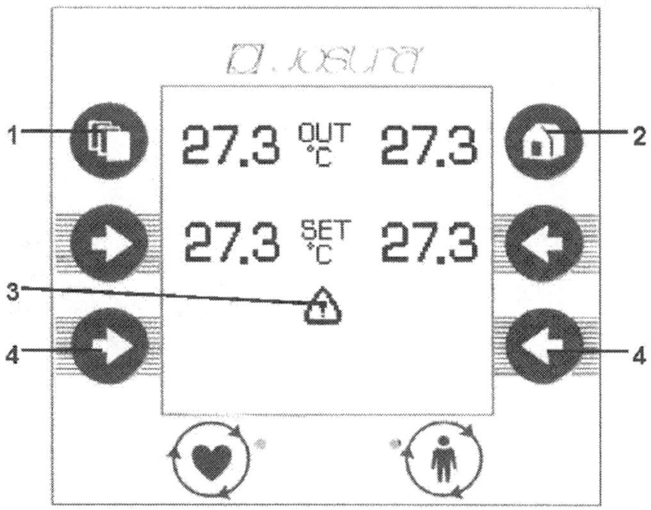

Fig. 12.

For errors where the HCU 30 continues to work, a small warning triangle stays at the bottom of the display.

NOTE

If there is too little water in the tank when switching on, the symbol above is shown in the place of the error symbol and it will not be possible to start the circulation. Fill water to approximately 1 cm above the cooling spirals.

If there already is enough water, appoint a service check on the level sensor. Press both error mute buttons to override the warning and continue to use the HCU 30 as normal.

HARD ERRORS

If any of the errors on the error pages is found, the pumps stop, the acoustic alarm sounds, and the display panel switches to the "Main menu," showing a warning triangle (the third error page is shown directly for the key stuck error). For an error under the heading "Main Pump" or "Card Pump," the pump stops the erroneous circulation only. Press both error mute buttons to see the error pages.

Press the menu button to switch between the error pages. An error is shown as "ERROR xx" (xx = error code) instead of "OK." Press the main menu button to return to the main menu.

Policy and Procedure Guidelines

CP35

ANTITHROMBIN III DEFICIENCY

Definition

Antithrombin III (AT III) deficiency may either be inherited or acquired. Inherited AT III deficiency follows an autosomal dominant transmission pattern. A reduced amount of AT III (usually below 50% of normal levels) constitutes the most common form. Most often, patients present between 15 and 30 years of age with lower limb thrombosis or pulmonary embolism. Other precipitating factors include pregnancy, surgery, and infection.

Acquired AT III deficiency is more common than inherited deficiency. Some causes of acquired AT III deficiency are:

a. Decreased synthesis of AT III from liver cirrhosis
b. Drug Induced: L-Asparaginase, estrogens, **heparin**
c. Increased excretion of AT III: Protein losing enteropathy, nephrotic syndrome, inflamatory bowel disease
d. Accelerated consumption of AT III: DIC, surgery
e. Dilutional: cardiopulmonary bypass (CPB), autologous blood removal

Operative Management

Antithrombin III deficiency in patients about to undergo CPB is largely a presumptive diagnosis based on substantial heparin resistance, e.g., failure to attain an ACT >400 s after administration of 600 U/kg of heparin. Failure to recognize and correct heparin resistance are the onset of CPB is likely to produce low-grade activation of coagulation with consumption of platelets and procoagulants. Although this can result in the formation of microemboli, a hemorrhagic diathesis is likely to follow the termination of CPB secondary to procoagulant consumption.

Cardiopulmonary Bypass

Are you certain the patient is really AT III deficient?

1 Make sure the heparin was administered to the patient.

a. IV line separation or loose connection?
b. If administered peripherally, has the IV infiltrated?

2. Check the heparin vial: has it expired or is the lot ineffective?

3. Attempt to redose the patient with 5,000 to 10,000 U of a different biologic source of heparin, e.g., from porcine mucosal heparin to bovine lung.

4. Once anesthesia has given 8–10 mg/kg of heparin, call the blood bank and order fresh frozen plasma (FFP). Antithrombin III deficiency has been shown to respond to the administration of FFP, which contains normal concentrations of AT III. The volume of FFP needed to raise AT III levels sufficiently to induce safe anticoagulation depends upon the magnitude of the deficiency, but 2–3 U appears sufficient for most adults.

Note: Always alert the surgeon to the potentiality of an AT III deficiency, and confirm with anesthesia your proposed treatment plan.

5. After the Administration of FFP, re-dose the patient with additional heparin. Often, an additional 10,000 U of heparin is sufficient to increase the ACT >480 s.

6. **Closely monitor your ACT values every 15 min.**

Food for Thought

ACT prolongation after administration of FFP does not establish that AT III deficiency caused the heparin resistance, because increasing plasma AT III levels should increase heparin-induced anticoagulation whether or not initial AT III levels are inadequate. This may be important if the cause of heparin resistance is heparin-induced thrombocytopenia, or marked thrombocytosis.

In heparin-induced thrombocytopenia, an interaction of heparin, platelets, and immunoglobulin G (IgG) antibody is the likely mechanism for heparin resistance. This would theoretically respond best to platelet-rich plasma pheresis accompanied by volume replacement with FFP before CPB. After CPB and neutralization of heparin, platelet concentrates would be needed. In marked thrombocytopenia, the treatment for heparin resistance would be the same, but the likely mechanism involved would be competitive heparin binding to platelets, inducing an acute release of platelet factor 4, an endogenous substance capable of binding and neutralizing heparin.

The use of FFP to replace AT III may become obsolete with the recent introduction of a human AT III concentrate, which has been used successfully to treat pregnancy induced AT III deficiency.

—Pooled from human plasma, but heat treated and should be free of infectious disease transmission risks.
—Half life of 22 h.
—Capable of raising adult AT III levels by 30% with 1,000 U.
—Cost: approximately $1800 for 1,000 U.
—Use for heparin resistance in cardiac surgery has been reported.

Policy and Procedure Guidelines

CP36

COLD AGGLUTININS

Introduction

Cold agglutinins, also called autoimmune hemolytic anemia, is a condition where immunoglobulins IgM, autoantibodies in plasma, react with antigens, mainly the Anti-I, on a patient's red blood cell or with exogenous red blood cells and cause agglutination or hemolysis. This condition results in a variety of symptoms, including intravascular hemolysis, hemoglobinuria, cold-induced vasoocclusive symptoms, hemolytic anemia, microvascular occlusion in renal, peripheral, and cardiac vasculature, myocardial infaction (MI), and cyanosis.

Testing for cold agglutinins is performed using the direct or indirect Coomb's test, and it is usually done at room temperature or 18–20°C with observation for the presence of clot in saline suspended red blood cells (RBCs). Test results include:

—Thermal amplitude: the temperature range *over* which the antibodies react. May be a narrow or broad spectrum or be close to 37°C.
—Titer: the percentage level of the blood's reactive antibody.
—Critical temperature: the temperature above which agglutination activity ceases.
—Indirect Coomb's: establishes the presence of antibodies in the serum that react with autologous or exogenous blood.
—Direct Coomb's: demonstrates complement component attached by the antibody to the patient's washed RBC membrane.

Cold agglutinins are found in all subjects, and normally only react at temperatures of 0–4°C. There is an exponential increase in antibody activity (titer) upon cooling below the threshold of thermal amplitude, and rapid reversal of antibody activation and RBC agglutination with rewarming above the thermal amplitude threshold. Agglutination is not affected by hemodilution or heparinization.

CPB Management

—Preoperative plasma pheresis to remove 90% of the antibodies. Replacement of volume with fresh frozen plasma.

—Maintenance of patient's temperature above the critical temperature at all times. Use mild or moderate hypothermic bypass, warm operating room environment, hypothermia blanket on warm, and radiant lights.
—Normothermic bypass with continuous normothermic coronary perfusion.
—Use of warm blood cardioplegia or warm crystalloid cardioplegia.
—Coronary washout with warm crystalloid cardioplegia, followed by administration of cold crystalloid cardioplegia.
—Warming of all solutions, medications, and blood products before adminstration to the patient.

Cold Agglutinins

If cold agglutinins are encountered during hypothermic bypass:

—Systemic rewarming to 32–37°C. ***This is the only immediate counteraction to reverse RBC agglutination.***
—Re-check activatal clothing time first to rule out insufficient heparinization.
—Administer only **warm** cardioplegia (either crystalloid or blood). If the surgeon wishes to give crystalloid cardioplegia, you will need to change out the MP-4 for a clear set.
—Use of a posterior pericardial insulating pad to insulate the heart from the underlying warm tissues.
—Snared bicaval cannulation to prevent warm systemic blood from entering the heart. Left heart venting to evacuate any warm bronchial or mediastinal return.
—Check a blood sample in a red top tube by placing in ice and observing for agglutination, then rewarming by hand and observing for disappearance of agglutination.
—Send complete lab screening for cold agglutinins with determination of critical temperature and titer (this lab result may take several hours). Send a sample for plasma-free hemoglobin.
—Administer microcirculatory enhancers (NTG, SNP) to alleviate central nervous system and kidney ischemia and dysfunction secondary to increased blood viscosity.
—Administer steroids to alter macrophage-complement receptor function (macrophages are unable to recognize RBCs in the presence of steroids).
—Washed RBCs should be used to avoid using fresh serum complement.

Cold blood or crystalloid cardioplegia administration may cause intracoronary hemaagglutination with poor distribution of solution, coronary thrombosis, subendocardial ischemia, and MI.

Administration of normothermic asanguinous cardioplegia to washout coronary circulation until sinus return is clear before infusion of cold cardioplegia is advisable. Before removal of the XCL, reperfusion of the heart with ***normothermic*** cardioplegia to prewarm the myocardium and prevent cooling of intracoronary blood by cold muscle tissues.

Note: Landymore states, "*Although the red cell population is temporarily removed by the first injection of normothermic crystalloid cardioplegia, and is subsequently followed by cold crystalloid injections, blood soon returns to the arrested heart through non-coronary collaterals.*"

Policy and Procedure Guidelines
CP37

DISSEMINATED INTRAVASCULAR COAGULATION

Definition

Disseminated intravascular coagulation (DIC) is a condition in which coagulation factors normally present in the blood are depleted or inactivated, resulting in the inability of the patient to form clots and maintain homeostasis. Simultaneous clotting followed by lysis occurs in a diffuse and widespread manner throughout the body.

DIC can be caused by the following factors:

***Inadequate heparinization**
*Acute hypotensive effect, shock
*Uncontrolled prolonged hemorrhage
*Total body washout with replacement of volume with banked blood products containing temporarily inactivated clotting factors
*Infection, sepsis, viremia
*Obstetrical complications
*Burns, crush injuries, trauma
*Liver disease.

When vascular integrity is lost, large amounts of phospholipids are released, resulting in activation of platelets and the coagulation cascade, followed by consumption of these factors. Phospholipids cause widespread formation of fibrin, leading to consumption of factors, with a decrease of labile factors 5, 8, and fibrinogen. These factors are used once in the coagulation process, and must be replenished. When clots are broken down, large amounts of fibrin split products (FSPs) are released into the circulation. With an increase in FSPs present, normal clot formation is inhibited, and platelets become dysfunctional.

***A first clue of DIC can be detected by observing a handheld activated clothing time (ACT) sample for formation of clot, followed shortly by lysis of the clot.**

Treatment

*If DIC is suspected, send sample to lab for STAT complete coagulation profile. A positive result is indicated by prolonged PTT and TT, thrombocytopenia, hypofibrinogenemia, and increased FSPs.

*Maintain or initiate complete heparinization with ACTs >480 s.

*Replace coagulation factors by administering FFP, RBCs, platelets, and cyroprecipitate if necessary. Continue factor replacement and platelet therapy post-operative for 24–48 h, as indicated.

*May be necessary to maintain cardiopulmonary bypass to assist in homeostasis, until coagulation factors are reactive (approximately 4 h).

Policy and Procedure Guidelines

CP38

PROCEDURE FOR MASSIVE GAS EMBOLISM AS OUTLINED IN "THE PRACTICE OF CARDIAC ANESTHESIA" LITTLE, BROWN; 1ST EDITION (1990)

1. **Stop** cardiopulmonary bypass (CPB) immediately.
2. Steep **Trendelenberg** position.
3. Remove aortic cannula vent air from aortic cannulation site.
4. **Deair** arterial cannula and pump line.
5. Institute hypothermic **retrograde operator vena cava (SVC) perfusion** by connecting arterial pump line to the SVC cannula with caval tape tightened. Blood at 20–24°C is injected into SVC at 1–2 L/min or more, and air plus blood is drained from aortic cannulation site to the pump.
6. **Carotid compression** is performed intermittently during retrograde SVC perfusion to allow retrograde purging of air from the *vertebral arteries*.
7. Maintain retrograde SVC perfusion for at least 1–2 min. Continue for an additional 1–2 min if air continues to exit from aorta.
8. In **extensive** systemic air injection accidents in which emboli to splanchnic, renal, or femoral circulation are suspected, **retrograde inferior vena cava perfusion** may be performed **after** head deairing procedures are completed. This is performed while the *carotid arteries are clamped* and the patient is in *head-up position* to facilitate removal of air through the aortic root vent, but prevent reembolization of the brain.
9. When no additional air can be expelled, **resume anterograde CPB**, maintaining hypothermia at 20°C for at least 40–45 min. Lowering patient temperature is important because increased gas solubility helps to resorb bubbles and because decreased metabolic demands may limit ischemic damage before bubble resorption.
10. Induce **hypertension** with vasoconstrictor drugs. Hydrostatic pressure shrinks bubbles; also, bubbles occluding arterial bifurcations are pushed into one vessel, opening the other branch.
11. Express coronary air by massage and needle venting.
12. **Steroids** may be administered, although this is controversial; the usual dose of methylprednisolone is 30 mg/kg.

13. **Barbiturate coma** should be considered if the myocardium will be able to tolerate the significant negative inotropy. Thiopental 10mg/kg loading dose plus 1–3mg/kg/h infusion may be used empirically. If EEG monitoring is available, titration of barbiturate to an EEG burst/suppression (1 burst/min) pattern is preferable.

14. Patient is weaned from CPB.

15. Continue ventilating patient with **100% O_2** for at least 6h to maximize blood-alveolar gradient for elimination of N2.

16. **Hyperbaric chamber** can accelerate resorption of residual bubbles. However, the risk of moving a critically ill patient must be weighed against the potential benefits.

Policy and Procedure Guidelines
CP39

HYPERKALEMIA

The Heart and Hyperkalemia

Most of the body's potassium is located intracellularly. Only a small fraction (≈2%) is found in the extracellular compartment. As serum potassium concentration increases, a decreased ratio of intracellular to extracellular K+ concentration occurs, and results in a decreased resting cell membrane potential. Increased serum Na+ and Ca+ concentrations limit depolarization of the cell membrane. In addition, there is shortening of the action potential duration from increased membrane permeability to K+. Mild hyperkalemia (6.0 mEq/L), with normal renal function generally needs no treatment. Moderate hyperakalemia (6.0–7.0 mEq/L), with normal renal function generally resolves with time and no therapy. Severe hyperkalemia (7.0 mEq/L), especially with EKG manifestations, requires immediate therapy. Renal excretion accounts for total maintenance of potassium balance.

Causes of Hyperkalemia

—Cardioplegia solutions
—Transfusion of overaged banked blood
—Renal dysfunction from any cause
—K from cell hemolysis
—Acidosis
—K sparing diuretics (Spironalactone,Triamterene, Amiloride)
—Ace inhibitors
—Digitalis in high doses
—KCL supplementation
—Drugs causing tumor lysis
—Low insulin production (DM)

Treatment of Hyperkalemia

1. If you get a lab value back that is questionable, be sure to send another sample for a repeat value. In the meantime, alert anesthesia to the possibility of true hyperkalemia, and the necessity for treatment of it.

2. Stop all infusions containing K+ (cardioplegic solution, priming solutions, IVs).
3. Increase the elimination of K+ from the extracelluar fluid:
   a. Infuse Dextrose and Insulin:
      1–2 g glucose/kg in children
      0.3 U R insulin/g glucose in children
      50 g glucose and 15 U R insulin in adults
   b. NaHcO3:
      1–2 mEq/kg children
      45 mEq adults
   c. Calcium:
      20 mg/kg calcium gluconate over 5 min in children
      500–1,000 mg of calcium chloride in adults
   d. Increase diuresis
   e. Hemoconcentration on CPB: Hemoconcentrate off as much pump volume as possible, adding normal saline (for injection) as needed for volume replacement. Recheck K+ and electrolyte levels often.
   f. Hemodialysis for persistent hyperkalemia.
   g. Emergency cardiac pacing if severe hyperkalemia is causing arrhythmia's.
   h. If you are aware preoperatively that your patient is hyperkalemic, during CPB you can scavenge the initial flush of cardioplegia to the cell saver.

*Note: All of the above listed procedures are contingent upon approval with both the surgeon and anesthesia.

How Treatment of Hyperkalemia Is Achieved

NaHcO3: Correction of acidosis by diminishing the extracellular hydrogen burden and transfer of K+ intracellularly, provides intracellular binding sites for K+ in the form of potassium carbonate; buffers dextrose; corrects acidosis from shift of H+ from intracellular to extracellular.

Hypertonic saline: Correct hyponatremia; counteracts cardiotoxicity; expands extracellular compartment and dilutes K+.

Glucose and insulin: Directly promotes the movement of K+ from extracellular to intracellular compartments.

Calcium: Activates receptor sites of potassium pumps on cell membranes; replaces serum Ca, which is driven intracellularly by administration of insulin.

Policy and Procedure Guidelines

CP40

MALIGNANT HYPERPYREXIA (HYPERTHERMIA)

Definition

Hypermetabolic state causing increased cellular activity within the muscle, especially the skeletal muscle. Hyperthermia doesn't appear to affect the myocardium directly.

Mechanism

There becomes an increased amount of calcium levels in the myoplasmic reticulum, resulting in escalated glycolytic pathway. The increased calcium levels cause muscle contracture, resulting in depletion of adenosine triphosphate (ATP) stores and production of heat, carbon dioxide, pyruvate, and lactate. The loss of calcium uptake is prevented due to the loss of ATP. The sodium/calcium pump is driven via the ATPase pump. Therefore, the efflux has increased levels of potassium, magnesium, phosphate, and enzymes myoglobin and calcium move intracellularly. Note that giving exogenous calcium intravenously will not work because the sodium/calcium pump is not able to function.

Triggering Factors

1. Depolarizing muscle relaxants, i.e., succinylcholine chloride and Gallamine.
2. Inhalation agents, i.e., all volatile anesthetics.

Agents that increase myoplasmic calcium levels include lidocaine, cardiac glycosides, caffeine, calcium salts, alpha agonists, and catecholamine.

Anesthetic Considerations

1. Disconnect vaporizers and change the tubing.
2. Pretreatment with Dantole4ne/Na oral preparation preoperatively.
3. It has been shown that Dantrolene blood levels have decreased with CPB, but it is not known whether additional Dantrolene is needed.

4. Drugs to use include-barbiturates, narcotics, benzodiazepines, and non-depolarizing muscle relaxants.
5. Hypothermia blanket.

Clinical Signs of Malignant Hyperthermia

1. Increased heart rate
2. Dysrythmias
3. Muscle rigidity (masseter muscle)
4. Increased temperature
5. Dissemmated intravascular coagulation
6. Tonic contracture of skeletal muscle.

Clinical Signs While on CPB with Aortic Cross Clamp On

1. Decreased venous oxygen saturation
2. Increased potassium and glucose
3. Decreased calcium levels
4. Increased temperature
5. Blood gas results reveal metabolic/respiratory acidosis

Treatment for Malignant Hyperthermia on CPB

1. Dantrolene/Na 1–10 mg/kg (2.5 mg/kg) immediately before muscle circulation is cut off; then increases the cardiac index
2. Cool the patient
3. Sodium bicarbonate administration for acidosis
4. Glucose and insulin for increased potassium levels
5. Mannitol and lasix for increased myoglobin levels to prevent acute renal failure
6. Disconnect oxygen tubing from the vaporizer on the pump
7. Avoid prime solutions with calcium

Policy and Procedure Guidelines
CP41

HEART SURGERY AND PERFUSION OF THE PREGNANT PATIENT

Two general categories of heart disease in pregnant women:

1. Women who have heart disease before pregnancy.
   a. valvular
   b. congenital
   c. coronary artery disease; **rare** in woman of child-bearing years
      1. severe insulin-dependent diabetes mellitus
      2. genetic hypercholesterolemia

2. Woman who have heart disease induced by pregnancy.
   a. preeclampsia
   b. cardiomyopathy
   c. thromboembolic disease
   d. aortic dissection

Associated with Low Rates of Maternal Complications But High Risk to the Fetus

Cardiovascular Changes

1. Cardiac output increases by 30–50% by the beginning of the third trimester, primarily due to stroke volume rather than heart rate.
2. Oxygen consumption increases by 10–15%.
3. Plasma volume increases 50–75%, but red blood cell volume increases only 40–50%, so the patient will seem anemic (estrogen mediated).

Cardiopulmonary Bypass

1. Both fetal heart rate and uterine contraction monitors provide valuable information for intraoperative management. Rate can be managed at either normothermia or mild hypothermia. A decrease in heart rate is associated with poor fetal perfusion.

2. The woman should be positioned in a **left lateral tilt** to avoid compression of the inferior vena cava or aorta.

3. Extracorporeal circuit should be able to accommodate a large blood volume, but employ a minimal priming volume.

4. Heparinization is well tolerated because the molecule is large and does not cross the placental blood barrier. Pregnancy tends to induce a hypercoagulable state with increases in factors VII, VIII, X, and XIII, as well as an increase in blood volume and metabolism. Theoretically, there should be an increase in heparin requirements. Therefore, a heparin assay should be done to determine a base requirement, and then ACTs should be monitored more frequently.

5. Mixed venous saturation will measure adequacy of perfusion.

6. **Temperature** should not fall below 32 degrees centigrade to avoid fetal fibrillation.

7. Uterine contractions are associated with hypothermia and rewarming.

8. Normal fetal heart rate is 120–140 beats/min. Maximize blood flow before giving vasopressors to achieve pressures of 60–70 mmHg. Ephedrine is recommended during pregnancy with indirect alpha and beta adrenergic activity. It appears to have the least effect on uterine blood flow due to the beta-2 stimulation.

9. Metabolic acidosis is treated with sodium bicarbonate.

10. Glucose is given to replenish decreased fetal glycogen stores.

11. Blood oxygen saturation is corrected by increasing perfusion flow, hemoglobin concentration, or oxygen flows, as indicated.

12. Note: sodium nitroprusside crosses the placenta in animals, it and may liberate free cyanide ions and result in metabolic acidosis.

Policy and Procedure Guidelines

CP42

SICKLE CELL ANEMIA

Definition

Sickle cell anemia is an alteration in the form and function of normal adult hemoglobin, which is replaced by Hb_s. In the normal adult, hemoglobin A is the predominant form of hemoglobin, comprising 96–97% of all hemoglobin. Sickle cell hemoglobinopathy is a single gene-recessive abnormality that may be present in a heterozygous recessive form, which is sickle cell trait, or in a homozygous form, which is expressed as the sickle cell disease. Patients with the homozygous form have a predominance of hemoglobin S, which may account for 80–98% of the hemoglobin. In contrast, patients with the sickle cell trait have a lower percentage of hemoglobin S, accounting for 20–45% of their total hemoglobin. Red blood cell sickling results from deoxyhemoglobin formation. The tendency toward sickling increases with hypoxemia, acidosis, increased concentrations of 2,3 DPG, infection, hypothermia, and capillary stagnation. A hypertonic environment that may cause crenation of normal blood cells will also lead to sickling in the abnormal cells. The abnormal hemoglobin changes properties of the cell membrane, increasing osmotic and mechanical fragility.

Operative Management

The operative strategy in sickle cell disease is to prevent sickling, and thereby prevent hemolysis or vasoocclusion phenomena.

Cardiopulmonary Bypass

1. Homozygous disease (exchange transfusion may be necessary).
2. Maintain adequate arterial oxygen tension/saturation.
3. Maintain adequate capillary perfusion, avoid low flow states.
4. Avoid low mixed venous saturations (maintain 80–85%).
5. Utilize moderate hemodilution to reduce blood viscosity.
6. Avoid acidosis shifts of the oxyhemoglobin dissociation curve.
7. Use moderate hypothermia (32°C) only.

8. Measure blood gases frequently, treat acidosis aggressively.
9. Use crystalloid cardioplegia (40 mEq/L is a high dose).
10. Minimize the use of cardiotomy suction to decrease mechanical trauma.

Policy and Procedure Guidelines
CP43

ABIOMED BVS 5000 PROTOCOL

Indications and Contraindications

The Abiomed BVS 5000 (device) is indicated for mechanical circulatory support for patients who develop ventricular dysfunction impairing hemodynamic stability after undergoing successful cardiac surgery.

A. Indications
   1. Patients 75 yr old or younger.
   2. Body surface area of over 1.3 m^2.
   3. Reasonable attempt to correct the ventricular dysfunction using pharmacological agents.
   4. Inability to wean from cardiopulmonary bypass (CPB) or significant unstable hemodynamics as follows: arterial pressure mean of less than 70 mmHg, cardiac index of less than 2 L/min/m^2, and pulmonary capillary wedge pressure or left atrial pressure of over 18 mmHg.
   5. Intraaortic balloon pump (IABP) may be tried at the discretion of the surgeon.
   6. The time between the first attempt to wean from CPB and the decision to implant the device should be within 6 h.
B. Contraindications for use
   1. Patients over 75 yr old.
   2. Patients with body surface area of less than 1.3 m^2.
   3. Preoperative cardiac arrest with prolonged resuscitation with good probability of permanent neurological damage.
   4. Major cardiac or extracardiac catastrophes occurring in the perioperative period that preclude survival. The examples of these are: uncontrolled hemorrhage, massive air embolism, interstitial pulmonary hemorrhage with an inability to maintain adequate ventilation, pump oxygenator or perfusion difficulties, massive transfusion reaction, significant hemolysis during CPB, and inadequate cannulation for the Abiomed BVS 5000.

5. Cerebral vascular accident (CVA) during or before the operation resulting in fixed, dilated pupils.

Equipment, Storage, and Maintenance

1. The console should be plugged in at all times in a designated location in the cardiac operating room area, the specific location should be agreed upon by the surgeons, cardiac OR nursing coordinator, and perfusion staff.

2. It is the responsibility of the Chief Perfusionist to arrange appropriate servicing of the console by the company, in cooperation with Biomedical Engineering.

3. The disposable sets of Abiomed BVS 5000 are located in the pump room. Three complete sets are available at all times. Please be sure to notify the Materials Manager when a device is used.

Systems Operation and Implantation of the Abiomed BVS 5000

A. Abiomed BVS 5000 Console Startup
   1. Turn on the console power switch that is located at the rear of the console. As soon as the power is turned ON, the console will perform self-diagnostic tests that require approximately 1 min to complete. The console flashes all indicators, sounds the audible alarm, and pumps air through the drive ports.
   2. Check the self-test; upon completion, the LCD display should read, "Left system ready for use" and "Right system ready for use." Caution: Do not depress the pump "ON" controls during the self-test. This will result in activation of the emergency system. In the event that the "ON" button was accidentally pushed during the self-test, turn the machine off and then start over by turning the power switch ON again.

B. Priming the Abiomed BVS 5000 Blood Pump
   1. The perfusionist will prime the blood pump.
   2. All the materials needed should have been brought into the operating room ready for use. The following items are needed: BVS blood pump (priming volume 600 ml) (a second blood pump may be necessary for biventricular support) one cardiotomy reservoir, 2 120-cm lengths of 3/8″ tubing, 4 tubing clamps, 2 IV infusion set, and 2 L of priming solution (Plasma Lyte).
   3. The perfusionist opens the blood pump and the accessory tubings. The scrub nurse takes them in her sterile field.
   4. The scrub nurse makes the proper connection of the blood pump tubing to the 3/8″ tubing. She then passes the blood pump, as well

as the other end of the extension tubings, to the perfusionist, keeping adequate length of the tubings in the sterile field with the connections. **Make sure the cloudy silicone connections stay securely in the sterile field.**

5. The perfusionist now connects the outlet of the cardiotomy reservoir to the inlet of the pump and the inlet of the reservoir to the outlet of the pump using the extension tubings that were passed to him by the scrub nurse.
6. Clamp the tubing on the outlet reservoir and fill the reservoir with priming solution using the infusion set.
7. The perfusionist inverts the blood pump and raises it above the reservoir, then releases the clamp and slowly lowers the blood pump in the inverted position, allowing it to fill. Once the blood pump is full and most of the air is displaced, turn it upright and place it in the BVS IV pole. Begin pumping.
8. During pumping, periodically invert the pump to dislodge any air in the valve sinuses. Allow the pump to run for approximately 5 min. Make sure all bubbles are removed from the valves.
9. After all the bubbles have been removed with 5 min of pumping, stop pumping. The scrub nurse clamps both latex adapters and blood pump lines.
10. The scrub nurse rolls back the latex adapters and keeps them in a sterile field to facilitate priming the second pump and repriming in the event of detection of air in the system. The pump is now ready to be connected to the primed cannulae when the surgeon is ready. Note: the perfusionist and the operating room nurses should periodically review these priming procedures with the help of the training manual, as well as the instruction tape.

C. Abiomed BVS 5000 Cannulation Techniques

1. Unpack the cannulae, which are in double-sterile packets. Take care to remove the accessory pack that contains the bullet, restraint, and tie wraps.
2. The next step is externalization of the atrial and arterial cannulae. To standardize the position of the cannulae, the left atrial cannula should be externalized just to the right of the midline; the aortic cannula is externalized more to the right, which is lateral of the left atrial cannula. For biventricular support, the right atrial cannula should be located to the left of the midline and the pulmonary artery cannula further to the left. Externalization is done first before suturing the cannulae to the heart, as a safety precaution. In tunneling the tubes, the skin incision is made, and a clamp is passed to create and dilate the tunnel. The clamp then grasps the heavy suture, which

is attached to the bullet that was previously inserted through the cannula. The cannula is then pulled from inside and through the skin.

3. **Left atrial cannulation**: The preferred site of left atrial cannulation is behind the interatrial groove. Depending on the surgical situation, the surgeon may elect to use the alternative sites of cannulation, which are through the left atrial appendage or through the left atrial dome between the aorta and superior vena cava. It is recommended to use double-pursestring sutures with pledgets using 1-0 or 3-0 Tycron or Prolene. Keepers are used to snag the sutures and are secured with multiple clips and ties to anchor the keepers to the cannula.
4. **Aortic cannulation**: The aortic cannula has been previously externalized. The surgeon trims the graft to fit with a slight bevel and performs and end-to-side anastomosis to the ascending aorta with continuous 4-0 or 3-0 Prolene. This anastomosis is best done with the ascending aorta cross-clamped with the patient still on CPB. Next, release the clamp, allow the cannula to fill gradually, tap the exterior of the graft to release any trapped air bubbles, release the clamp and allow back-bleeding into a basin to complete the venting process. Note: the IABP, if previously inserted, is removed when BVS support is utilized. The device has pulsatile flow, and IABP is not necessary.
5. **Right atrial cannulation**: Right atrial cannulation is often performed through the midfree wall of the right atrium. The right atrial appendage may be used also; however, this may not be available, since this is the usual site for the conventional right atrial cannulation for CPB. The same double-pursestring technique with pledgets is recommended with keepers. The atrial cannulation is allowed to be filled by maneuvers to increase the venous pressure, clamp the cannula, and fill the rest of the tubing with saline solution and reclamp.
6. Pulmonary artery cannulation: pulmonary artery cannulation is similar to the aorta.

D. CONNECTION OF THE BLOOD PUMP AND CANNULAE

1. Scrub nurse removes latex adapters at the tips of the blood pump tubings. The latex adapters are only for priming purposes. Keep these in the sterile field for possible later use.
2. Slide the restraint well on the cannula, away from the open end.
3. Blood pump connectors are then inserted into the cannula under irrigation. Make a bubble-free connection.
4. Pulling the restraint down over the connection and application of the tie wraps should be delayed until the pump is started. This

will facilitate disconnection of the pump if repriming becomes necessary.

E. STARTING THE BLOOD PUMPS

1. The preferred method of starting pumping is with the foot pump. Push the off button **twice** within 13 s. Open the rear cover and move the transfer lever up so that it is in the horizontal position. Grasp the foot pump, squeeze the pedal, and remove it from the compartment.
2. Place patient in Trendelenburg, turn table to the right so that the cannulation sites are in the dependent positions, and submerge the cannulation sites with saline.
3. Position pump level with patient's atria. Reduce CPB, and fill patient's atria (10–12 mmHg).
4. Begin foot pumping slowly, watching carefully for air. Be ready to clamp line immediately if any air is witnessed. If air is detected, stop foot pumping, locate origin of air. Are connectors tight? Are atria full? Are cannulae sufficiently deep? Remove air using saline and back-bleeding if necessary, and reconnect cannulae.
5. Replace foot pump in its compartment and be sure to return the transfer lever to the verticle position. The console will not be able to drive the pump if the transfer lever is not returned to the verticle position. If the console is off, then be sure to replace the foot pump before starting the console; failure to do this will result in self-test failure.
6. When pumping is turned on, the blood pump level can be adjusted so that it is lower than the atrial level, to allow adequate venous return. At this time, conventional CPB is discontinued and the patient is now on ABIOMED BVS 5000 support.

F. ANTICOAGULATION

1. The heparin should be reversed in the operating room according to protocol.
2. Upon admission to the cardiothoracic intensive care unit, a baseline activated clotting time (ACT), prothrombin time (PT), partial thromboplastin time (PTT) should be performed.
3. When chest tube drainage decreases and bleeding stops, wait another 2 h to be sure, then start anticoagulation. This is usually within 24 h of implantation of the device. Give a bolus of 5,000 U heparin first.
4. Start heparin titration to maintain ACT between 180–200 s. During the weaning period, as soon as the pump flow is 3 LPM or less, the ACT should be increased to 300 s until decannulation of the device.

G. BACKUP SAFETY SYSTEMS
   1. The console incorporates a fixed rate control system that will take over the console function if the computer-based control system fails. The emergency system pumps at approximately 35 beats per minute.
   2. "EMERGENCY SYSTEM ON" is displayed whenever this backup system is engaged. A pulsing audible alarm is sounded if the emergency system is on.
   3. Depression of the "ON" switch during self test is intended to activate the emergency system. To reset the system, turn the power switch off (at the back of console), and then on again.

H. WEANING FROM THE ABIOMED BVS 5000
   1. Weaning should be attempted when there is reason to believe that cardiac recovery has occurred, which can be assessed by :
      a. the appearance of ventricular ejection on the arterial wave form.
      b. transesophageal echo to assess ventricular wall motion changes and comparison of LV function.
   2. **Weaning Methods**
      a. reduce flow in .5 LPM decrements. In biventricular support, right pump flow should be reduced in advance of left pump flow.
      b. Assess patient's hemodynamic stability at a reduced level of support for at least 30 min before continuing to the next reduction.
      c. Increase ACT to 300 s when flow is 3 LPM or lower.

VV Hemoconcentration Right Ventricular Assist Device ([RVAD] Support Only!!!!)

To remove excessive volume in heart failure patients on RVAD support, access needs to be made for the employment of a hemoconcentrator. This needs to be accomplished by the surgical staff before priming the Abiomed circuit. After the Abiomed device is passed up to the surgical field, the following supplies are to be passed up to the sterile field, allowing for hemoconcentrator access. The surgeon or scrub nurse will cut in the following, one connector each on the inlet and outlet tubing:

1. 2 – 1/2″ × 1/2″ luer lock connectors
2. 2 – pigtails with three-way stopcocks

When the hemoconcentrator is not in use, each pigtail is to be flushed with clear saline to prevent clotting.

If clot is noted, do not flush the pigtail. Notify surgeon before removing.

ABIOMED BVS 5000 CONSOLE AND CANNULA CHARACTERISTICS

Console Flow and Pressure Parameters

Device	Side	Max. pressure	Max. flow
BVS 5000	right	200 mmHg	5.5 LPM
	left	250 mmHg	5.5 LPM
BVS 5000i	right	200 mmHg	5.5 LPM
	left	320 mmHg	6.5 LPM

Abiomed Cannula Flow Characteristics

Cannula Type	Ven. (device inflow)	Arterial (return to patient)
32 F right angle 4–5 LPM	RA, RV, LA	—
36 F malleable 4–5 LPM	RA, RV, LA, LVapex	RVOT-PA
42 F right angle 5.5–6.5 LPM	RA, LA	—
42 F maleable 5.5–6.5 LPM	RA, LA, LV apex	RVOT-PA
10-mm hemashield 5.5–6.5 LPM	—	PA, Ao anastamosis

Note: when receiving incoming patients, be sure to remove pneumatic drive line extensions used for transport.

Abiomed Assist Devices

The AB 5000 console (Fig. 1) can be used to operate either BVS blood pumps or AB 5000 ventricles. The console automatically adjusts the beat rate and systolic/diastolic ratio based on air flow into and out of the blood pump.

Mechanical System

Compressor system drives independent pressure-regulated systems. Switching from a pressurized to a nonpressurized state in the BVS blood pump and the AB5000 ventricle is via independent three-way solenoid valves. Return air is allowed to vent to atmosphere or vacuum.

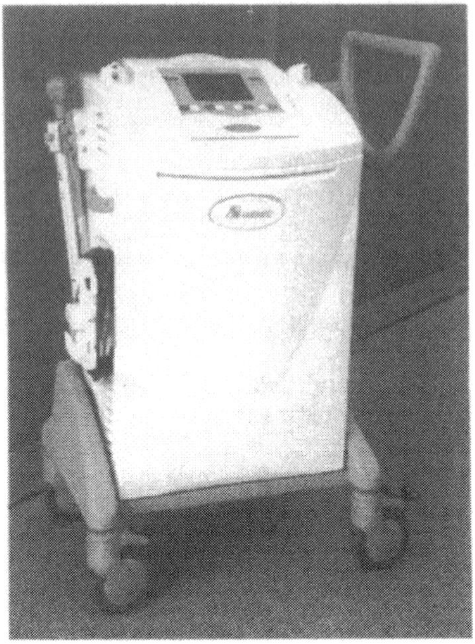

Fig. 1. AB 5000 console.

For the BVS blood pump, left line pressure is regulated to 320 mmHg, right line pressure is regulated to 200 mmHg, and the left and right line vacuum are regulated to −35 mmHg.

For the AB5000 Ventricle, left line pressure is regulated to 420 mmHg, right line pressure is regulated to 300 mmHg, and left and right line vacuum are regulated to −100 mmHg.

Operation

Plug in console and turn it on with power switch located on side panel (Fig. 2). Allow console to automatically perform its self-test. Left and right system ready for use signs will illuminate when system is ready for use. If self-test failure illuminates, do not use the console; get backup console and contact service personnel. The default blood pump type selection is BVS blood pump. Verify that left and right pump types displayed are "BVS pump." For AB5000 ventricle pump, you must plug in the electrical/pneumatic connector into the receptacle on the rotating driveline turret. Verify that the corresponding pump type displayed is "AMB. PUMP." For AB5000 ventricle only: pump type selection will be latched once the pump ON button is pressed. Removing the electrical/pneumatic connector while pump is on will trigger an

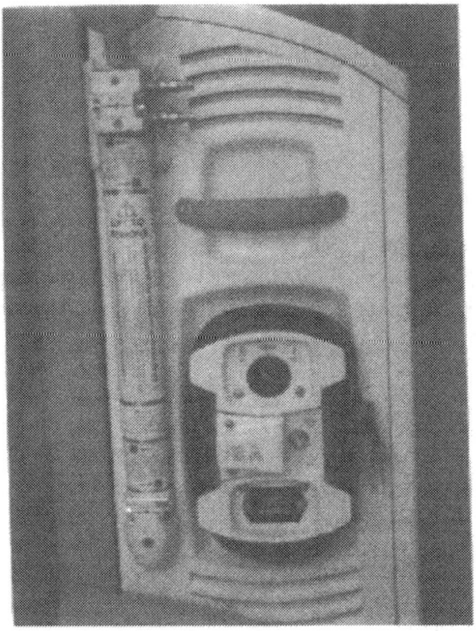

Fig. 2A. Left side of Abiomed console displaying on and off switch and hand pump.

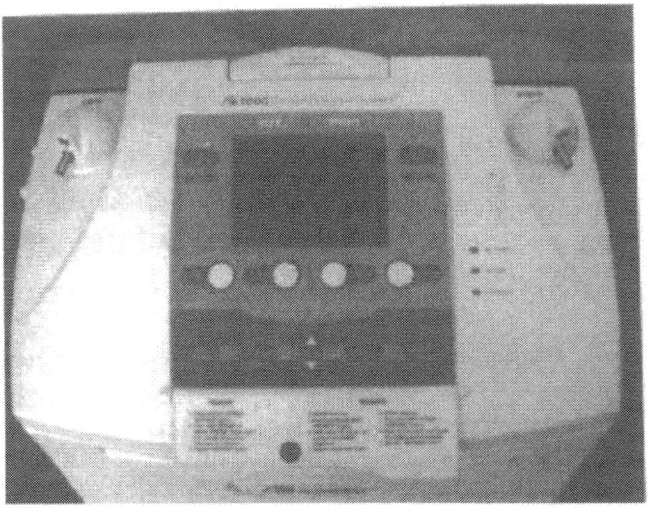

Fig. 2B.

alarm. If the electrical/pneumatic connector is not attached before pressing pump on, attach the connector and turn the pump off (press twice within 13 s), then on again. The new pump type will then be latched (Fig. 2B).

Weaning

When the Patient is to be weaned from the AB5000 system, the blood pump output may be set at any desired flow from 2 L/min to full flow (in 0.1-L/min increments). To begin weaning, open the door marked "Weaning and priming controls." Press and hold the appropriate ACTIVATE button. The ACTIVATE message will appear on the display. While continuing to hold the activate button, press the up or down arrow to set the selected weaning target flow. Release the activate button to achieve set flow (takes several beats). To return to normal operation, press and hold the activate button and press the up arrow until the target flow stops increasing. Release the ACTIVATE button and the console will automatically return to full available flow.

Battery Operation

As long as the console is plugged into an AC power source, the internal battery will be kept in a charged state. A column of labeled LED indicators to the right of the control panel shows the status of the battery. Internal 24 V battery provides 1 h operating time when fully charged. Charging time is 16 h to full charge after 1 hour of use.

AC POWER (LED GREEN) plugged in with line voltage present

BATTERY (LED yellow) line cord disconnected, console operating on battery. A periodic two beep audible signal also indicates battery is on.

BATTERY (LED red) line cord disconnected, <30 minutes battery operation remains, 3 beep audible tone reminder. Plug in console or obtain backup console.

CHARGING (LED yellow) console is plugged in, and the battery charge is <80% capacity.

Hand Pump Operation

Remove the blood pump drive lines from the connectors at the top of the console and attach them to the hand pump, left pump to the left connector, and right pump to the right connector. The hand pump may be operated while mounted on the console, or may be removed and held during operation. Check shuttle mechanism position for BVS or AB5000 pump (Figs. 3–6).

Abiomed AB 5000 Ventricle

The Abiomed AB 5000 circulatory support system (CSS) therapy is intended to treat patients suffering from reversible ventricular dysfunc-

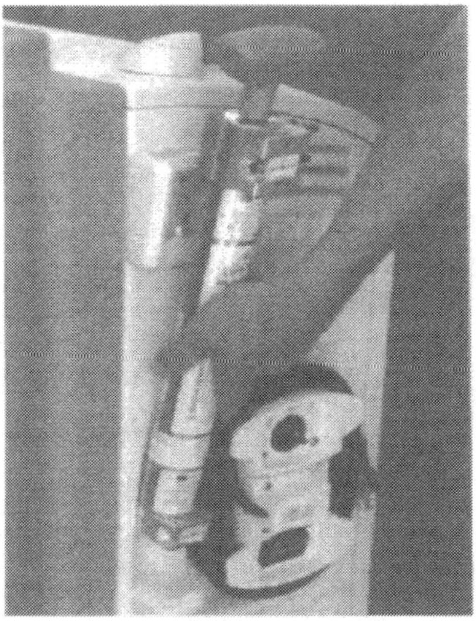

Fig. 3. Hand pump removal.

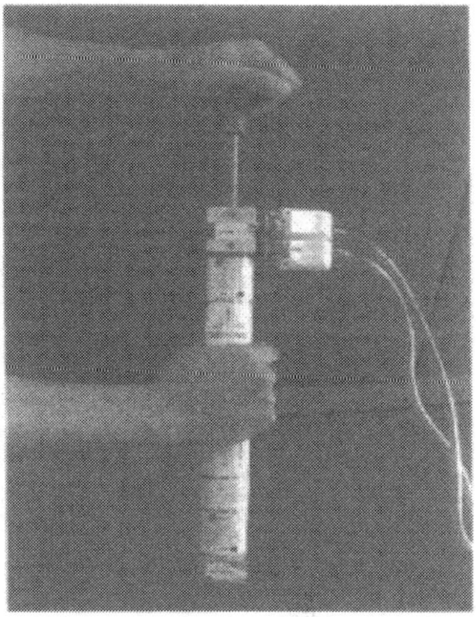

Fig. 4. Hand pump operation.

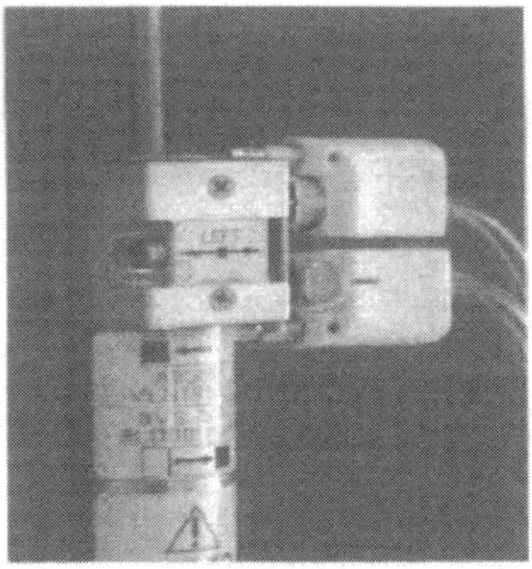

Fig. 5. AB5000™ ventricle position.

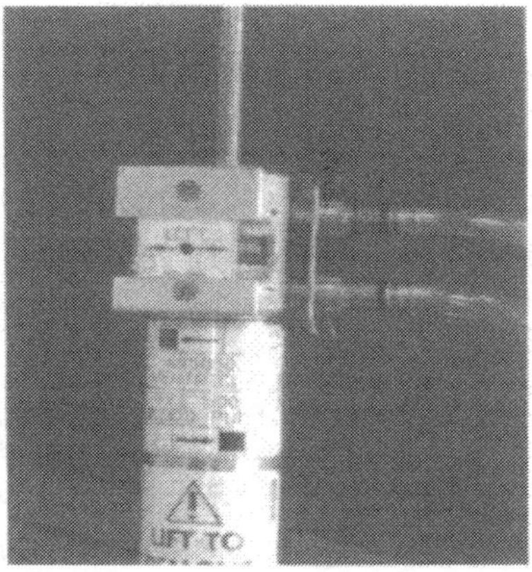

Fig. 6. BVS® Blood pump position.

tion. The intent of the system is to provide circulatory support, restore normal hemodynamics, reduce ventricular workload, and allow the heart time to recover adequate mechanical function.

PRIMING

Materials

Deep basin
Warmed priming solution (Normasol, lactated Ringers, or Plasma-Lyte)
Large bulb syringe
AB 5000 hand pump

Procedure

Fill large basin with warm prime solution (warm solution may help prevent formation of bubbles). Remove the cap tubing (with open clamps) from the arterial and atrial connectors of the ventricle. Set these lengths of tubing aside to be used as connector caps after priming. Pass the end of the driveline of the ventricle out of the sterile field. Secure the sterile portion of the driveline to the sterile drape. Connect the AB5000 hand pump to the driveline. Use the hand pump to evaluate the expansion and contraction of the ventricle bladder. Leave the bladder fully expanded. Fill the ventricle using the bulb syringe by slowly pouring priming solution into the atrial connector, which is marked with a blue arrow indicating direction of flow. Be careful not to touch the inflow or outflow valves of the device with the bulb syringe, as damage to the valves may occur. With the atrial and arterial connectors facing upward, submerge the ventricle in the basin. Rotate the ventricle, tapping gently to dislodge bubbles while keeping the ventricle submerged. Using the AB 5000 hand pump, begin pumping at approximately 40–60 strokes per minute to remove any trapped air (Fig. 7). The last stroke should leave the ventricle bladder fully expanded. Inspect for trapped air and remove if found. The Ventricle housing may contain small, trapped bubbles. These are normal and can be ignored. Submerge the two lengths of cap tubing in the priming solution. Make sure all air is removed, and then close the clamps. Push the clamped tubing onto the atrial and arterial connectors. This will prevent air from entering the ventricle when it is removed from the priming solution. Remove from priming solution and inspect to insure all air has been removed. The ventricle is now ready for connection to the arterial and atrial cannulae.

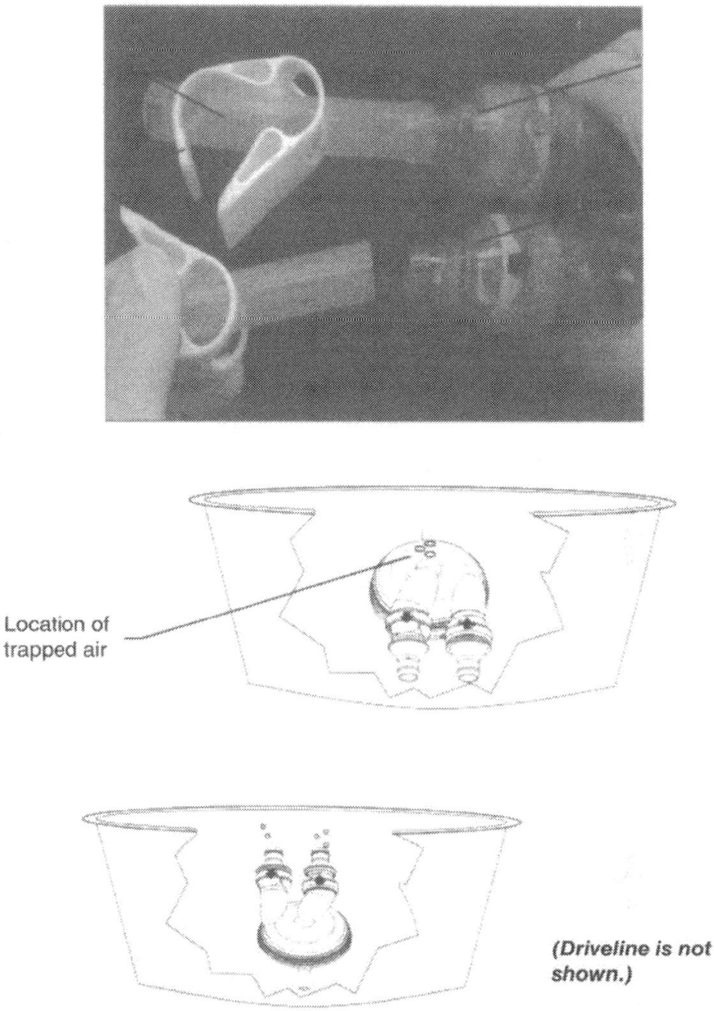

Fig. 7.

Cannulation

Percutaneous cannula exits should be 5 cm apart as measured from the center of each cannula. Cannulae should be positioned to minimize stress at the exit site and prevent kinking. Ventricle flow is dependent on cannula size. 36F atrial, flow >4.0 L/min. and 42F atrial, flow >4.8 L/min. When using LV apex cannulation, A 36-F malleable is often used (the bevel is to be positioned away from the septal wall to prevent entrapment).

Only threaded cannula restraints provided with the ventricle should be used. Do Not use the BVS5000 nonthreaded cannula restraints (cannula may become disconnected during use!!). **Please note: Only use the threaded cannula restraint marked with a red arrow with a hemashield cannula.**

If the cannulae are not of equal length and cannot be cut, a tubing adaptor provided with the ventricle may be used. Push the barbed connector of the tubing adaptor fully into the shorter cannula. Slide the cannula restraint towards the connector until it is snug against the fitting (Fig. 8). Hold the adaptor connector and finger tighten the threaded restraint. Make sure the restraint is not cross threaded. Position the remaining cannula restraint on the tubing, and then the tubing can be cut to length. This tubing is the treated as the cannula for connection to the AB5000 ventricle. Care must be taken by the surgical team to confirm proper direction of flow and correct connection to the ventricle. All connections must be air free.

Initiating Support

Caution: do not attach the right ventricle driveline to the left drive port. Damage to the ventricle can result due to overdriving. Turn on the console and allow the complete self-test to run. Place the patient in Trendelenberg position. Reduce or stop CPB to allow the patient's atria

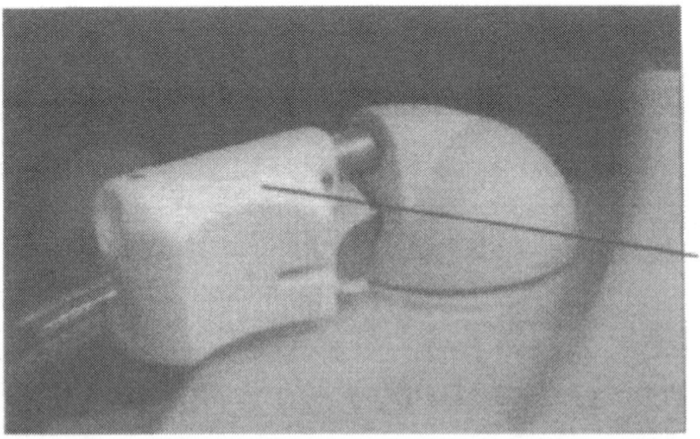

Fig. 8.

to fill with blood. Use saline or blood to submerge the the atrial cannulation sites. Slowly press the AB500 hand pump, or activate the single-stroke feature. Inspect for air and remove if necessary. Connect the drive line to the AB500 console. The drive line must be connected to the console before the on button is pressed. Press on button and observe beat rate.

Policy and Procedure Guidelines
CP44

BIO MEDICUS VENTRICULAR ASSIST PROTOCOL EQUIPMENT

1. Bio-Medicus pump console
2. Sterile disposable pump head (2)
3. Electromagnetic flow probe
4. Sterile custom tubing pack (heparin bonded)
5. Tubing clamps
6. 1 L double-spiked bag balanced electrolyte solution

Preparation of the left ventricular assist device by the perfusionist is begun by inserting the 3/8″ × 3/32″ wall tubing with spike into the bag of solution. Debubble the circuit up to and including the Bio-Medicus pump head by gently applying positive pressure to the bag of solution while venting through the other spike. Once the pump head is filled with solution, a clamp is placed on the tubing distal to the outflow of the pump head. Hang the solution on an IV pole and engage pump head to console. When the pump is turned on, spike the solution bag with the other 3/8″ × 3/32″ tubing, completing the recirculation loop. Continue recirculating the circuit until all air is removed. The system is now ready to be passed into the sterile field, divided, and connected to appropriate cannulae.

CANNULATION (LEFT)

1. Left atrial cannula (typically venous-appropriate size for patient) (see cannula chart)
2. Aortic cannula previously placed for cardiopulmonary bypass

Purse string sutures are placed in the left atrium, and the cannula is tied securely to avoid air entrainment into the assist circuit. The left atrial cannula is connected to the inflow of the bio-pump, carefully avoiding air bubbles. The outflow from the bio-pump is then connected to the aortic cannula previously used for cardiopulmonary bypass, and air again is evacuated.

CANNULATION (RIGHT)

1. Right atrial cannula
2. Pulmonary artery cannula (similar to type used for aortic cannulation)

Cannulae are brought out through the superior or inferior aspect of the incision. The skin is approximated, whereas the sternum is not. The perfusion lines are secured to the drapes.

INITIATION OF VENTRICULAR ASSIST

After weaning from cardiopulmonary bypass, and once the decision has been made to support the patient on ventricular assist, flow is initiated and increased incrementally. The total systemic blood flow (native ventricular output + ventricular assist pump flow) should be maintained at $2.2\,L/min/m^2$. If the left ventricular assist pump cannot maintain $2.2\,L/min/m^2$ with good cannula placement and adequate volume, then right heart failure is significant and right heart assist may also be required.

ANTICOAGULATION

The patient weaned from cardiopulmonary bypass should have heparin neutralized with the appropriate dose of protamine. The first 24 h of ventricular assist will require no heparin therapy; after the initial 24 h, a heparin drip should be started to maintain an activated clotting time of 180–200 s. The ventricular assist device unit is never decreased below 500 cc/min, regardless of the level of anticoagulation.

DISCONTINUATION FROM VAD

After 24 h, if the patient's clinical picture is stable, the left assist pump flow rate is decreased to a level that causes the left atrial pressure to rise to 20–25 mmHg. Cardiac output calculations should be assessed to determine the function of the ventricle. When the surgeon has decided that the native ventricle can support the required cardiac output, the assist device may be removed. Removal of the device should be in the cardiac surgery intensive care unit or the operating room.

Policy and Procedure Guidelines
CP45

ASSEMBLY AND IMPLANTATION OF THE HEARTMATE IP LVAS DEVICE

Device Description

The Heartmate IP LVAS is a pulsatile ventricular assist system intended for ciculatory and hemodynamic support and consists of an implantable blood pump (or left ventricular assist devices [LVAD]), an interconnecting drive line, implant components, and external drive console, which is microprocessor controlled. The LVAS is surgically implanted in either the preperitoneal or intraabdominal locations.

The blood pump, composed of a rigid titanium housing, is a pusher plate type device, capable of producing a stroke volume of 83 ml, generating up to 10 LPM blood flow, and a beat rate up to 140 bpm. Displacement of the blood pump diaphragm with pulses of air delivered by the external console via the drive line results in pumping of the blood.

Indications for Use

The Heartmate LVAD is indicated for use in patients who are on the cardiac transplant list, as temporary mechanical circulatory support for nonreversible left ventricle failure as a bridge to cardiac transplant. The patient should meet all the following criteria.

1. Approved cardiac transplant candidate.
2. On inotropes.
3. On intraaortic balloon pump, if possible.
4. LA pressure or PCWP equal to or greater than 20 mmHg with either:
   a. Systolic BP equal to or less than 80 mmHg, or
   b. Cardiac Index of equal to or less than 2.0 L/min/m^2.

Contraindications

BSA less than 1.5 m^2.

Implantation Procedure

Open the box containing the implantation kit. Make sure the following parts of the system are present:

ventricular assist device
outflow graft
thread protectors (1 set)
apical sewing ring
nonabsorbable suture
inflow valve conduit
outflow valve conduit
interconnecting cable
apical coring knife
return box with handling and return instructions

Note: save box for return of explanted pump to TCI.

In addition, 2 drive consoles with fully charged batteries and carts, console operating manual, and Heartmate IP LVAS directions for use, should be present.

Equipment Needed for Implantation

—3 sterile basins.
—2 L sterile normal saline for valve rinse procedures.
—sterile injectable saline for filling of blood pump.
—50 cc nonheparinized blood for clotting of outflow graft.
—1–2 U cryoprecipitate, to be aspirated into sterile 20-cc syringe with blunt needle
—Thrombin-glue kit, aspirated into sterile 20-cc syringe with blunt needle.
—sterile prep sponge
—1 sterile scissors, 2 sterile kelly clamps, 2 small sterile bowls
—2 sterile nonpowdered glove fingertips.

Assembly Instructions

—Ask circulating nurse for back table with sterile drapes and basin set.
—Individual assembling LVAD must be scrubbed, masked, gowned, and gloved in a sterile fashion. The LVAD is to be assembled using a strict aseptic technique.
—Open onto the sterile field: sewing ring with holder, dacron outflow graft with attached screw connector, and coring knife. Give sewing ring and holder and the coring knife to scrub nurse. Make sure a sterile banding gun and sterile nylon tie band are available for the procedure.

—Obtain 50 cc nonheparinized blood from anesthesia, and place in a small cup.
—Remove loose metal sewing ring from outflow graft and reserve for use after preclotting procedure.
—Pull the outflow graft taut by clamping the end to your sterile drape and holding on to the ring connector end. Coat the graft with the blood using the sterile prep sponge. Ensure the graft is well coated, while making sure blood does not come in contact with the threads of the metal ring connection or drip into the graft. (It will be helpful to have a square flat basin under your graft during this procedure to avoid saturation and contamination of your sterile field). Do not bake the metal sewing ring.
—Unclamp distal end of graft and use kelly to secure around body of graft near ring connection. Give to circulating nurse, in sterile manner, to bake.
—Run flash sterilizer and dry the graft in an autoclave using residual heat and standard protocol. Allow graft to cool after autoclaving.

Directions for Preclotting of TCI Heartmate and Thoratec Dacron Arterial Grafts

Immerse arterial graft in 2 U of cyoprecipitate (50 ml/U) and massage into graft for 5 min. Remove graft from cryoprecipitate and place in basin of 50 ml of thrombin (1,000 U/ml). Massage thrombin into the graft for 3–4 min. A gel should form on the graft. If not, repeat the process. Finally, flush out the graft carefully with saline to remove any remaining thrombin. Note: Spray thrombin may be used in place of soak method on the outside of graft material.

If preclotting BIVAD arterial grafts, cryopreciptate both grafts before thrombin procedure to prevent cross contamination and possible thrombin inside the graft. Thrombin will be on your gloves when you move to the second graft. Caution: Care must be taken not to contaminate the inner surface of the Dacron with thrombin to prevent the generation of thrombus in the bloodstream.

—Once cooled, replace the metal sewing ring on outflow graft, and place open-ended thread protector onto the outflow graft connector.
—Remove porcine xenograft valves from shipping jars by clamping white, plastic sleeves and placing onto sterile field onto blue towel. Give sleeves back to the circulator. Cut serial number tags off of valves and carefully remove all attached string.
—Simultaneously rinse both valves by gently agitating in sterile saline (rinse 10 min in basin one, 3 min in basin two, and 3 min in basin three). Inspect valve leaflet integrity during process.

—Give 2 syringes containing cryo and thrombin glue to nonsterile assistant. Hold the valves horizontally over a blue towel. Have assistant dispense equal amounts of cryo and thrombin over openings on exterior of graft conduits. Rotate the conduits to ensure even coating. Stand valves upright on sterile field without disturbing the cryo/thrombin coating. (Care must be taken to prevent cryo or thrombin from entering or collecting in the lumen of the valve conduits).

—Before attaching valves and filling of LVAD, a self-test of the console and calibration of the blood pump must be performed. You will require assistance from a second nonsterile person.

—Open the blood pump and drive cable onto the sterile field. Have assistant turn on the console and observe the proper self-test. Connect the interconnecting cable to the LVAD using the key in the cable connector as a quide to align it with the keyway in the LVAD percutaneous drive line.

—Pass the console end of the interconnect cable from the sterile field to the console operator, using minimal length of cable possible. Note that the cable bifurcates to air and electric connectors.

—Connect the pneumatic portion of the cable by attaching the white wing nut on cable end to the pump air drive out on the drive console rear panel. Attach the grey electrical connector by aligning and pushing it into the keyway labeled pump sensor in.

—Set the console to Fixed Rate 20 bpm, and Ejection Duration to 450 ms. Hold the LVAD parallel to the ground (Blood side up), and run a vent cycle, followed by 1 or 2 cycles at fixed rate. Observe that the stroke display is functional. (An LVAD that cannot be calibrated should not be implanted).

—The console must now remain "on" or stroke signal will be lost for deairing procedure.

—Disconnect the interconnect cable from the LVAD percutaneous drive line connector. Preserve sterility of maximum length of interconnect cable possible for reconnection during LVAD implantation.

—Attach preclotted inflow and outflow valve conduits to LVAD blood pump. Follow arrows on pump for proper orientation. Be sure to grasp valve connectors properly so that grafts or valves are not twisted or damaged. Hand tighten securely.

—Hold the LVAD in a vertical position. Fill the blood pump with sterile normal saline (for injection) through the inflow conduit. Tap and rotate pump with the outflow valve conduit at the highest point to expel all air. Once the pump is filled completely, attach a nonpowdered sterile glove fingertip over the inflow and outflow valve conduits. The pump is now ready for implantation.

—Confirm that:
Outflow graft has connector properly in place and oriented before surgeons begin anastomosis.
Outlet connector/graft connection is secure (firmly hand tightened).
LV vent is removed before pump strokes are initiated.
Aortic cross clamp is in place during pump deairing and initial pump strokes with hand crank.
Aortic clamp is off before normal pumping begins.
Observe proper pump filling/ejection and report flows.

Deaeration of the LVAD

Once the LVAD is in place and the inflow and outflow anastomoses are completed, residual air must be completely evacuated from the LVAD blood pumping chamber before initiating LVAD activation.

—Lower patient's head to a Trendelenburg position. A cross clamp should be on the outflow graft and the graft vent needle in place.
—Securely attach the hand crank to the actuation point located on the rear panel of the drive console. Slowly turn the hand crank in a clockwise direction to manually cycle the LVAD. The first cycle will pressurize the LVAD and force the priming saline and residual air out through the pores of the outflow graft and through the vent needle. At the end of ejection, blood will flow into the LVAD from the left ventricle. Hand cranking through both the eject and fill phases of the LVAD cycle should be done very slowly. LVAD filling is represented by the bar graph on the front panel display.
—When appropriate, the surgeon will remove the outflow graft cross-clamp while you continue to manually cycle the LVAD. Blood volume should be shifted from cardiopulmonary bypass (CPB) to the patient to allow for adequate LVAD filling.
—Continue turning the hand crank slowly to evacuate all air from the system and to allow the LVAD to fill completely as indicated on the bar graph of the console.
—Remove the hand crank and begin Fixed Rate pumping at a rate of 20 bpm with an Ejection Duration of 450 ms. This should produce a flow of approximately 1.6 LPM. Continue weaning CPB while increasing the LVAD rate at 5-bpm increments, until CPB is terminated.
—When the LVAD rate is 45 bpm or greater, and the stroke volume is 70–80 ml, adjust the ejection duration to 250–300 ms. The Auto mode may now be used.

Warnings and Precautions

—A complete backup Heartmate IP LVAS (LVAD, interconnect cable, and drive console) must be available on-site and in close proximity to the patient for use in emergency.

—All entrapped air must be evacuated from the LVAD blood pumping chamber and conduits to reduce the risk of air embolus. Prolonged deairing may be caused by inadequate blood being supplied to the LVAD.

—Right heart failure can occur after implantation of the device. RV dysfunction, especially when combined with elevated pulmonary vascular resistance, may limit LVAS effectiveness due to reduced filling of the LVAD.

—The patient electrical lead (identified as "Pump sensor in") should be disconnected from the back of the console whenever defibrillation paddles are used.

—In the event the LVAS stops operating and blood is stagnant in the pump for greater than a few minutes, there is a risk of stroke or thromboembolism should the device be restarted.

—Although a non-calibrated LVAS may provide adequate hemodynamic performance, the "Low Flow" alarm will be inactive. Therefore, an LVAS which cannot be calibrated should not be implanted.

—If "XXX" is displayed for stroke volume, confirm that the blood side of the LVAD is facing up, and repeat the vent cycle to observe functional stroke volume. If the inability to calibrate persists, replace the interconnect cable and console and recalibrate.

—Do not allow the percutaneous drive line to become wet or contaminated.

—Heparin is not be used after device implantation, unless low flow conditions (stroke volume less than 30 cc) arise for longer than 30 min, or if medically indicated.

—Once the device is successfully implanted, administer protamine to reverse heparin.

—Always remove the hand crank before initiating console pumping. Failure to do so may result in the crank becoming airborne, and may cause injury.

Policy and Procedure Guidelines
CP46

VENTRICULAR ASSIST PROTOCOL WITH ROTAFLOW CENTRIFUGAL PUMP OR CENTRIMAG CENTRIFUGAL PUMP

Equipment

1. MaQuet Rotaflow pump console or CentriMag console
2. Rotaflow or Centrimag sterile disposable pump head (2)
3. Cardiotomy reservoir (if perfusionist primes)
4. Sterile tubing (2–6′ lengths) or (RVAD loop pack [Fig. 1]) (if coated use tie bands)
5. Tubing clamps
6. 1 L bag balanced electrolyte solution
7. 3/8″ Cobe sat/Hct cell with 2 pigtails (if CVVH is needed, check with surgeon?)

Procedure

1. The perfusionist or surgeon may prime the Rotaflow or CentriMag centrifugal blood pump.

2. All the materials needed should have been brought into the operating room ready for use. The following items are needed: Rotaflow or CentriMag

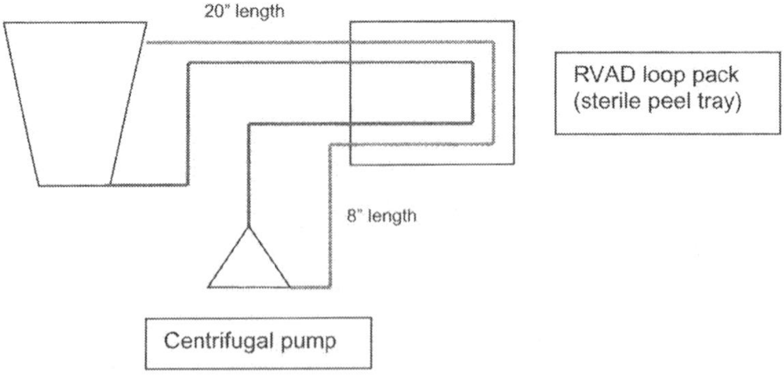

Fig. 1. RVAD loop pack.

console, Rotaflow or CentriMag disposable sterile tubing (2 6′ lengths 3/8″ × 3/32″ or RVAD loop pack) cardiotomy reservoir, rapid prime line and 2L of priming solution, and lactated Ringer's if perfusionist is priming outside sterile field.

3. The accessory tubings are aseptically handed to the scrub nurse in the sterile field. The surgeon will cut desired tubing lengths and connect them to the pump inlet and outlet allowing enough length for connection to the extracorporeal cannulae. The surgeon will prime the centrifugal head and tubing with a bulb syringe. The centrifugal pump head is handed off to the perfusionist for proper insertion into the drive unit. The pump outflow tubing is clamped until all tubing/cannulae connections are made and the circuit is confirmed air free. Confirm proper flow direction with the surgical team. (**THIS LINE IS OUT OF THE PATIENT AND INTO THE CETRIFUGAL PUMP, etc.**)

RPMs are set to ensure forward flow, clamp is released, and support is established upon the surgeons command.

Alternate Method

Using the RVAD table loop, connect the short blue end to the Rotaflow or CentriMag pump inlet and the short red end to the Rotaflow or CentriMag pump outlet. Next, connect the long blue end to the bottom of the cardiotomy reservoir and the long red end to the top of the cardiotomy reservoir and prime pump.

4. Clamp the tubing on the reservoir outlet and fill the reservoir with priming solution using the rapid prime line. The Perfusionist inverts the blood pump and raises it above the reservoir, then releases the clamp and slowly lowers the blood pump in the inverted position allowing it to fill. Once the blood pump is full and most of the air is displaced, turn it upright and place it in the drive unit. Begin pumping. Make sure all bubbles are removed.

5. Stop recirculation by clamping the pump outflow tubing in preparation for connection to the cannulae. The surgical team will clamp and divide each tubing, confirming proper flow direction with the perfusionist (i.e., **THIS LINE IS OUT OF THE PATIENT AND INTO THE CENTRIFUGAL PUMP**)

Note: Use the long, black Rotaflow drive line to position the pump head close to the patient allowing short tubing lengths while maintaining enough drive line and tubing length to facilitate safe transport to the ICU.

Cannulation

1. Right/left atrial cannula, lighthouse tip, right angle, or malleable.
2. Pulmonary artery/aortic cannula (similar to type used for arterial cannulation), Hemashield graft sewn to the PA/Ao (Abiomed cannula), or RVOT cannulation with appropriately sized malleable cannula.
3. May use coated cannulae and connectors if possible.

Initiation of Ventricular Assist

After weaning from cardiopulmonary bypass, and once the decision has been made to support the patient on ventricular assist, flow is initiated and increased incrementally. The total systemic blood flow (native ventricular output + ventricular assist pump flow) should be maintained at 2.2 L/min/m^2.

Anticoagulation

The patient weaned from cardiopulmonary bypass should have heparin neutralized with the appropriate dose of protamine. The first 24 h of ventricular assist may require no heparin therapy; after the initial 24 h anticoagulation therapy and modalities will be determined by the attending surgeon. The VAD flow should not be decreased below 500 cc/min, regardless of the level of anticoagulation, to avoid possible stagnation and thrombus formation.

Discontinuation from VAD

After 24 h, if the patient's clinical picture is stable, the assist pump flow rate is decreased to a level that causes the atrial pressure to rise. Cardiac output calculations should be assessed to determine the function of the ventricle. When the surgeon has decided that the native ventricle can support the required cardiac output, the assist device may be removed. Removal of the device should be in the cardiothoracic intensive cave unit (CTICU) or the operating room.

Rotaflow

When using the Rotaflow (Fig. 2) as a standalone be sure the console is plugged into an emergency outlet (red) and make sure the rear mains circuit breaker is in the on position. Always have a backup console and drive unit available. Use extreme caution when moving patients on VAD support. If transporting with rotaflow on the stretcher, do not allow the fan or air intakes to become blocked.

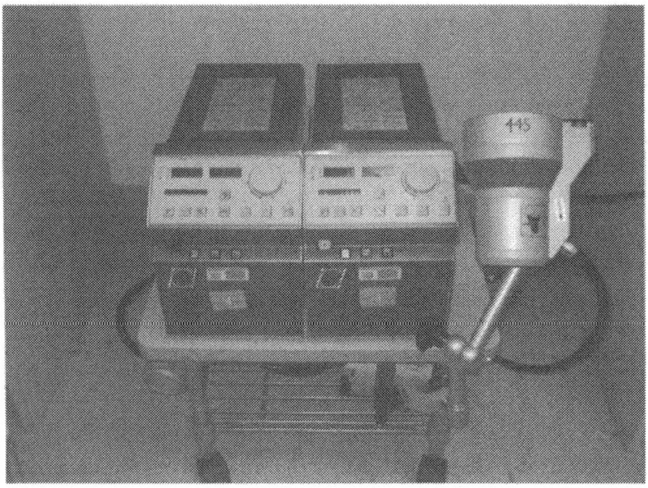

Fig. 2. The Roteflow.

POLICY AND PROCEDURE MANUAL

Date issued:	
Approved:	Approved:

Centrimag/Rotaflow VAD with Quadrox "D" ECMO

On occasion, it may be necessary to provide pulmonary support after Centrimag or Rotaflow ventricular assist device placement. This support should only be used on right side ventricular assist. The Quadrox D diffusion membrane oxygenator from MaQuet should be used.

The perfusionist should prime the Quadrox D oxygenator using a cardiotomy reservoir, 3/8″ tubing, a roller pump, and prime solution. After priming and debubbling the oxygenator, the inlet and outlet tubing should be clamped and divided approximately 6–8″ from the oxygenator. The Quadrox D is then inserted into the RVAD pump outflow tubing utilizing 2 3/8″ × 3/8″ connectors. In some circumstances, pigtails may be attached to the luer locks on a 3/8″ Cobe sat/Hct cell connected to the blood inflow side of the Quadrox D oxygenator for CVVH for VV extracorporeal membrane oxygenation (ECMO), but should not be used for VA ECMO (Figs. 3 and 4). **Confirm with surgeon before setup**.

Use caution and confirm proper direction of flow out of the centrifugal pump into the oxygenator and then out of the oxygenator and into

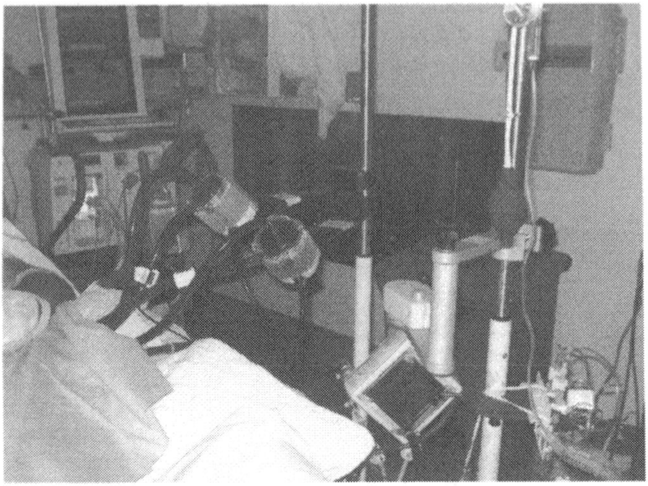

Fig. 3. In extenuating circumstances pigtails may be attached to the luer locks on a 3/8″ Cobe sat/hct cell connected to the blood inflow side of the Quadrox D oxygenator for CVVH for VV ECMO, but should not be used for VA ECMO.

the patient (PA cannula). The oxygenator should be placed at or below the level of the patient.

Oxygenator inlet and outlet pressures should be monitored using Transpac pressure transducers and a pressure bag. Do not use pressure domes because stagnation of flow will allow clot formation in the pres-

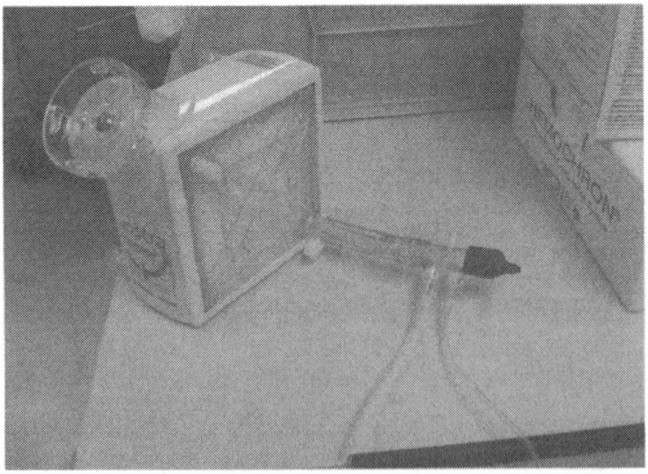

Fig. 4. Quadrox blood inlet with 3/8″ sat/Hct cell and pigtails for CVVH.

sure monitoring lines. Positive pressure lines and coated tubing should be tie banded at the second barb back to secure extracorporeal tubing without causing pockets and possible areas of thrombus formation.

A Sechrist blender is used to provide adequate sweep and appropriate FiO_2 during ECMO support. An oxygen tank may be used for transport to the CTICU. A heater–cooler is used to maintain normothermia during ECMO support. Continuous temperature and pressure monitoring should be used during ECMO support.

Charting with an adult ECMO flow sheet/checklist should begin immediately upon ECMO initiation and continue into the ICU. Once in the ICU, pre- and postoxygenator pressures should be monitored on the CTICU patient monitor. The perfusionist must confirm with the CTICU nursing staff that pressure alarms are set at 50–75 mmHg above and below the baseline values. This will allow us to track changes over time as well as acute events which may require immediate attention. Continuous patient temperature monitoring should also be tracked on the CTICU patient monitor, and alarm parameters should be set within 0.1–1.0 degrees above and below normothermia.

Upon arrival in the CTICU and when rounding, the perfusionist should, inservice nursing, record appropriate patient parameters, including blood gases, RPMs, flow, BP, CVP, PA, pre/post pressures, SVO_2, heparin rate, ACT, temperature, and major events, and review the checklist, including careful inspection of the oxygenator, heater–cooler, blender, tubing connections, lines, centrifugal pumps, consoles, pressure transducers, and any perfusion-related parameters or equipment.

Policy and Procedure Guidelines
CP47

PROCEDURE FOR THORATEC VENTRICULAR ASSIST DEVICE

Description

The Thoratec ventricular assist device (VAD) System consists of three major components: a blood pump, cannulae, and a drive console. The device is designed to support the circulation of blood in the pulmonary circulation (right sided support) and/or the systemic circulation (left sided support) in patients meeting the criteria for VAD support.

1. Equipment. Verify that all VAD components needed for the procedure are present.

Ventricular assist blood pump
Dual drive console
Pneumatic lead
Electrical lead
Hand pumping bulb
VAD accessory kit
Thrombin spray and cryoprecipitate for graft preclotting
Cannulae (Fig. 1):
Arterial cannula, long straight, 18 cm graft 14812-2558-000
18 cm long straight tube + 30 cm long graft (14 mm ID)
Ventricular cannula, blunt tip 14114-2572-000
27 cm long straight tube + 2.5 cm long, 16 mm OD velour-covered tip (no side holes)
Ventricular cannula, extra long, blunt tip 14816-2569-000
29 cm long straight tube + 2.5 cm long, 16 mm OD velour-covered tip (no side holes)
Atrial cannula, short 14120-2563-000
25 cm long with right angle bend and 10 cm velour cuff
Atrial cannula, long 14121-2562-000
30 cm long with right angle bend and 13 cm velour cuff

2. Pass VAD equipment to sterile field (inspect for any defects).

3. VAD preparation. Prime VAD using 100 U sodium heparin in 250 ml 5% albumin. Once filled (approximately 150 ml), cap outlets of

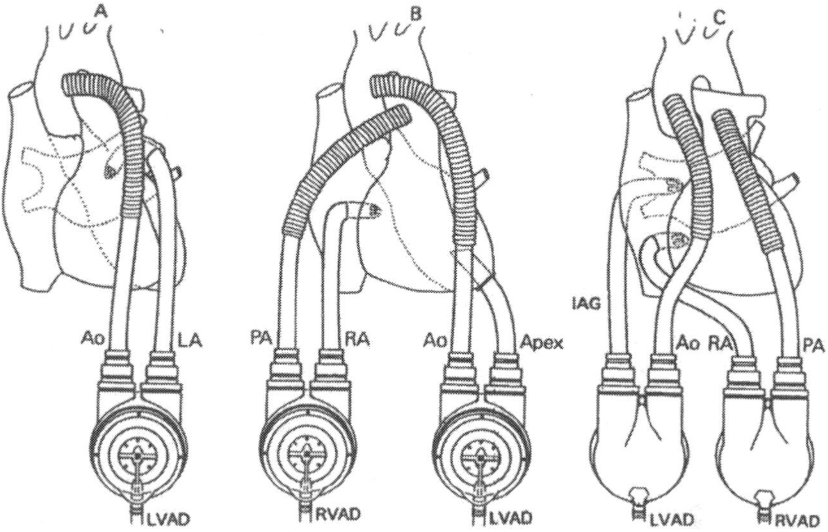

Fig. 1. Typical cannulation sites for right or left ventricular assist.

device with luered valve housing caps found in accessory kit. Cap pump dual-lead drive line with blue cap found in accessory kit. This connector must be protected from fluids.

4. Confirm that colored ring collets correspond with cannulae connections (Figs. 2 and 3):

White collet nuts (smaller) are used for the arterial and ventricular cannulae.

Black collet nuts (larger) are used for the cage-tip atrial cannula.

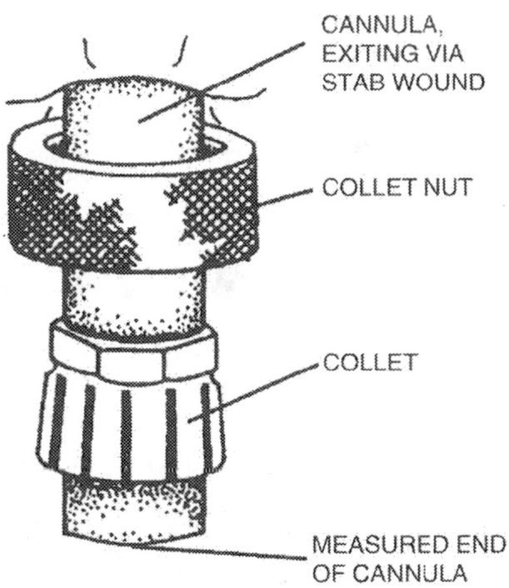

Fig. 2. Schematic of collet nut and collet over cannula that will be conneted to VAD.

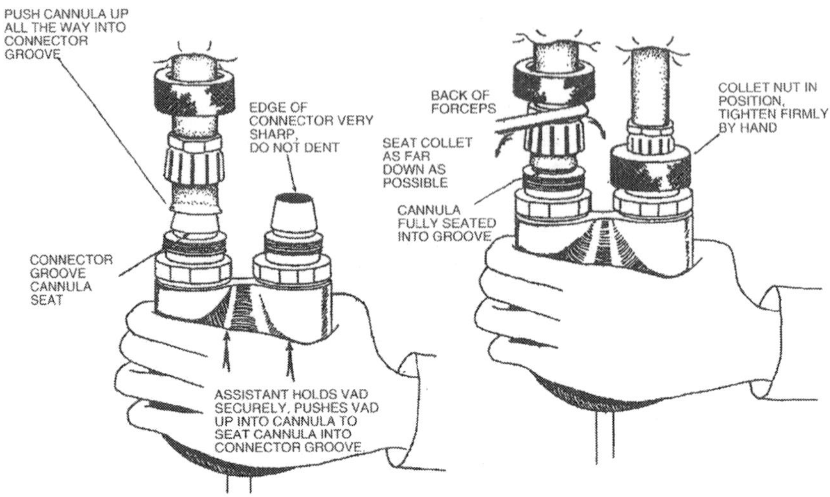

Fig. 3. Schematic discription of attachment of the cannula to VAD.

5. Arterial cannula preparation. Put 2 U (50 cc/U) of cryoprecipitate in a basin and massage into graft for 5 min. Remove graft from cryoprecipitate and place in basin of 50 ml thrombin (1000 U/ml). Spray thrombin may be preferred on the outside of graft material in place of soak method. Massage thrombin into the graft for 3–4 min.

CAUTION: Care must be taken not to contaminate the inner surface of the Dacron with thrombin to prevent the generation of thrombus in the bloodstream.

A gel should form on the graft. If not, repeat the process. Finally, flush out the graft carefully with saline to remove any remaining thrombin. If preclotting BIVAD arterial grafts, cryoprecipiate both grafts before thrombin procedure to prevent cross contamination and possible thrombin inside the graft.

DUAL DRIVE CONSOLE OPERATION

Refer to red quick reference sheet attached to console and as follows:

Thoratec Dual-Drive Console Quick Reference

A. STARTUP PROCEDURE (Before Connecting to Patient)

1. Verify that **Power** switch is **On** (on back door)

2. Open back door and verify that UPS is **On** (on rear surface of uninterruptable power supply, "UPS").
3. Turn top and bottom module **Power** switches to **On** (to **Operation** on older units) and verify that **Calibration** switch is **Off** (on rear drive modules).
4. Turn **On** compressor switches (on compressor tray) for top and bottom modules.
5. **Check that Emergency Selector Valve is in normal position (central position, located on inside of back door).** Close back door.
6. Set initial console settings for operating room:
   a. **Mode** **Async**
   b. **Set rate:** 40 bpm
   c. **Set % systole:** 20%
   d. Pressure: 100–110 mmHg
   e. Vacuum: 0 to −4 mmHg

B. <u>INITIAL PUMPING IN THE OPERATING ROOM</u>

1. Surgeon will remove blue protector from the dual-lead drive line and attach pneumatic and electrical leads.
2. Start hand pumping slowly, check suture lines and removal of all air from VAD.
3. Connect VAD **Drive Lines** and **Fill Switch In (Hall Switch** in older units) cables to driver (on back door).
4. Initiate VAD pumping (**Pump On**) after VAD is de-aired in Async (fixed rate mode) at 40 bpm. (To stop VAD pumping, press **Pump On**, light will blink, press **Enter** to stop pump. Press **Clear** to silence alarm). To reinitiate pumping, press **Pump On.**
5. Observe for air, check for intact suture lines, then:
   a. Gradually increase drive pressure to over 200 mmHg (LVAD) and over 140 mmHg (right VAD [RVAD]).
   b. Apply vacuum carefully to approximately −10 to −25 mmHg.

      <u>**CAUTION: When the chest is open, excessive vacuum increases the risk of air embolism.**</u>

   c. Wean the patient from CPB.
   d. Increase set rate/% systole, or change to **Volume** mode once VAD is filling and ejecting completely.
6. Troubleshooting for inadequate VAD filling and flow output.
   a. Increase drive pressure and/or vacuum (with caution).
   b. If required, decrease set rate and % systole to allow more time for filling.
   c. Administer fluids or blood products.

d. Provide inotropic support and vasodilators as needed.
e. Insert RVAD for RV failure with high right atrial pressure and poor left VAD (LVAD) filling.

C. EASIEST SETTINGS FOR AUTOMATIC PUMPING

1. Recommended settings:
   a. **Mode: Volume** (full-to-empty)
   b. **Set Value Rate: 50–60** bpm
   c. **Set Value % systole: (Always use one half of Set Value Rate), i.e., 25–30%**
   d. Drives Pressures
      LVAD: 230–245 mmHg
      RVAD 140–160 mmHg
   e. Vacuum –25 to –40 mmHg
2. Few or no adjustments should be required with a stable patient. No fine-tuning is required.
3. If the **sync** alarm comes on (no fill signal), indicating that the VAD is not filling at this rate, lower the **Set Value Rate** to 40 bpm, and lower the **Set Value % systole** to 20%.
4. Refer to Detailed Descriptions in the Dual-Drive Console Directions for Use for more information.

D. ALARMS AND TROUBLESHOOTING

For all alarm conditions—first assess the patient, then observe the VAD to insure that it is filling and emptying, then assess the console.

1. SYNC alarm in Volume mode (No fill signal received; VAD output displays –E-): Check cables and connections, vacuum level, patient volume, and cannula position. **If required, lower set (backup) rate, and set % systole to allow more time for filling.**
2. Pressure alarm (Drive pressure (Eject) is <100 mmHg or >250 mmHg): Adjust regulator. Check compressors, pneumatic connections, and transducer calibration.
3. Vacuum alarm (Drive pressure (Fill) is >+4 mmHg or <–99 mmHg): Adjust regulator. Check compressors, pneumatic connections and transducer calibration.
4. Low Battery alarm (<30 min remaining on module battery): Plug console into AC electrical outlet to recharge batteries; replace battery if required.
5. External Alarm. Connect external alarm output (one for each VAD) to hospital remote alarm (nurse call) system. (Alarms when no fill signals received from VAD for 8 s or longer); same troubleshooting as Sync alarm.

ALWAYS KEEP HAND PUMPING BULBS WITH THE CONSOLE

In the event of console failure, disconnect pneumatic driveline from console and connect to hand bulb. Squeeze the hand bulb about once per second. Connect VAD to back-up console as soon as possible.

Typical Dual-Drive Console Settings for Automatic Operation

Mode:	Volume
Set rate:	50–60 bpm
Set % systole:	25%–30% (1/2 Set Rate = 300 ms)
Drive pressure:	LVAD: 230–245 mmHg RVAD: 140–160 mmHg
Vacuum:	–25 to –40 mmHg

It is important to maintain:

- VAD index >2.0 L/min/m^2
- Complete VAD filling (green fill light)
- Complete VAD ejection (confirm with Flash Test—transmission of light through the opposite side of the VAD, using a flashlight)

THORATEC DUAL-DRIVE CONSOLE TROUBLESHOOTING GUIDE

Condition	Possible Cause(s)	Corrective Action
No fill light when VAD observed to be full	Module not receiving fill signal, faulty fill cable (VAD to console)	Check cable connection. Replace cable (VAD to driver)
Vol output display read –E-	Pressure not above 100 mmHg range, no fill signal received, ms eject not greater than 250 ms	Check for fill signal, confirm adequate drive pressure, confirm ejection duration >250 ms **(Press % Systole twice to read eject time ms)**
Pressure alarm sounds; Red light is ON	Pressure is less than 100 mmHg or greater than 250 mmHg (an–E- Appears instead of VAD output)	Adjust regulator; check compressors, UPS, pneumatic connections, or calibration.

(Continued)

(*Continued*)

Condition	Possible Cause(s)	Corrective Action
Vacuum alarm sounds; Red light is ON	Vacuum is outside acceptable range of +4 to −99 mmHg	Adjust regulator; check compressors, UPS, and pneumatic connections, or calibration.
Sync alarm sounds in VOLUME mode	No fill signal is received (an –E- appears instead of VAD output)	Check fill switch cables and connections, vacuum level, Patient volume, and cannula positions. If required, lower Set Rate (back-up rate) and Set % Systole to increase Time for VAD filling.
Low battery alarms sounds; Red light is on	Module batteries have less than 30 min of power remaining	plug Dual Drive Console into electrical outlet to recharge batteries or replace batteries if required.
Incomplete VAD filling	Vacuum too low	Increase Vacuum (50 mmHg)
	Set rate or set % systole too high	Decrease set rate (until fill signal appears) and decrease set % systole (>250 ms to 300 ms).
	Poor cannula position; cannula or pneumatic hose may be kinked	Check cannula position; check cannula and pneumatic hose for kinks.

(*Continued*)

Condition	Possible Cause(s)	Corrective Action
	Patient-related reasons: hypovolemia, right ventricular failure, ventricular recovery, tamponade, inadequate pharmacologic support	Volume loading to increase preload (atrial pressure) may improve VAD filling; medication may improve VAD filling by increasing ventricular contract-Ility or right ventricular output to an LVAD.
Incomplete VAD ejection	Drive pressure too low	Increase drive pressure (LVAD <250 mmHg and RVAD <170 mmHg).
	Set % systole too low	Increase set % systole (<320 ms).
	Patient's systolic blood pressure or pulmonary pressure too high	Lower patient's systolic pressure (if hypertensive).
	Outflow cannula may be kinked	Check outflow cannula.
How to Increase VAD Output	If no hypovolemia, cardiac tamponade or right ventricular failure and adequate pharmacological support	Increase Vacuum (<–50 mmHg) or decrease set % systole (>250 ms or an –E- will be displayed).

ANTICOAGULATION PROTOCOL*

Phase 1

Heparin at 10 U/kg/h

When chest tube drainiage falls to 50 ml/h for 2–3 h, with stable hematocrit and hemoglobin levels without transfusion of blood products, and coagulation factors (prothrombin time [PT], partial thromboplastin time [PTT], fibrinogen, and platelet count) approaching normal.

Several centers use low molecular weight dextran at 25 ml/h in the first 24–72 postoperative hours, instead of heparin. However, the use of dextran is controversial because its effectiveness and mechanism of action in VAD patients is unclear.

Phase 2

Increase heparin dose to maintain the PTT approximately 1.5 times control.

After at least 72 h post-op, when the risk of bleeding is diminished by the healing of raw surfaces and the repair of hemostatic abnormality associated with cardiopulmonary bypass.

Phase 3

Warfarin administration to maintain International Normalized Ratio (INR) range 2.5–3.5.

Once the patient is extubated and tolerating oral medication, start warfarin (overlapping with heparin). Warfarin administration is similar to patients with a mechanical heart valve. After obtaining an acceptable INR, discontinue heparin or dextran.

Several centers administer aspirin (80 mg) every day for patients supported >30 d or for platelet counts >300 (TH/mm^3) to help prevent platelet aggregation on the artificial surfaces.

*Significant drops in the hematocrit (Hct) and hemoglobin (Hbg) levels, possibly requiring blood transfusions, or the inability to stabilize Hct or Hgb levels may require modification of anticoagulation (i.e., lower heparin or warfarin dosage, or discontinuing aspirin administration).

Directions for Preclotting of TCI Heartmate and Thoratec Dacron Arterial Grafts

Immerse arterial graft in 2 units of cyoprecipitate (50 ml/unit) and massage into graft for 5 minutes. Remove graft from cryoprecipitate and place in basin of 50 ml of thrombin (1,000 units/ml). Massage thrombin into the graft for 3–4 minutes. A gel should form on the graft. If not, repeat the process. Finally, flush out the graft carefully with saline to remove any remaining thrombin.

Note: Spray thrombin may be used in place of soak method on the outside of graft material.

If preclotting BIVAD arterial grafts, cryoprecipitate both grafts prior to Thrombin procedure to prevent cross contamination and possible thrombin inside the graft.

Thrombin will be on your gloves when you move to the second graft.

Caution: Care must be taken not to contaminate the inner surface of the Dacron with thrombin to prevent the generation of thrombus in the bloodstream.

Policy and Procedure Guidelines
CP48

THE DEBAKEY VENTRICULAR ASSIST DEVICE

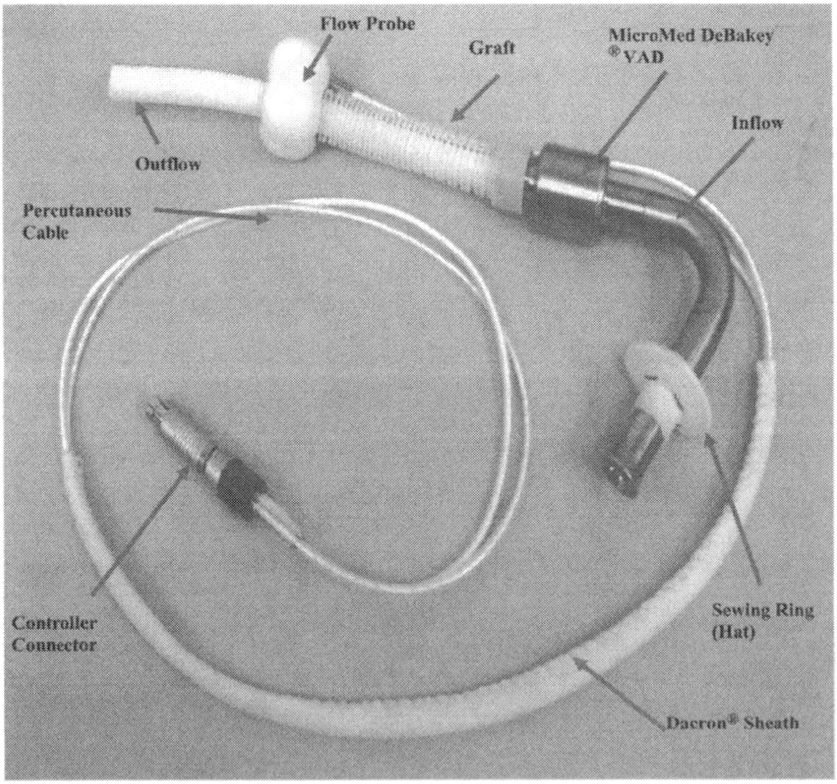

Fig. 1.

STERILE PUMP SETUP

Preliminary Procedures

Order 3 L of D5W, gather CDAS, surgical suitcase, 4 charged batteries, plug in CDAS, program controllers.

Remove round coring blade and white plastic tip from suitcase (small plastic cylinder, supplied new with each Ventricular assist device [VAD]) and give to nurses to flash.

Preparing the Pump for Surgery–Sterile Assistant

1. Remove contents from the sterile pump pouch **(note: the foil wrap around the pump is not sterile, remove this wrap first, then make an aseptic handoff to the sterile field, peeling open the inner clear plastic wraps)** and the surgical accessories, which include (Fig. 2):

- VAD (with attached sterile wedge and sterile wedge nut)
- Accessory bag (sterile items: sewing ring, cable cap, wedge nut wrench, Surgilube, and graft protector)
- Trocar handle (2 plastic pieces and 1 metal piece)
- Trocar blade (2 12-mm pieces: 1 metal circular blade and 1 plastic tip)
- Percutaneous introducer (4 pieces: plastic handle and cover and metal point and shaft)
- Dummy pump (2 pieces: plastic pump body and metal inlet cannula)
- VAD sterile extension cable (gray, approximately 0.8 m)
- Sterile 12-mm Sulzer Vascutek graft.

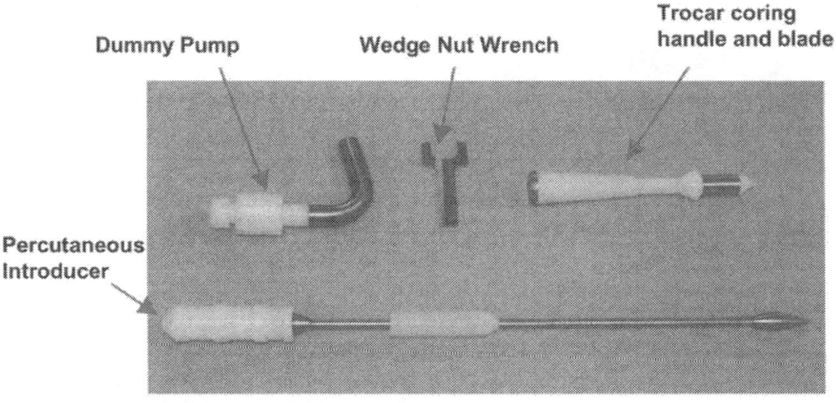

Fig. 2. Assembled Surgical Tools.

2. Carefully unscrew nut and inner compression ring from pump. Be careful this ring doesn't fall off the table when removing the nut. Attach the graft to the pump (tighten with wedge nut wrench) (Figs. 3–8).

3. Slide on graft protector until it snaps into place (Fig. 9).

4. Slide the flow probe onto the graft; the wire points in the direction of the pump, parallel with the pump motor wires (Fig. 10).

5. Attach the pump cable to the sterile gray extension cable.

6. Hand off the open end of the extension cable to the non-sterile perfusionist or technician.

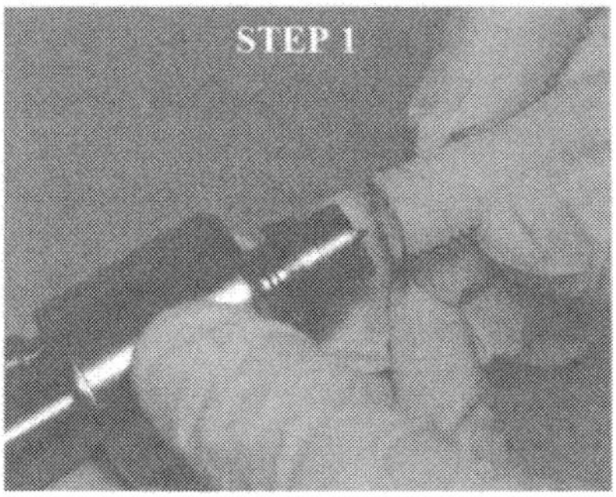

Fig. 3. Slide graft on outlet of pump.

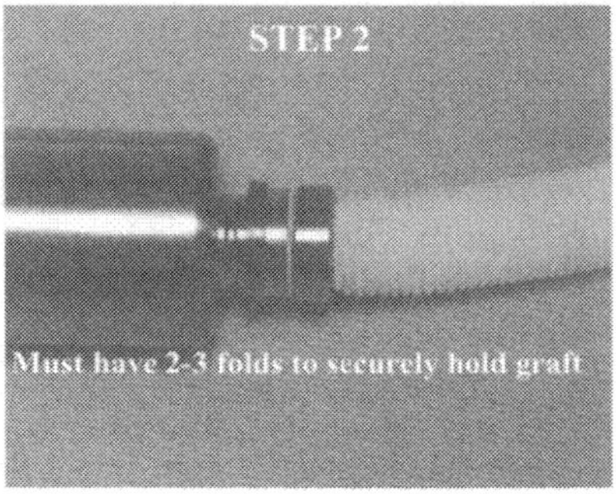

Fig. 4. Slide wedge over graft, trapping 2 or 3 folds of graft. If graft creases, hold wedge while gently pulling graft until crease is pulled out.

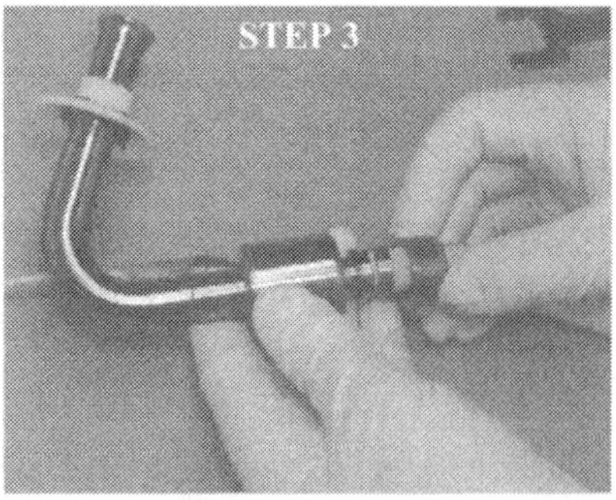

Fig. 5. Slide nut over graft and wedge and tighten to a "loose," finger-tight condition.

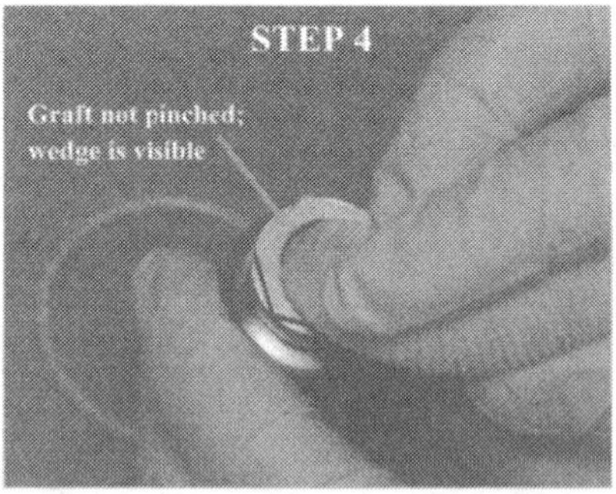

Fig. 6. Gently pull any pinched graft that may occur between nut and wedge. When graft is installed correctly and not pinched, the wedge will be visible when the graft is gently pulled away from the nut.

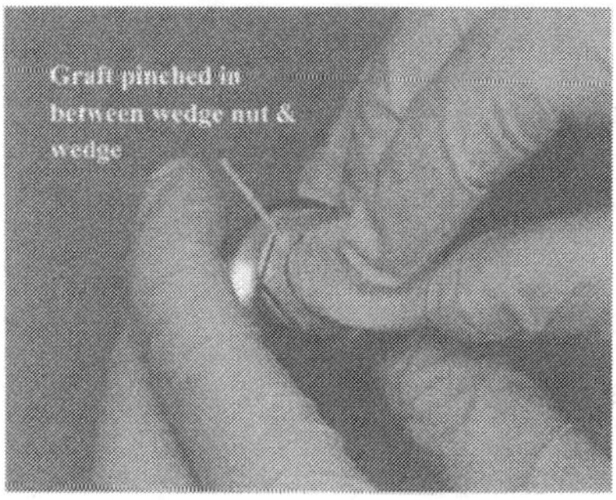

Fig. 7. Pinched graft. **INCORRECT**

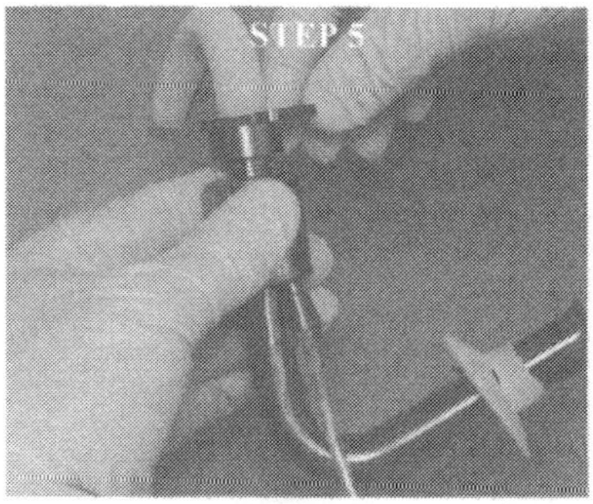

Fig. 8. When assured that graft is not pinched, tighten wedge nut with wrench. Do not hold inlet cannula when tightening nut; only hold pump housing as illustrated.
Caution: Do not press on power cable connection!

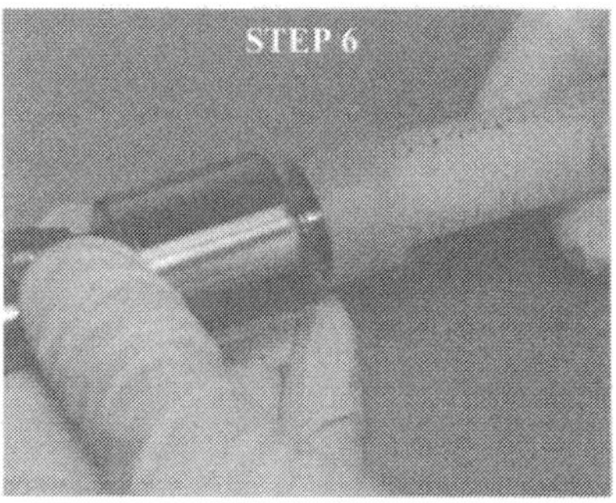

Fig. 9. Slide graft protector over nut. Make sure graft protector slides fully on nut and snaps into place.

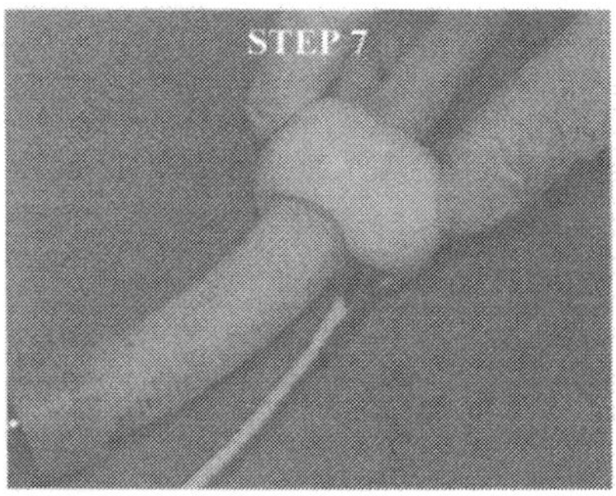

Fig. 10. Slide on the flow probe; the wire points in the direction of the pump parallel with the pump motor wires. **Note:** Make sure the flow probe is close against the graft protector when given to the surgeon and implanted.

7. Place the pump in a bowl of sterile D5W (10 cm deep; approximately 3 liters), and manipulate the pump to remove air (Fig. 11).

8. Place your finger over the inlet of the pump to partially occlude inflow by approximately 80% (Fig. 12). Always maintain pump inlet below the fluid level.

9. Instruct nonsterile perfusionist or technician to start the pump (Box 1). (The pump may require several start/stops to completely remove the

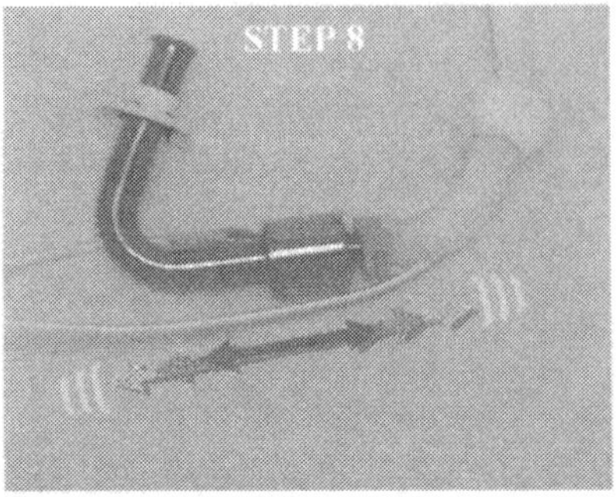

Fig. 11. Place the pump in a bowl of sterile 5% dextrose in water (10 cm deep; approximately 3 L) and manipulate the pump to remove air. Gently shake pump axially to wet bearings and remove air bubbles. Repeatedly tilt the pump to allow D5W to wash completely through the pump.

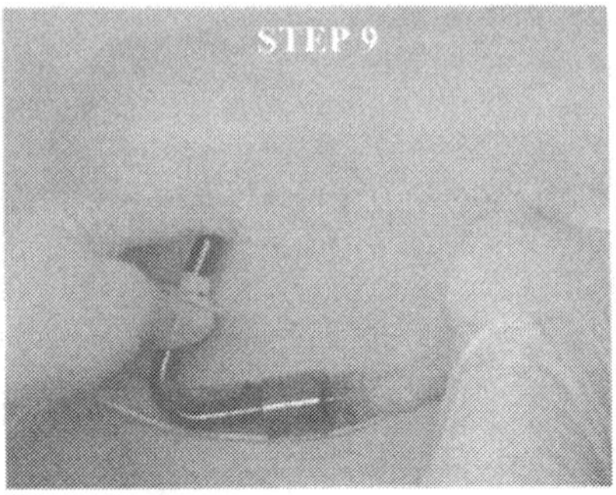

Fig. 12. Place finger over the inlet of the pump to partially occlude inflow. Always maintain pump inlet below saline.

air entrapped in the bearings.) Use backup controller and 2nd clear lexan battery holder in drawer of CDAS. See last figure for detailed instruction.

10. Let the pump run for several seconds. Observe strong flow from pump outlet.

11. Disconnect the gray extension cable from the VAD cable and:

BOX 1. TEST PUMP

1. Use 2nd clear lexan battery holder and connect to back up controller. Do not connect battery yet.
2. Have sterile tech connect gray extension cable to the device. Hand the other end of the gray extension cable off the field and connect to the backup controller.
3. While the sterile tech keeps the pump submerged and 80% of the inflow occluded, put the battery into the clear lexan holder and test pump flow.
4. Remove battery and repeat to confirm deairing and proper pump operation.
5. Cover basin with sterile towel and leave pump submerged until ready for use, disconnect extension cable and keep electrical connections dry.

a. Discard the extension cable from the surgical field

–or–

b. Ask the nonsterile perfusionist or technician to disconnect the test extension cable from the controller and retain the test extension cable in the surgical field, with protection over the now nonsterile connector.

12. Place the protective cap over the VAD cable to protect it during the surgery. Leave pump in the basin of D5W and cover with a sterile towel.

13. At the request of the surgeon, hand him or her the pump with the protective cap in place.

14. When the surgeon tunnels the percutaneous lead through the skin, retain the percutaneous introducer in the sterile field and hand off the VAD connector to the nonsterile perfusionist or technician.

15. Instruct sterile scrub nurse to set up the surgical tools as shown in Fig. 2.

DEBAKEY VAD, NONSTERILE TASKS, CONTROLLER SETUP

Surgical Suitcase

- Verify the contents of the suitcase with the packing list. A backup suitcase must be present and complete before surgery may proceed.
- Remove new coring blade and plastic tip (small plastic cylinder, new with each device) from suitcase and give to nurses for sterilization. Steam or ETO sterilize nonsterile components while disassembled: percutaneous introducer, dummy pump, coring trocar handle, new coring blade, and plastic tip.
- Fully charge VAD batteries using the PHSS.

Controller (prepare both controllers)

1. Power up CDAS first and then laptop, power switches on rear of each.

2. It will power up and ask for password. Enter "**boot**", then click on pump control screen. It will ask for password. Enter "**minman**" and hit enter.

3. Plug 1st controller into CDAS. It will say "directory not found please enter pt. data." Click "**ok**", then click "**ACCEPT**" and "**SAVE**" until the screen clears and allows you to click on "**STOP PUMP.**" Then click on "**ACKNOWLEDGE ALARMS**" box and the alarms will silence.

4. Go to **set up display screen**, find box, and click on **patient data**. Enter patient data, (patient name, 3 initials, patient ID, hospital ID, implant date DD/MM/YY, and pump ID [this # is found on the outside of the big gray suitcase). Do not alter Controller ID or Flow Probe data. Save and accept the patient data.

5. Download language to controller. **English** is the default language, but must be entered.

6. Run All VAD controller tests from CDAS (set up display screen). Select "**TEST**" then click "**EXECUTE TEST.**" Repeat until all tests are complete.

7. Stay in set up display screen and

A. set alarm parameters to maximum to avoid alarms during surgery

- **a. excess current threshold amps to 3.0**
- **b. set low rpm threshold to 7,500 and press set**
- **c. set low flow threshold to –4.0**

B. click on **synch with CDAS time**

8. Set "pump speed preset" to **7,500 RPM**

9. Disconnect controller, mark it with a patient white sticky label, and place it in the draw of CDAS for backup.

10. Repeat above procedure with second controller. When done place 9 V battery in 2nd controller and leave this controller hooked up to CDAS.

Immediately Before Surgery (if performed as above move to step 6)

1. Power up the *primary* controller by connecting to the CDAS.
2. "Stop Pump" from Pump Control screen on CDAS (once startup sequence is finished).
3. Synch controller time to CDAS time (setup screen).
4. Verify alarm values are at extremes (setup screen).
5. Install internal 9 V battery into *primary* controller.
6. Connect battery pocket to primary controller and install a fully charged battery. Prepare surgical pouch, set up small surgical pouch with 1 fully charged battery inserted into clear lexan battery holder, plug clear plastic battery holder cable into primary controller port #2 (leave CDAS connected to port #1). Place battery behind controller and insert into flexible material surgical pouch. Place 2 tie bands around pouch to hold battery and controller together. Extend cord from CDAS and hang pouch with a Kelly clamp from the table at the patient's right hip.

Connection of Pump to Controller

1. At the instruction of the sterile assistant or surgeon, take the percutaneous cable (just tunneled through the skin) and inspect the connectors for liquid debris.
2. Fully slide on the white defibrillation insulator.
3. Connect the cable to the *primary* controller hanging below the operating table.
4. At the request of the surgeon, start and stop the pump.

Immediately After Starting the Pump

1. Take a snapshot of the pump performance on the Pump Control screen (optional).
2. Report the pump performance at the request of the surgeons.
3. If the flow signal is noisy (tracing is not smooth), verify that the received voltages are above 1 V (pump control screen). Add Surgilube or saline if necessary at graft probe site.
4. Set the pump RPM conservatively slow (7,500–9,000 RPM).

After Surgery

1. Adjust the pump speed on the Pump Control screen.

2. Adjust the alarm values (usually approximately 20% from the nominal values; set excess current to 1.2).

3. Attach the retention clip to the connector barrel (optional) and screw the white defib insulator onto the controller nut (Fig. 13).

4. Assemble VAD Pack, and place two fully charged batteries into P1 and P2 in the VAD pack. Disconnect the P2 from the controller at the patients right hip **(Make sure the CDAS remains plugged into the contoller and still powered up at this point or the VAD will stop).** Plug the P2 wire from the VAD pack (with fully charged batteries installed) into the P2 port on the controller at the patient's right hip. Now the VAD pack with batteries will power the device and you can disconnect the CDAS wire from port P1 on the controller. Immediately plug the P1 wire from the VAD Pack into the P1 port on the controller for battery back up. The CDAS wire can be plugged into the covered CDAS connection port on the outside of the VAD Pack to confirm communication.

5. Check and record performance of the flow probe/meter by evaluating received amplitude on Pump Control screen of CDAS (should be >1 V).

6. Reset these same alarm values (using setup display screen) on the backup controller.

7. **NEVER POWER DOWN CDAS WHEN CONNECTED TO THE PATIENT**. To shut down CDAS, disconnect CDAS from patient (unplug from VAD Pack, exterior connection, make sure two charged batteries are plugged in VAD Pack and connected to controller). After you have disconnected the CDAS from the patient, hit control-alt-delete and click shut down, wait until the screen says safe to shut down. Power down the laptop first, then power down CDAS, then unplug from wall.

8. In **CTICU** unit, plug in CDAS, power up CDAS, power up laptop, wait unitl patient display screen comes up, and then **CDAS wire must be plugged into the covered CDAS connection port on the outside of the VAD Pack to supply wall power to the device and prevent the backup batteries from draining**. Go to "exit tech mode" and click. This prevents anyone from making changes without knowing the password.

9. When a device event occurs, notify the Vice President, Clinical Affairs at MicroMed Technology, Inc. at 713-838-9214 or Vice President, Engineering at 281-236-7738.

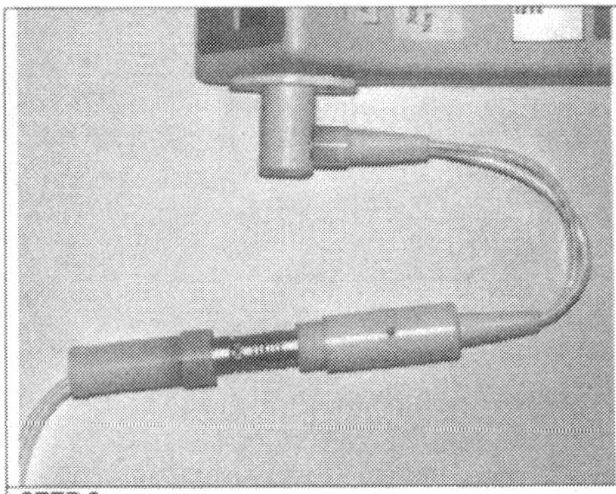

STEP 1:

The white defibrillation insulator should be placed on cable at time of implant. The threaded end should point towards the VAD controller.

STEP 2:

Install the C-clip into the connector verifying it is completely seated in the groove between the sliding barrel and the barrel stop. OPTIONAL

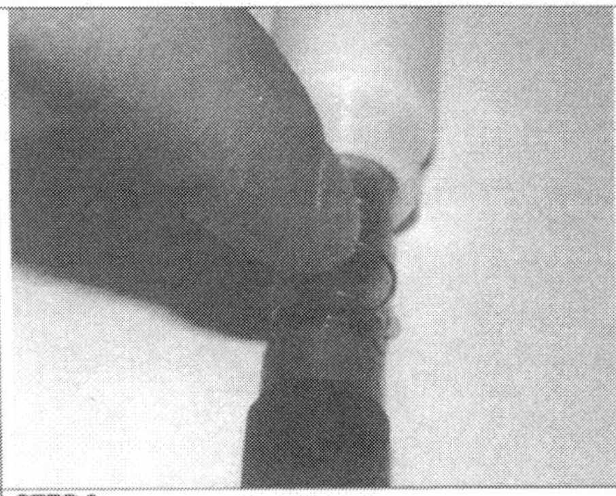

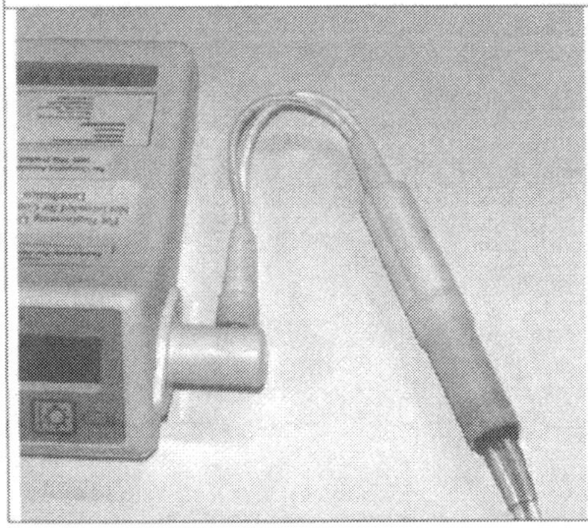

STEP 3:

Screw the white defibrillation insulator onto the controller using finger tight pressure.

Fig. 13.

Policy and Procedure Guidelines

CP49

IMPELLA VAD

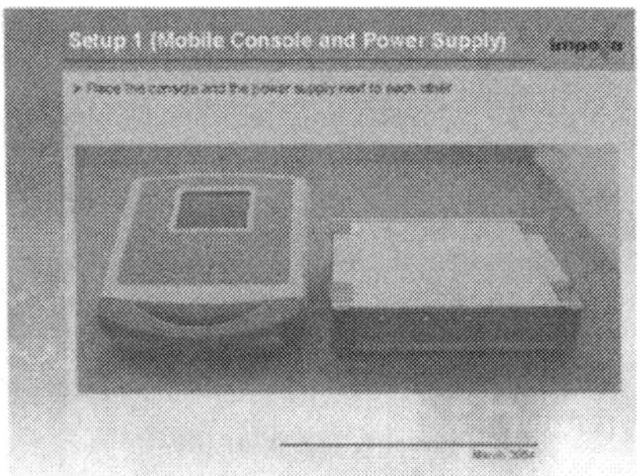

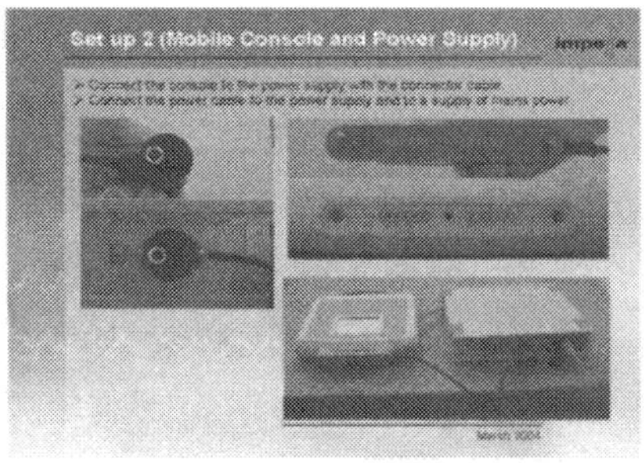

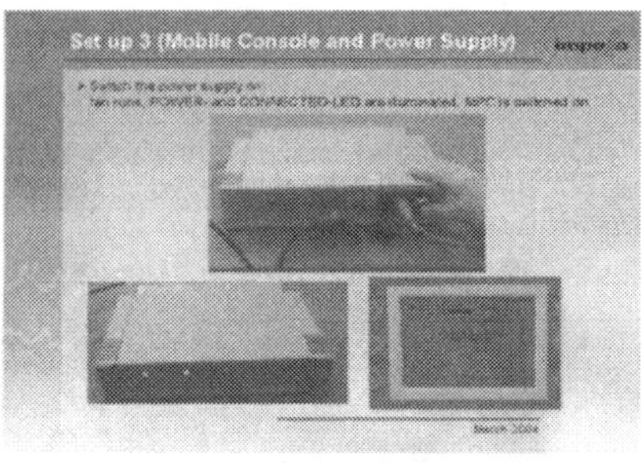

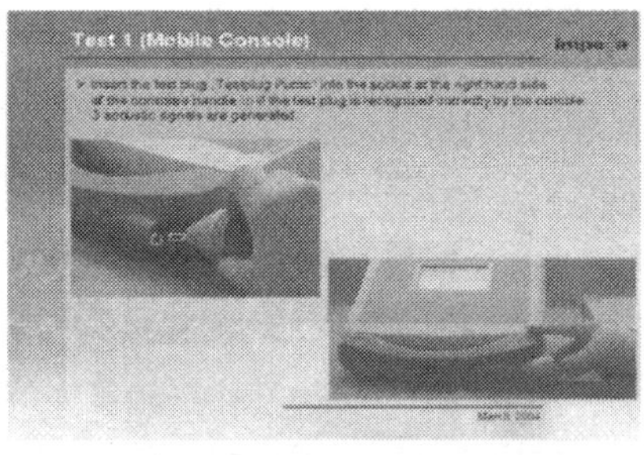

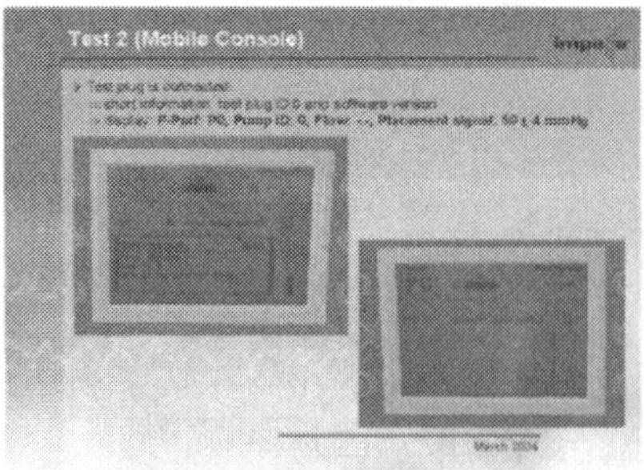

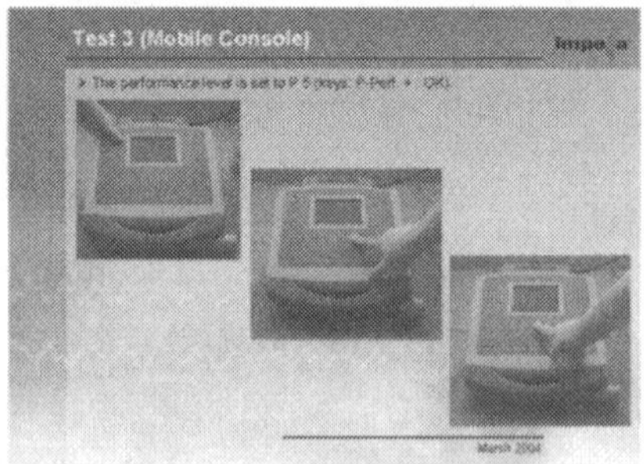

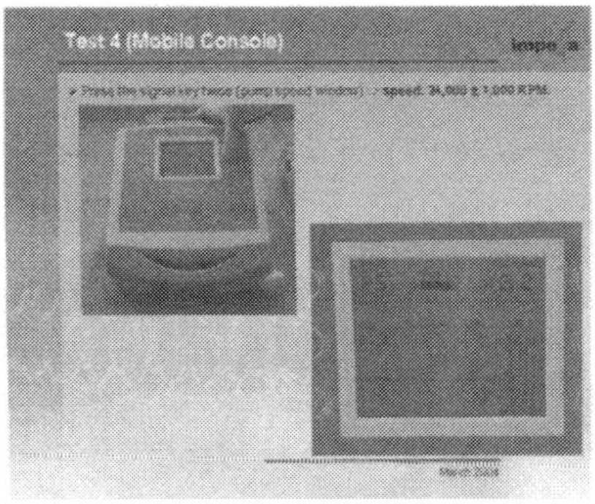
Test 4 (Mobile Console)
March 2004

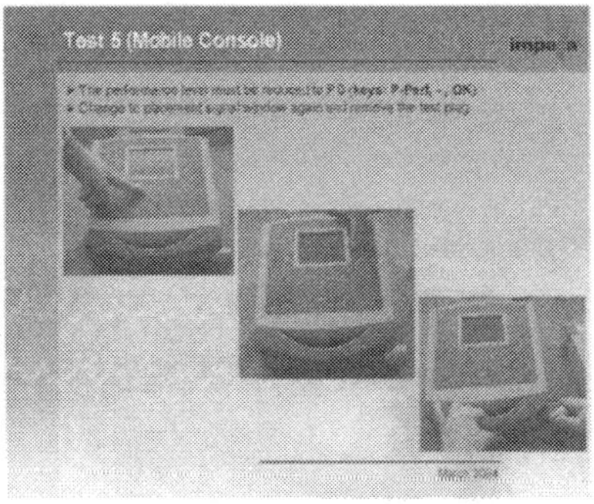
Test 5 (Mobile Console)
March 2004

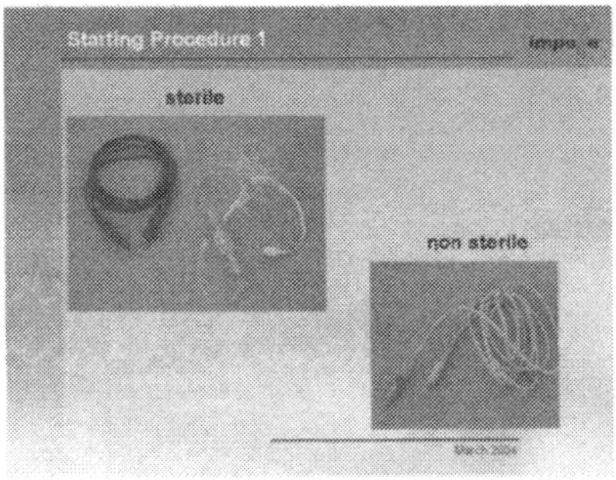
Starting Procedure 1
sterile
non sterile
March 2004

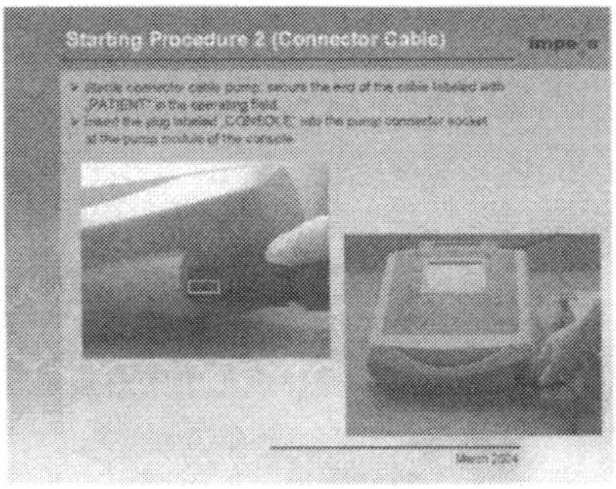
Starting Procedure 2 (Connector Cable)
March 2004

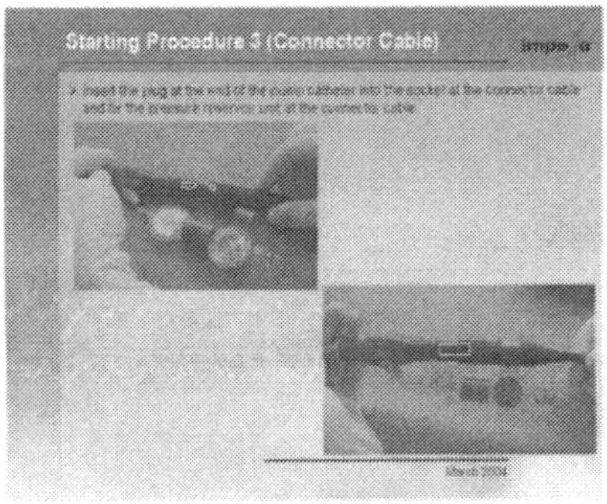
Starting Procedure 3 (Connector Cable)
March 2004

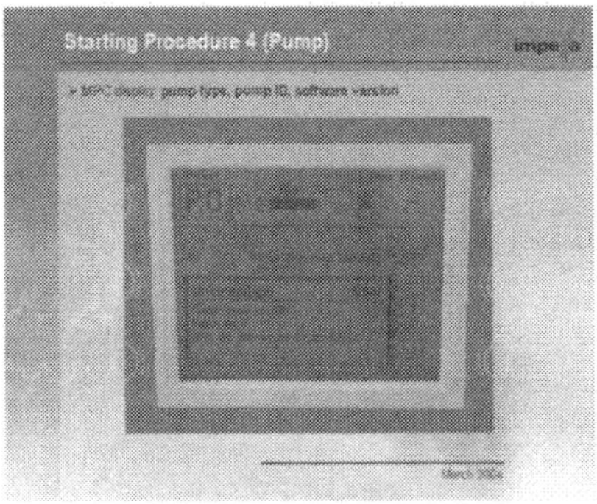
Starting Procedure 4 (Pump)
March 2004

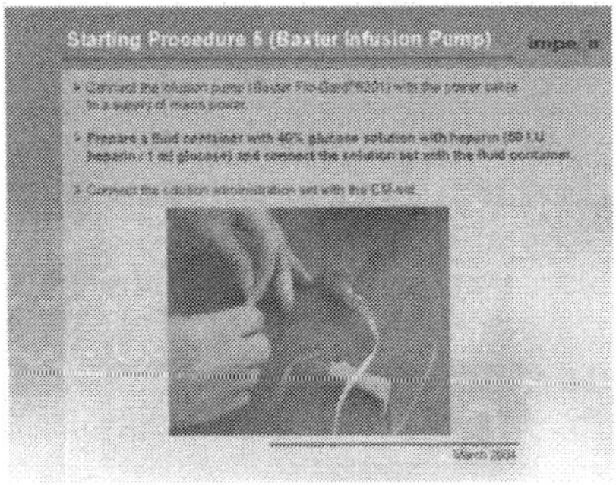
Starting Procedure 5 (Baxter Infusion Pump)
March 2004

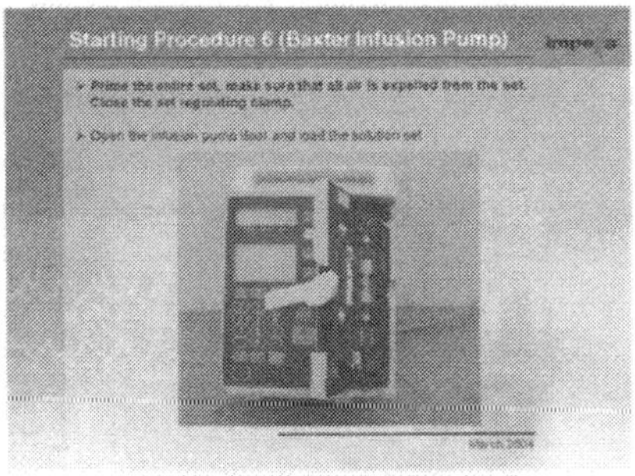
Starting Procedure 6 (Baxter Infusion Pump)
March 2004

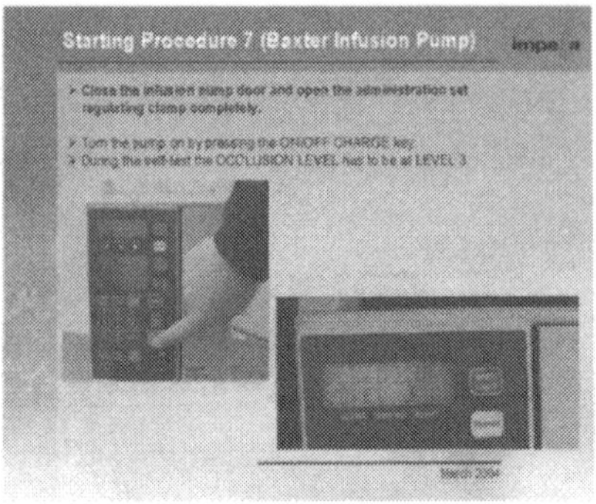
Starting Procedure 7 (Baxter Infusion Pump)
➢ Close the infusion pump door and open the administration set regulating clamp completely.
➢ Turn the pump on by pressing the ON/OFF CHARGE key.
➢ During the self-test the OCCLUSION LEVEL has to be at LEVEL 3.
March 2004

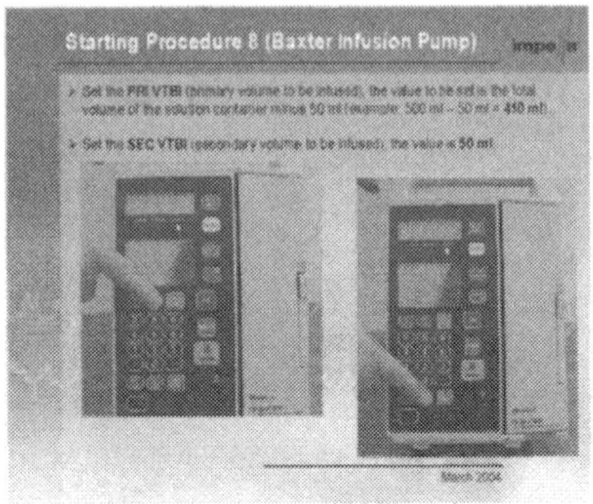
Starting Procedure 8 (Baxter Infusion Pump)
➢ Set the PRI VTBI (primary volume to be infused), the value to be set is the total volume of the solution container minus 50 ml (example: 500 ml – 50 ml = 450 ml).
➢ Set the SEC VTBI (secondary volume to be infused), the value is 50 ml.
March 2004

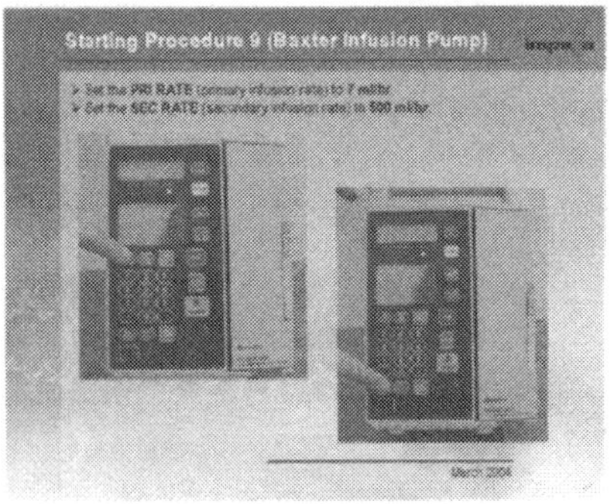
Starting Procedure 9 (Baxter Infusion Pump)
➢ Set the PRI RATE (primary infusion rate) to 7 ml/hr.
➢ Set the SEC RATE (secondary infusion rate) to 500 ml/hr.
March 2004

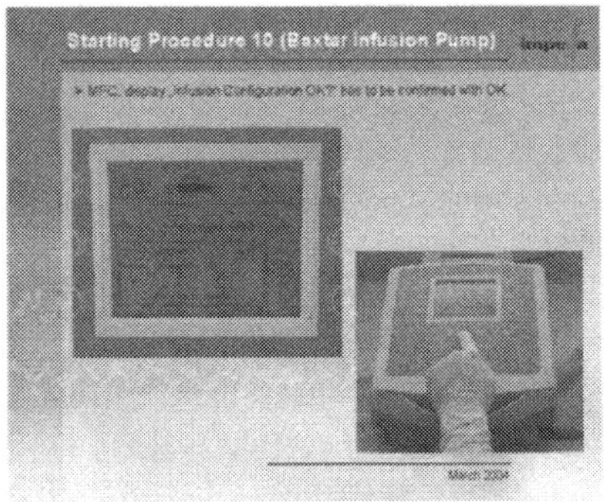
Starting Procedure 10 (Baxter Infusion Pump)
➢ MPC: display „Infusion Configuration OK?" has to be confirmed with OK.
March 2004

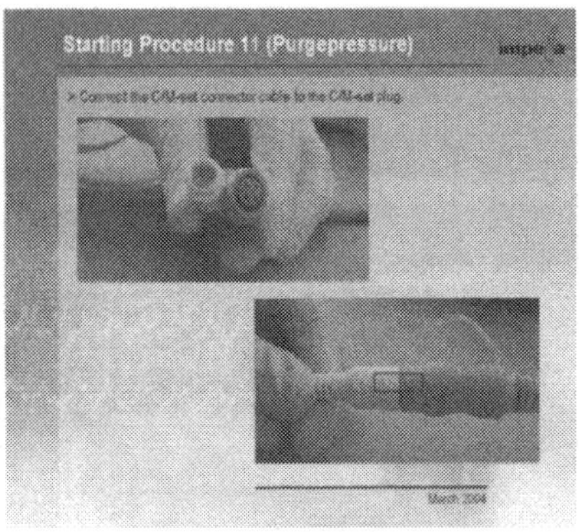
Starting Procedure 11 (Purgepressure)
➢ Connect the C/M-set connector cable to the C/M-set plug.
March 2004

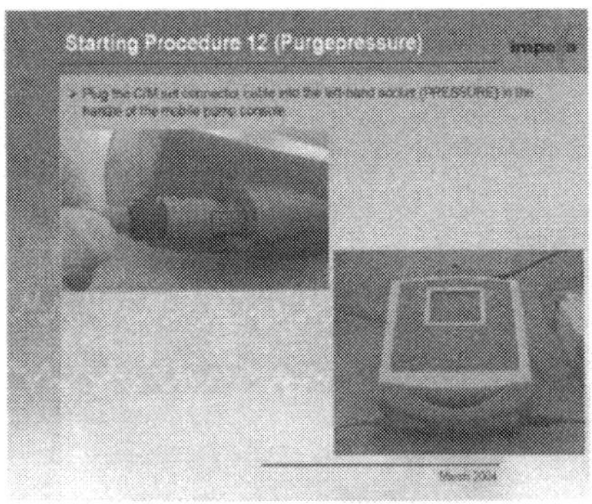
Starting Procedure 12 (Purgepressure)
➢ Plug the C/M set connector cable into the left-hand socket (PRESSURE) in the handle of the mobile pump console.
March 2004

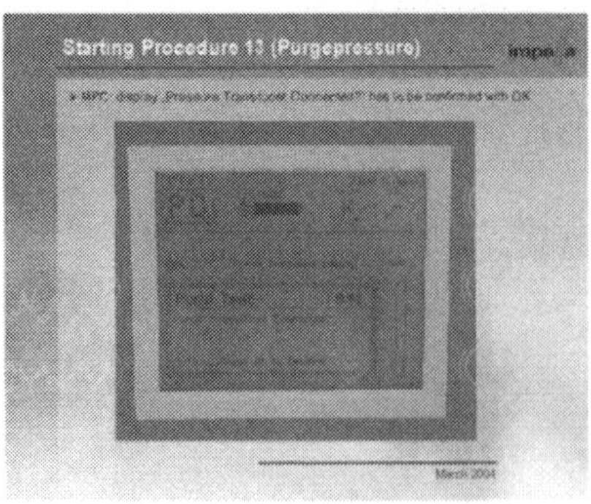
Starting Procedure 13 (Purgepressure)
➢ MPC: display „Pressure Transducer Connected?" has to be confirmed with OK.
March 2004

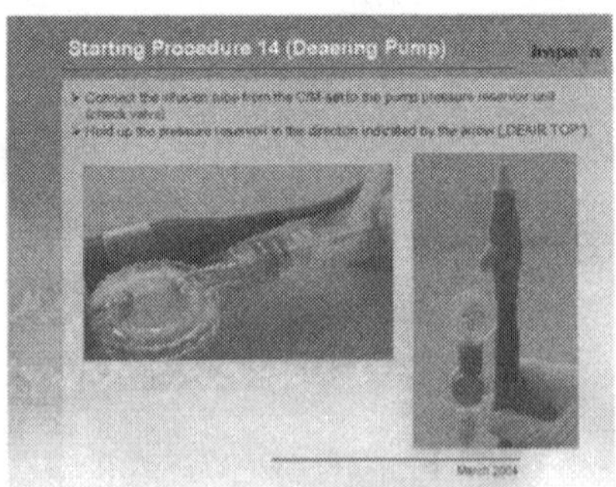
Starting Procedure 14 (Deaering Pump)
➢ Connect the infusion tube from the C/M set to the pump pressure reservoir unit (check valve).
➢ Hold up the pressure reservoir in the direction indicated by the arrow („DEAIR TOP").
March 2004

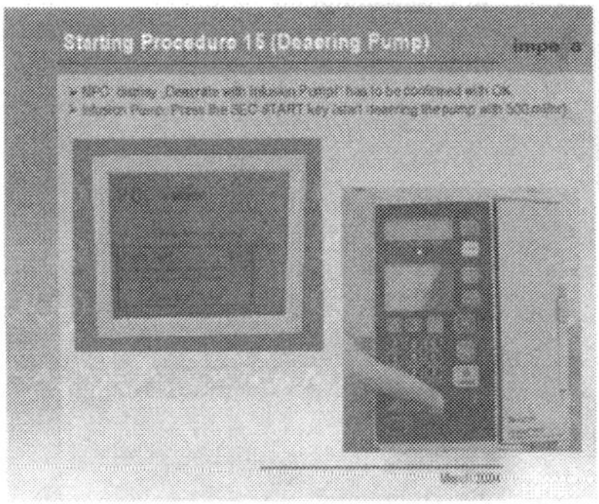
Starting Procedure 15 (Deaering Pump)

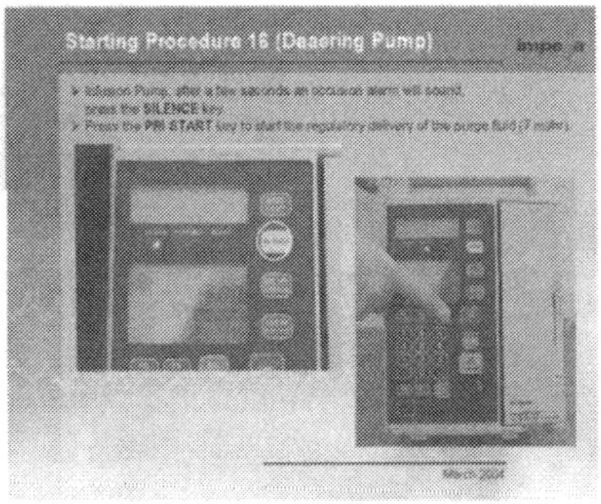
Starting Procedure 16 (Deaering Pump)

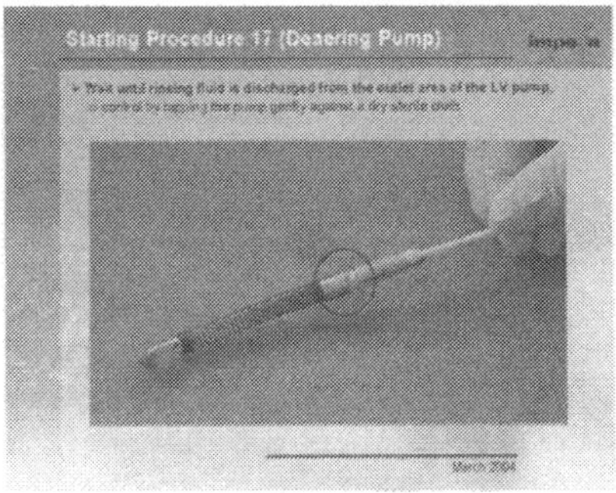
Starting Procedure 17 (Deaering Pump)

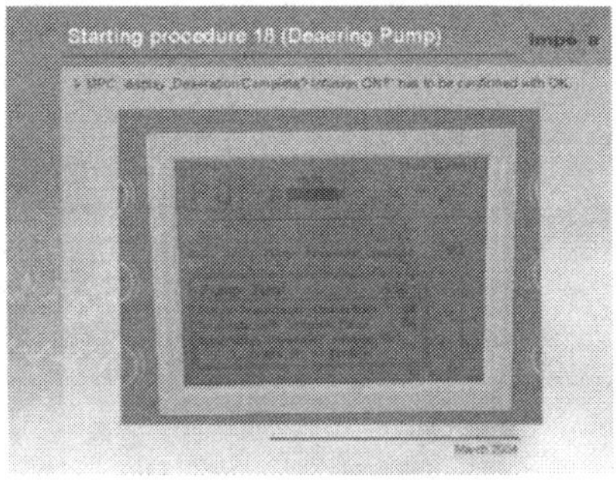
Starting procedure 18 (Deaering Pump)

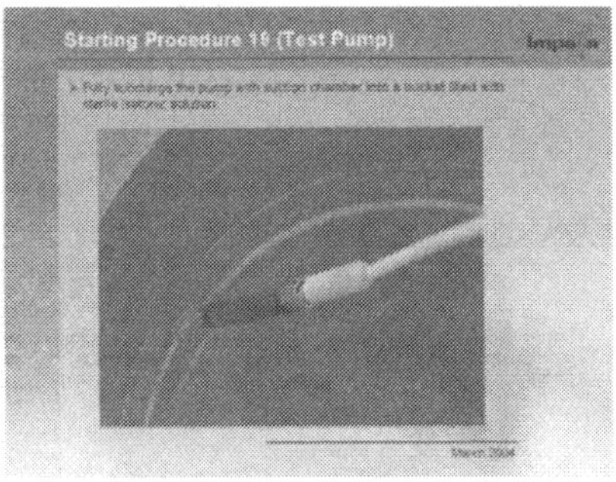
Starting Procedure 19 (Test Pump)

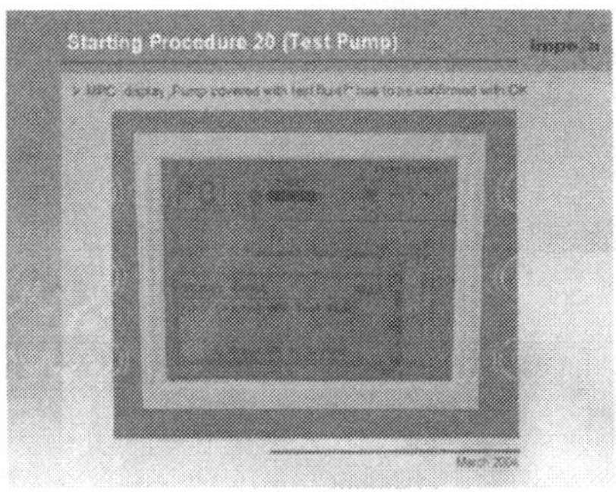
Starting Procedure 20 (Test Pump)

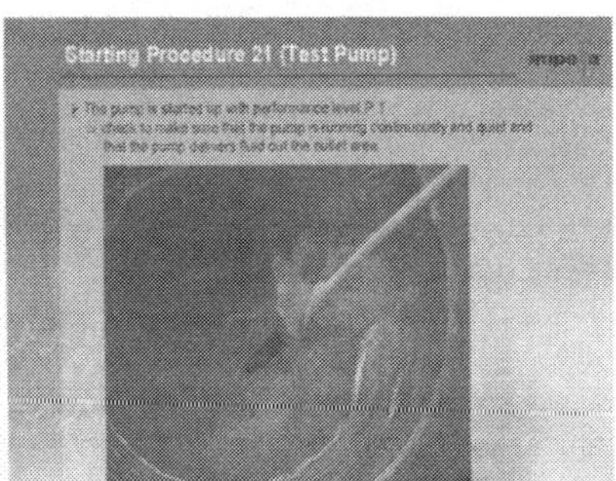
Starting Procedure 21 (Test Pump)

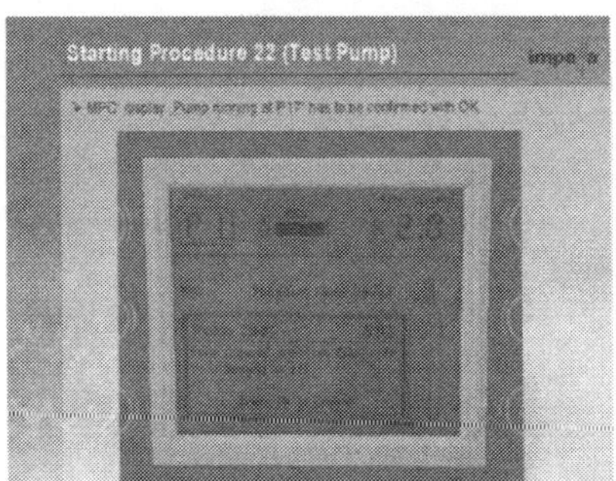
Starting Procedure 22 (Test Pump)

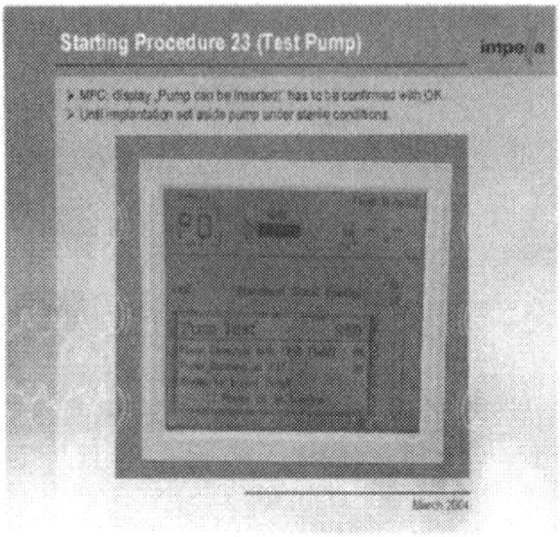
Starting Procedure 23 (Test Pump)
MPC: display „Pump can be inserted" has to be confirmed with OK
Until implantation set aside pump under sterile conditions
March 2004

Policy and Procedure Guidelines

CP75

Table 1
Children's Hospital of New York (CHONY) Bypass Circuits

Flow cc/L per min	*Oxygenator*	*Loop*	*Prime**	*Filter*	*Boot*
		Inches			
< 650 cc	**Baby RX**	1/8–3/16	Q-180 cc	none	3/16-
			RM-220 cc	AFO2	3/16-
> 650 cc–1.3 L	**Baby RX**	3/16–1/4	270 cc	AF02	1/4-
> 1.3 L–1.5 L	**Baby RX**	1/4–3/8	375 cc	AF02	1/4-
> 1.5 L–2.5 L	**SX-10**	1/4–3/8	610 cc	AF02	<2 L–1/4 2 L–2.5 L–3/8
> 2.5 L–3.5 L	**SX-10**	3/8–3/8	850 cc	AL-8	3/8-
> 3.5 L	**SX-18**	3/8–1/2	1150 cc	AL-8	1/2-

Dr. Quaegebeur circuit size.
Use a 2.2 CI to calculate the patient's bypass flow.
Dr. Mosca and Dr. Chen
Use a 2.5 CI for 0–13 kg and a 2.4 CI for >13 Kg

Table 2
Chony Venous Cannulae

DLP Single-Stage Straight	*Max Flow (ml/min)*	*Venous Line*
14	300	3/16-
16	450	3/16-
18	800	3/16
18	1,000	1/4
20	1,200	1/4
22	1,600	1/4
22	1,800	3/8
24	2,200	3/8-
28	2,800	3/8-
30	3,100	3/8-
32	3,500	3/8-
32	4,000	1/2-
34	4,400	1/2-
36	5,000	1/2-
38	5,500	1/2-
40	6,000	1/2-

Table 3
Chony Venous Cannulae

Bio-Medicus	*Max Flow*	*Augmented Flow (ml/min)*
8	300	
10	600	
12	900	
14	1,200	
15	750	2,000
17	1,100	2,600
19	1,500	3,500
21	2,000	4,500
23	2,500	
25	3,000	
27	3,500	
29	4,500	

Table 4
Chony Venous Cannulae (bicaval)

Angled DLP		*Max Flow (ml/min)*
12	12	500
12	14	750
14	14	1,000
12	16	1,000
14	16	1,200
16	16	1,500
16	18	1,800
18	18	2,100
18	20	2,500
20	20	2,800
20	24	3,200
24	24	4,000
24	28	5,000
28	28	6,000

Table 5
Chony Arterial Cannulae

Terumo	*Max Flow (ml/min)*
7.0 soft flow	5,000
8.0 soft flow	7,000
Medtronic EOPA	*Max Flow*
18	4,700
20	5,700
22	7,000

Table 6
Chony Arterial Cannulae

Bio-medicus	*Max Flow*
8	650
10	1,100
12	2,200
14	2,900
15	3,000
17	4,000
19	5,500
21	6,500
23	8,000
DLP WIRE	*Max Flow*
6	400
8	650
10	1,100
12	2,200
14	2,900
16	4,000

Policy and Procedure Guidelines

CP76

PRIME CONSTITUENTS

All circuits are initially primed with plasmalyte, which is partially chased out by the albumin, blood, or fresh frozen plasma (FFP), then the drugs are added, so the balance of all prime volumes is plasmalyte. All packed red blood cells (PRBCs) are washed with the Cell Saver.

A blood prime is often not necessary (*see* Blood Protocol).
*Calcium is added only if blood is used.
^An equivalent dose is given immediately after cross clamp removal.

Prime constituents	*Albumin*	*FFP*	*PRBCs*	*Heparin*	*CaCl*	*$NaHCO_3$*	*Mannitol*	*Total prime*
Circuits								
Micro <3 kg Baby RX	**coat circuit with 50 cc of 25%**	**60 cc**	**125 cc**	**500 U**	**75 mg**	**(10 mEq + 1 mEq/kg)/2**	**(250 mg/kg)/2**	**220 cc**
Micro >3 kg Baby RX	50 cc of 25%	none	125 cc	500 U	50 mg	(10 mEq + 1 mEq/kg)/2	(250 mg/kg)/2	220 cc
Micro 1/4-3/16	**50 cc 25%**	**none**	**#180 cc**	**700 U**	***75 mg**	**(10 mEq + 1 mEq/kg)1.5**	**(250 mg/kg)1.5**	**270 cc**
1/4-3/8 Baby RX 1/4 boot	**50 cc 25%**	**none**	**#250 cc**	**1,000 U**	***100 mg**	**(10 mEq + 1 mEq/kg)1.5**	**(250 mg/kg)1.5**	**375 cc**
SX-10 1/4-3/8	100 cc 25%	none	#350 cc	1,200 U	*100 mg	10 mEq + 1 mEq/kg up to a total of 25 mEq	250 mg/kg	610 cc
SX-10 3/8-3/8	**150 cc 25%**	**none**	**#350 cc**	**1,700 U**	***100 mg**	**25 mEq**	**250 mg/kg**	**850 cc**
SX-18 3/8-1/2	200 cc 25%	none	#350 cc	2,200 U	*100 mg	25 mEq	250 mg/kg	1,150 cc

Policy and Procedure Guidelines
CP77

CARDIOPLEGIA

The Sorin Vanguard Cardioplegia System has been modified to a 1:1 ratio of blood to cardioplegia (CP) (Q shot). The system consists of 3/16″ raceway tubing and a 1/8″ delivery line. This system will be used with the low-dose CP solution for all patients perfused with the Micro, B, or C packs. All CP solution that is used with the 1:1 system is filtered with a 0.2 μm filter. The 4:1 blood to CP set (also the Sorin Vanguard) is used for all patients perfused with the D or E packs. It consists of 1/4″ over 1/8″ raceway tubing, a pump bypass bridge, and a 1/8″ delivery line. This system utilizes both the high and low dose CP solutions.

THE CARDIOPLEGIA SOLUTION

Low dose			High dose		
D5W		900 cc	D5W		430 cc
KCl	60 mEq	)	KCl	60 mEq	)
$NaHCO_3$	30 mEq	) 100 cc	NaHCO3	15 mEq	) 76.3 cc
Mannitol	12.5 g	)	Mannitol	6.25 g	)
Total		1,000 cc	Total		506.3 cc

DOSE

Dr. Q.

1:1: 15 cc/kg for an arrest dose then 5 cc/kg at 30-min intervals.

4:1: 7 cc/Kg of high dose, then an additional 8 cc/kg of low for the initial dose, then 5 cc/kg of low dose at 30-min intervals.

If circulatory arrest is utilized, then the second dose is given 40 min after the first.

Dr. Mosca and Dr. Chen

1:1: 15 cc/kg for an arrest dose, then 7 cc/kg at 20-min intervals.

4:1: 7 cc/kg of high dose, then an additional 8 cc/kg of low for the initial dose, then 7 cc/kg of low dose at 20-min intervals.

No additional cardioplegia is given during circulatory arrest.

Policy and Procedure Guidelines

CP78

COMMON CANNULAE AND ASSOCIATED FLOWS

CHONY VENOUS CANNULAE

DLP® single stage straight	*Max Flow cc/min*	*Venous line*
14F	300	
16F	450	
18F	800	3/16
18F	1,000	1/4
20F	1,200	1/4
22F	1,600	1/4
22F	1,800	3/8
24F	2,200	3/8
28F	2,800	3/8
30F	3,100	3/8
32F	3,500	3/8
32F	4,000	1/2
34F	4,400	1/2
36F	5,000	1/2
38F	5,500	1/2
40F	6,000	1/2

Bio-Medicus®	*Max Flow cc/min*	*Aug flow*
8 Fr	300	
10 Fr	600	
12 Fr	900	
14 Fr	1,200	
15 Fr	750	2,000
17 Fr	1,100	2,600
19 Fr	1,500	3,500
21 Fr	2,000	4,500
23 Fr	2,500	
25 Fr	3,000	
27 Fr	3,500	
29 Fr	4,500	

Bi-caval Angled DLP® or Angled Edwards®		*Max Flow cc/min*
12F	12F	500
12F	14F	750
12F	16F	1,000
14F	14F	1,000
14F	16F	1,200
16F	16F	1,500
16F	18F	1,800
18F	18F	2,100
18F	20F	2,500
20F	20F	2,800
20F	24F	3,200
24F	24F	4,000
24F	28F	5,000
28F	28F	6,000

CHONY ARTERIAL CANNULAE

DLP® wire	*Max Flow cc/min*
6 F	400
8 F	650
10 F	1,100
12 F	2,200
14 F	2,900
16 F	4,000

Bio-Medicus®	*Max Flow cc/min*
8 F	650
10 F	1,100
12 F	2,200
14 F	2,900
15 F	3,000
17 F	4,000
19 F	5,500
21 F	6,500
23 F	8,000

Policy and Procedure Guidelines

CP79

BLOOD ADMINISTRATION

The addition of packed red blood cells (PRBCs) to the bypass prime depends on the type of defect being repaired and how low the postdilution hematocrit (hct) will be.

If the procedure is relatively quick, such as an ASD repair, and you calculate that your hct at the discontinuation of bypass will be approximately 25%, then your strategy should be to avoid exogenous blood (*see* MUF and CLEAR PRIME REPLACEMENT protocols.). If the postdilution hct is <25%, then a blood prime or the administration of PRBCs on cardiopulmonary bypass (CPB) may be necessary.

For most defects, the patient should be weaned from CPB with a hematocrit that is at least 30%. For the first stage of the Norwood and the Arterial Switch, a weaning hct of 35% is expected.

All PRBC units should be washed by the cell saver to ensure a physiologic potassium level in the prime. (*see* PRBC Cell Saver/autotransfusion protocol.)

All blood is leukodepleted by the New York Blood Center. If it is not, then it should be filtered with a leukodepleting filter before processing by the cell saver.

All patients <4 mo of age will only receive irradiated/CMV-negative blood.

All DeGeorge patients will only receive irradiated blood.

Policy and Procedure Guidelines

CP80

APROTININ (TRASYLOL) DOSING

Always consult the Surgeon and Anesthesia when considering aprotinin. In general, it is used for all reoperations and for all cases utilizing deep hypothermic circulatory arrest.

TEST DOSE

Administered by anesthesia after heparinization.

<15 kg = 0.3 cc
15–30 kg = 0.6 cc
>30 kg = 1 cc

PATIENT DOSE

Load: Administered by anesthesia after heparinization.

<51 kg———20,000 KIU/kg (2 cc/kg)
>50 kg———100 cc

Pump: Added to the pump prime after the load is started.

<21 kg———40,000 KIU/kg (4 cc/kg)
21–50 kg——80 cc
>50 kg———100 cc

MAINTENANCE

Run by anesthesia until the patient leaves the operating room. 25% of the pump prime dose in cc/h.

Policy and Procedure Guidelines
CP 81

MODIFIED ULTRAFILTRATION SETUP AND PROTOCOL

Setup

See diagram (Fig. 1)

1. Connect the modified ultrafiltration (MUF) inflow stopcock to the arterial port on the manifold.
2. Place pump boot tubing in twin pump head tubing guides without threading it through the roller pump, then connect free end to the HPH 400.
3. Connect outflow tubing to HPH 400. Connect stopcock to leured port on Vanguard.
4. Connect shunt line from stopcock/Vanguard to venous reservoir.
5. Connect effluent line to HPH 400 and close Roberts clamp. Connect distal end of effluent line to a collection reservoir.

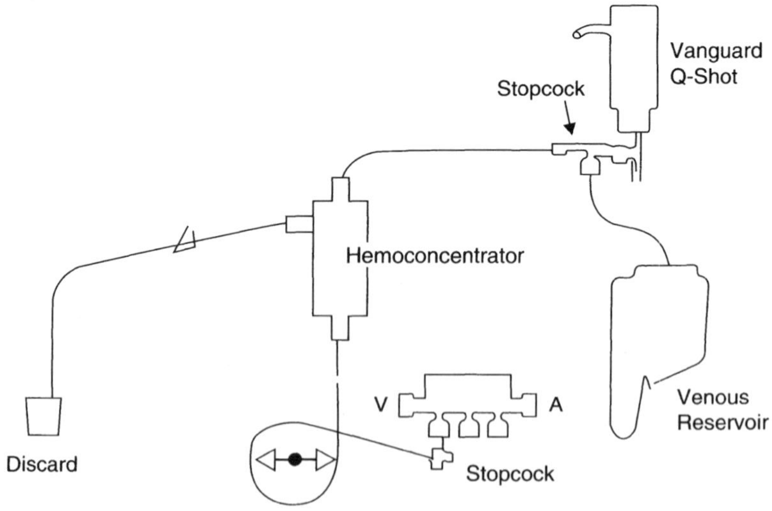

Fig. 1.

Priming

1. Turn distal stopcock to divert flow to venous reservoir.
2. Turn proximal stopcock/manifold to divert flow to HPH 400.
3. Turn stopcock on arterial filter to divert CO_2 through HPH 400.
4. Prime the MUF circuit from this position (after bypass circuit is primed).
5. Burp distal stopcock on Vanguard, then shut off to vanguard.
6. Turn manifold stopcock off to the MUF circuit.

Hemoconcentrating on CPB

1. Open all stopcocks/manifolds on MUF circuit to divert flow to the cardiotomy reservoir.
2. Increase cardiopulmonary bypass (CPB) flow to compensate for MUF shunt.

Muffing

1. Hand duckbill cannula to surgical field.
2. After cross clamp removal and during rewarming, turn cardioplegia (CP) temp to 36°C.
3. Turn on MUF pump and load tubing into raceway.
4. Turn stopcock on Vanguard to divert MUF flow through the CP set.
5. Flush MUF circuit to field until warm (30°C is ok). Flush out any residual CP.
6. After discontinuing CPB, keep arterial line **unclamped**. (You are pulling from this line.)
7. After the venous cannulae are removed, drain the venous line into the venous reservoir.
8. Upon direction from the surgeon, begin MUF procedure. Run MUF pump no higher than 15 cc/kg/min.
9. Open the effluent line.
10. Run arterial head as necessary to maintain central venous pressure and blood pressure.
11. When the venous reservoir volume is drained down close to the level shutoff sensor, add Plasma-Lyte to maintain MUF.
12. Discontinue MUF after 10 min, or when your pump volume becomes too dilute. Target MUF effluent volume should at least be equivalent to the pump prime.
13. After MUF, reset your cardioplegia temperature to 2°C.

Policy and Procedure Guidelines

CP82

ABO INCOMPATIBLE HEART TRANSPLANT PERFUSION PROTOCOL

Circuit

1. Use either the 3/16–1/4″ loop or a larger circuit (if necessary). Do not use the 1/8″–3/16″ loop.
2. Connect a stopcock to the venous leur and connect the venous manifold line to the end of this stopcock. Then, connect a rapid prime line to the sidearm of the stopcock and spike an empty Plasma-Lyte bag.
3. The circuit reservoir should be large enough to accommodate two times the patient's estimated blood volume, so you may need to upsize the circuit.

Blood Products

Cardiology will already have ordered the appropriate type put you need to make sure of the amount. Use the prime calculations to determine how many units of packed red blood cells (**PRBCs**) and CCs of fresh frozen plasma (**FFP**) you need for the procedure and inform the blood bank.

Blood Product Compatibility for ABO Incompatibility

Donor	*Recipient*	*Indicated*	*Transfusion*	*Product*
Group	**Group**	PRBC	**Plasma**	Platelets
AB	**O**	O	**AB**	AB
B	**O**	O	**AB or B**	AB or B
A	**O**	O	**AB or A**	AB or A
AB or A	**B**	O or B	**AB**	AB
AB or B	**A**	O or A	**AB**	AB

Priming

1. Prime the circuit with Plasma-Lyte and de-air as usual.

2. Chase the Plasma-Lyte with enough washed PRBC's, FFP, and drugs to attain two times the patient's blood volume in the reservoir, with a hematocrit of 30%.
3. Check prime gas, and correct as necessary.

Prime Calculations

EBV (estimated blood volume), **DPV** (desired prime volume), **RCV** (red cell volume), **WaRBCV** (washed red blood cell volume), 0.65 (average hct of cell saver blood), **PV** (prime volume), **TPV** (total plasma volume), **CPV** (calculated prime volume), **TCPV** (total calculated prime volume).

Age	*cc/kg*
Adult	65
3 years	70
1 year	75
6 months	80
1 month	85
Newborn	90

kg × cc/kg = EBV	______
2 × EBV + PV = DPV	______
DPV × .30 = RCV	______
DPV × .70 = TPV	______
RCV/0.65 = WaRBCV	______
TPV + WaRBCV = CPV	______
CPV + Drugs = TCPV	______

DRUGS (PRIME) (SEE NEXT PAGE)	
CaCl	
For blood	______
For FFP	______
Total	______
$NaHCO_3$	______
Heparin	______

Drugs

50 mg CaCl per 125 cc WaRCV

75 mg CaCl per 250 cc of FFP **To a Total OF 1 g of CaCl, then check level with ISTAT**

5 mEq $NaHC0_3$ for every 125 cc of WaRBCs) **to a total of 50 mEq, then check level with I-STAT**

3 U heparin per cc of caculated prime volume.

Give the usual dose of Mannitol AFTER you go on bypass.

Give the entire aprotinin dose (load plus pump) AFTER you go on bypass.

Example prime (3 kg child)

3 kg × 85 cc per kg = 255 cc

2 × 255 + 260 = 770 ccDPV

770 × .30 = 231 ccRCV

770 × .70 = 539 ccTPV. **Approximately 2 U FFP, but tell the blood bank that you need 539 cc.**

231/0.65 = 355 ccWaRBCV. **Each unit of PRBCs yields about 300 cc of WaRBCV.**

So, 539 cc + 355 cc = calculated prime volume (CPV).
894 cc = CPV

Drugs

304 mg CaCl (355/125 = 2.84 × 50 = 142 mg **for WaRBCs**) (539/250 = 2.16 × 75 = 161.7 mg **for FFP**) 142 + 161.7 = 303.7 mg

17 mEq $NaHCO_3$ (355/125 = 2.84 × 5 = 14.2 mEq)

2,680 U heparin (3 × 894 = 2,680 U)

So, 894 cc + 23 cc (drugs) = total calculated prime volume (917 cc TCPV)

Prebypass Hemoconcentration

The difference between the DPV and TCPV is caused by the extra volume incurred by the addition of washed RBCs and drugs. If time allows, you should hemoconcentrate your prime to remove an amount of effluent that is equal to the extra volume.

Example: TCPV (917 cc) – DPV (770 cc) = 147 cc extra volume.

RUN AN ISTAT TO CONFIRM A PHYSIOLOGIC PRIME SOLUTION

Initiation of Bypass

1. The patient should only be heparinized for cannulation with 50 U/kg (this heparin will be washed out).
2. Keep the pump suckers **off** until the exchange is complete.
3. Upon initiation, quickly drain the patient's blood volume into the transfer bag, while simultaneously transfusing the circuit volume to the

patient. Attempt to maintain relative hemodynamic stability while exchanging.

4. When the minimum operating level of the oxygenator is reached, begin draining only into the venous reservoir and initiate bypass as usual.

5. Wash collected exchanged volume with the Cell Saver and return to the patient as needed.

6. Hemoconcentrate to maintain a hct of 30–35%.

7. Isohemagglutinin Anti-A and Anti-B titers will be sent to the blood bank for a QUICK SPIN 10 min after the initiation of bypass and before the aortic cross clamp is removed (pink top tube). If A plasma is used, then you will always have a slightly positive Anti-B, and if B plasma is used, then you will always have a slightly positive Anti-A. If AB plasma is used, then there should not be any positive result. Refer to the following chart to determine the Anti-A and Anti-B titers that need to be avoided.

Perform any subsequent exchanges by translocating volume equal to the patient's EBV to the cell saver and replacing this volume with FFP and WaRBCs. **Confirm Negative Antibody Titers Before XCL Removal.**

Donor	*Recipient*	*Antibodies to Aviod*
AB	O	ANTI-A (vs GRAFT)/ANTI-B (vs GRAFT)
B	O	ANTI-B
A	O	ANTI-A
AB	B	ANTI-A (vs GRAFT)/ ANTI-B (vs GRAFT AND RECIPIENT)
A	B	ANTI-A (vs GRAFT)/ ANTI-B (vs RECIPIENT)
AB	A	ANTI-B (vs GRAFT)/ ANTI-A (vs GRAFT AND RECIPIENT)
B	A	ANTI-B (vs GRAFT)/ANTI-A (vs RECIPIENT)

Policy and Procedure Guidelines
CP83

APHERESIS POLICY AND PROCEDURE

Apheresis will be used intermittently during extracorporeal membrane oxygenation (ECMO), when indicated, to remove antibodies to donor hearts in rejecting posttransplant patients.

A total plasma exchange is performed by the Plasma Pheresis department.

The Pheresis access line (Fig. 1) should be connected to the ECMO circuit at the most proximal venous line leured connection, and the Pheresis return line should be connected to the venous line on the low-pressure side of the pump (Fig. 2). So, both connections are on the low pressure side of the venous line.

Perfusion Setup (First Pheresis Treatment)

A large bore stopcock will be placed on the most proximal leured port on the venous line.

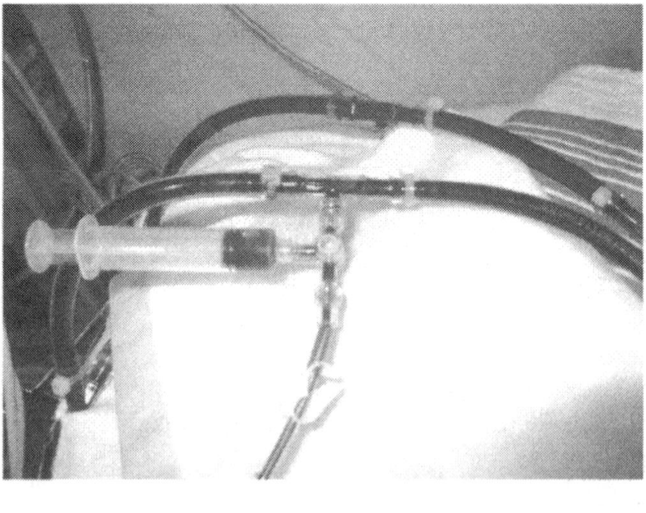

Fig. 1. Pheresis access line setup.

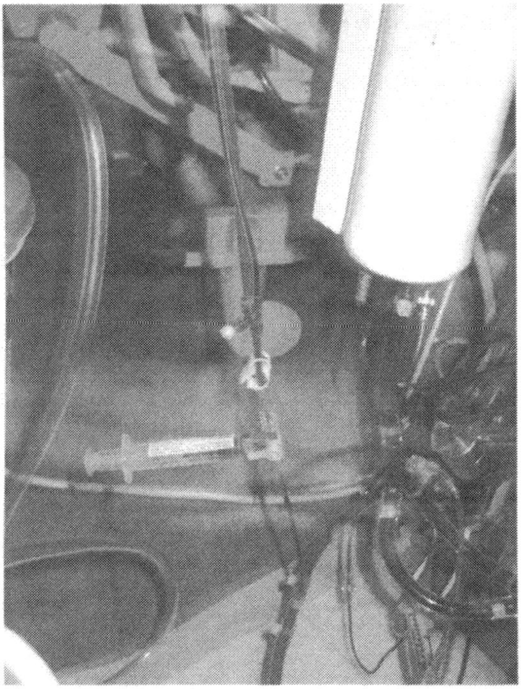

Fig. 2. Pheresis return line setup.

1. Turn off the ECMO flow and clamp above and below the leured port.
2. Remove the PRN adapter, and connect a stopcock to the leur.
3. Connect a 10 cc syringe to the end of the stopcock.
3. Open the most proximal clamp and aspirate 2 cc of blood from the patient to remove any clots at the connection.
4. Make sure the stopcock is now turned off to the patient.
5. Remove the remaining clamp and reestablish ECMO flow.
6. Put a new stopcock on the pigtail, which will be utilized for Pheresis return (usually the ACT access line). Make sure the line is free of air.

Connecting the Pheresis Lines to the ECMO Setup (First Treatment)

1. Move the 10-cc syringe on the stopcock on the pheresis access port to the sidearm of the stopcock.
2. Connect the pheresis access line to the end of the stopcock.
3. Open the white finger clamp on the Pheresis line and ask the pheresis nurse to flush her access line while you aspirate any air with your 10 cc syringe. Close white fingerclamp.

4. Open the stopcock so that flow can be established with the pheresis access line via the venous line.
5. Keep the white access line finger clamp closed until you are ready to establish pheresis flow.
6. Connect the pheresis return line to the return stopcock.
7. Have the pheresis nurse flush the return line into a 10-cc syringe on the sidearm of the return stopcock. Clamp the white finger clamp and open the stopcock to the return line.

Connecting the Pheresis Lines (Subsequent Treatments)

1. Connect a new large bore stopcock to the Pheresis return line.
2. Place a 10-cc syringe on the end of the Pheresis access stopcock.
3. Aspirate to remove any clots.
4. Connect a 10-cc syringe to sidearm of this stopcock.
5. Follow lines 2–7 of connecting the Pheresis line to the ECMO pump (first treatment).

Establishing Pheresis Flow

1. When the Pheresis nurse is ready to start flowing, open the white finger clamps on the pheresis access and return lines.

2. Pherisis flow is based on the patient weight and on the amount of negative pressure generated by the pheresis machine.

3. The Pheresis negative-pressure alarm should be set to shut off the pheresis machine at a negative pressure that is lower than the ECMO negative-pressure shutoff is set at; i.e., ECMO negative shutoff set at −120 then Pheresis negative shutoff set at −110 or lower.

4. Increase Pheresis flow rate until the target flow is reached or until the negative-pressure maximum is reached.

Concerns

1. If the ECMO shuts off due to a bubble, then you should ask the Pheresis nurse to manually pause her machine while you are off. (The Pheresis machine has a bubble detector, so any macro air from this machine should be caught.)

2. The calcium levels in the patient could fall for two reasons: because the pheresis anticoagulant is citrate, and because of the citrate in the FFP. The calcium chloride levels should be monitored every 20 min during Pheresis.

3. The Pheresis machine is programmed for a positive fluid balance. If flow is not an issue, then it can be set for a zero balance.

4. You will need to increase your heparin drip because some of your heparin will be removed by the pheresis procedure, so check ACTs 15 min at the start of the procedure.

Policy and Procedure Guidelines
CP84

CARDIOPULMONARY BYPASS PROCEDURES FOR PEDIATRICS (ALL CASES PERFORMED IN THE CHILDREN'S HOSPITAL OF NEW YORK)

General Description

Cardiopulmonary bypass is used to support the patient's circulation during the oxygenator period of surgical intervention. This can be achieved with various pump combinations, and the system used in this hospital will be described. The bypass system will be evaluated and periodically upgraded whenever new and improved equipment and techniques become available.

Indications

Cardiopulmonary bypass is indicated for patients requiring extracorporeal perfusion during heart, lung, or major vessel surgery. Hypothermia and hemodilution provide safe periods of low flow and/or circulatory arrest when necessary. This is determined by the attending surgeon, depending on the complexity of the operation.

Procedure

Blood flow is determined by the patient's body surface area (BSA). A calculated blood flow at a cardiac index of 2.2–2.5 L/min/m^2 is used to determine the size of the circuit.

Circuit Design and Safety Considerations

The pediatric perfusion circuit has been designed to maintain adequate blood flow with minimal hemolysis and prime volume, while providing maximal safety for the patient. The latter is achieved by the use of pressure, air bubble, and level and temperature alarms. The level and pressure alarms will servoregulate the arterial pump to further protect the patient from sudden cessations of blood flow, and the bubble detection system will shut off the arterial pump head in the instance of inadvertent air in the arterial line. A vented arterial filter is also used at the surgeon's discretion. To ensure the proper direction of blood flow in all shunts that arise from the arterial side of the circuit, one-way valves are used. Also, one-way vacuum relief valves are used on the suction lines to guard against reverse pump direction and to reduce hemolysis.

All equipment is maintained within operating specifications by the manufacturer, and preventive maintenance is carried out according to their schedule. Preventive maintenance contracts are maintained on all equipment, and periodic monthly inspections by the CPMC Bioengineering department are completed before expiration to insure electrical safety.

Documentation of the Perfusion Procedure

At the beginning of each procedure, the following forms are necessary:

- Perfusion record (original + 3 copies)
- Perfusion Summary Record
- NY State form
- Transfusion Record
- Drug administration form

Each form will be properly labeled with the patients name, date of birth, and MRN.

After calculating the patient's BSA, flow rate, heparin dose, and postdilutional hematocrit, the rest of the preoperative data and history should be recorded on the appropriate forms. Serial numbers for disposables and equipment should be noted, and the prebypass checklist completed. During bypass, at 15-min intervals, documentation of the blood flow rate, arterial blood temperature, esophageal temperature, axillary or rectal temperature, mean arterial blood pressure, and central venous pressure (if available) must be made on the perfusion record. Additional information is recorded in the "Events" column.

In addition to continuous monitoring of the venous oxygen saturation by the perfusionist, blood gases and electrolytes should be monitored at least once during hypothermia, and once during rewarming. Blood gas and electrolyte values are obtained by use of the I-STAT handheld blood gas analyzer. Blood gases and electrolytes should be adjusted by the perfusionist to maintain normal levels, as determined by the attending physicians. For longer bypass procedures, these studies should be done at least once an hour and recorded on the perfusion record.

Priming the Circuit

After setting up the circuit and flushing the circuit with 100% CO_2 through a sterile gas filter, priming of the circuit can begin. For all circuit prime constituents, refer to Prime Constituents protocol. The circuit is then debubbled and recirculated before use. A postdilutional pump hematocrit (*see* Blood Protocol) may require that packed red cells (PRBCs) be added to the perfusion circuit. This decision is surgeon directed, and usually based on the complexity of the surgical procedure and preoperative condition of the patient.

Blood products (fresh frozen plasma and PRBCs) should be kept in the blood refrigerator after being checked by the perfusionist and a physician. Proper identification of the blood with the patient's name, birth date, hospital number, blood type, donor number, and expiration date is mandatory before addition to the pump. This must be witnessed by another member of the open heart team, and both signatures must be recorded on the transfusion form. One copy of the blood transfusion form is placed on the patient's chart, the other is returned to the blood bank.

Anticoagulation

A prebyass Kaolin activated clotting time (ACT) is obtained before heparrrinization to determine the baseline coagulation before initiating bypass. Adequate heparinization is achieved when the ACT reaches 480 s. On bypass, the ACT should be maintained for greater than 480 s with additional heparin administration when necessary. If Trasylol is used (*see* Trasylol protocol), then 600 s is the on-bypass ACT goal. An ACT should be monitored every 20 min on bypass, and more frequently during rewarming, when the ACT may decrease rapidly. After the end of bypass, a protamine dose is calculated by measuring the heparin level with an automated protamine titration using a Hepcon HMS System. If the Hepcon machine is unavailable, then 1 mg of protamine is given by the anesthesiologist for every 100 U of heparin that was administered during the bypass procedure. Ten minutes after protamine, an ACT and heparin level are performed to assure complete neutralization of the heparin and that the ACT has returned to within 10% of the prebypass baseline.

Cardioplegia

Cardioplegia delivery is accomplished at a 1 : 1 or 4 : 1 ratio (blood to cardioplegia). All patients who are perfused with the micro, B, or C packs will receive 1 : 1 blood cardioplegia. All others will receive 4 : 1 blood cardioplegia. For a better description of the solutions, refer to the Cardioplegia protocol.

Priming

The 1 : 1 cardioplegia system is antegrade primed. The 4 : 1 system is initially retrograde primed via the open bridge; the bridge is then clamped, and antegrade priming of the cardioplegia conducer is accomplished. The system is subsequently pressure checked to ensure adequate occlusion. The cardioplegia solution is delivered in an antegrade fashion, with back pressure in the system maintained between 130 mmHg and 200 mmHg.

Clinical Blood Gases

In conjunction with in-line venous saturation and hematocrit monitoring, as well as with visual assessment of "arterialized or desaturated blood," blood gases, as measured by the I-STAT, will be utilized as follows:

1. An arterial and venous blood gas will be checked within the first 5 min of cardiopulmonary bypass.
2. Subsequent arterial and venous blood gases will be checked every hour while on cardiopulmonary bypass or whenever a relevant clinical change is encountered.
   Examples of relevant clinical changes are:
   —cooling to circulatory arrest
   —anticipated aortic cross clamp removal
   —rewarming
   —anticipated removal from cardiopulmonary bypass

Intraoperative Blood Gas Strategy

The current blood gas strategy at CHONY is Alpha Stat. It is important to attempt to avoid hypocapnea during all procedures, especially when cooling to and rewarming from circulatory arrest.

Recovery of Pump Volume

At the end of bypass, all blood is recovered from the perfusion circuit. This is accomplished by clamping the arterial line and translocating the bypass circuit volume to the Cell Saver reservoir via a 1/8″ PVC line. Additional crystalloid solution is added to the pump to replace this volume, thereby maintaining the integrity of the primed circuit, until the pump is completely diluted and red cell recovery is no longer possible. Once the aorta is decannulated, then aggressive flushing of the circuit via the AV bridge through the venous limb of the circuit with a balanced electrolyte solution can be carried out. All blood is then processed in the autotransfusion device, properly lableled, and given to anesthesia. *See* Protocol for Intraoperative Autotransfusion.

Circuit Breakdown/Disposal

Pump circuit breakdown should not begin until all lines have been separated from the patient and surgical field. This includes arterial lines, all venous lines (i.e., central, femoral, neck, etc.) and cardioplegia lines (i.e., central, aortic, coronary sinus, steerable neck cannula, etc.). Once all lines have been disconnected from the patient and returned to the perfusionist, pump circuit disassembly may begin when directed by the surgeon. The HCU 30 takes approximately 5 min to prime and achieve a normothermic operating temperature should reinitiation of cardiopulmonary bypass become necessary. The HCU 30 heater–cooler should remain connected and recirculating until instructed to discard the pump circuit, at which time the lines may be deprimed, valves closed, and cardioplegia system lines removed from the delivery set.

Policy and Procedure Guidelines

CP85

OXYGEN FLUSH SETUP (TO REMOVE NITROGEN DIOXIDE AND TO CHECK NITRIC DELIVERY)

—Run oxygen through this system at 15 LPM with nitric oxide (NO) set at 40 PPM (Fig. 1).

—When NO_2 is less than 1.5 PPM, and NO is +/– 8 PPM of 40 PPM, then you are ready to administer NO therapy.

NO DELIVERY SETUP

—Set NO to the prescribed PPM (Fig. 2).

—Anesthesia's sweep gas must exceed minute volume, (the sweep needs to be over 6 LPM).

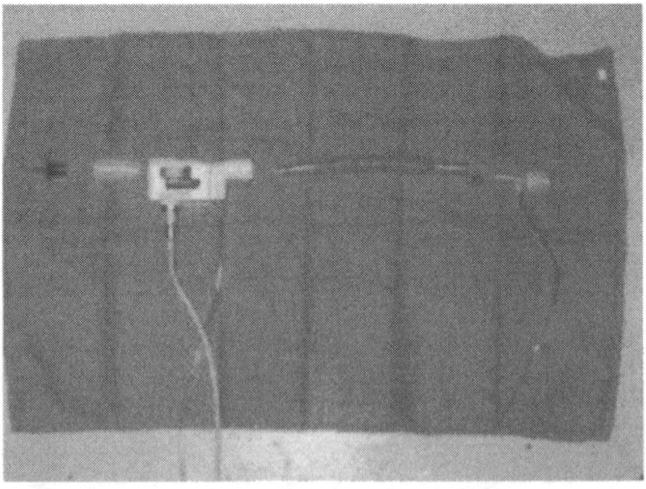

Fig. 1.

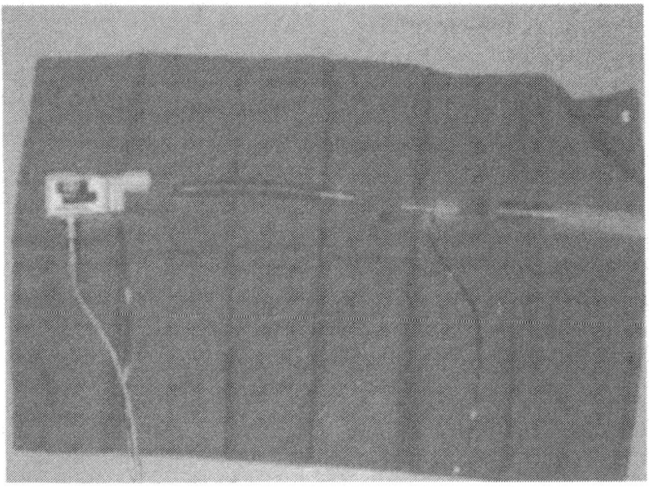

Fig. 2.

NO TRANSPORT SETUP

—Set portable O_2 tank to >6 LPM and connect to oxygen tubing (Fig. 3).
—Use ambu bag in normal fashion for transport.
—You will often get a monitor failure alarm when you unplug the unit. If this happens you won't see an NO_2 or NO readout, but you will still be delivering NO.

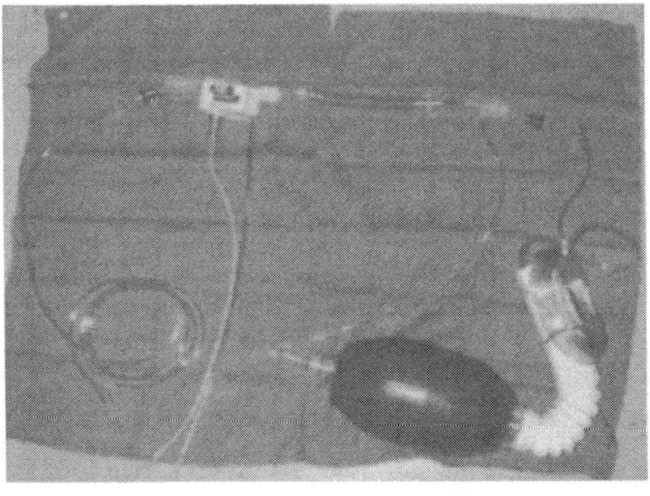

Fig. 3.

Policy and Procedure Guidelines
CP86

EXCHANGE TRANSFUSION PERFUSION PROTOCOL FOR SICKLE CELL DISEASE AND ISOANTIBODY TITER REDUCTION

Circuit

1) Use either the 3/16″–1/4″ loop or a larger circuit (if necessary). Do not use the 1/8″–3/16″ loop.
2) Cut a Y connector into your venous line, then connect a rapid prime line to the Y and spike an empty Plasma-Lyte or 3 L saline bag.
3) The circuit reservoir should be large enough to accommodate 1.5 times the patient's estimated blood volume. (You may need an E-Pack for a 20-kg child.)

Priming

1) Use 1.5 times the patient's blood volume for the calculations.
2) Choose a circuit that EASILY accommodates the needed volume based on your calculations. It is OK to use the next larger circuit.
3) Prime the circuit with Plasma-Lyte and deair as usual.
4) Chase the Plasma-Lyte with enough washed packed red blood cells (PRBCs) fresh frozen plasma (FFP), and drugs to attain 1.5 times the patient's blood volume in the reservoir with a hematocrit of 30%.
5) Check a prime gas and correct as necessary.
6) No albumin is necessary for priming.
7) Circulate your prime from the oxygenator to the top of your reservoir via the bypass line.

Blood Products

To ensure receiving enough PRBCs and FFP units from the blood bank, you need to do the following calculations and then order appropriately. Ask for FFP in cc in an amount at least equal to the total plasma volume.

Ask for PRBCs based on the amount of units you will need to wash to receive enough blood to cover the WaRBC amount.

Prime Calculations

EBV (estimated blood volume), **DPV** (desired prime volume), **RCV** (red cell volume), **WaRBCV** (washed red blood cell volume), 0.65 (average hct of Cell Saver blood), **PV** (prime volume), **TPV** (total plasma volume), **CPV** (calculated prime volume), **TCPV** (total calculated prime volume).

Age	*cc/kg*
Adult	65
3 years	70
1 year	75
6 months	80
1 month	85
Newborn	90

kg × cc/kg = EBV	______
1.5 × EBV + PV = DPV	______
DPV × .30 = RCV	______
DPV × .70 = TPV	______
RCV/0.65 = WaRBCV	______
TPV + WaRBCV = CPV	______
CPV + Drugs = TCPV	______

Drugs (prime)	
(See next page)	
CaCl	
For blood	______
For FFP	______
Total	______
$NaHCO_3$	______
Heparin	______

Drugs

50 mg CaCl per 125 cc WaRCV

75 mg CaCl per 250 cc of FFP, **to a total of 1 g of CaCl, then check level with I-STAT.**

5 mEq $NaHCO_3$ for every 125 cc of WaRBCs **to a total of 50 mEq, then check I-STAT.**

3 heparin per cc of cal culated prime volume.

Give the usual dose of Mannitol AFTER you go on bypass.

Give the entire aprotinin dose (load plus pump) AFTER you go on bypass.

Example Prime (14 kg Child)

14×80 cc per kg = 1120 cc
$1.5 \times 1120 + 610 = 2290$ cc DPV
$2290 \times .30 = 687$ cc RCV
$2290 \times .70 = 1603$ cc TPV
$687/0.65 = 1056$ cc WaRBCV
So, 1056 cc + 1603 cc = CPV.
2659 cc = CPV

Drugs

mg CaCl ($1056/125 = 8.4 \times 50 = 422$ mg **for WaRBCs**) ($1603/250 = 6.4 \times 75 = 481$ mg **for FFP**) $422 + 481 = 903$ mg

42 mEq $NaHCO_3$ ($1056/125 = 8.4 \times 5 = 42$ mEq)

7977 Uheparin ($3 \times 2659 = 7977$)

So, 2659 cc + 59 cc (drugs) = TCPV (2718 cc TCPV)

Prebypass Hemoconcentration

The difference between the DPV and TCPV is caused by the extra volume incurred by the addition of WaRBCs and drugs. If time allows, you should hemoconcentrate your prime to remove an amount of effluent that is equal to the extra volume.

Example: TCPV (2718 cc) – DPV (2290 cc) = 428 cc extra volume. **Run an I-STAT to confirm a physiologic prime solution.**

Initiation of Bypass

1) Keep the pump suckers **off** until the exchange is complete.

2) Upon initiation, quickly drain the patient's blood volume into the transfer bag while simultaneously transfusing the circuit volume to the patient. Attempt to maintain relative hemodynamic stability while exchanging.

3) When the minimum operating level of the oxygenator is reached, begin draining only into the venous reservoir and initiate bypass as usual.

4) Discard removed volume appropriately; do not wash it.

If Clear Cardioplegia is Necessary (Sickle Cell Disease Only)

1. Instead of connecting the blood line of the cardioplegia set to your circuit, use a perf adapter and/or a stopcock to connect this line to a liter of Plasma-Lyte.

2. Begin delivering warm cardioplegia at 30°C and immediately dial down to 2°C to cool the dose. This gives you a warm washout followed, by a semicold dose.
3. Subsequent doses should be delivered cold.

Policy and Procedure Guidelines
CP87

JOSTRA HL-20 PUMP CALIBRATIONS

Single Pump

Tubing (inches)	*RPM*	*Flow*	
1/2	100	4.5 L	
3/8	100	2.6 L	
1/4	100	1.28 L	
3/16	100	0.75 L	
Cardioplegia Ratios	*Tubing (inches)*	*RPM*	*Flow*
8 : 1	3/32× 17/164	100	1.55 L
4 : 1	1/4× 1/8	100	1.60 L
1 : 1	3/16× 3/16	100	1.35 L**
1 : 1	1/8× 1/8	100	0.72 L**

Twin Pump

Tubing	*RPM*	*Flow*
1/4	250	1.5 L
3/16	100	.35 L**
1/8	100	.15 L

**Flows tested with a graduated cylinder at 100 RPM.

Policy and Procedure Guidelines

CP88

WASHING PACKED RED BLOOD CELLS (PRBCS) WITH THE CELL SAVER

All units of PRBCs will be prewashed with the Cell Saver to remove excess potassium from the blood.

PROCEDURE

1. All donor blood must be checked by the primary perfusionist and an MD. Common practice cross-check procedure will be followed.
2. After ensuring the proper blood/patient match, translocate the blood to the Cell Saver cardiotomy.
3. For every unit of PRBCs to be processed, 750 cc of Plasma-Lyte should be mixed with it.
4. Fill the Cell Saver bowl at a rate of 250-cc/min.
5. Once the bowl is filled, wash at the same speed.
6. Wash with 250 cc, of Plasma-Lyte.
7. Empty the bowls contents into a transfer bag via a 40 μm blood filter.
8. Use the washed blood to displace the clear prime in your cardiopulmonary bypass circuit.

The New York Presbyterian Medical Center

Policy and Procedure Manual

Date issued:	
Approved:	Approved:

PROCEDURE FOR ADULT EXTRACOPOREAL MEMBRANE OXYGENATION (ECMO) USING ROTAFLOW PUMP, QUADROX "D" & "E" PACK CIRCUIT

Purpose

To provide long-term cardiopulmonary support for patients requiring ECMO.

Supplies and Equipment Needed

1. ECMO cart, which includes the Rotaflow pump console and hand crank, oxygen blender, and O_2 tank.
2. 1 ea—"E" tubing pack, which includes a coated tubing pack; rotaflow disposable centrifugal head; Quadrox D diffusion membrane oxygenator (Fig. 1).
3. Heater–cooler device.
4. Cardiotomy reservoir (for priming).
5. Backup of all the above, including an additional oxygenator, pump head, and tubing pack.
6. Transducers.

Procedure

1. The system is assembled by attaching the circuit lines to the oxygenator and recirculating with priming solution after flushing with CO_2. Follow usual priming technique. After complete deairing, disconnect the venous side of the loop from the cardiotomy, clamp the cardiotomy outlet, and separate the centrifugal pump inlet line at the 3/8″ × 3/8″ connector. Using an air-free technique, connect the venous side of the patient loop to the 3/8″ × 3/8″ leur connector on the inlet side of the centrifugal pump to

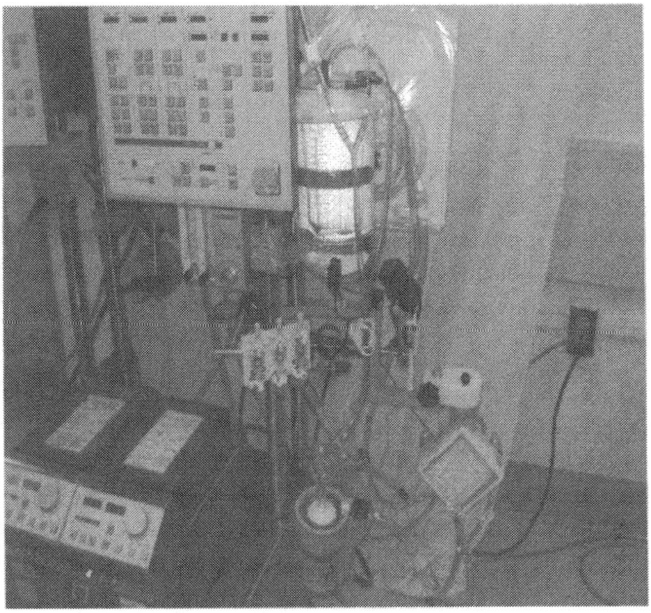

Fig. 1. ECMO circuit with rotaflow and Quadrox D.

create a closed-loop ECMO circuit without the cardiotomy. (No albumin in the prime because it may decrease the activity of the bonded tubing).

2. All connections must be tie banded because the coating makes the tubing slippery on the connectors.

3. For peripheral cannulation, see the vascular access cannula selection.

4. If central cannulation will be continued from cardiopulmonary bypass, then conversion to ECMO will be made using the arterial and venous cannulas already in place.

5. In postcardiotomy patients, no heparin will be given for the first 24 h.

6. Activated clotting time (ACT) will be monitored hourly.

7. After 24 h, if the PT is below 15 s, the platelet count is greater than 75,000, and the chest tube drainage has decreased to less than 1 ml/kg/h, then heparin may be started on order of a physician to maintain the ACT at target 180–200 s.

8. Oxygenator replacement. Because the Quadrox D is a nonmicroporous membrane, progressive failure over time due to fluid accumulation within the gas phase of the device is greatly reduced. However, oxygenator

performance and line pressure trends should be monitored. The following guidelines are for documenting oxygenator failure that requires replacement:

With Venous O_2sat >65%

FIO_2 of 100%—post oxygenator $pO_2 < 200$ mmHg
gas flow 10 L/min—arterial $pCO_2 > 40$ mmHg

Procedure for Oxygenator Changeout

1. Notify physician and nursing staff. Tell them that the patient will be off ECMO for 1–2 min. Increase ventilator FiO_2 to 100%.
2. Volume load the patient if necessary.
3. Increase the ACT to >200 s.
4. Setup a new oxygenator using 3/8″ tubing, pigtail, and 1/4″ recirculation line to existing cardiotomy. Flush with CO_2 and prime oxygenator.
5. Come off bypass by clamping postcentrifugal pump and postoxygenator, and turn console speed control to 0. Isolate patient by clamping the arterial and venous lines to the table.
6. Remove tubing from both oxygenator inlet and outlet.
7. Connect new oxygenator into circuit, remove clamp from recirculation line, and purge air from the oxygenator into the cardiotomy reservoir. Recirculate until the system is debubbled. Turn off pump and clamp recirculation line and double clamp cardiotomy outlet line. Attach O_2 gas line to the new oxygenator. Clamp oxygenator outlet tubing. Remove clamps from the arterial and venous lines to the table.
8. Turn on the pump, remove the clamp from the oxygenator outlet, and resume ECMO flow rate. Add additional volume as necessary to reach the desired flow rate.

Alternate method:
Preprime oxygenator using the small single pump stand alone base with a cardiotomy reservoir and 3/8″ tubing. Recirculate, deair, and clamp oxygenator inlet and outlet tubings approximately 4″ from oxygenator. Using aseptic technique, divide the lines leaving 6″ inches of tubing on oxygenator inlet and outlet. Use 3/8″ × 3/8″ connectors, insert new oxygenator into circuit using an air-free technique (either leured connectors with pigtails and 60 cc fluid-filled syringes or two man technique with saline syringe filling and flooding during air-free tubing connection). Confirm air-free connections and air free circuitry, properly reposition clamps, connect gas line, connect water lines, confirm gas flow, and resume ECMO flow and support.

LUNG TRANSLANTS: CARDIOPULMONARY BYPASS: DR. SONNETT

Procedure for Adult ECMO

PURPOSE

ECMO for the adult patient provides various methods of cardiac and respiratory support, depending on the location of the cannulation sites. In the VV mode, respiratory support is accomplished with the patient's own heart producing pulsatile aortic pressure. In the VA mode, both cardiac and respiratory support is achieved with a nonpulsatile aortic blood pressure. Cannulation can be either perepheral or central, depending on operative status.

EQUIPMENT SELECTION AND SETUP

An adult ECMO bypass tubing pack (E-Pack) is used with a Rotaflow centrifugal pump and a Quadrox D diffusion membrane oxygenator. Please refer to the figures (Figs. 2–4) for proper set-up of the E-Pack circuit. In extenuating circumstances, pigtails may be attached to the leur locks between the centrifugal pump the inlet of the Quadrox D oxygenator for CVVH for VV ECMO, but should not be used for VA ECMO. Pre- and postmembrane pressures should be monitored. The setup is then flushed with CO_2 before priming. The priming volume of 1200–1500 ml consists of 6% Hextend and lactated Ringer's. 2000 U of heparin and 25 ml of sodium bicarbonate is added to the prime. Blood prime should be used if the estimated postdilutional hematocrit is below 20%. A blood gas on the prime should then be performed, and

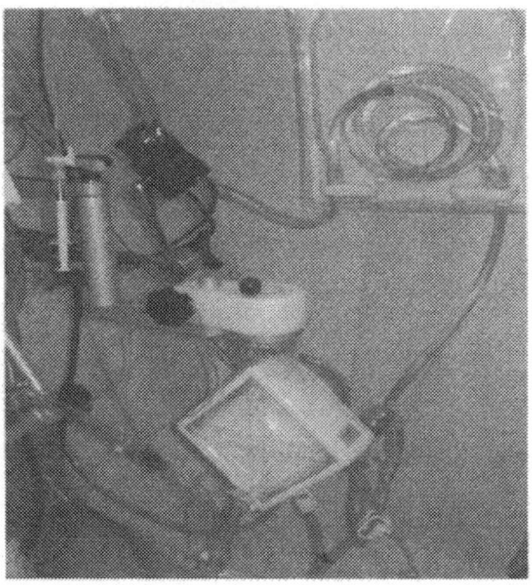

Fig. 2. QUADROX D oxygenator.

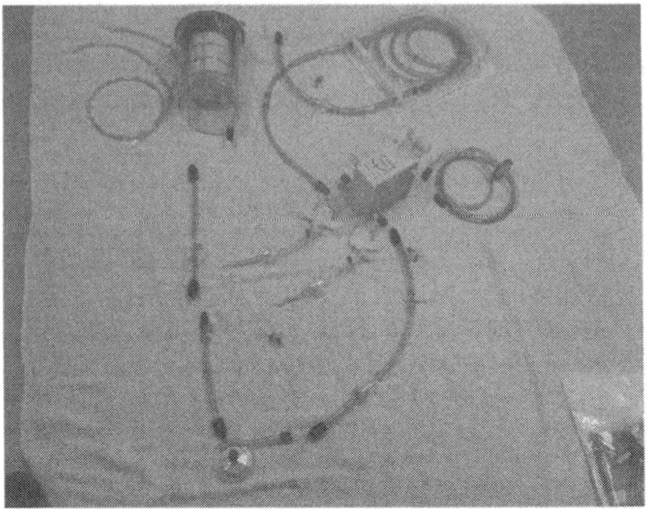

Fig. 3. E-PACK setup for priming, adult ECMO.

the prime should be adjusted as close to normal physiologic values as possible. After deairing the circuit, the venous inflow tubing to the cardiotomy reservoir is removed and connected to the inflow of the centrifugal pump. Recirculation is continued until just before attachment to the cannulae. The cardiotomy reservoir MUST be double

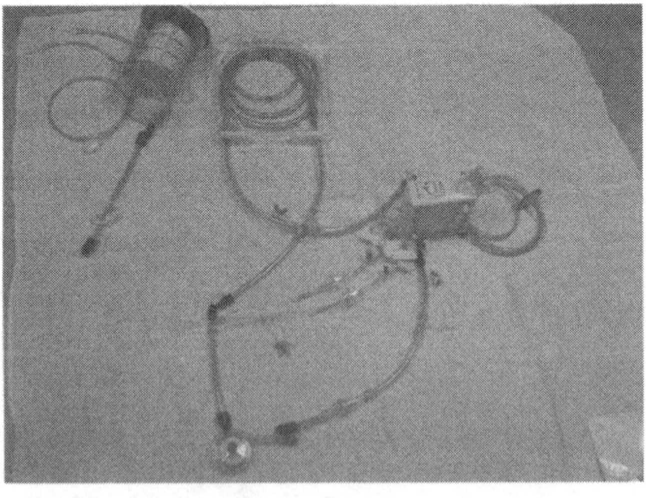

Fig. 4. E PACK ECMO setup after priming. Cardiotomy removed.

clamped, or preferably removed from the circuit, before bypass to ensure a closed system and prevent exsanguination, stagnation with thrombus formation, or possible air entrainment.

Vascular Access and Cannula Selection

VV cannulation is the method of choice, as long as there is proper cardiac function. Choose cannulae sizes that allow for the greatest range of flow for a given body surface area. Discuss cannula choices with the surgeon before insertion. Peripheral venous drainage can be accomplished via a Bio-Medicus cannula inserted into the femoral vein, through the inferior vena cava, and into the right atrium for adequate venous drainage. Pump return to the patient may be accomplished using a Bio-Medicus cannula via the internal jugular vein or various femoral cannulae. Consult the cannula flow selection chart for appropriate sizing of cannulas.

VA cannulation is used when there is combined cardiac and respiratory failure. Venous drainage may be accomplished via femoral vein, internal jugular, or direct right atrial cannulation. Arterial inflow may be accomplished via femoral artery, internal carotid artery, or the ascending aorta. Other cannulation sites may be required as per surgeon's request. Consult cannula flow chart for appropriate cannulas.

Distal limb perfusion may be necessary, and this can be accomplished be using a luered connector with a short piece of tubing and small distal cannula connected to the primary cannula luered port.

ECMO Initiation and Management During Bypass

Before cannulation, the patient should be systemically heparinized with 100 U/kg of sodium heparin, with ACTs >300 s. The sterile AV loop is passed off to the surgical field, and recircluation is discontinued. Tubing clamps are placed distal to the centrifugal head and distal to the oxygenator. Upon adequate anticoagulation, cannulation is performed by the surgeon. ECMO is initiated by removing both arterial and venous clamps and increasing blood flow to the desired rate. Gas flow is then immediately instituted to the recomended gas to blood flow ratio of 1 : 1 for the oxygenator used as per the manufacturer's recomendations. Line pressures should be checked immediately to ensure adequate venous drainage and arterial return and to rule out the possibility of arterial dissection. Volume may be given through the ECMO circuit via the pigtail lines, if necessary. However, volume management through patient access lines is preferred. Blood gases are sampled routinely at the bedside, and the patient is managed using an alpha-stat protocol to maintain values within normal acceptable ranges. ACTs are sampled hourly and maintained at >180 s. All ACT and blood gas samples should be obtained by the nurse via the patient's arterial line. Blood gases should not be drawn from the pump, except for the purposes of checking oxygenator performance or for calibrating the oxygen saturation analyzer. The perfusionist is required to document patient and ECMO pump parameters on the pump record on an hourly basis and all significant events as they occur.

Weaning and Decannulation from the ECMO Circuit

Weaning from the ECMO circuit is performed by decreasing pump flow with appropriate ventilator settings, under the authorization of the attending MD. Upon weaning, the heparin drip should be increased to maintain ACTs >200–250 s. Pump flow is discontinued by clamping distal to the centrifugal head, and oxygenator and cannulas are removed by the surgeon.

REFERENCE

ECMO: Extracorporeal Cardiopulmonary Support in Critical Care 2nd ed. JB Zwischenberger, RH Steinhorn, RH Bartlett. eds Ann Arber, MI: Extracorporeal Life Support Org; 2000.

INDEX

C

E

F

G

I

W

Made in the USA
Monee, IL
13 September 2026

62976952R00326